HYPERBARIC SURGERY

HYPERBARIC SURGERY

DIRK JAN BAKKER, MD, PhD

FREDERICK S. CRAMER, MD

EDITORS

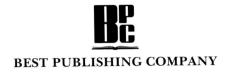

BEST PUBLISHING COMPANY

Cover Photos: Dirk J. Bakker, MD, PhD

Cover and Text Design: Jill McAdoo
                        Vanessa Palacio

Editorial: James T. Joiner
           Stephanie Karles

International Standard Book Number:1-930536-08-9
Library of Congress catalog card number:2002109044

Published by:
Best Publishing Company
Post Office Box 30100
Flagstaff, AZ 86003-0100, USA

Tele: 800.468.1055 or 928.527.1055
Fax: 928.526.0370
Web: www.bestpub.com
E-mail: divebooks@bestpub.com

CONTENTS

DEDICATION

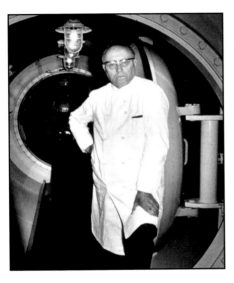

Dedicated to
Professor Dr. med. Ite Boerema
1904-1980

Boerema was born on October 10th, 1904, in Uithuizen in the province of Groningen, the Netherlands. His father was a skipper on a trading barge on regular routes within the Netherlands and on the former Zuiderzee. Boerema initially preferred to have a career in the Royal Dutch Navy but he was considered unfit because of his eyesight. He studied Medicine at the University of Groningen (MD), and specialized himself in General Surgery. He served as a staff surgeon in the University Clinic of Groningen under prof. Eerland, from 1927 until 1946. In 1928 he got his degree as doctor medicinae (PhD) at the same University, in Anatomy and Embryology. From 1946 until 1974 Boerema was professor of Surgery at the University of Amsterdam. During this time he received many honorary doctorates from Universities all over the world. Boerema died in London on June 28, 1980 after open heart surgery, possibly due to cerebral air embolism (!).

In 1948 Boerema got the idea that hypothermia might be an aid in cardiac surgery. In an extensive experimental study he proved that indeed moderate hypothermia (28° C) was a safe method to lengthen the time of circulatory arrest, which in those days increased distinctly the surgical possibilities in open heart surgery. Both Boerema and Bigelow, who worked independently on the same concept in Toronto, Canada, were credited for the introduction of this new principle in surgery. In 1962 Boerema received an important and large research grant from the U.S. Department of Health, Education and Welfare (Public Health Service) for further experiments with hypothermia in combination with hyperbaric oxygen in open heart surgery. The title of the research proposal was: "Surgery in an operating room with high atmospheric pressure." The further history of this is described in detail in the chapter "History of Hyperbaric Medicine and Surgery" in this book.

In 1963 Boerema organised the First International Congress on Hyperbaric Medicine in the Surgical Clinic of the University of Amsterdam. Participation was strictly on invitation. Many famous names can be found on the list of participants, for instance Chris Lambertsen, Philadelphia; Owen Wangensteen, Minneapolis; Claude Hitchcock, Minneapolis; Charles

Illingworth, Glasgow; Herman Rahn, Buffalo; W. Trapp and R. Adams Cowley, Vancouver; Albert Behnke, San Francisco; Ed Lanphier, Buffalo; Julius (Jack) Jacobson, New York; George Crile, Cleveland; Gray, Northwood, UK; William Blakemore, Philadelphia; Seymour Schwartz, Rochester; and many others from all over the world. This marked the beginning of the International Congresses that have taken place since.

Boerema was a teacher of extraordinary qualities. "He had a passionate love for his profession, an innate feeling of mission, long experience, clear conceptions and above all, the ability to speak simply and in a clear and vivid way, an ability to reduce problems to their essential core, a feeling for the maintenance of tradition and continuity, and an interest in those being taught," to quote his oldest pupil, Kuyer professor of surgery from the Groningen University. He was teaching by the example he was setting in his work, his writings and, more particularly, in his lectures and demonstrations.

Boerema was the first in the Netherlands to introduce the systematic preoperative case discussion of all patients with the entire surgical and anaesthesiological staff of the Department, together with the consulting specialists of Internal Medicine, Radiology and other consultants, important for the case. This was maintained during the 28 years of his professorship in Amsterdam and taken over by his successors. His words became famous: "Participation in the discussion by all, final judgement by only one," meaning himself of course. His regimen had something of military rigidity about it. However, this was not in any way inconvenient during our period of training. This hierarchy is both natural and indispensable at the operating table.

He also introduced special patient demonstrations for General Practitioners. From the "School" of Boerema many also attained the rank of professor in all surgical specialities: Orthopedics, Traumatology, Vascular surgery, Cardiopulmonary surgery, Urology, Plastic and Reconstructive surgery, Oncologic surgery and Experimental surgery.

Besides hyperbaric oxygen therapy, Boerema invented the Boerema button, with which a safe anastomosis was possible after a total gastrectomy. He also developed a new tool to close relapsing incisional hernias, the sc. railroad plasty of Ton. He found a method to interrupt bleeding varicose veins in the oesophagus in hepatic cirrhosis. Furthermore, a special operating technique, the gastropexia anterior geniculata, to treat hiatal hernias, was developed by him. Last but not least he published and lectured on decompression illness.

With his self discipline, energy, devotion, genuine interest in his pupils, even long after their training was finished and they had attained their own position, readiness to sacrifice himself in the interest of his task, Boerema will long be remembered.

We thought it most appropriate to dedicate this book to his memory.

Dirk Jan Bakker MD, PhD
Frederick S. Cramer, MD

FOREWORD

About two years ago Fred Cramer and myself got the idea to write a book. Since we are both surgeons and have for many years been involved in hyperbaric oxygen therapy (HBOT), we decided that a book about Hyperbaric Surgery would be most appropriate, not in the least because such a textbook does not exist.

Not that much surgery is done nowadays under hyperbaric conditions, like it used to be, but surgeons have always been very much involved in HBOT and there are still many indications in the field of Surgical Specialties for HBOT.

We like to show the way surgeons are thinking when using HBOT in their daily practice in a wide variety of indications: Traumatology, Orthopedics, Plastic and Reconstructive Surgery, Urology, Surgical Oncology, in Wound Healing, the treatment of Burns, the treatment of serious Soft Tissue Infections, Cardiothoracic Surgery, Intensive Care Medicine, etc.

In reading the history of hyperbaric medicine it is obvious how much surgeons have contributed to the development of both the scientific aspect and the practical application of HBOT in Medicine.

After a period when hyperbaric medicine was synonymous with medical problems in diving and in caisson workers, an upsurge took place in the early fifties when open heart surgery was performed under hyperbaric conditions in the Amsterdam University Clinic by one of the pioneers of HBOT, prof. Ite Boerema. I myself, involved in hyperbaric medicine since the end of 1968, performed heart surgery inside the chamber under pressure until 1972, mainly involving palliative procedures in newborn children with congenital heart diseases (sc. blue babies).

Much basic research was done and when this indication in open heart surgery disappeared because of the development and perfection of the possibilities for cardiorespiratory bypasses during surgery, many things were learned about the physiology and pathophysiology of congenital heart diseases and the influence of oxygen under increased pressure in general and in various other diseases.

In the "backwash" of the clinical application of HBOT much research was done. That was the normal order of things in those days. Some professor had an idea and after a short time of animal and laboratory research this idea was applied in clinical practice. The stature of the clinical professor who applied the technique guaranteed the validity of the method and the good results as well. We believed in what they wrote and did, and tried to follow them.

These times are long gone by now. We have entered the fascinating new era of Evidence Based Medicine (EBM), in which another way of scientific proof of clinical therapeutical methods is asked for. It is indeed a healthy challenge, and not so much a threat, to be asked to show the best existing evidence to underline our accepted indications. Within the hyperbaric community both the Undersea and Hyperbaric Medical Society and the European Committee for Hyperbaric Medicine go to great pains in order to adhere to today's scientific standards.

Also EBM is evolving, which is proven by the more central role clinical expertise and patients' choices are playing in weighing the evidence and deciding the best way to go with an individual patient.

At the same time, it is clear that the possibilities of prospective randomized clinical trials as practised in the evaluation of medicines can never be reached in some of the very complicated surgical indications like chronic osteomyelitis, crush injuries, and soft tissue infections with an enormous individual variation.

It is an excellent thing that, nevertheless, randomized prospective trials with HBOT are performed even in these difficult diseases.

It is not so much the problem that there are controversial indications in HBOT, but the problem is sometimes more the way we are dealing with these indications.

If we clearly show in a methodological accepted trial that in a certain disease there is no place for HBOT, do we stop using HBOT for this disease? Do we argue on the basis of trials or on the basis of anecdotal reports and what we call "eminence or experience based" medicine? On the other hand, we must always defend the crucial role of clinical expertise in patient treatment. Evidence based medicine asks for experienced doctors and not only epidemiologists and biostaticians.

When we discussed the idea of publishing a book about Hyperbaric Surgery with Jim Joiner of Best Publishing Company, we met enthusiastic approval and support. Together we selected, from a wide range of HBOT physicians and scientists, the foremost experts and invited them to contribute a chapter for this book. We were extremely grateful to notice the same enthusiasm in their willingness to contribute to this work. The authors are, without exception, experts in their own medical specialty and are also practicing HBOT, where appropriate, in their field of medicine.

Another goal of this book is to show that we are standing on the shoulders of our famous predecessors in HBOT. Therefore we decided that any financial profit coming out of the publication of our book would be used to reprint Proceedings of older Congresses that are not available anymore but from which a lot still can be learned. We will start with the First International Congress in Amsterdam in 1963, and go on from there. We were very happy to notice that everyone who contributed to this book wholeheartedly agreed with this goal.

We sincerely hope that this publication may serve the best interest of HBOT in clinical medicine and that we are able to show that HBOT has a definite and respected place in medicine and is not a therapy in search of a disease. We like to be judged by the same and well-respected scientific standards that are valid nowadays when establishing medical indications is involved.

We, as editors, hope that your pleasure in reading and studying this book equals theirs in compiling and editing it.

D.J.Bakker, MD, PhD, Senior Editor

PREFACE

It is both an honor and pleasure for me to write this brief preface for the new textbook on *Hyperbaric Surgery*. To the best of my knowledge this is the first text to be devoted to the subspecialty of "Hyperbaric Surgery."

The application of intermittent high-dose oxygen as a drug in the management of the surgical patient has been at the core of the specialty since the very beginning. Professor Boerema of Amsterdam is the recognized pioneer in the field and the host of the first International Congress on Hyperbaric Medicine, which was held in Amsterdam in 1963.

It is most appropriate that Professor Bakker, the Senior Editor of this text, has chosen to dedicate the book to the memory of Professor Boerema. Dr. Boerema was an internationally known cardiac surgeon who pioneered the use of hyperbaric oxygen (HBO) in the management of complex surgical infections, most notably gas gangrene.

Dr. Bakker has compiled a distinguished group of international experts, all of whom have made significant contributions to the textbook. A total of 20 authors from 6 countries have contributed their time and expertise to this project. The book is a total volunteer effort with proceeds going to the Foundation for the International Congress on Hyperbaric Medicine.

The book is intended for the practicing surgeon who has the availability of a hyperbaric chamber facility for the treatment of his/her patients. For those surgeons who are actively involved with the facility itself, the chapter on decompression illness (DCI) will be most useful. A large number of scuba divers are active in all parts of the world. They will frequently present themselves to HBO facilities for treatment at locations not adjacent to diving venues.

Finally, this textbook would not be possible without the total dedication and support from Jim Joiner, President of Best Publishing Company. Jim is a personal friend and colleague. His contribution to this textbook and his support of the International Congress on Hyperbaric Medicine is most appreciated.

Fred Cramer, MD, Editor
President, XIV International Congress on Hyperbaric Medicine
San Francisco, California, USA — October 2002

CONTRIBUTORS

DIRK J. BAKKER, MD, PhD
Medical Director, Academic Medical Center, University of Amsterdam, Amsterdam, The Netherlands

Medical Director Suite J1-153
Academic Medical Center
University of Amsterdam
PO Box 22700
1100 DE Amsterdam
THE NETHERLANDS
Tele: (31) 020 56 63 468
Fax: (31) 020 56 64 440/020 69 19 854
Email: D.J.Bakker@amc.uva.nl

PAUL CIANCI, MD, FACP
Director, Department of Diving & Hyperbaric Medicine, Doctors Medical Center, San Pablo, California, John Muir Medical Center, Walnut Creek, California, and Saint Francis Memorial Hospital, San Francisco, California, Professor Emeritus of Medicine, University of California, Davis

2000 Vale Road
San Pablo, California 94806
Tele: (510) 235 3483
Fax: (510) 970 5770

FREDERICK S. CRAMER, MD, FACS
Associate Clinical Professor of Surgery, Uniformed Services University of the Health Services, Bethesda, Maryland, USA

1592 Union Street
San Francisco, California 94123
Email: fscramer@xit.net

JOHN J. FELDMEIER, DO
Professor and Chairman, Medical College of Ohio

Department of Radiation Oncology
3000 Arlington Avenue
Toledo, Ohio 43614-5807
Tele: (419) 383 4541
Fax: (419) 383 3040
Email: JFeldmeier@mco.edu

MICHAEL L. GIMBEL, MD

Deptartment of Surgery
UPMC
677 Scaife Hall
3550 Terrace Street
Pittsburgh, Pennsylvania 15261
Tele: (412) 683 1516
Fax: (866) 254 0719

THOMAS K. HUNT, MD, DMHC, FACS, FRCS
Professor of Surgery, Director Lab/Clinic Wound Healing Research Laboratory,University of California, San Francisco, California

513 Parnassus Avenue HSW-1652
San Francisco, California 94143-0522
Tele: (415) 476 0410
Fax: (415) 476 5190
Email: huntt@surgery.ucsf.edu

ALESSANDRO MARRONI, MD
President, Divers Alert Network Europe, Vice President, European Committee for Hyperbaric Medicine, Secretary General, European College of Baromedicine

PO Box 77 - DAN
64026 Roseto Abruzzi
ITALY
Tele: (39) 085 893 0333
Fax: (39) 085 893 0050
Email: alexnu@daneurope.org

DANIEL MATHIEU, MD, PhD
Professor in Critical Care Medicine

Intensive Care and Hyperbaric Medicine Department
Hospital Calmette
Lille University Hospital Center
Boulevard du Prof. Leclercq
Lille 59037
FRANCE
Tele: (33) 320 445491
Fax: (33) 320 444317
Email: dmathieu@chru-lille.fr

CLAUS-MARTIN MUTH, MD
Assistant Professor of Anesthesiology, Consultant in Hyperbaric Medicine,
DMO German Navy

Sektion APV
Universitätsklinik für Anaesthesiologie
Universität Ulm
Parkstrasse 11 • D-89073 Ulm
GERMANY
Tele: (49) 731 50025145
Fax: (49) 731 50025143
Email: claus-martin.muth@medizin.uni-ulm.de

BARBARA L. PERSONS, MD
Surgery Resident, Department of Surgery
University of Nevada School of Medicine, Las Vegas, Nevada

2040 West Charleston Blvd.
Suite 301
Las Vegas, Nevada 89102
Tele: (702) 671 2278
Fax: (702) 671 2245
Email: barbarapersons@yahoo.com

PETER RADERMACHER, MD
Professor of Anesthesiology, DMO German Navy,
Consultant in Hyperbaric Medicine

Sektion APV
Universitätsklinik für Anaesthesiologie
Universität Ulm
Parkstrasse 11 • D-89073 Ulm
GERMANY
Tele: (49) 731 50025140
Fax: (49) 731 50025143
Email: Peter.Radermacher@medizin.uni-ulm.de

JÖRG SCHMUTZ, MD
Foundation for Hyperbaric Medicine

177 Kleinhüningerstrasse
Basel, CH-4057
SWITZERLAND
Tele: (41) 61 6313013
Fax: (41) 61 6313006
Email: joerg.schmutz@hin.ch

ERIK S. SHANK, MD
Board Certified in Undersea and Hyperbaric Medicine by the American Board of
Preventive Medicine (2002 Diplomat)

Department of Anesthesia and Critical Care
MGH, Clinics 3
32 Fruit Street
Boston, MA 02114
Fax: (617) 726 7536
Email: eshank@etherdome.mgh.harvard.edu

PAUL J. SHEFFIELD, PhD, CHT
Board Certified Aerospace Physiologist, Board Certified Hyperbaric Technologist,
Fellow, Aerospace Medical Association, President, International ATMO, Inc.,
School of Aeronautics Board of Advisors, Florida Institute of Technology

International ATMO Inc.
414 Navarro, Suite 502
San Antonio, TX 78205
Tele: (210) 614 3688
Fax: (210) 223 4864
Email: Psheffield@milx.net

ADRIANNE PS SMITH, MD, FACEP

Medical Director, Wound Care Center, Texas Diabetes Institute,
Assistant Professor, University of Texas Health Science Center of San Antonio

15607 Rose Crest Circle
San Antonio, Texas 78248
Tele: (210) 358 7250
Fax: (210) 358 7251
Email: smithap@uthscsa.edu

MICHAEL B. STRAUSS, MD, FACS, AAOS, ABPM/UHM

Medical Director, Baromedical Department, Long Beach Memorial Medical Center,
Long Beach, California, Clinical Professor, Orthopaedic Surgery, University
of California, College of Medicine, Irvine, California, Orthopaedic Consultant,
Preservation-Amputation, Care and Treatment Clinic (PACT), Veterans
Administration Medical Center, Long Beach, California

2888 Long Beach Blvd. #235
Long Beach, California 90806
Tele: (562) 595 6944
Fax: (562) 427 2135
Email: mstrauss@memorialcare.org

A.J. VAN DER KLEIJ, MD, PhD

Academic Medical Center
Department of Surgery
Universtiy of Amsterdam

Meibergdreef 9
1105 AZ, Amsterdam Z-O
THE NETHERLANDS
Tele: (31) (020) 56 65 740
Fax: (31) (020) 56 64 440
Email: A.J.vanderKleij@amc.uva.nl

J.P.R. VAN MERKESTEYN, DDS, MD, PhD

Associate Professor

Department of Oral and Maxillofacial Surgery
Leiden University Medical Center
Postbox 9600, 2300 RC, Leiden
THE NETHERLANDS
Tele: (31) 715 262 372
Fax: (31) 715 266 766
Email: J.P.R.van_Merkesteyn@lumc.nl

WILBUR T. WORKMAN, MS, CHT

Director, Quality Assurance and Regulatory Affairs,
Undersea and Hyperbaric Medical Society

18111 Copper Ridge Drive
San Antonio, Texas 78259
Tele: (210) 404 1553
Fax: (210) 404 1535
Email: UHMSQARA@aol.com

WILLIAM A. ZAMBONI, MD, FACS

Professor and Chairman, Department of Surgery, Chief, Division of Plastic Surgery,
University of Nevada School of Medicine, Las Vegas, Nevada

2040 West Charleston Blvd.
Suite 301
Las Vegas, Nevada 89102
Tele: (702) 671 2278 ext. 24
Fax: (702) 671 2245
Email: wzamboni@med.unr.edu

CHAPTER 1

HISTORY OF HYPERBARIC MEDICINE AND SURGERY

D.J. Bakker

INTRODUCTION

Hyperbaric medicine has its roots in the history of diving and diving medicine. There are roughly five different periods (and subjects) to describe when summarising history of hyperbaric medicine and surgery.

1. Diving, diving medicine, and the invention of diving apparatuses
2. Pressurised air and the treatment of certain diseases
3. Caisson work, work under pressure, and related problems
4. Pneumatic centers and patient treatment
5. Hyperbaric surgery and hyperbaric medicine
   (incl. international developments)

Diving and Diving Medicine

Far back in history, as far as 4500 BC, diving was already recognised as a human occupation. At that time diving had advanced to an industry that provided the community with shells, pearls, food, and sponges. Since men cannot hold their breath for more than a few minutes, it was tried to extend these limits by various diving equipment. Breath-hold diving only existed until the nineteenth century; after that helmet diving and other equipment was invented and developed.

The first to whom diving in an underwater vehicle is attributed in history is Alexander the Great, who was lowered, as the story goes, into the Bosporus Straits in a glass barrel with lighted candles inside. An illustration of this can be found in the Burgundy Library in Brussels, Belgium (62). Aristotle also mentions this diving bell. He was also the first one who mentioned ruptured eardrums in divers (2).

Jain (1990) gives some important benchmarks from the history of diving medicine in relation to hyperbaric medicine (39).

In 1531, de Marchi (4), who lived from 1490 until 1574, described an instrument to raise the galleys of Caligula from the bottom of Lake Nemi. He claimed a one-hour's stay under water to be possible.

Fraisnier (1562) called attention to two Greeks who dived in a bell to the bottom of the river Tagus in 1538, an event watched by Charles V of Spain (31, 37).

In 1620, the Dutchman Cornelis Jacobsz Drebbel (1572-1634) constructed the first "one atmosphere submarine" or a forerunner of such, moved forward by rowers. It is said that this boat could reach depths of 12-15 feet in the river (52, 67).

The first modern records of diving bells used in practical salvage started in 1640 when Von Treileben used a primitive bell for salvaging 42 canons from the sunken Swedish warship Vasa from 132 feet of water in the bay of Stockholm (Sweden). The next reports are by Halley in 1690 and Smeaton in 1790 (43).

Sir Robert Boyle provided the first indication as to the aetiology of decompression sickness in 1670, when he produced symptoms of decompression sickness in a snake, which he had placed in a vacuum cleaner (43). Triger (1841) gave the first description of the symptoms of decompression sickness in man.

August Siebe, a German coppersmith working in London, invented a copper diving helmet riveted to a leather jacket (1819). A force pump for the necessary compressed air was connected to it. He designed a full and completely closed diving dress in 1837. This suit remained more or less unchanged until 1945, when lightweight diving masks became available.

SCUBA (self-contained underwater breathing apparatus) was invented in 1943 by the Frenchmen Gagnon and Cousteau.

The present-day medical use of hyperbaric oxygen treatment started in fact as a result of naval research on the physiologic effects of raised pressure on humans in diving. Behnke and Shaw were the first to use hyperbaric oxygen in the treatment of decompression sickness in naval divers (9).

In 1947 the following conclusions were drawn as to the toxicity of oxygen:

1. The harmful effect of oxygen on the nervous system manifests itself at a pressure of 3 ATA and higher.
2. The nervous systems are concomitant with the elevation of oxygen tension in central venous blood flow.
3. Acidity of venous blood is increased.
4. Increasing the carbon dioxide tension in the lungs greatly enhances the toxicity of oxygen.
5. Adverse pulmonary and nervous effects observed in man are reversible and are not followed by gross residual injury (10, 60).

Further developments in diving and diving medicine are beyond the scope of this chapter and can be found in numerous textbooks on these subjects (see also *A Pictorial History of Diving*) (1).

Pressurised Air and the Treatment of Certain Diseases

The first attempt to treat patients with air under pressure was done by the English clergyman Henshaw. He had only an idea but absolutely no scientific background for this. He constructed between 1662 and 1664 a pressure chamber, which he called "Domicilium." In this chamber he could change climate and pressure conditions. High pressures were used for the treatment of acute diseases and "hot stages of fever"; low pressures for chronic diseases and diminishing the "shivering state of fever."

...In time of good health this domicilium is proposed as a good expedient to help digestion, to promote insensible respiration, to facilitate breathing and expectoration, and consequently, of excellent use for the prevention of most affections of the lungs....

Henshaw used a pair of bellows for pressurisation, which prevented him, no doubt, from too high pressures (34, 37).

Probably independent from each other Priestly (1775) and Scheele (1777) discovered oxygen (56, 59). Priestly pointed already to a possible therapeutic use when he wrote:

*... From the greater strength and vivacity of the flame of a candle in this pure air, it may be conjectured that it might be peculiarly salutary to the lungs in certain morbid cases, when the common air would not be sufficient to carry off the phlogistic putrid effluvium fast enough. But perhaps we may also infer from these experiments, that though pure dephlogisticated air might be very useful as a medicine, it might not be so proper for us in the usual healthy state of the body; for as a candle burns out much faster in dephlogisticated than in common air, so we might, as may be said, live out too fast and the animal powers be too soon exhausted in this pure kind of air; but I fancied that my breast felt peculiarly light and easy for some time afterwards. Who can tell but that in time, this pure air may become a fashionable article of luxury. Hitherto only two mice and myself had the privilege of breathing it....*and continued:.... *A moralist, at least, may say, that the air, which Nature has provided for us, is as good as we deserve....*

Lavoisier (Fig. 25) and Sequin in 1789 observed toxic effects (44) while Paul Bert (Fig. 27) in 1878 considered pure oxygen as particularly dangerous, even at normal pressure (11). The only therapeutic indication, according to Bert, was acute carbon monoxide poisoning. (Claude Bernard reported in 1857 on the chemical affinity of CO and haemoglobin.) Bert used "enriched air" containing 60% oxygen and not pure oxygen. He also demonstrated that inhalation of pure oxygen by skylarks produced oxygen seizures. Everyone will have a grand mal seizure when he or she is breathing oxygen at three atmospheres for three hours or more. This is called the "Paul Bert effect." The so-called Lorrain-Smith effect (inhalation of pure oxygen at 1 ATA or 1,013 bar, causes pulmonary damage) is known since the early 1900s (45). Jain and Fischer give a review of the history of oxygen in 1989 (38).

The Dutch Society of Sciences (Hollandsche Maatschappij der Wetenschappen) awarded in 1782 a prize for the best apparatus to study the influence of compressed air ("dikke lucht") on animals and plants. This challenge could not be met in 1782, or in 1785, 1788, or 1789. It lasted until 1970 when Boerema presented his experiences to the General Meeting of the Society. However, he did not get the prize. The final date had long expired (21). (Fig. 5)

Caisson Work and Related Problems

The use of caissons for industrial purposes started in 1839 when Triger, a French mining engineer, constructed a steel ring-shaped shaft in Chalonnes (France) to enable coal mining from the bottom of the Loire River. The shaft, with a 5-foot diameter, was lowered over 25 feet through quicksand to the coal underneath. The upper part of the shaft was closed with an airlock and the shaft was pressurised to 25 feet of water pressure (3,5 ATA). In this way "dry" coal mining was possible (29). Triger also published some physiologic findings, for instance "that one is unable to whistle at 3 ATA" and "everyone speaks through the nose in pressurised air." As we mentioned already, the first description of decompression illness in man is also from Triger in 1841.

These same techniques were used in England for building bridges over rivers (1851) and the Rhine-bridge between Kehl and Strassbourg in 1859 (between Germany and France). In 1862/1863 the Seine bridge near Argenteuil (France) was finished. After this a little monograph by Foley on medical aspects of caisson work was published (29).

It was, however, not until 1885 that tunnel workers suffering from caisson disease were successfully treated in a hyperbaric chamber with pressurised air, not yet with oxygen. This pressure chamber was operated in connection with the construction of the Hudson tunnel in New York. It lasted until 1917 that the first decompression tables were published, after much research guided by Haldane in England (33).

Caissons were also used at the bridge building activities over the Mississippi in St. Louis (1869-1874) and at the Brooklyn Bridge in New York (1867-1876). The biggest caissons however, were used in 1898 with the building of two gigantic dry docks for the Imperial Wharf in Kiel, Germany.

Meesters published a thesis on caisson disease in 1958 (46) and Faesecke (1997) published a very thorough and extensive study on "work under pressure" (29). From then on pressure chambers or pneumatic centres were gradually established all over Europe and the United States. In North America the first chamber was built in Rochester (USA) and in Ashawa (Canada) in 1860, which was later moved to Toronto. In the Netherlands chambers were built and used for medical purposes in Haarlem by Pyan (1882) (who claimed that he performed 27 operations under hyperbaric conditions in three months' time), in Amsterdam by Arntzenius (1885), and in Hilversum by Tresling in 1887 (3).

Pneumatic Centres

In the early 19th century, Beddoes, a professor of chemistry in Oxford, investigated the effects of different gas mixtures on the treatment of a variety of diseases such as hydrocephalus, gout, melancholia, and scurvy. He called his efforts to treat these patients "pneumotherapy" (6).

The first pressure chamber after Henshaw was built by Junod in 1834. The diameter was five feet and the pressure ranged from 2,5 to 4 ATA. The chamber was made of copper. Good results were obtained, as Junod claimed, in the treatment of vasoconstriction of the peripheral blood vessels and vasoconstriction in the internal organs. He also treated many lung diseases (41). Pravaz built a chamber in 1837 and reported his results in 1840. He treated 12 patients simultaneously and he called this le bain d'air comprimé (which is French for "pressurised air bath"). He reported on bronchial dilation and he had favourable results primarily in bronchial tuberculosis but also in a number of other anomalies (54, 55).

According to Arntzenius, the first who developed pneumatic therapy in Europe, even before Junod, was Tabarié who built a chamber in

Montpellier (France) in 1840. But before that, as the story goes, he handed a sealed package containing a detailed description of pneumatic therapy to the French Academy of Sciences in 1832. Later, in 1840, he reported improvement in 49 cases of respiratory diseases, which he treated in Montpellier (3, 4, 54, 55).

Bertin operated a chamber in 1855, which was constructed as a vertical cylinder with a rectangular door, windows, and comfortable seats. Kelly (USA) constructed a similar installation in 1876. This chamber had an outside lock, controlled by the system operator and not by the occupants (33).

In 1861 Corning used the first hyperbaric chamber in the USA to treat nervous diseases. These chambers were placed in his private consulting rooms.

Fontaine built a mobile pressure chamber with a capacity of ten seats in 1879 (31). (Fig. 28)

In 1848 a centre was started in Marseille (France) by Debreuilh (the third in France) followed by Lyon (Milliet) and two more in Nice.

After 1860 the centres spread quickly over Europe. (Fig. 16) Through a generous gift of the Swedish Government, Sandahl was able to start a pneumatic centre in Stockholm in 1860. Gindrod opened an Institue in London in the same year, followed by Jacobsson in Altona (Germany) in 1862 (Fig. 15) and Carlo Forlanini, the pioneer of artificial pneumothorax in the treatment of tuberculosis, in 1875), Copenhagen (Denmark), Munchen, Stuttgart, Bad Reichenhall-Ems (in Bavaria where von Liebig employed five chambers with room for 50 patients in total) and Dresden (Germany), Wien (Austria), Odessa and Moscow (Russia), New York (USA), and Brussels in Belgium. (Fig. 26 & 31)

Beigel founded in London the first society with the goal of establishing pneumatic centres in 1867.

The Russian government subsidised the centre of Simonoff in St. Petersburg with the amount of 2200 roubles yearly. Dr. Simonoff was appointed as professor of air therapy at the Imperial Academy in the same St. Petersburg. In 1873 he got a governmental contract to treat sick soldiers.

Many books and papers were published. In France by Bertin, Pravaz, Junod, Tabarié, Fontaine, and especially Paul Bert (Bert 1878); in Germany by von Vivenot, Knauthe; Simonoff in Russia and others (3).

A very extensive study on pneumatic therapy and a review of the literature is given by Arntzenius in 1887 (with over 300 references) (3). Arntzenius operated a pneumatic centre in Amsterdam and gave in his book a detailed description of the working mechanism of pressurised air on the human organism as he saw it; besides that he described many clinical patients with their diseases and the results of his treatment. Diseases that he claimed to have treated successfully are asthma, emphysema, pleuritis, tuberculosis, anaemia, whooping cough, chlorosis, and feeding disorders. He distinguished a general effect of pressurised air, on the organism as a whole, and a local effect, especially on the lungs.

The most remarkable but also controversial chambers in the USA in the 20th century were, no doubt, built and/or inspired by Orville Cunningham, an anaesthesiologist working in Kansas City, Missouri, in 1921. (Fig. 29) The Kansas City chamber was a large horizontal cylinder, about ten feet in diameter and nearly ninety feet in length. The tank was equipped with air locks, toilets, shower baths, compartments, and Pullman car equipment (58). Intensive treatment took ten and a half days. Cunningham treated a variety of diseases, including diabetes mellitus, from 1921 on and in 1925 his chamber was the only one operational in the USA. Unfortunately, tragedy struck one night when a mechanical failure resulted in complete loss of compression in the hyperbaric chamber, and all patients inside died. After this Cunningham began treating diseases like syphilis, hypertension, diabetes mellitus, and cancer on the assumption that anaerobic conditions played a role in all these diseases (60).

Mr. Timken, an engineer and businessman in Cleveland, Ohio, built the most "famous and/or notorious" chamber in 1928. The large steel ball was meant to be a new "tank" and a sanatorium, controlled by Cunningham. (Fig. 30) This construction contained 72 rooms in six stories with "all the amenities of a good hotel."

The American Medical Association approached Cunningham very carefully, asking repeatedly and politely for an explanation about the therapy and the results, but Cunningham never answered. He published one article in 1927 (26).

The result of all this was that the Bureau of Investigation of the American Medical Association condemned the Cunningham "tank treatment" in 1928 (22). The chamber was dismantled in 1937 and the scrap metal was used for building tanks in the Second World War ("Tank for Tanks") (68).

Hyperbaric Oxygen, Hyperbaric Medicine, and Hyperbaric Surgery

After the discovery of oxygen by Priestly in 1775 and Scheele in 1777 (56, 59), Lavoisier and Sequin already observed toxic effects of oxygen in 1789 (44). Paul Bert (1878) considered pure oxygen as particularly dangerous, even at normal pressures; he advocated the use of normobaric oxygen in decompression sickness. In his view the only therapeutic indication was carbon monoxide poisoning. This was shown already by Haldane in animal experiments with CO-poisoned mice. The first patient with CO-poisoning was treated with hyperbaric oxygen by George Smith from Aberdeen (Scotland) and the first thesis on this subject appeared in Amsterdam by Sluyter in 1963 (61, 63).

The first report on hyperbaric surgery, an operation performed under pressure, is from Paul Bert (1879). The aim was to give pure nitrous oxide anaesthesia, but Bert realised that this was impossible at a normal pressure because of the lack of oxygen. He than proposed to give 50% nitrous oxide with 50% oxygen at 2 ATA. In this way he gave the same amount of nitrous oxide as in 100% at 1 ATA. The description of the operation can be found in the paper by Rendell-Baker and Jacobsson (57). "An ingrown toenail was removed in an extremely nervous girl of 20 years. The operation was performed in the large chamber of the aerotherapeutic establishment of Dr. Daupley with an excellent result."

Fontaine developed a mobile hyperbaric operating room based on (Fig. 28) the ideas of Bert in 1879. "With this chamber," he wrote, "one can do surgery in hospitals, sanitaria and private homes." It was moved from hospital to hospital in Paris wherever it was needed. Pean, a well-known French surgeon, performed twenty-seven operations in three months' time helped by five or six assistants. Unfortunately Fontaine had an accident in his pneumatic institute and died (31).

With the intention to exploit the enhanced potency of nitrous oxide anaesthesia at raised pressures, E.P. Howland from the USA built an apparatus as "an inhaling air chamber for dental and surgical operations" (57).

The third report on hyperbaric surgery is given by Pyan from Haarlem, the Netherlands, who claimed to have performed twenty-seven operations under pressure in his pneumatic centre within a three-month period (3). (Since more or less the same story goes for Pean in France, the question remains if Arntzenius did not mean to write Pean instead of Pyan from Haarlem.)

In the early 20th Century, Sayer Bruch from Berlin, used a hypobaric chamber for lung surgery. (Fig. 17)

Mosso (1900) used oxygen at 2 ATA in animal experiments with monkeys (51). In the beginning of the 20th century, publications on clinical or experimental work on hyperbaric oxygen treatment were not very numerous. Behnke et al. (7, 8, 9), working in the U.S. Navy, studied the influence of oxygen under pressure on the human physiology and recommended the use in "compressed air illness" (decompression sickness).

Ozorio de Almeida and Costa (1934), investigated the toxic effects of high-pressure oxygen (1934), the influence on experimental cancer in rats (1934), experimental gas gangrene (1934), and leprosy (1938) (4, 39). End and Long (1942) studied the effect of hyperbaric oxygen on carbon monoxide poisoning experimentally in dogs and guinea pigs (28).

Churchill-Davidson and his colleagues, working at St. Thomas Hospital in London, used hyperbaric oxygen to enhance the radiosensitivity of malignant tumors. He irradiated patients in an monoplace hyperbaric oxygen chamber (23, 24). The results in those days, however, were disappointing (1978). (Fig. 12-14)

A true upsurge in hyperbaric surgery followed in 1956 in Amsterdam when Boerema and his co-workers used this in cardiovascular surgery. The main purpose was to determine the value of this method in cardiac surgery. The idea of using oxygen under increased pressure was closely related to the idea of hypothermia. By lowering the body temperature to 28°C, oxygen consumption was reduced to 50% of its level at 37°C. A period of complete circulatory arrest for seven to eight minutes was well tolerated.

Hypothermia or artificial cooling as a therapy has a long history. Amputation under cold anaesthesia was done as early as 1832 by Larrey, a front surgeon in the French army under Napoleon who, during the Russian campaign, performed operations on exhausted, half-frozen and sometimes drunken soldiers (48). Smith and Fay (30, 65) treated patients with carcinoma in the expectation that growth of the tumors would be slowed down or even stopped by cooling. Talbot, Dill, and Forbes used it in the treatment of mental disorders (42). Blalock and Crossman were the first to use cooling to diminish the metabolism thus lowering the oxygen demand of the body or a part of the body (16, 25). Bancroft used this in the treatment of diabetic gangrene (5).

Boerema, very interested in heart surgery, tried to extend the possible duration of cardiac arrest in order to be able to perform open-heart surgery, meaning performing repairs inside the heart. He started his experiments in 1948 and published his results in 1951 (17). He used extracorporeal cooling (arterial blood was cooled and reinfused in a vein). Very soon it became obvious that cooling below 26°C was poorly tolerated by the heart.

Independent from Boerema, Bigelow had the same idea and published his results in 1950-1954 (13, 14, 15). Swan reported about 100 clinical cases and hypothermia in 1955. They used surface cooling (66). Numerous problems can be read in a great many publications. Keuskamp (1960) gives an excellent review (42). (Fig. 10)

The best way of cooling a patient was finally found to be through the method of surface cooling. (Fig. 11) A special apparatus was developed and Boerema published his results with this in 1956 (18). In 1951, Boerema wrote (17):

With the help of considerable cooling, the metabolic rate in animals dropped so far that the brain could dispense with the circulation of blood for a much longer time than would be normally the case. In consequence of this the circulation could be interrupted for a period of time three times as long as normal. There was ample time to open the heart, which had been practically drained of blood by clamping the venae cavae, and to perform a vue an intracardial operation. It is possible that this method may eliminate the necessity for an artificial heart in cardiac surgery.

Henry's law states that the physical solution of a gas in a liquid increases in a linear fashion with increasing the pressure of that gas above that liquid. Boerema found that by inhaling 100 % normobaric oxygen the amount of physically dissolved oxygen in the plasma was five times higher than when air was breathed at the same body temperature. He found that the amount of oxygen in physical solution increased greatly when the atmospheric pressure is raised. It is of interest to read his analysis of the problem of open-heart surgery and his, at that time theoretical, solution.

From a purely technical point of view, open intracardial surgery offers no difficulties; splitting of valves, excision of tumours and closure of defects can be carried out in the same way as has been done for many years in various parts of the body. The problem, however, is how to approach the lesion? If industry is taken as an example, the ideal would be stopping the motor during repairs. However, unlike the situation in industry, stopping the heart causes damage to all organs, including the heart itself. In other words the difficulty of the whole problem lies in the impossibility of stopping the circulation for any great length of time. The drawback to the normal oxygen supply in the body is the absence of a reservoir where oxygen can be stored. With hyperbaric oxygen the amount of oxygen in physical solution increases greatly when the atmospheric pressure is raised. If oxygen is inhaled at three atmospheres absolute pressure, then the amount of oxygen in physical solution is probably fifteen times as much as is found in blood normally (18).

Boerema thought that in this way every cell in the body could be supersaturated with oxygen before cardiac arrest; every cell could have its own large oxygen reservoir. (Fig. 4, 6-9)

Now the Amsterdam surgical clinic did not have a hyperbaric chamber. At the end of 1955, arrangements were made with the relevant department of the Royal Netherlands Navy at Den Helder, about 60 miles north of Amsterdam, for the start of animal experiments at the diving unit. Boerema with a team of volunteers went to be tested for the job in December 1955. Quite a few of the staff hesitated at the thought of the unknown risks.

By lowering the body temperature to 28°C, a period of complete circulatory arrest for seven to eight minutes was well tolerated and it was possible to perform small intracardial repairs in this way. Lower temperatures were not well tolerated and resulted in arrhythmias.

From 1956 until 1959 the main object of study was inflow and outflow occlusion of the heart, with and without hypothermia. This was followed by experiments on life without blood ("Haemoglobin itself was no longer necessary") (19). (Fig. 1-3, 20, & 22-24)

In 1959 a large hyperbaric chamber, a pressurised operating theatre, was finished on the grounds of the Wilhelmina Gasthuis in Amsterdam. A lot of research, very much stimulated by Boerema, was done on the possible value of "hyperbaric oxygen drenching" on many diseases both clinically and experimentally. Unfortunately, or maybe fortunately the first and only indication at that moment, being cardiac surgery, rapidly disappeared with the development and perfection of the heart-lung machine. At first, because of the priming volume necessary for the heart-lung machine, it was not possible to operate on small children with the help of extracorporeal circulation.

In palliative cardiac surgery of blue babies, hyperbaric oxygen remained of value initially. The first operation was carried out on December 18,1960. Until 1972, a total number of 143 cardiac operations in the Amsterdam hyperbaric chamber were carried out.

The value of the treatment of gas gangrene was also found and the first patient was treated in November 1960. Boerema described the results as follows (20):

Another disease in which hyperbaric oxygen therapy does indeed influence the enzymatic processes in a miraculous life-saving way is anaerobic infection, especially with Clostridium Welchii. Forty patients, mostly completely hopeless cases, often deeply jaundiced, or already comatose were sent to my department. In all cases but one cure (of the anaerobic infection) was complete in twenty-four hours. The temperature immediately dropped to normal, the patients woke up from coma, asking for food, talking and behaving normally. No primary amputations were done. After several weeks we only removed, very economically, the dead tissue, or the dead foot. So we not only saved lives, but also limbs. Originally we thought this miraculous result might be explained by killing of the clostridia by the oxygen, that is by disturbing important enzymatic processes. However, we soon found out that in many proved cases, while the patients were clinically cured, there were still clostridia present in the tissues. Van Unnik (Amsterdam) then found that oxygen at three-atmosphere pressure stopped completely the production of necrotising a-toxin of the clostridia, apparently by influencing some of their enzymatic processes. This action on the necrotising a-toxin was present only during the session in the hyperbaric chamber, not between the sessions. However, we must accept that this intermittent arrest of the a-toxin production prevents the damaging of the tissue of the host enough to eliminate the condition necessary for the clostridia to multiply. The host then wins the battle. Furthermore van Unnik proved that oxygen saturation at three atmospheres stops the production of a-toxin, but that two atmospheres does not. So for the treatment of infection with Clostridium welchii hyperbaric oxygen at two atmospheres pressure will probably not help the patients.

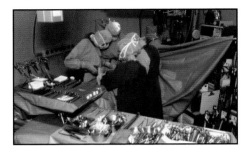

1. Operation inside the hyperbaric chamber. (See page 9)

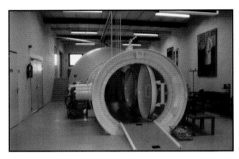

2. Multiplace hyperbaric chamber in the University Hospital "Academic Medical Center" of the University of Amsterdam (my hospital so to speak). (See page 9)

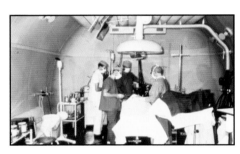

3. Preparation for an open-heart operation in 1964 in Amsterdam. (See page 9)

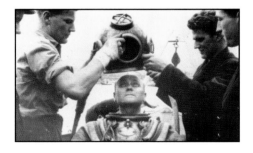

4. Period of experimental surgery with the Dutch Royal Navy in Den Helder, 1956. Prof. Boerema prepared for diving in a "standard diving suit." (See page 8)

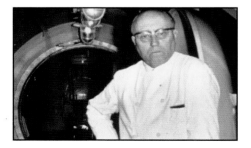

5. Professor Boerema at the entrance of the large hyperbaric chamber in the "Wilhelmina Gasthuis" in 1972. (See page 3)

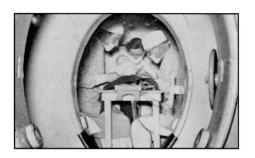

6. Experimental surgery (heart operation in rabbits) in the old recompression chamber of the Royal Navy in Den Helder. (See page 8)

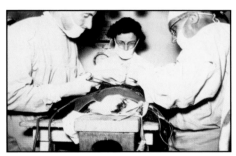

7. The same picture as in photo 6, but enlarged. On the left professor N.G. Meyne; in the middle Professor Vermeulen-Cranch, the first prof. of anaesthesiology in the Netherlands; and on the right side Professor Boerema. (See page 8)

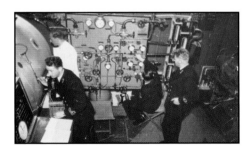

8. Supervision outside the chamber while experiments were done inside. (See page 8)

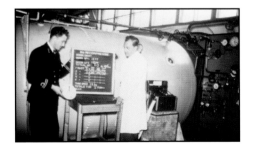

9. Supervision outside the chamber by both navy and medical personnel. (See page 8)

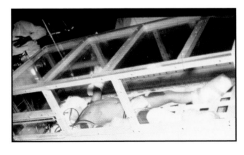

10. Cooling device for open-heart surgery in children. Primitive version from 1956. (See page 8)

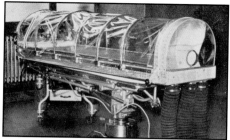

11. Improved cooling device, especially built by us for the use of surface cooling. Cold air was blown over the anaesthesized patient until the core temperature was 30 - 31 °C. Then the device was opened and put in the chamber. The operation started and when at 3 ATA the heart was arrested and the intervention performed.
(See page 8)

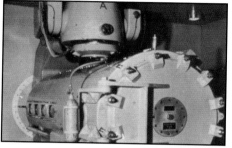

12. Hyperbaric oxygen in combination with radiotherapy. The original chamber and radiation device used by Dr. Churchill-Davidson in St. Thomas Hospital in London in 1964.
(See page 7)

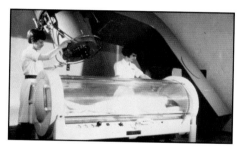

13. A more modern radiation device and a Vickers chamber in an English hospital in 1967.
(See page 7)

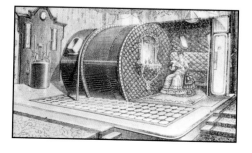

14. An old-fashioned Vickers monoplace chamber.
(See page 7)

15. Forlanini's "pneumatic institute." First treatment chamber constructed as a horizontally positioned chamber.
(See page 5)

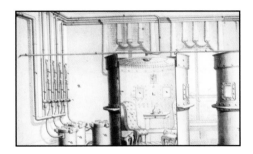

16. **Pneumatic center in Stockholm, Sweden in 1867.**
    (See page 5)

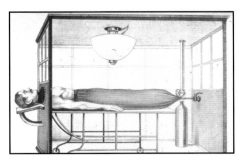

17. **Hypobaric chamber in use for lung diseases by professor Sauerbruch in the "Charité" hospital in Berlin last part of the 19th and first half of the 20th century.   (See page 7)**

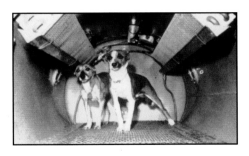

18. **Experimental animal chamber of Owen H. Wangensteen (USA). (See page 17)**

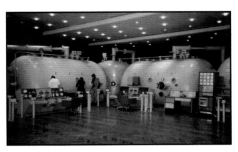

19. **All Union Hyperbaric Center in the Surgical Research Institute, Abrikosovsky Street in Moscow in 1975 (demolished in the nineties). (See page 18)**

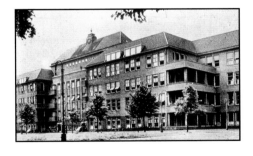

20. **Surgical clinic of Prof. Boerema at the "Wilhelmina Gasthuis" in Amsterdam. (See page 9)**

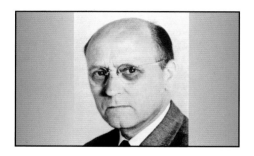

21. Prof. Dr. med. Ite Boerema, the "Father of Modern HBO." (See page 7)

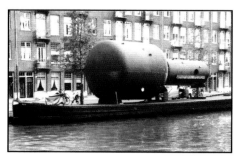

22. The giant Boerema-chamber on one of the famous Amsterdam "Grachten" (= canals). (See page 9)

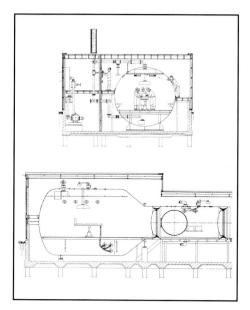

23. Cross-sections of HBO chamber in the Wilhelmina Gasthuis show clearly the great dimensions of this early system. (See page 9)

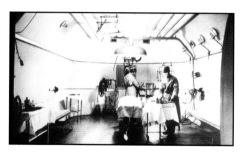

24. The HBO operation theater in the Wilhelmina Gasthuis at Amsterdam. This compartment has a length of nearly 8 m and a diameter of 4.6 m. The windows are comparatively small and it's impossible to look out of them. (See page 9)

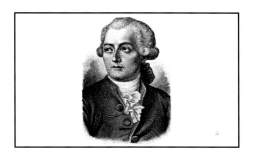

25. Antoine Laurent Lavoisier, one of the greatest scientists ever. (See page 3)

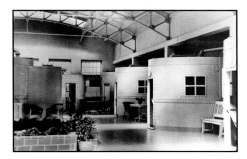

26. "Pneumatic Chambers" in the Dianabad at Bad Reichenball. (See page 5)

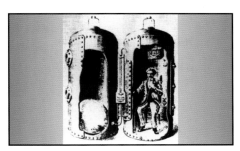

27. Paul Bert during a test in his hyper/hypo chamber. As in coal mines a bird was used for indicating bad gases in the breathing air. (See page 3)

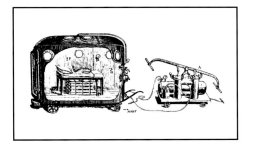

28. The very first "Mobile Hyperbaric Chamber" developed by the French surgeon Fontaine. (See pages 5 & 6)

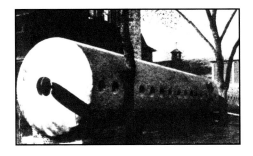

29. Cylindrical HB-treatment chamber of Orville J. Cunningham at Kansas City, USA. (See page 5)

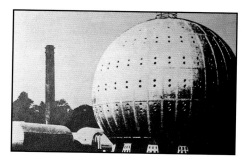

30. **Cunningham knew no limits. Here the monstrous sphere of Cleveland. It is most likely the biggest hyperbaric chamber ever built. It had a volume of 3,880 m³. (See page 6)**

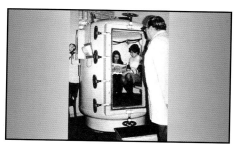

31. **First medical treatment chamber in Germany. Owned by Dr. med. Josef Reush at Nittel on the Mosel. (See page 5)**

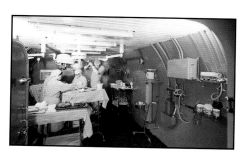

32. **Prof. Dr. med. G. Friehs built the second biggest HBO operation theater in Europe at Graz, Austria. Only Prof. Boerema's unit at Amsterdam was bigger. (See page 17)**

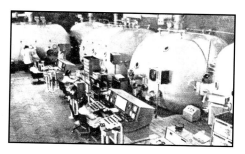

33. **Most likely the biggest HBO-center ever built in the world: The hyperbaric unit at the All Union Center for Surgical Research, Moscow. (See page 18)**

Other indications that were studied were carbon monoxide poisoning, tumor growth, effects of cytostatics under pressure, experimental cancer in mice, impaired diffusion capacity of the lungs, ergot foot, Meleney's ulcers, vascular insufficiency of the retina and chronic vascular insufficiency of the extremities, rheumatic diseases, tetanus, sepsis, wound healing, cerebrovascular insufficiency, asphyxia neonatorum, organ preservation, diabetes mellitus and its complications, and gas emboli.

Many expectations were not fulfilled and gradually the true indications for hyperbaric oxygen treatment emerged. Meyne gave a complete review of all the work of the Amsterdam surgical clinic in this field between 1956 and 1972 (48, 49).

The surgical uses of the hyperbaric chamber were summarised by Trippel et al. in 1966 (69). They mentioned the treatment of ileus by Wangensteen in 1955 (70). (Fig. 18) Indications were:

1. Protection during induced circulatory arrest
2. Homotransplantation
3. Clostridial infection
4. Acute arterial insufficiency
5. Chronic arterial insufficiency
6. Hypovolemic shock

They concluded that overenthusiasm had subsided and that, at that time current, interest was acquiring "a healthy attitude of cautious acceptance."

Smith, also in 1966, discussed respiratory disease of the newborn, carbon-monoxide poisoning, cyanide poisoning, open heart surgery, acute coronary occlusion, chronic and acute arterial insufficiency, cold injuries, cerebrovascular disease, malignant disease, and anaerobic and aerobic infections, and considered these all more or less important indications for hyperbaric oxygen therapy (64).

Pascale and Wallyn (53) reported their surgical experience in infectious diseases (clostridial myonecrosis or gas gangrene and tetanus), chronic osteomyelitis, cardiac surgery, peripheral arterial insufficiency, vascular surgery, and burns. They studied the possible value of hyperbaric oxygen experimentally in dogs in massive pulmonary embolism and in hemorrhagic, septic, and traumatic shock. More or less the same indications were discussed by James Watt from the Royal Navy (71).

Surgical experiments in a hyperbaric oxygen chamber, mainly cardiac surgery and traumatic amputations, were performed and reported by Friehs in 1971 (32). (Fig. 32)

Another important indication, however rare, has been reported from the Amsterdam center. They performed whole-lung lavage under hyperbaric oxygen conditions for alveolar proteinosis with respiratory failure with good results (40).

International Developments

In 1963 the First International Congress on Hyperbaric Oxygenation under the presidency of Prof. Boerema took place in the surgical clinic of the Wilhelmina Gasthuis in Amsterdam. Participants were present only on invitation by Boerema. This meant the start of the still existing International Congress on Hyperbaric Medicine (ICHM), which is the oldest organization in the field and has a permanent office in Amsterdam.

The field was judged so important that the international meetings initially followed in quick succession; Glasgow 1964 (Illingworth, McAledingham) and Duke University 1965 (Saltzmann, Brown, and Cox). The progress then slowed down because many researchers left the field and the next congress was held in 1969 in Sapporo, Japan (Wada, Iwa, and Sakakibara). Subsequently, congresses were held every four years in 1973 in Vancouver, Canada B.C. (W.G.Trapp); 1977 Aberdeen, Scotland (G. Smith); 1981 Moscow, (Fig. 19 & 33) USSR (S. Yefuni). Then on a tri-annual base in Long Beach, California, 1984 (J.H. Jacobson II); Sydney, Australia in 1987 (I. Unsworth) and back in Amsterdam in 1990 (D.J. Bakker). In 1996 in Milan, Italy (A. Marroni); 1993 Fuzhou, China (Wen Ren Li); 1999 Kobe, Japan (H. Takahashi) and 2002 in San Francisco, USA (F.S. Cramer). The 2005 meeting is planned in Barcelona, Spain (J. Desola) together with the EUBS. An excellent review of all scientific presentations at the first five congresses is given by Davis in 1977 (27).

Between the second and the third International Congress, a significant conference on hyperbaric oxygenation was held in January 1965 and the papers were published in the *Annals of the New York Academy of Sciences*. Conference chairmen were C.J. Lambertsen, George Bond, and J.H. Jacobson II (35).

U.S. Navy Diving and Submarine medical officers founded in 1967 the Undersea Medical Society (UMS), later, in 1986 during a meeting in Kobe, Japan, converted to the Undersea and Hyperbaric Medical Society or the UHMS. Originally the UMS was dedicated to diving and undersea medicine but later also clinical hyperbaric medicine was recognised and included in the society.

An important achievement was reached in 1976 when the UMS authorised an *ad hoc* Committee on Hyperbaric Oxygenation. E.P. Kindwall was made chairman and he selected 18 international members from the field of hyperbaric medicine. The task of the committee was to evaluate the clinical and scientific evidence for the various indications claimed to benefit from hyperbaric oxygen treatment. The first report was published in May 1977. This was accepted as a source document by the Blue Cross/Blue Shield organisation in the USA. The *ad hoc* character of the committee was changed a few years later in a Standing Committee called Hyperbaric Oxygen Therapy Committee with the same task. Their report is updated regularly and the committee meets at least yearly.

Meanwhile in Europe the need was felt for a European society for diving and underwater medicine. In 1965 the European Undersea Biomedical Society was founded (EUBS). In 1993 the name was changed to European Undersea and Baromedical Society to also include clinical hyperbaric medicine.

As far as the indications for hyperbaric oxygen therapy were concerned, the European centers followed more or less the indications of the USA determined by the HBO Committee. The various European centers were very much oriented on the USA, not in the least by the annual conferences organised by George Hart in Long Beach, California, that were a great source for improving knowledge in the field and meeting many colleagues.

This changed when in February 1989 in Milan, Italy, the European Committee for Hyperbaric Medicine was founded (72). The first chairman was Prof. Wattel from Lille, France. This committee acts as an organised Hyperbaric Medicine Scientific Body. The first plenary meeting was held in August 1990 in Amsterdam. One of the goals is to organize consensus meetings on the various indications or groups of indications for hyperbaric oxygen therapy. The first was held in Lille, France in 1994 on acute and chronic indications; the second in Marseille, France in 1996 on recreational diving; the third in Milan, Italy in 1999 on indications in orthopaedic surgery and traumatology; the fourth was held in London, UK on the diabetic foot in 1998; and the fifth in Lisbon, Portugal in 2001 on the role of hyperbaric oxygen treatment in radiation damage of normal tissues. In between these meetings a workshop on safety and wound healing was held in Belgrade, Yugoslavia in 1998.

Regular meetings are planned between the UHMS Committee and the European Committee to reach consensus about the various indications in hyperbaric medicine.

The era of experience-based or even eminence-based hyperbaric medicine left some time ago. By consenting to and participating in modern methods to establish evidence-based hyperbaric medicine, much credibility has been gained world-wide for our speciality. This book will hopefully prove our point.

REFERENCES

1. "A pictorial history of diving". Bachrach AJ, Desiderati BM, Matzen MM eds. 1988 Best Publishing Co., San Pedro Calif.

2. Aristotle. De historia animalium. Lib VII, Cap 7; 300 BC

3. Arntzenius AKW. De Pneumatische Therapie. Scheltema Holkema, Amsterdam 1887

4. Bakker DJ. The use of hyperbaric oxygen in the treatment of certain infectious diseases especially gas gangrene ansd acute dermal gangrene. Drukkerij Veenman BV Wageningen 1984; 15-16, 29-32

5. Bancroft FW, Fuller AG, Ruggiero WF. Improved methods in extremity amputations for diabetic gangrene. Ann Surg 1942; 115: 621

6. Beddoes SB, Watt J. Considerations on the medical use and the rpoduction of factitious airs. Bristol 1796: 9.

7. Behnke AR, Johnson FS, Poppen JR, Motley EP. The eefect of oxygen on man at pressures from one to four atmospheres. Am J Physiol 1935; 110: 565-572

8. Behnke AR, Forbes HS, Motley EP. Circulatory and visual effects of oxygen at 3 atmospheres pressure. Am J Physiol 1936; 114: 436-442

9. Behnke AR, Shaw LA. Use of hyperbaric oxygen in treatment of compressed air illness. Nav Med Bull 1937; 35: 1-12

10. Behnke AR. A brief history of Hyperbaric Medicine. In Davis JC, Hunt TK. Hyperbaric Oxygen Therapy. Bethesda (Md): Undersea and Hyperbaric Medical Society; 1977: 3-10

11. Bert P. La pression barométrique. Recherches de physiologie experimentale. Paris, Masson Cie 1878.

12. Bert P. C R Acad Sci (Paris) 1879; 89: 132-135

13. Bigelow WG, Greenwood WF, Lindsay WK. Hypothermia. Its possible role in cardiac surgery: an investigation of factors governing survival in dogs at low body temperature. Ann Surg 1950; 132: 849

14. Bigelow WG, Callaghan JC, Hopps JH. General hypothermia for experimental intracardiac surgery. Ann Surg 1950; 132: 531

15. Bigelow WG. Hypothermia. Surg 1958; 43: 683

16. Blalock A, Mason MF. A comparison of the effect of heat and cold in the prevention and treatment of shock. Arch Surg 1941; 42: 1054

17. Boerema I, Wildschut A, Schmidt WJH, Broekhuyzen L. Experimental researches into hypothermia as an aid to surgery of the heart. Arch Chir Neerl 1951; 3: 25

18. Boerema I, Kroll JA, Meyne NG et al. High atmospheric pressure as an aid to cardiac surgery. Arch Chir Neerl 1956; 8: 193-211

19. Boerema I, Meyne NG, Brummelkamp WH et al. Life without blood. A study of the influence of high atmospheric pressure and hypothermia on dilution of the blood. J Cardiovasc Surg 1960a; 1: 133-146

20. Boerema I. High tension oxygen therapy. Proc Royal Soc Med 1964; 57 (9): 817-818

21. Boerema I. Surgery under high atmospheric pressure. Haarlemse Voordrachten no XXX. Algemene Verg van de Hollandse Sociëteit der Wetenschappen te Haarlem. Bohn NV Haarlem 1970: 13-14

22. Bureau of Investigation. The Cunningham "Tank treatment". JAMA 1928; 90 (18): 1494-1496

23. Churchill-Davidson I, Sanger C, Thomlinson RH. High pressure oxygen and radiotherapy. Lancet 1955; i: 1091-1095

24. Churchill-Davidson I. Oxygen effect on radiosensitivity. Conf on Research on Radiotherapy of Cancer. Cancer 1961 (suppl): 122

25. Crossman LW, Ruggiero WF, Hurley V, Allen FM. Reduced temperature in surgery. Amputations for peripheral vascular disease. Arch Surg 1942; 44: 139

26. Cunningham OJ. Oxygen therapy by means of compressed air. Anaesth Analg 1927; April: 64-66

27. Davis JC. Background. In Davis JC, Hunt TK (eds). Hyperbaric Oxygen Therapy. Undersea Medical Society Inc. Bethesda MD, 1977: XIII-XXII.

28. End E, Long CW. HBO in carbon-monoxide poisoning. I. Effect on dogs and guinea pigs. J Ind Hyg Toxicol 1942; 24: 302-306

29. Faesecke KP. Arbeit in (berdruck- Die Forschungsarbeiten von Arthur und Adele Bornstein beim Bau des ersten Hamburger Elbtunnels 1909-1910. Dissertation Universität Hamburg. Hamburg University Printing 1997

30. Fay T. Observations on prolonged human refrigeration. N Y State J Med 1940; 2: 1351

31. Fontaine JA. Emploi chirurgical de láir comprimé. Union Méd 1879: 28; 445

32. Friehs G. Experimentelle Chirurgie unter hyperbarem Sauerstoff. Wiener Med Wchschr 1971; 16: 334-339

33. Haux GFK. History of Hyperbaric Chambers. Best Publ Comp Flagstaff Az 2000

34. Hoff EC. Bibliographical sourcebook of compressed air, diving and submarine medicine. Washington DC, Res Division, Project X-427, Bureau of Medicine and Surgery, Navy Dept, 1948,6.

35. Hyperbaric oxygenation. Ann N Y Acad Sci 1965; 117: 647-890

36. Jacobson JH II, Morsch JHC, Rendell-Baker L. The historical perspective of hyperbaric therapy. In: Boerema I, Brummelkamp WH and Meyne N (eds): Clinical application of hyperbaric oxygen. Proceedings of the First International Congress in September 1963. Elsevier Publ Cie Amsterdam, London, New York; 1963: 7-19

37. Jacobson JH II, Morsch JHC, Rendell-Baker L. The historical perspective of hyperbaric therapy. In: Whipple HE (ed) Hyperbaric Oxygenation. Ann N Y Acad Sci 1965; 117: 651- 670

38. Jain KK, Fischer B. Oxygen in Physiology and Medicine. Charles C Thomas Publ Springfield Ill; 1989: 3-13

39. Jain KK. Textbook of hyperbaric medicine. Hogrefe & Huber Publ Toronto, Lewiston NY, Bern 1990;4

40. Jansen HW, Zuurmond WW, Roos CM et al. Whole-lung lavage under hyperbaric oxygen conditions for alveolar proteinosis with respiratory failure. Chest 1987; 91: 829-832

41. Junod VT. Recherches physiologiques et therapeutiques sur les effets de la compression et de la rarefaction de l'air tant sur le corps que sur les membres isolés. Rev Méd Franc Etrang 1834 ; 3 : 350.

42. Keuskamp DHG. De ervaringen met luchtkoeling ten behoeve van operaties aan het hart (Experiences with air cooling for heart operations) Thesis University of Amsterdam. Rototype/Broos, Amsterdam 1960

43. Kindwall EP. History of diving and diving medicine. In : Strauss RH (ed.) Diving Medicine, Grune Stratton, Inc Orlando, New York 1976 :2, 4

44. Lavoisier AL, Sequin A. La respiration des animaux. Med Acad Sci 1789; 566

45. Lorrain-Smith J. The pathological effects due to increase of oxygen tension in the air breathed. J Physiol 1989; 24: 19-35

46. Meesters JN. Caissonziekte (Caisson disease). 1958 Thesis, University of Amsterdam. Erven Bohn, Haarlem.

47. Medical Research Council Working Party. Radiotherapy and Hyperbaric Oxygen. Lancet 1978; ii: 881-884

48. Meyne NG. Hypothermia and cardiac surgery. Review and preview. Arch Chir Neerl 1973; XXV (II); 227-244

49. Meyne NG. Hyperbaric oxygen and its clinical value. Charles C Thomas Publ. Springfield Ill., 1970

50. Meyne NG. Hyperbaric oxygen, increased pressure and the activities in this field in Boerema's department in the period 1956-1972. Arch Chirur Neerl 1973; XXV (fasc II): 195-213

51. Mosso A. Action physiologiques et applications thérapeutiques de l'oxygéne comprimé. C R Acad Sci (Paris) 1900 ; 131: 483

52. Naber HA. De Ster van 1572. Uitg. Wereldbibliotheek Amsterdam 1907: 58-59

53. Pascale LR, Wallyn RJ. Surgical applications of the hyperbaric chamber. Surg Clin N Am 1986; 48: 63-70

54. Pravaz CHG. Mémoire sur l'emploi du bain d'air comprimé associé a la gymnastique dans le traitement du rachitisme, des affections strumeuse et des surdités catarrales. L'Experience 1840 ; 5 : 177

55. Pravaz CHG. Observations relatives aux effects thérapeutiques des bains d'air comprimé. C R Acad Sci (Paris) 1840 ; II : 910

56. Priestly J. The discovery of oxygen (1775). Alembic Club Reprints, University of Chicago Press, Chicago 1906

57. Rendell-Baker L, Jacobson JH II. Hyperbaric oxygenation. Int Anaesthesiol Clin 1999; 37(1): 137-167

58. Saturday Evening Post, March 5, 1921

59. Scheele CW. Chemische Abhandlung von der Luft und dem Feuer. In: Engelmann W (ed). Ostwalds Klassiker der Exakten Wissenschaften Leipzig 1894; 58: 87

60. Shah SA. Healing with oxygen. A history of hyperbaric medicine. Pharos of Alpha Omega Alpha Honor Med Soc 2000; 63(2): 13-19

61. Sluyter ME. The treatment of carbon-monoxide poisoning by administration of oxygen at high atmospheric pressure. Thesis University of Amsterdam, 1963

62. Smith EB. Priestley lecture: on the science of deep sea diving-observations of the respiration of different kinds of air. Chem Soc Rev 1986; 15: 503-522

63. Smith G, Sharp GR. Treatment of carbon-monoxide poisoning with oxygen under pressure. Lancet 1960; i; 905-908

64. Smith G. Current therapeutics. CCXXVI- The present status of hyperbaric oxygen therapy. The Practitioner 1966; 197: 553-561

65. Smith LW. Refrigeration in cancer. N Y State J Med 1940; 40: 1355

66. Swan H, Virtue RW, Blount SG, Kircher LT. Hypothermia in surgery; analysis of 100 clinical cases. Ann Surg 1955; 142: 382

67. Tierie G. Cornelis Drebbel (1572-1633) H.J.Paris Amsterdam 1932

68. Trimble VH. The uncertain miracle - hyperbaric oxygen . Doubleday, New York 1974

69. Trippel OH, Jurayj MN, Staley CJ, van Elk J. Surgical uses of the hyperbaric oxygen chamber. Surg Clin N Am 1966; 46(1): 209-221

70. Wangensteen OH. Intestinal obstruction. 3rd ed. Charles C Thomas, Springfield, 1955: 190.

71. Watt J. Surgical Applications of Hyperbaric Oxygen Therapy in the Royal Navy. Proc Roy Soc Med (United Services Section) 1971; 64: 877-881.

72. Wattel F, Marroni A, Mathieu D. European Committee for Hyperbaric Medicine (ECHM) to coordinate, promote and study the development of clinical hyperbaric medicine in Europe. Minerva Anaesthesiol 2000; 66: 733-748.

CHAPTER 2

AIR EMBOLISM

F.S. Cramer

INTRODUCTION

Air embolism is a major cause of death following diving accidents as well as in intensive care units of major acute care hospitals. The practicing surgeon is involved with the care of patients exposed to the risk of air embolism on a daily basis. Although prevention is the most important issue, air embolism will continue to occur despite everyone's best efforts. This chapter will endeavor to help the surgeon establish a prompt diagnosis and transfer the patient to the nearest hyperbaric chamber on an emergency basis. For those surgeons working closely with a hyperbaric facility, the management of pulmonary overpressure (diving accidents) must also be well understood.

The major problem with this clinical disorder is one of early diagnosis and definitive treatment. Time is the most critical factor in determining the eventual outcome in most cases. This chapter will concentrate on the importance of early diagnosis and therapy. Treatment is based upon solid physiological principles. Therapy involves both compression of the air bubbles (Boyle's Law) and oxygenation of ischemic (hypoxic) tissue with hyperbaric oxygen (HBO).

The problem with air bubbles in the circulation began 300 million years ago during the Mississippian Period of the Paleozoic Era, when the first amphibians left the sea to take up a terrestrial (air-breathing) lifestyle. During the eon that has passed since then, humans have developed a number of important defense mechanisms to prevent the inadvertent entry of air bubbles into the bloodstream. For example, if the lung is punctured from without, the elastic lung tissue produces a rapid collapse (Figure 1). If an artery is lacerated it bleeds briskly, thereby precluding the entry of air. Likewise, with certain important exceptions, veins collapse which tends to prevent air entry. The dural sinus is an important exception to this rule and a major risk factor for air embolism with the patient in a sitting position during neurosurgery.

Because of the important natural factors mentioned above, air embolism was not a major clinical problem prior to this century. However, with the advent of modern technology, such as compressed air diving and submarines, man has introduced a significant opportunity for air entry into the systemic circulation following pulmonary overpressure accidents. In addition, the modern use of invasive devices during surgery and intensive care of the critically ill patient offer numerous opportunities for the entry of air into the circulation, with death and stroke resulting (1).

ETIOLOGY

The first published report of a death resulting from air embolism was published in France in 1821 (2). The patient was undergoing an operation on his clavicle and suddenly cried out "my blood is falling into my heart–I'm dead." This was coincident with a hissing sound noted by the surgeon during the operation. Fifteen minutes later the patient died–presumably from a major venous air embolism with cardiac arrest.

Air embolism may be categorized as either venous or arterial in nature (2). Venous emboli are the most common, while arterial are the most serious. The lungs are an excellent filter of air emboli. However, they may be overwhelmed by a massive embolism or bypassed via a patent foramen ovale in the heart. Approximately one-third of the population may have a probe-patent foramen. This may easily open, when the pulmonary outflow tract is obstructed with a large venous embolism, thereby creating a right-to-left shunt via the atrial septum.

A classic example of air embolism, one which has been seen since the very early days of compressed air diving, is defined as "pulmonary overpressure." This occurs when the person is exposed to a rapid and sudden decrease in ambient pressure with a closed glottis. It is generally agreed that if the pressure differential between the alveoli and the outside of the lung exceeds 80 mm of mercury, the potential for rupture of the delicate tissue of the air sac becomes a realistic possibility.

Rupture pressure can be attained by breath-holding from depths as shallow as four feet or slightly over one meter of water. Clinical cases have been reported with scuba (self contained underwater breathing apparatus) diving accidents during shallow water breathing by untrained individuals in a swimming pool environment. A similar situation may occur in an altitude chamber, or high-flying aircraft, during a rapid decompression if conscious breath-holding takes place. This is unusual due to the naturally open glottis during normal respiration. However, when the diver's face is in the water and a rapid ascent carried out under emergency conditions, the natural response is complete breath-holding.

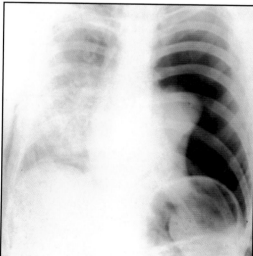

Figure 1. Chest X-ray of Pneumothorax

The United States Navy has described their extensive experience with air embolism during submarine escape training at their facility in New London, Connecticut (3) + (Figure 2). The cerebral air embolism produced under this circumstance is rapidly life threatening if not treated immediately in a compression chamber. The chamber at the training facility was initially located at the base of the 200 foot water tower. When the student surfaced at the top and became unconscious, it was necessary to transfer him to the ground level chamber via elevator. Due to the time delay in recompression, the clinical outcome was not always satisfactory. The chamber was then relocated to the top of the training tower with excellent clinical results. This relocation serves to dramatically demonstrate the critical time factor in the successful management of arterial air embolism.

Other results of pulmonary overpressure accidents which are frequently seen are pneumothorax (Figure 1) and pneumomediastinum. When seen alone, neither of these require intervention with compression therapy. However, they should alert the physician to a possible occult neurological deficit, which may progress and require hyperbaric chamber treatment.

An examination of the extensive literature on the subject of air embolism reveals a number of etiological mechanisms, both venous and arterial (Table 1). A brief review of the situations listed reveals that even a low incidence of medical accidents can result in a significant number of clinical air embolism cases. This is due to the common occurrence of the events listed in Table 1. For example, central venous catheterizations are a routine daily event in acute care hospitals. The list is not exhaustive, but merely serves to point out the many different methods which may interrupt the integrity of the vascular system, thereby allowing the inadvertent entry of air into the circulation.

PATHOPHYSIOLOGY

Time is the first and single most important factor in the ultimate outcome of a clinical case of air embolism. The bubble is immediately identified as a foreign body by the platelets, thereby unleashing a cascade of complex biochemical reactions. Platelets are activated and undergo the release of multiple vasoactive amines and prostaglandins. Dr. Philp and his co-workers in Canada have demonstrated the platelet response to air bubbles with elegant electron microscopy (4).

An immediate effect of the bubble is to lodge distally in the smaller arterioles of the brain and obstruct the flow of blood (Figure 4). The mechanical effect of this obstruction is easy to understand. It is also readily apparent that ischemia with resultant hypoxia of the distal tissue occurs. With the passage of time, edema progressively develops due to cellular hypoxia and swelling.

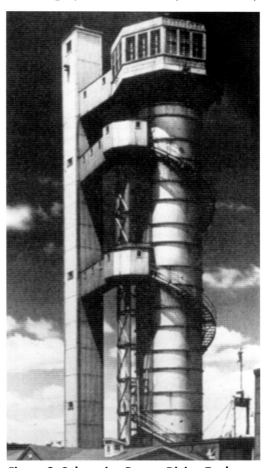

Figure 2. Submarine Escape Diving Tank

TABLE 1. ETIOLOGY OF SURGICAL AIR EMBOLISM

ETIOLOGY—AIR EMBOLISM ARTERIAL

1. Pulmonary Overpressure-
   SCUBA, Chamber, etc.
2. Lung Biopsy
3. Arterial Catheter
4. Angiography
5. Operative Surgery
6. Paradoxial - Patent Foramen Ovale
7. Chest Trauma - Penetrating
8. Neonatal Respiratory Distress
   Syndrome
9. Pneumothorax - Artificial
10. Cardiopulmonary Bypass
11. Autotransfusion
12. Dialysis

ETIOLOGY—AIR EMBOLISM-VENOUS

1. Catheters - Central Venous-
   Swan-Ganz
2. Laparoscopy
3. Neurosurgery
4. Liver Transplantation
5. Umbilical Venous Catheters
6. Necrotizing Enterocolitis
7. Lumbar Disk Surgery
8. Infusion Pump
9. Air Contrast Salpingogram
10. Retroperitoneal Air-
    Duodenal Injury
11. Pelvic Surgery-
    Trendelenburg Position

TABLE 2. SURGICAL AIR EMBOLISM– PRESENTATION

18 PATIENTS

SYMPTOM	NUMBER
1. Focal Motor Deficit	12
2. Loss of Consciousness	7
3. Coma	6
4. Disorientation	5
5. Visual Defect	3
6. Focal Sensory Deficit	3
7. Respiratory Arrest	2
8. Nausea	2
9. Seizure	1
10. Headache	1
11. Abdominal Pain	1
12. Chest Pain	1
13. Ventricular Fibrillation	1

Some patients may have demonstrated one or
more symptoms.

TABLE 3. SURGICAL AIR EMBOLISM

18 PATIENTS
Age: 18-78 years (mean 57)
Sex: Male 16 – Female 2

PRIMARY DIAGNOSIS	NUMBER
1. Cardiovascular Disease	7
2. Gastrointestinal Disease	6
3. Pulmonary Disease	2
4. Experimental Subject	1
5. Other	2

TABLE 4. SURGICAL AIR EMBOLISM- PATIENT RESULTS

18 PATIENTS

RESPONSE	NUMBER	PERCENTAGE
Complete	10	55
Partial	5	28
None	3	17
Expired	2	11

Average time to reach chamber: 8 hours

The bubble is subsequently transformed into a sausage shape due to vasoconstriction of the vessel and edema of the tissue (5). Once the bubble is compressed and absorbed, reflow may still not occur into the damaged tissue due to the edema and fibrin formation (6).

Direct damage to the endothelial cells may also occur due to the mechanical effect of the bubble. This damage is worsened by further decompression of the patient once air embolism has occurred. An example of this happening is the helicopter transport of a patient, even at altitudes as

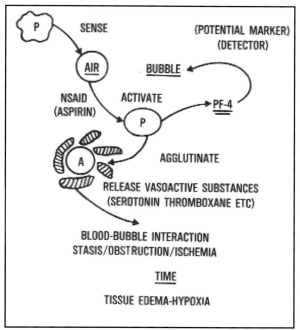

Figure 3. Platelet/Bubble Interaction

low as 1000 feet. Exposure of the underlying collagen following mechanical disruption of the endothelial lining of the blood vessel rapidly leads to further thrombosis and obstruction. Air bubbles may persist for remarkably long periods (days) in the tissue. Fibrin forms around the bubble in conjunction with a clump of platelets. This fibrin matrix covering leads to stabilization of the bubble and persistent symptoms.

DIAGNOSIS

Sir William Osler, the father of differential diagnosis, once stated that "A diagnosis not thought of is difficult to make." It could not be better said with regard to the clinical diagnosis of air embolism. Pulmonary overpressure is usually considered promptly, since the diving and aviation medical community is well versed in this area. In clinical medicine the opposite is true, as very few physicians are trained in these operational areas. The possibility of air embolism from surgical procedures must be considered, if it is to be diagnosed promptly.

Any patient with a history of exposure to pressure change, trauma, or an invasive surgical procedure–who suddenly suffers an acute neurological event–should be suspected of having a cerebral air embolism until proven otherwise. Air bubbles may be visualized in the ophthalmic vessels which is diagnostic for the disorder. The presence of air has been described on computer tomography scanning, but time should not be wasted on sophisticated diagnostic studies. Immediate treatment is critical to a successful outcome and even minutes may make a difference.

The onset of cerebral air embolism is sudden and dramatic. For example, the patient may be postoperative in the intensive care unit and doing well. Both arterial and central venous catheters are routinely in place for monitoring. With no prior neurological history, a grand mal seizure is typically seen–followed by focal motor and/or sensory neurological defects. Once urgent supportive steps are taken, to include cardiopulmonary resuscitation, the diagnosis of a possible air embolism should be entertained.

In the United States Air Force experience with cerebral air embolism, eighteen arose from invasive procedures, seven of which involved a central venous catheter. The lung may not be a completely perfect filter of venous air bubbles when large amounts are injected (7). The possibility of a patent foramen ovale may also allow transit of the venous bubbles to the arterial circulation.

TREATMENT

The initial steps of cardiopulmonary resuscitation are undertaken in the standard manner if either cardiac or respiratory arrest has occurred. If a cardiac machinery murmur is present with a low flow state, the patient should be immediately placed on the left side and aspiration of the air from the right atrium with a central venous catheter carried out.

Once the cardiac status is stable and patient's ventilation under control, the patient should be placed in a head-down position. A maximum of 30 degrees of Trendelenberg is recommended to allow the impacted bubbles to flow retrograde due to the forces of buoyancy. Animal studies have demonstrated that in an obstructed (no-flow) vessel, this simple maneuver is remarkably effective in restoring flow.

One hundred percent oxygen should be administered with a tight-fitting anesthesia mask or endotracheal tube. This surrounds the air bubble with oxygen at a high partial pressure. The size of the bubble will diminish due to the diffusion of nitrogen out of the bubble (Dalton's Law). Hypoxic and ischemic distal tissues are also oxygenated as much as possible while at ambient pressure.

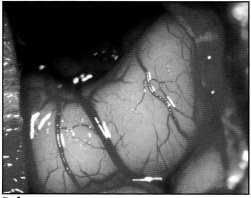 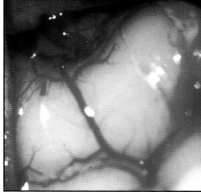

Before   **After**
Figure 4. Brain of a Cat Before and After Pulmonary Overpressure

If the patient is conscious or has a nasogastric tube in place, aspirin should be given. All non-steroidal anti-inflammatory drugs (NSAID) have an immediate and potent anti-platelet effect which is irreversible for the life of the platelet.

Intravenous steroids are routinely used as bolus (Decadron–10 mg) and repeated at 6-hour intervals for at least 24 hours. Steroids are not used for longer than 72 hours to avoid adrenal suppression. The role of steroids remains controversial. They have been used routinely in the author's experience without apparent complication. The theory that steroids may increase the patient's sensitivity to oxygen toxicity has not been demonstrated.

Heparin should be avoided due to the risk of a possible hemorrhagic stroke and subsequent worsening of the condition due to intra-cerebral bleeding.

Hydration with isotonic saline solutions is important if cerebral edema is not a prominent symptom. Hemoconcentration secondary to intravascular dehydration is a common problem in diving cases where concomitant fluid loss is frequently present.

Emergency transportation to the nearest hyperbaric chamber should be carried out by either ground ambulance or at sea level pressure in an appropriate aircraft. Even the slightest decrease in ambient pressure is harmful and should be avoided. In mountainous terrain the hyperbaric chamber facility should not be located at a higher elevation than the patient's initial location. The use of unpressurized helicopters should be restricted to overwater transportation, where low flying (less than 50 feet) can be done safely. The time of surface (watercraft) transportation may be significantly longer, thereby contraindicated if a helicopter is readily available.

Definitive treatment of serious air embolism can only be given in a hyperbaric chamber, where the entire patient is pressurized to greater than one atmosphere absolute (ATA).

Either a multiplace or monoplace chamber may be utilized. The choice is dependent primarily upon the type of chamber that is the most readily available.

If a multiplace chamber is used, immediate compression of the patient to 6 ATA is the standard initial approach. Bubbles will be immediately reduced to one-sixth of their previous volume (Boyle's Law) (Figure 5). During the time at this depth, either chamber air or a mixture of nitrox (50% nitrogen-50% oxygen) may be used. The time at this depth is thirty minutes on a standard U.S. Navy Table 6a (Figure 6). The time at 6 ATA may be extended to maximum of two hours if the clinical situation warrants. Decompression is then carried out on a Table 4 to 60 feet of seawater (2.8 ATA), where an extended Table 6 is accomplished (Figure 7).

Upon reaching 60 fsw (2.8 ATA) on the Table 6a, if the patient's symptoms worsen, a saturation treatment may be instituted at 100 feet of seawater (4 ATA). This is a demanding technique and few multiplace chambers are likely to have the necessary resources. The author has personal experience with saturation treatment on two occasions and remains less than enthusiastic about its indication and efficacy.

When a monoplace chamber is used, treatment is begun at either 2.8 or 3.0 ATA with 100% oxygen breathing on a U.S. Navy Table 6. Research has shown that this may be as effective as an initial compression to 6 ATA (8). Immediate oxygenation of ischemic tissue is accomplished by the hyperbaric oxygen and cerebral edema may also be lessened (9).

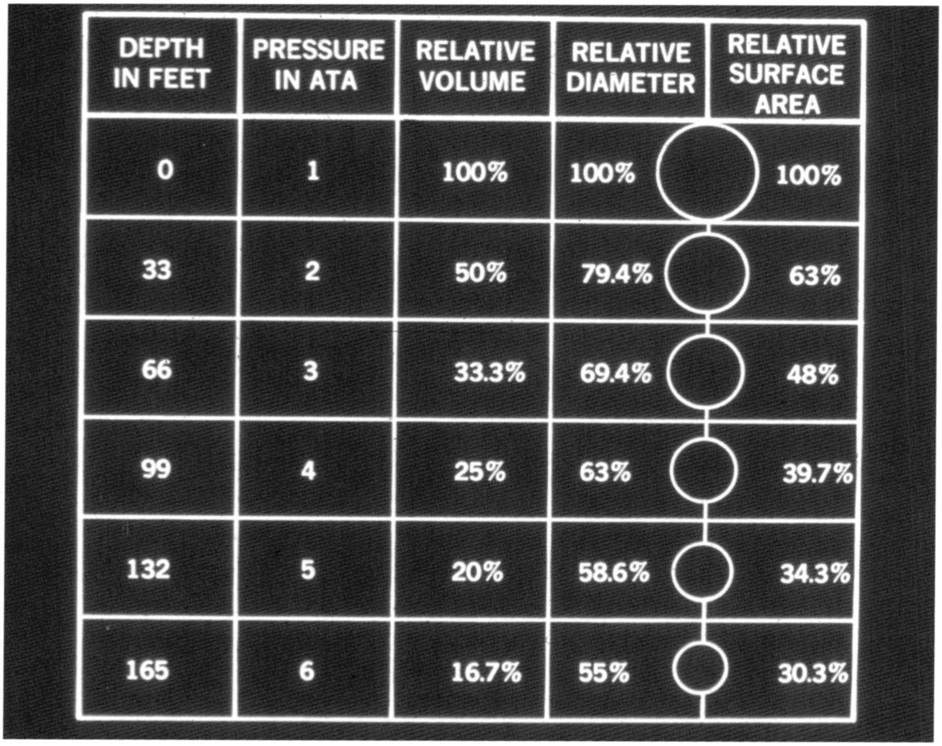

DEPTH IN FEET	PRESSURE IN ATA	RELATIVE VOLUME	RELATIVE DIAMETER	RELATIVE SURFACE AREA
0	1	100%	100%	100%
33	2	50%	79.4%	63%
66	3	33.3%	69.4%	48%
99	4	25%	63%	39.7%
132	5	20%	58.6%	34.3%
165	6	16.7%	55%	30.3%

Figure 5. Surface Area

Repetitive treatment with a daily Table 6 is recommended for those cases where a neurological defect persists. The end-point to hyperbaric therapy is a failure for the symptoms to improve objectively, either during or immediately following the treatment on two successive days of therapy.

CASE REPORTS

The following five brief case reports are discussed to illustrate the type of patients who experience air embolism. Case #5 is actually an example of decompression illness (DCI) with severe chokes. It is included to emphasize the critical role of ambient pressure change during transportation. The first four cases were treated at the United States Air Force School of Aerospace Medicine, Hyperbaric Medicine Division, Brooks Air Force Base, San Antonio, Texas. The author participated in the care of each of the case reports.

Case #1: The patient was a 48-year-old female who had a coin lesion noted on chest X-ray. She was a heavy smoker and bronchoscopy was indicated to rule out malignancy. An endobronchial biopsy was done on the left side. Immediately following the biopsy, the patient had a seizure and became unconscious. A CT scan of the brain demonstrated generalized edema and air in the cerebral vessels with spasm. She was transferred to the ICU for supportive care. The neurologist in charge observed the patient for the next 24 hours with a diagnosis of probable cerebral air embolism.

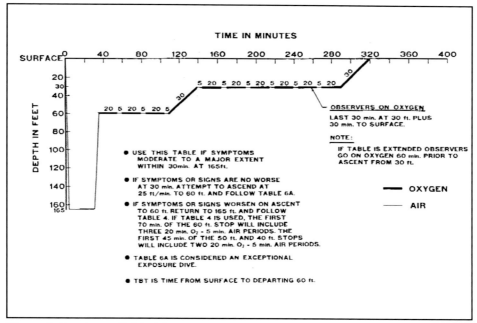

Figure 6. Treatment Table 6A

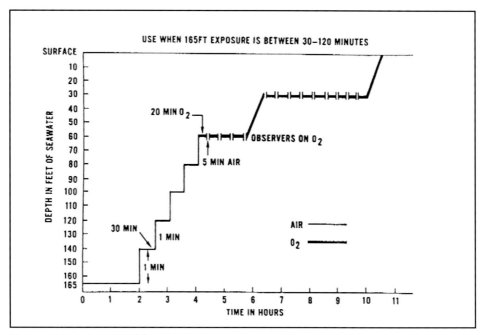

Figure 7. Treatment Table 4-6

When the patient remained in coma she was transferred to San Antonio by air ambulance at sea level pressure breathing 100% oxygen. She was immediately placed in the hyperbaric chamber and treated on a Table 6a. With no improvement after 30 minutes at 6 ATA the time was extended to 2 hours. The patient was then brought to 100 feet on a Table 4 and saturation was established at 4 ATA. She demonstrated progressive neurological improvement at that depth after 24 hours. At 48 hours she was awake and alert with recent memory loss as the only persistent symptom. She exited the chamber after a 72 hour treatment with minimal residual neurological symptoms. Unfortunately, the biopsy revealed carcinoma of the lung and she died of this disease one year later.

This case represents the efficacy of HBO therapy in a patient who was delayed 24 hours in reaching the hyperbaric facility. The role of saturation therapy in this case is unclear. The use of extended (back-to-back) Table 6s may also have been of benefit.

Case #2: This patient was a 56-year-old male undergoing open-heart valvular replacement surgery at a major medical center a few hundred miles north of San Antonio. The patient sustained a pump accident when coming off bypass. The circulatory system was completely drained of blood and replaced with pump oxygen, greater than 95%. When the femoral artery was cut-down upon, to place a large bore catheter, no blood was present. Blood was subsequently replaced and the chest wall closed. The patient remained in coma and was transferred to San Antonio via air ambulance at sea level pressure. Upon arrival he remained in a coma and was immediately taken to 165 feet of seawater (6 ATA). Since he was immediately postoperative from open-heart surgery two observers were inside the chamber. A fully trained, board-certified general surgeon (author) and a senior nurse anesthetist participated in the direct care of the patient while pressurized.

After two hours at 6 ATA without improvement, he was brought to 100 fsw on a Table 4 and saturation therapy begun. After 48 hours there was only minimal neurological improvement noted. The other major organ systems remained stable and functioning satisfactorily. The patient exited the chamber with only slight further improvement in his neurological condition. He was transferred to the intensive-care unit and over the next few weeks gradually awakened. The long-term prognosis was poor with probable severe neurological impairment.

This case is an example of major gas (oxygen) entry into the circulation. In spite of heparin and pump oxygen, as the gas involved, serious sequelae developed. Time was also a risk factor since a hyperbaric center was not available in the city where the surgery was carried out. This situation has now been rectified as HBO facilities become more readily available.

Case #3: The patient was a 62-year-old male who was undergoing coronary angiography at a San Antonio Medical Center for suspected coronary artery disease. Air was inadvertently injected into the coronary arteries, when the syringe was filled with air instead of dye. The error was immediately noted by the cardiologist on the fluoroscopy screen. The heart went into a ventricular fibrillation rhythm and was successfully defibrillated. The patient had a mild grand mal seizure but awoke promptly. He complained of total blindness in his right eye and a complete hemiparesis of his left side. This was consistent with a large air embolism to his right carotid artery.

Fortunately, the second cardiologist (Fellow) previously served as a flight surgeon. He was knowledgeable regarding the treatment of cerebral air embolism with hyperbaric oxygen therapy. The patient was immediately transferred to Brooks AFB via ground ambulance. He arrived approximately 60 minutes after the event. His eyesight had returned, but his left hemiplegia remained the same.

He was immediately taken to 165 fsw on a U.S. Navy Table 6a. After 15 minutes on air he began to spontaneously move his left leg. He completed the standard Table 6a with progressive improvement in his paralysis. He exited the chamber five hours and twenty minutes later with no significant neurological impairment. Subsequently, he underwent coronary artery surgery four weeks later without further complication.

Case #4: The patient was a 68-year-old male with a large abdominal aortic aneurysm. He was undergoing aortic angiography via a translumbar needle/catheter. In a manner similar to Case #3, air rather than contrast dye was placed in the power syringe. A massive aortoiliac air embolism was immediately noted by the radiologist. Fortunately, the vascular surgeon involved with the case was knowledgeable in hyperbaric medicine and frequently functioned as an inside observer at the Brooks Air Force Base chamber. The patient was immediately transferred via ambulance to the hyperbaric facility.

Upon arrival the patient was complaining of severe abdominal pain with distention. Both of his legs were cold and painful. The pain was controlled with parenteral narcotics. He was placed in the chamber and a descent to 165 fsw was begun within one hour of the incident. He was treated on an extended Table 6a with immediate amelioration of his abdominal distention and pain. He exited the chamber essentially asymptomatic. He underwent successful repair of his aneurysm two weeks later.

Case #5: The patient was a 22-year-old male who was undergoing physiological training as a part of his Flight Engineer School for the KC-135 aircraft. This was being held at Fairchild Air Force Base, Spokane, Washington. The altitude chamber training consisted of a rapid ascent to 35,000 feet, after 30 minutes of 100% oxygen breathing at the surface. Following hypoxia drills at this altitude, a sudden decompression to 41,000 feet was carried out. The students were then returned to the surface. All students were advised to avoid strenuous exercise for the remainder of the day.

The patient had a normal lunch and then ran a brisk five miles, which was his daily custom. He later told physicians that he didn't believe this exercise was strenuous, since he did it every day. Approximately four hours later he presented to the emergency room at the local Air Force Base hospital complaining of sub-sternal chest pain, shortness of breath, and a dry non-productive cough. He was afebrile and the chest X-ray was normal.

Because of his recent altitude chamber exposure, the flight surgeon on-call (author) contacted the Hyperbaric Medicine Unit in San Antonio. A diagnosis of decompression illness (DCI) with "chokes" was made and arrangements made for the emergency transfer of the patient to the nearest hyperbaric facility. The local hyperbaric chamber was inoperative at the time. A KC-135 was diverted from a training mission over Seattle for air evacuation of the patient to Castle Air Force Base in Merced, California.

The aircraft was on the ground within the hour and the patient transported to the flight line by ground ambulance. He was breathing 100% oxygen by aviator's mask and an isotonic intravenous fluid was being administrated. He was resting comfortably with stable vital signs. However, he continued to complain of sub-sternal chest pain which was moderate to severe.

The altitude of Fairchild Air Force Base is 2750 feet above sea level. Immediately after take-off the cabin pressure of the KC-135 was increased to 500 feet below sea level. This represented an increase of pressure of 3,250 feet. There was an immediate and dramatic change in the patient's symptoms, with a total and complete cessation of his chest pain. He fell asleep for the remainder of the 90-minute flight to California. The aircraft flew at 19,500 feet, which allowed the cabin pressure to be maintained at 500 feet below sea level.

Upon descent to land the engine power was reduced. This allowed the cabin pressure to rise to 3000 feet above sea level. Once again the patient's substernal chest pain recurred, although it was less severe. The patient was promptly treated with an extended Table 6 and exited the hyperbaric chamber without further problems.

Although this case is not one of air embolism, it does involve the evolution of nitrogen gas bubbles which became trapped in the lung. This is a very serious type of DCI and can rapidly progress to vascular collapse and death. The dramatic change in his symptoms, with relatively slight changes in ambient pressure, point out the need to avoid any negative pressure change when dealing with air embolism or other bubble-related disorder.

CONCLUSION

Air embolism is a dramatic and life-threatening clinical disorder. It is a common problem in intensive care units and acute care hospitals due to invasive surgical procedures. The diagnosis must be made promptly and definitive treatment in a hyperbaric chamber carried out on an emergency basis. The prognosis depends primarily upon the elapsed time from onset to treatment.

A high index of suspicion on the part of the clinician is important if significant mortality and morbidity is to be avoided. The surgeon must know the location of the nearest hyperbaric chamber facility, so that immediate consultation can be obtained. The details of the United States Air Force experience with cerebral air embolism are listed in Tables 2, 3, and 4. The recent increase in availability of hyperbaric chambers in the medical community makes the early recognition of the problem of air embolism even more important to a successful outcome.

REFERENCES

1. Murphy, B.P., Harford, F.J., Cramer, F.S., Cerebral Air Embolism resulting from Invasive Procedures, Annals of Surgery, 201(2): 242-245, 1985.

2. Muth, C.M., Shank, E.S., Gas Embolism (Review), New England Journal of Medicine, 342: 476-482, Feb 17, 2000.

3. Kinsey, J.L., Air Embolism as a result of submarine escape training. U.S. Armed Forces Medical Journal, 5:243-255, 1956.

4. Philp, R.B., A review of blood changes associated with compression-decompression: relationship to decompression sickness. Undersea Biomedical Research, 1(2): 117-50, June 1974.

5. Coulter, et al, Gas Embolism-Correspondence, New England Journal of Medicine, 342:2000-2002, June 29, 2000.

6. Leitch, D.R., Greenbaum, L.J., Hallenbeck, J.M., Failure to recover with treatment and secondary deterioration, Undersea Biomedical Research, 11(3): 265-274, 1984.

7. Butler, B.D., Hills, B.A., The lung as a filter for microbubbles, Journal of Applied Physiology, 47: 537-543, 1079.

8. Leitch, D.R., Greenbaum, L.J., Hallenbeck, J.M., Cerebral arterial air embolism, Is there benefit in beginning HBO treatment at 6 Bar?, Undersea Biomedical Research, 11(3): 221-235. 1984.

9. Sukoff, M.H., Hollin, S.A., Espinosa, O.E., J.H. Jacobson, II, The protective effect of hyperbaric oxygenation in experimental cerebral edema. Journal of Neurosurgery, 29: 236-239, 1968.

NOTES

THE ROLE OF HYPERBARIC OXYGEN IN THE SURGICAL MANAGEMENT OF CHRONIC REFRACTORY OSTEOMYELITIS

M.B. Strauss

INTRODUCTION

Chronic refractory osteomyelitis (CROM) is defined as osteomyelitis, that is infection of both the cortical and medullary portions of bone, that has persisted or recurred after treatment has been given. Chronic refractory osteomyelitis needs to be differentiated from osteitis where involvement is limited to the superficial portion of cortical bone such as is found at the base of pressure sores. Specific treatments for CROM may include one or more of the following: antibiotics, debridement, ostectomy, segmental bone resection, antibiotic impregnated beads, and hyperbaric oxygen (HBO). It is easy to ascribe failure in CROM to inadequate and/or incomplete prior treatment(s). For the purposes of this chapter, the definition of CROM given above is sufficient to define when HBO should be used for the surgical management of this problem.

Since the indications for HBO were delineated by the Undersea [and Hyperbaric] Medical Society in 1977, CROM has been an approved use for this therapy.[1,2] However, in the intervening 25 years, the focus and utilization of HBO for CROM has changed markedly. Now HBO is rarely used for CROM of long bones. In contrast, it is used frequently for CROM of the feet especially in the patient with the hypoxic wound, host compromising factors, or both. Hyperbaric oxygen is always an adjunct to orthopaedic management and antibiotics for CROM.

The reason HBO is rarely used for CROM of long bones is threefold. First, the incidence of CROM of long bones has decreased due to improved management of open fractures with organism-specific antibiotics, early coverage with flaps, improved stabilization techniques, dead space management with antibiotic impregnated beads, and recognition of the need for immediate amputation of the severely mangled extremity. Second, the use of microvascular free flaps after aggressive debridement of long bone CROM provides both coverage and improved blood supply to the involved bone.[2-5] Finally, segmental resection of non-viable, infected bone and then osteotomy and callotaxis of the remaining healthy bone to bridge the gap (Ilizarov technique) is used to eliminate the focus of bone infection.[6] When they fail and the decision to salvage the limb is made, then HBO should be used as an adjunct to management in the repeat attempt to eradicate infection in long bones.

PATHOPHYSIOLOGY

The pathophysiology of CROM includes infiltrates, chronically infected bone, edema, and blood vessel occlusion.[7] The consequence is impaired vascularity and hypoxia in the infected bone. The host, in response to the infection, tries to isolate the involved area from its healthy tissues by forming scar tissue around the infection focus. This scar tissue becomes an interface (Figure 1). On the infection side of the interface, organisms are protected from the host's infection fighting responses and the delivery of antibiotics. On the other side of the interface healthy host tissues are present, but are unable to penetrate the interface to "fight" the infection. The extent of dead bone (sequestrum and/or diffuse sclerosing involvement) and

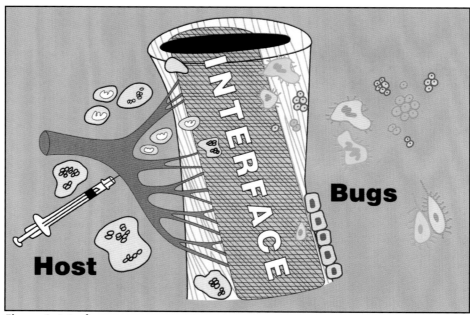

Figure 1. Interface

The interface acts as a barrier between the host infection controlling mechanisms (including antibiotic delivery) and the organisms causing the infection. Teleologically, it is the body's method to isolate and keep the infection focus from spreading to healthy body tissues. Most commonly the interface is cicatrix (dense, impermeable scar tissue) but cartilage, dead bone, inspisated pus, bone cement, and orthopaedic hardware can also be impenetrable barriers.

the amount of the interface varies in each case of CROM. This complicates the comparison of management interventions, since each case is a unique problem in itself.

MANAGEMENT PRINCIPLES

Management of CROM is simple in principle. First, dead, infected bone is removed by debridement and/or segmental resection. Next, the interface is eliminated to reestablish a blood supply to the infection site and thereby provide access for leukocytes and antibiotics to kill bacteria. Third, hypoxia in the wound environment is corrected so angiogenesis, osteoclast resorption of dead and infected bone, and neutrophil oxidative killing will occur. Hyperbaric oxygen is an intervention that helps host responsiveness by correcting wound hypoxia in two stages (Figure 2). First, there is markedly improved diffusion of oxygen into hypoxic tissues from the elevated tissue fluid oxygen tensions that result from HBO. Second, the improved tissue oxygen tensions provide an environment for angiogenesis, fibroblast activity, leukocyte oxidative killing of bacteria, and osteoclastic resorption of dead bone to occur. Tissue oxygen tensions of 30 to 40 mmHg pressure are required for these responses.[8,9] The hyperoxygenation effect of HBO may stop the multiplication of or kill bacteria, especially anaerobes.[10]

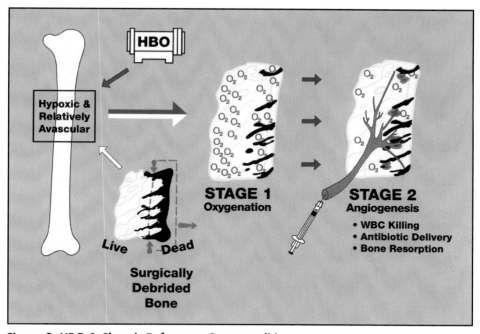

Figure 2. HBO & Chronic Refractory Osteomyelitis

For conceptual purposes hyperbaric oxygen acts in two stages for chronic refractory osteomyelitis. Although surgery may remove the bulk of dead bone (dashed red rectangle), microscopic residuals (black) are likely to remain. In Stage 1 HBO raises the oxygen tensions of the tissues around the infection site. This provides an environment (Stage 2) for angiogenesis, leukocyte oxidative killing, osteoclasis, and antibiotic delivery to occur.

Finally, HBO helps certain antibiotics enter bacteria especially in hypoxic environments.[11] Antibiotics such as the aminoglycosides, amphoteracin, and possibly Vancomycin require active, oxygen-dependent transport across bacteria cell walls to penetrate and kill the organisms. Active transport of these bacteria does not occur if tissue oxygen tensions are below 20-30 mmHg.

Failures with surgery and antibiotics in the management of CROM occur because the demarcation between healthy and involved bone is not always clear. Even with extensive debridement, residuals of osteomyelitis are likely to remain. This may be the reason antibiotics fail to sterilize the bone. Ultimate success in arresting CROM depends upon the reestablishment of vascularity to the margins of the bone infection and the enhancement of host responses to eliminate the residuals and prevent the spread of infection to adjacent non-involved bone. This defines the justification for HBO. In addition, when flap surgeries are done with injured tissues, in compromised hosts, and/or redone, there is concern about sloughs because of compromised perfusion. Hyperbaric oxygen helps preserve flap viability.[12-15]

Wound hypoxia is almost always a contributing factor to CROM. The most frequent cause of wound hypoxia is diabetes with associated occlusive vascular disease, capillary basement membrane thickening, impaired red blood cell deformability, auto sympathectomy, capillary hypoxia with chemically mediated ischemia-reperfusion injury, and osmotic and glycosylation effects of hyperglycemia.[16] Other causes of impaired host responses, wound hypoxia, or combinations include arteriosclerotic (non-diabetic) peripheral vascular disease; trauma; collagen vascular disease; use of steroids, immunosuppressors, and/or antimetabolites; smoking; radiation; vasculitis; steal syndromes from arteriovenous shunts; venous and/or lymph fluid stasis disease; and coagulopathies. In summary, HBO's role in CROM is to increase tissue oxygen tensions to levels where host factors will function and complement surgery and antibiotics for managing the infection.

CLASSIFICATION OF CROM

Classification systems for osteomyelitis are useful for guiding management and determining which cases require HBO as an adjunct. The classification most familiar to orthopaedic surgeons and hyperbaric medicine specialists is that of Cierney and Mader.[17] The classification not only stages osteomyelitis into four types but it defines three types of hosts (Table 1). A Type A host is a normal host and competent for handling infection. A Type B host has impaired host responses to infection either systemically such as the diabetic or locally such as post-traumatic vascular injury to an extremity. A Type C host is minimally infected with osteomyelitis and/or the cure would cause more complications than the disease itself. What makes the Cierney-Mader classification helpful for hyperbaric medicine is that it provides guidelines for using HBO in CROM. Hyperbaric oxygen is recommended as an adjunct to the management of Stage-3 (discrete sequestrum) CROM in impaired (Type B) hosts and in all stage 4 (diffuse, sclerosing) CROM cases.

My recommendation for using HBO as an adjunct for managing CROM is based on the clinical finding of chronic osteomyelitis that has persisted or recurred after treatment. If the bone infection meets this

TABLE 1. THE CIERNEY-MADER CLASSIFICATION OF OSTEOMYELITIS[17]

Stage	Findings (Site of Osteomyelitis)	Host Status
1	Medullary	**A = Normal**
2	Superficial, (Cortical involvement i.e., osteitis)	**B = Compromised** Systemic = S Local = L
3	Defined, well-demarcated sequestrum	**C = Inappropriate** (The treatment could be worse than the disease.)
4	Diffuse, sclerosing	

Consider HBO as adjunct to management

    1. Stage 3, Host Status B

    2. Stage 4, Host Status A or B

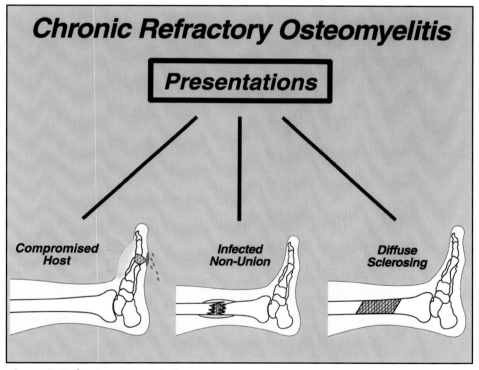

Figure 3. Refractory Presentations

Once the definition of chronic refractory osteomyelitis is met (bone infection that has persisted or recurred with/after treatment), three clinical presentations are apparent. Although HBO is an adjunct to the management of all three, each has specific findings and optimal treatment protocols (see text and Table 2).

definition and the decision is made to arrest the infection, then HBO should be used in the management. From this information three clinical presentations for using HBO in CROM become apparent (Figure 3): First, CROM in the compromised host; second, CROM associated with a septic nonunion of a long bone fracture; and third, CROM of the diffuse-sclerosing type.

CLINICAL PRESENTATIONS OF CHRONIC REFRACTORY OSTEOMYELITIS AND THE ROLE OF HYPERBARIC OXYGEN

The Compromised Host

The major use of HBO for CROM is in the patient who is a compromised host. The specific features of CROM in the compromised host are threefold: (1) Wound hypoxia, (2) Mixed infection with aerobic and/or anaerobic organisms, and (3) Failure of the host to develop an inflammatory response. Management of CROM in the compromised hosts is first directed at improving the host status through optimizing cardiovascular function, renal function, nutrition, and antibiotic selection; and using HBO as adjunct to correcting wound hypoxia. Next, the wound environment needs to be made as optimal as possible for controlling the infection. Dead and infected bone is removed. Cicatrix which is prone to form in the hypoxic environment must be excised to the point that there is no longer any fibronodular material in the debrided wound. Plain x-rays of chronic osteomyelitis often show patchy (moth-eaten appearance) osteolysis, erosion of cortical margins and/or periosteal new bone formation. Nuclear scans and magnetic resonance imaging can augment the information derived from plain films, but may be difficult to interpret due to bone remodeling and Charcot arthropathy changes.

Consequently, the judgement about the extent of dead bone that needs to be debrided is largely a clinical one which is determined during surgery. The finding of bleeding bone is the best indication of bone viability. Any osteomyelitis involvement of a metatarsal head dictates that the entire head and adjacent neck be debrided to obtain a healthy margin. Bone devoid of periosteal or other soft tissue attachment is assumed to be nonviable. Likewise, for bone that has a chalk-like consistency and is brittle when debrided. If unsure whether or not the bony margins are viable after debridement, the wound should be left open and wound care measures instituted post-operatively. Healthy granulation tissue over the margins of the debrided bone during post-operative management confirms the adequacy of the debridement. If granulation tissue does not form over the exposed portions of bone in the open post-debridement wound, then additional debridement is required. Hyperbaric oxygen generates an inflammatory response through angiogenesis, leukocyte mobilization, and osteoclastic activity.

Post-debridement, the wound is managed with physiological dressings until it is ready for coverage and/or closure. In CROM of the foot, the closure, coverage options usually become obvious as the inflammatory response with granulation tissue formation appears. Techniques such as partial foot amputations, ray resections, composite skin grafts and flaps, skin grafts over a bone and/or the plantar surface of the foot, and unconventional flaps may be needed to achieve closure and preserve as much of the mechanics of the foot as possible. Once the infected bone has been removed and the inflammatory response has been generated, successful wound healing almost always occurs (see Problem Wound chapter).[16]

The functional goals of this group of patients are usually simple. They want to preserve as much of their foot as possible in order to maintain their ability to ambulate independently for activities of daily living. Consequently, even proximal midfoot amputations and sub-total calcanectomies can achieve these goals, and should not be dismissed because of cosmetic considerations or concerns that function might not be what it was before the CROM developed.

The patient who is a marginal ambulator even with these levels of amputation usually are able to maintain a level of functional ambulation. In contrast, a below knee amputation may end the patient's ability to be independent because of the difficulty of donning the prosthesis, the weight of the prosthesis, balance and proprioception problems, and weakness in the upper extremities such that the use of walking aids in combination with a prosthesis is unsafe. Spacers in shoes can fill voids left by missing foot parts. Custom-designed shoes are made to accommodate almost any type of foot amputation. Thus, preservation of the foot is justifiable for functional reasons. For economic reasons it is cost-effective, also. Costs of a lower limb amputation and associated care approached $50,000.00 when revascularization failed.[18]

Although adequate descriptions of standard amputation levels in the foot exist, they may not be appropriate for the patient who is a compromised host. Unconventional amputations may be required. Standard levels of foot amputations in this group of patients should be eschewed in favor of eliminating the CROM site, preserving as much bone and foot architecture as possible, and making the foot mechanically sound. Combination forefoot-midfoot amputations (in contrast to a complete midfoot amputation) oftentimes meet these goals. The removal of bony prominences (ostectomies) and partial ray resections are other techniques used to preserve as much foot architecture as possible. In general, through ankle (i.e., Symes) amputation is not recommended for this group of patients due to limb shortening, which makes walking without a prosthesis unsafe in a population with muscle weakness and balance problems. Also, the patient with occlusive vascular disease, peripheral neuropathy, or both is at increased risk of end stump breakdown with weight bearing. Finally, the Symes prosthesis tends to be bulky and not well matched to the shape of the patient's other leg.

With the above interventions success in arresting CROM in the compromised host is 80% or better when comprehensive management including HBO is given.[19-23] Failures do occur because of new vascular occlusive events, residual foci of bone infections, development of new wounds from mechanically unsound foot architecture, and vasculitis associated with collagen vascular diseases. A particularly difficult group of patients to eradicate CROM are a subset of diabetics with Methicillin resistant *Staphylococcus aureus* infections. It appears that even with antibiotics, surgery, and HBO the bone never becomes sterile perhaps because of deficiencies in their immune responses. Once antibiotics are stopped, the bacteria suppressed by the antibiotics begin to multiply and the infection flourishes. Consequently, surgical considerations for this group of patients require bone resection at least one joint proximal to the infected bone, which in the foot and ankle may mean a lower limb amputation is needed in order to eradicate the infection.

The Septic Nonunion

Septic nonunions of long bones occur infrequently due to improved management of patients who have open fractures with crush injury components. Nonetheless septic nonunions can be anticipated in approximately 50% of the high energy and/or artery laceration open fracture group (see Crush Injuries and Compartment Syndrome chapter). When a septic nonunion develops and there is the justification to preserve the leg, that is, there is the potential for useful function and intractable pain is not present, then HBO should be used as an adjunct to surgery and antibiotics for limb salvage. Problems characteristic of the septic nonunion include: (1) Infection, (2) Instability, and (3) A fibrocartilaginous interface with dead bone at the fracture site.

Orthopaedic management includes debridement of the dead, infected bone at the fracture ends and the fibrocartilaginous interface. In addition, the fracture site must be rigidly stabilized. The presence of motion at the nonunion site shears off new blood vessels bridging the fracture site, promotes bacterial growth, and proliferation of fibrocartilaginous tissue. Managing this problem with rigid external fixation stabilizes the fracture, keeps hardware out of the wound, and allows access for wound care and surgeries. Often skin flaps in this group of patients are threatened due to the effects of the initial injury and/or the previous surgical interventions. Hence, preservation of threatened skin flaps is another benefit of HBO for these problems.[12-15] Once the wound base appears vascular, then bone grafting and flap coverage are done to heal the fracture and cover the wound.

In my management of 30 patients with septic nonunions using adjunctive HBO, fracture healing occurred in 100%. One patient had a small residual focus of osteomyelitis which was eliminated with a second debridement and muscle flap coverage (Case Report 3). In this group of patients approximately one-third developed stress fractures at some time during their convalescence after HBO treatments. This suggests that HBO enhanced the osteoclast function for bone remodeling so much so that the bone was temporarily weakened enough for a stress fracture to occur when ambulation resumed. Typically, the stress fractures were adjacent to rather than at the old septic nonunion sites. All these post-HBO treatment stress fractures healed either without interventions or with ambulatory cast treatment.

Diffuse Sclerosing Chronic Refractory Osteomyelitis

Diffuse sclerosing CROM is a difficult problem because there is usually extensive involvement of cortical and underlying medullary bone, but demarcation between live and dead bone is not clear and the interface may not be well defined. The difficulty in eradicating diffuse sclerosing CROM is further compounded by the compactness of cortical bone. Cancellous bone has 45 times as much surface area per gram of bone for antibiotic, leukocyte, osteoclast, and fibroblast contact as cortical bone. Thus, host responses and antibiotic delivery to the infected bone is severely limited. The approach to this problem includes: (1) Improvement of vascularity to the involved bone, (2) Removal of obviously dead and infected bone, and (3) Optimization of host responses.

Hyperbaric oxygen treatments should be given for approximately two weeks before surgical debridement to improve vascularity to the bone and stimulate osteoclast function. This helps with demarcation of infected from healthy bone although the margins are rarely as clear as with discrete sequestra and well-established interfaces. Stability is usually not a problem as in the septic nonunion. The only sure method to ascertain bone viability is observing the growth of granulation tissue on the debrided bone surfaces during post-operative wound care. If granulation tissue is not observed, then additional debridements must be done. Once the debrided bone surface is covered with granulation tissue, coverage is achieved with healing by secondary intention, skin grafting, or flap surgery.

Unfortunately, HBO is often overlooked as an adjunct in the initial management of diffuse sclerosing CROM even though it meets the Cierney-Mader as well as my criteria for its use. The surgical approach is directed at aggressive debridement of bone almost to the point of risking a pathological fracture and concurrent coverage with a rotational muscle or microvascular free flap. Antibiotic impregnated beads may be temporarily placed under flaps to sterilize the bone.[24] Antibiotic impregnated beads are usually removed after three weeks by which time almost all the antibiotic has eluded out of them. After six weeks the flaps are usually stable enough for bone grafting to be done underneath them if there is concern that the remaining bone may fracture. Although these approaches are frequently successful, HBO should be used when the host is compromised, when a previous debridement and closure were unsuccessful, and/or infection persists after placement of antibiotic beads, rotational flaps, or microvascular free flaps.

Case Reports

Case 1. A 30-year-old blind, diabetic male with profound peripheral neuropathy status post renal transplant on immunosuppressors developed a malpeforans ulcer in the right forefoot. This was managed with debridement and antibiotics at another hospital. After approximately one month of antibiotics and several debridements, the infection continued leading to the recommendation for a Symes or possibly below knee amputation (Figure 4a). The patient refused these options and was transferred to our facility to add HBO treatments to his care. After one week of adjunctive HBO treatments the cellulitis and edema resolved in his forefoot. The wound became healthy except for clear demarcation of a necrotic area under the 2nd metatarsal head (Figure 4b). New x-rays showed lysis of the metatarsal head confirming the presence of osteomyelitis (Figure 4c). With removal of the infected bone the wound healed rapidly by secondary intention (Figure 4d). The patient resumed community ambulatory activities and, in fact, became an instructor for the use of guide dogs for the blind.

The following figures are of a 30-year-old blind male diabetic with profound peripheral neuropathy and uncontrolled infection in his left foot:

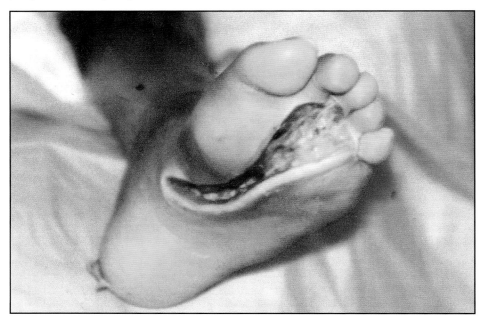

Figure 4a. Presentation after one month of antibiotics and debridements. Note induration around skin margins of the lower third of the wound.

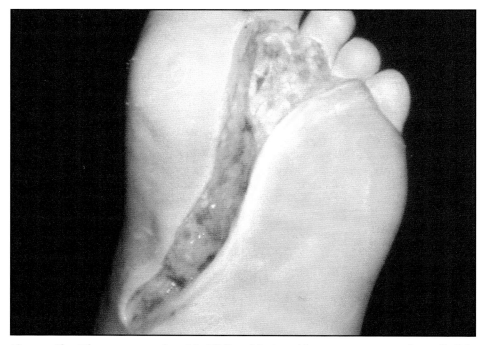

Figure 4b. After one week with HBO added to his management, the cellulitis resolved, the wound became smaller due to contraction and edema reduction, and a focus of sepsis localized over the 2nd metatarsal head.

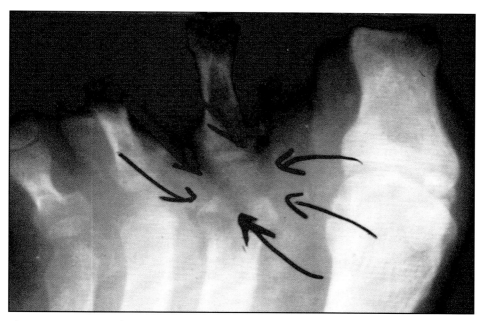

Figure 4c. X-rays after ten days of HBO showed lysis (a new finding) of the 2nd metatarsal head.

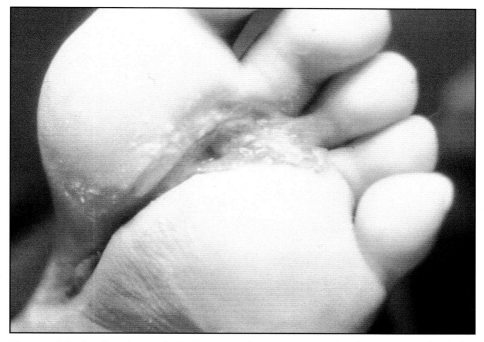

Figure 4d. At the time of discharge, about one week after removal of the metatarsal head, the wound was almost healed.

Comment: Three effects were realized with the addition of HBO. First, the infection began to improve. Second, sharp demarcation of necrotic from healthy tissue occurred. Third, osteolytic changes developed in the metatarsal head confirming the diagnosis of CROM. Whether my definition and classification (CROM in a compromised host) or the Cierney-Mader classification (Stage 3, B-Host) is used, HBO was indicated. In the presence of blindness, preservation of his leg allowed the patient to remain a community ambulator. The patient's healed foot remained functional for 15 years at which time he died from a silent myocardial infarction while hospitalized for another diabetic problem.

Case 2: A healthy 27-year-old male had a hindfoot fusion to manage a tarsal coalition. A post-operative infection developed. After four debridements, appropriate antibiotics, and removal of most of the lateral column of his mid- and forefoot the infection was not arrested (Figure 5a). The patient requested a below knee amputation, but was persuaded to try HBO by his referring orthopaedic surgeon as an adjunct to an additional course of antibiotics and surgery to save his foot. At the time of hospital admission, the foot was swollen. A 10-centimeter-wide area of skin around a tract that coursed to the underlying bone had a verrucuous-eczematoid, cellulitic appearance (Figure 5b). In preparation for surgery, HBO treatments were given for two weeks in conjunction with wound cleansing, elevation, and rest. Antibiotics were withheld at this time. Foot tomograms showed a discrete sequestrum

The following figures are of a 27-year-old male that developed an uncontrollable wound infection after a hindfoot fusion:

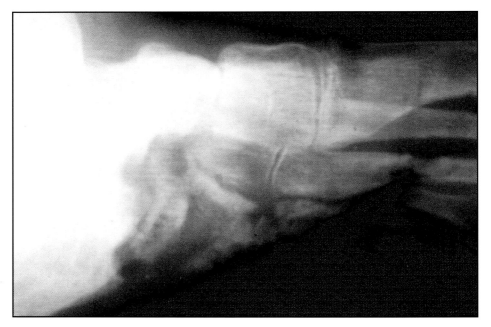

Figure 5a. An x-ray after four debridements and courses of antibiotics showed extensive destruction of the lateral column of his midfoot and forefoot.

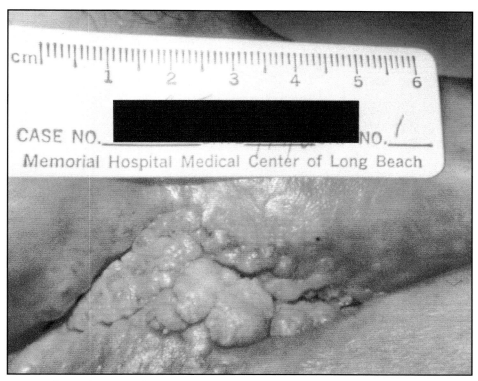

Figure 5b. At the time of starting HBO the wound on the lateral side of his midfoot had an "angry" appearance.

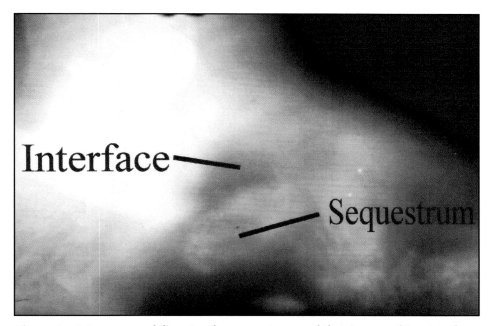

Figure 5c. A tomogram delineates the sequestrum and the circumscribing interface.

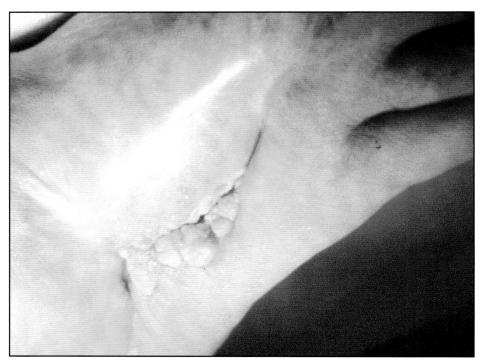

Figure 5d. After two weeks (the patient did not receive antibiotics during this time) the wound appearance was greatly improved and now amendable to establishing healthy surgical margins with debridement in the operating wound.

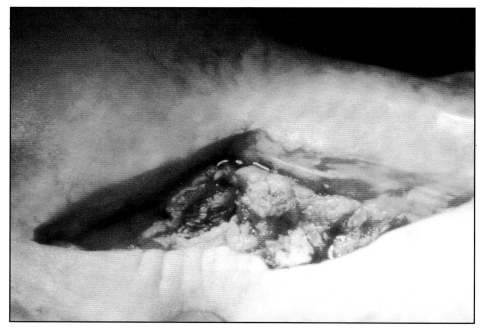

Figure 5e. After excising the sinus tract the sequestrum (black) and the surrounding interface (white glistening cicatrix) were clearly demarcated.

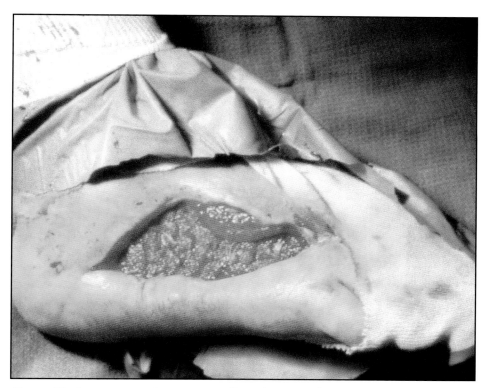

Figure 5f. An open autologous cancellous bone graft (Papineu technique) was used to fill the defect and provide stability for the lateral column of the foot.

surrounded by a fibrous interface (Figure 5c). During this time the skin around the tract became healthy (Figure 5d). The wound was then debrided and remarkably sharp demarcation between the sequestrum and its interface and the adjacent healthy tissues was observed (Figure 5e). After an additional week of HBO treatments, organism-specific intravenous antibiotics, normal saline dressing changes, a healthy granulating wound base developed. The wound was then filled with autologous cancellous bone (Papineu technique[25]), left open to heal by granulation tissue invasion, consolidation of the bone graft, and secondary epithelialization (Figure 5f). The wound healed with solid fusion of the lateral column and arrest of the infection.

Comment: This patient also met the criteria for using HBO, but in contrast to the first case report was a locally vs. systemically compromised host. The local compromise was due to scar formation and interference with circulation around the infection site from infection and repetitive surgeries. The two weeks of preparatory HBO treatments made the tissues in the infection site much more amendable to establishing healthy margins at the time of debridement. This was attributed to resolution of edema, induration, and the egzematoid appearance of the skin as well as the angiogenesis effect in the wound.

Case 3: A healthy 59-year-old male sustained a severe open proximal tibia fracture extending to the subchondral bone of the tibial plateaus following a motorcycle vs. car accident. The patient underwent open reduction and internal fixation with medial and lateral stainless steel buttress plates. The flaps sloughed and the entire anterior cortex of the proximal tibia became avascular (Figure 6a). Before an above the knee amputation was done the attending orthopaedic surgeon elected to use HBO as an adjunct to salvage the leg. The fracture was stabilized with rigid external fixation using transfixing pins in the distal femur and below the fracture site in the proximal tibia. Dead bone was debrided from the proximal tibia leaving an enormous cavity bounded by metal plates, medially and laterally, and bone cortex posteriorly. Hyperbaric oxygen, antibiotics based on the bone cultures, and wound care continued. After three weeks the cavity became lined with granulation tissue (Figure 6b). It was then filled with autologous cancellous bone graft and covered with a medial gastrocnemius muscle flap (Figure 6c). After six months the bone graft consolidated. However, a small draining sinus from the lateral aspect of the proximal leg persisted. A second stage debridement was done about a year later with removal of the plates and covering the wound with a lateral gastrocnemius flap. This arrested the infection. The patient has remained a community ambulator (Figure 6d).

Comment: Although this injury might not meet the Cierney-Mader criteria for using HBO for osteomyelitis, it met the definition I proposed previously and fits the clinical presentation of a septic nonunion. In this

The following figures are of a 59-year-old male that sustained a severe proximal tibia fracture:

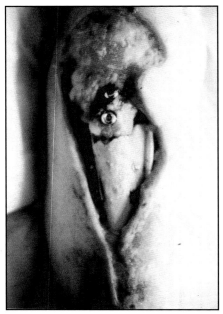 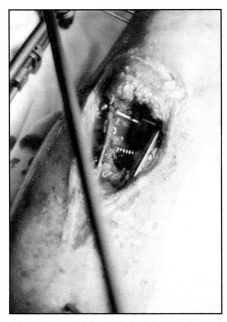

Figure 6a. Large skin slough over dead (white, chalky appearance) fracture fragments in proximal leg. Note the edematous skin margins.

Figure 6b. After debridement and stabilization with external fixation and two weeks of HBO, healthy skin margins and a granulating wound base developed.

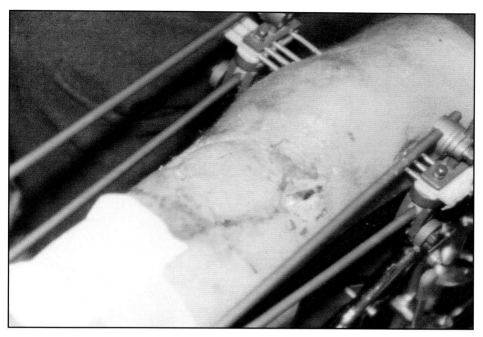

Figure 6c. After autologous cancellous bone grafting and a medical gastrocnemius flap, the wound was completely covered except for a minute draining tract (crusted over in photo) from the upper lateral portion of the wound.

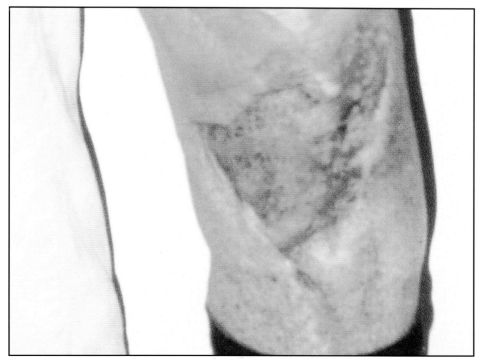

Figure 6d. Clinical follow-up 17 years later. The patient had 60° of motion in his knee. He stopped motorcycle riding.

challenging case success was attributed to the patient's host status (A-host in the Cierney-Mader system) and the integration of orthopaedic and plastic surgery interventions with HBO. Contributions that can be attributed to HBO in this case included angiogenesis of the debrided cavity, enhancement of the vascular invasion of the bone graft, control of infection, ossification of the bone graft, survival of the muscle flaps, and demarcation of residual bone infection focus.

Case 4: A 27-year-old male sustained a high-energy comminuted proximal tibial shaft fracture with complete bone displacement in a pedestrian vs. car bumper accident (Figure 7a). A primary amputation was recommended, but the patient refused. The fracture was reduced and stabilized with internal fixation. Over a one-year period the fracture healed, but the patient had persistent drainage and slough of the skin over the leg in spite of antibiotics. A split thickness skin graft was used to cover the wound, but a draining sinus persisted. With any ambulatory activity cellulitis flared in the leg. X-rays showed that the fracture had healed, but there were lytic areas and periosteal new bone formation from the proximal tibial metaphysis to the distal third of the leg consistent with diffuse sclerosing CROM (Figure 7b). Two weeks of HBO treatments were given without antibiotics before saucerization of the wound. The wound was left open post-operatively (Figure 7c). A healthy granulating base developed. Hyperbaric oxygen

The following figures are of a 27-year-old male that sustained a limb threatening proximal tibia fracture following a pedestrian vs. car bumper accident:

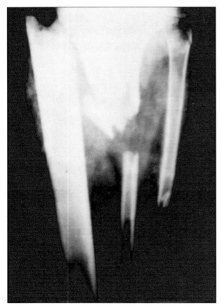

Figure 7a. X-rays showed a complete displacement, commun-ition, and bayoneting of the fracture fragments. Gas was present in the soft tissues (consistent with an open fracture).

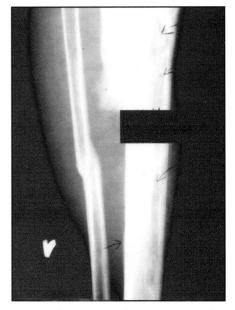

Figure 7b. X-rays about nine months after injury were consistent with diffuse sclerosing chronic refractory osteomyelitis. The fracture had healed. Note the lytic areas (arrows) and periostial new bone formation along almost the entire diaphysis of the tibia.

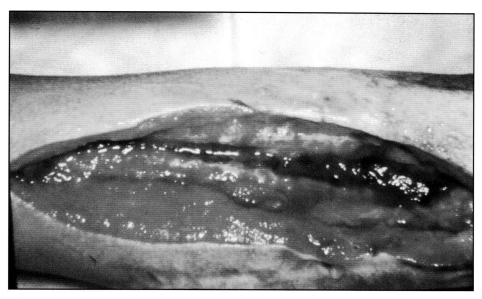

Figure 7c. Wound appearance after saucerization with a trough of bone removed from the anterior tibial diaphysis.

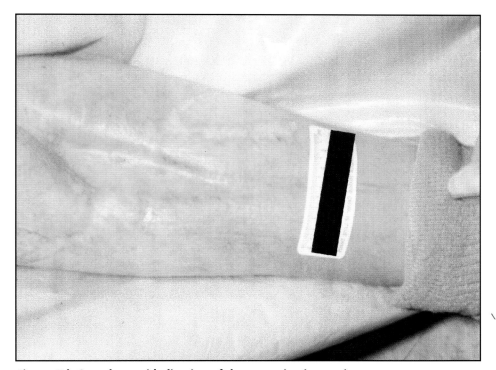

Figure 7d. Complete epithelization of the saucerization cavity.

treatments continued for a total of 60. The healing saucerization cavity was managed with normal saline dressing changes. After the saucerization, organism specific antibiotics continued for six weeks. Over a six-month period the wound granulated and epithelialized (Figure 7d). During follow-up an occult asymptomatic stress fracture was noted on x-ray below the original fracture site. This healed spontaneously. Seventeen years later the patient returned requesting a statement saying his bone infection was cured in order to clear him for a lung transplant.

Comment: The patient's condition met the criteria for HBO from both the Cierney-Mader and my recommendations. From the extent of the infection, as it appeared on x-ray, it is unlikely that saucerization alone with antibiotics would have eradicated it. To eradicate the infection using Illizarov techniques and/or bone grafting would have required removal of the majority of the tibial shaft. The extensive bone loss would make successful outcomes using those techniques unlikely. The benefits from using HBO were likely due to stimulation of angiogenesis, neutrophil oxidative killing, and osteoclastic activity. The delayed stress fracture attests to the active bone remodeling effects of HBO. Although other alternatives such as microvascular free flaps, and antibiotic impregnated bead techniques could have been used to manage this problem, is unlikely they could have achieved more durable and more functional results than the combination of HBO, simple saucerization surgery, and antibiotics.

DISCUSSION

Even though the role of HBO in the surgical management of CROM is better defined now than at anytime in the past, it still is not utilized to its fullest potential. The reasons for this are not clear. Costs of HBO are one consideration. Availability of HBO chambers is another. Although the lack of randomized control trials is often cited as the reason for not using HBO, the irony of this is twofold. First, the orthopaedic surgeons, endocrinologists, and infectious disease consultants who make the decisions about what interventions to use for the management of CROM, by-and-large make their decisions based on observed outcomes, laboratory studies, and their personal experiences rather than randomized controlled trials. Second, even with randomized control trials such as in Bouachour's fracture-crush injury report, traumatologists have not notably changed their utilization of HBO for these conditions.[26] Nonetheless the pathophysiologic basis for using HBO is sound and the outcomes are predictable as attested by several hundred reported patient experiences.[23]

During my 25 years' experience utilizing HBO as an adjunct to orthopaedic surgery I have made the following observations regarding the usefulness of HBO in CROM:

1. **Pretreatment with HBO improves the environment around the CROM infection site:** This is the rationale for recommending two weeks of HBO before surgery and starting antibiotics especially in the septic nonunion and diffuse sclerosing CROM presentations. Effects observed include decreased wound edema, induration, and drainage; improved quality of the skin around the wound; and better demarcation of infected from non-infected tissues.

2. **Hyperbaric oxygen helps demarcate live from dead, infected bone:** Presumably this is a consequence of the angiogenesis and osteoclast stimulation effects of HBO. The vascularity of the tissues adjacent to the interface and dead bone seem to be preferentially affected, but little change is expected in the avascular infection focus (i.e., sequestrum) itself from pre-debridement HBO treatments. This effect helps the surgeon establish viable infection-free margins at the time of debridement.

3. **Hyperbaric oxygen preferentially stimulates the osteoclast:** The osteoclast, a macrophage derivative that generates phosphatases, etc. to dissolve bone, is highly oxygen dependent. Its metabolic activity is 100 times greater than the osteocyte, the structural cell of bone embedded in the mineralized matrix.[27] The osteoclast removes residual dead and infected bone that remains after debridement. The osteoclast cannot function in a hypoxic environment. Strong evidence to support the osteoclast remodeling process after HBO treatments is seen in the high incidence of stress fractures when patients resume ambulation after CROM has been arrested in long bones.

4. **Optimal protocols using HBO must be followed to achieve success (Table 2):** Protocols must be individualized to the patient's presentation (i.e., compromised host, septic nonunion, or diffuse sclerosing CROM). For the latter two presentations pre-surgical, pre-antibiotic HBO treatments are given to improve the CROM infection site environment and stimulate angiogenesis. This usually requires two weeks. Next, infected bone is surgically debrided. Re-debridements may be required if granulation tissue formation is not observed on the exposed bone post-debridement. For septic nonunions and diffuse sclerosing CROM, six weeks of organism-specific antibiotics are needed once the last wound debridement and/or after coverage, reclosure is done. Usually, two additional weeks of HBO treatments are given for these presentations after wound coverage, closure to enhance host factor removal of the remaining vestiges of dead, infected bone. This may require a total of 60 HBO treatments.

5. **The duration of CROM does not have an adverse effect on the outcomes:** When HBO is used as an adjunct to surgery and antibiotics, the outcomes appear independent of the duration of the problem. This observation takes exception to a previous report.[19] The 80% arrest rate I have observed when HBO was used as an adjunct to surgery and antibiotics has been independent of the duration of CROM.

6. **Advancing age is not a cause for poorer outcomes if HBO is used for CROM:** Aging is recognized as a negative predictor for good outcomes, especially in trauma and fracture management.[26,28] If the patient's bone infection meets the definition of CROM and the decision is made to avoid amputation of the extremity, our outcomes were equally good in older compromised host patients as in younger ones. Other factors such as ambulation status, cardiovascular condition, smoking, etc. should be considered when evaluating host status

TABLE 2. HYPERBARIC OXYGEN (HBO) PROTOCOLS FOR CHRONIC REFRACTORY OSTEOMYELITIS

Presentation and Findings	Recommended HBO Treatments*		Total HBO Treatments	Comments
	Pre-OP HBO**	Post-OP HBO**		
Compromised Hosts 1. Hypoxia 2. Mixed infection 3. Lack of inflammatory response	Zero to 7	7-14	14-21	If infection is eradicated with surgery, HBO is stopped: 1. After the angiogenesis effect is initiated (~ 14 days) 2. Flaps are stable (~ 5 days)
Septic Non-Union 1. Infection 2. Instability 3. Fibro-cartilage interface at fracture site	14	16-46	30-60	Usually surgeries staged e.g. 1. Debridement and stabilization with external fixation 2. Bone grafting and flap coverage. 3. HBO should be continued for 2 weeks after flap coverage or for a total of 60 treatments.
Diffuse Sclerosing 1. Diffuse involvement 2. Poor demarcation 3. Extensive	14	46	60	Because of diffuse involvement a full 60 HBO treatments are recommended to optimize angiogenesis and osteoclastic activity.

Notes: * HBO treatments are usually given for 90 to 120 minutes at 2 to 2.4 Atmospheres Absolute Pressure once (outpatient) or twice (inpatient) a day.
  ** OP = Operative

(see Host Score in Crush Injuries and Problem Wound chapters). Hyperbaric oxygen appears to signal fibroblast activity and mediate the effects advancing age have on fibroblast function.[29,30]

7. **Outcomes with HBO are equally good regardless of synergistic infections with mixed aerobic and anaerobic organisms:** Compromised hosts frequently have cultures with mixed flora. This has been reported as a cause for poor outcomes with surgery and antibiotics in this group of patients.[31] With HBO, outcomes (80% arrest of infection) appear to be independent of the bacteria-causing the infection. The single exception is in a sub-group of diabetics with Methicillin resistant *Staphylococcus aureus* (MRSA) infections in their bones.

8. **Once CROM has been arrested using HBO, the results are durable:** This observation is ascribed to the "jump start" effects HBO has on host factors, and the continuation of these effects after surgery and

antibiotic treatments are completed. For the compromised host with arrested CROM, strategies to present new and recurrent infections must be followed.[32] An indirect seemingly negative effect that supports this observation is the high incidence of stress fractures attributed to ongoing osteoclastic activity after HBO is stopped and ambulation is resumed in this group of patients.

9. **If the decision is made to arrest the infection, and if the definition of CROM is met, management must be done as if the patient's CROM is a new case regardless of what was done before:** This requires that the protocols described before (see Observation 4) are followed. Antibiotic selection must be based on bone cultures from the debridement surgery regardless of what had been cultured before. The extent of debridements is based on what needs to be done now rather than what was done in the past. Hyperbaric oxygen needs to be given according to the protocols described.

10. **Not every case of CROM will be arrested with the adjunctive use of HBO:** Failures, that is, amputations proximal to the infection site, have been observed in several circumstances. These include: (1) Methicillin resistant *Staphylococcus aureus* infections in a subset of compromised hosts, (2) Patients with collagen vascular diseases, especially those requiring steroids and/or antimetabolites, (3) New vascular occlusive events, (4) Intractable pain, and (5) Insufficient patient compliance to follow the required wound care, antibiotic, HBO, and reinjury prevention protocols.

Finally, how does HBO measure up as an Evidenced Based Indication for CROM? Since it is an adjunct to surgery and antibiotics and is used when prior management fails, it needs to be judged differently than a primary treatment modality is. Nonetheless using the American Heart Association 1999 Guidelines, HBO is a Class-II (probably useful and effective with a favorable risk/benefit ratio) Evidence Based Indication.[33] The absence of a randomized control trial keeps it from being a Class I indication. Another approach to determining evidence based indications is based on a 10-point, five criteria evaluation system that I devised (Table 3).[34] Each criteria is graded from 2 to 0. Two points indicate overwhelming evidence for the criteria exists. One point indicates that evidence is consistent with the criteria. Zero points indicate that the evidence shows that there is no information, no benefit or possible harm would result with using the intervention. Half points are used when the information is between the scoring points used for each criterion. The criteria of no other treatment available takes into account that previous treatments for CROM have failed. A score of five or greater suggests the intervention meets the criteria of an Evidence Based Indication. For CROM, HBO is awarded a score of 6 based on 1-1/2 points for observed outcomes, 2 points for mechanisms, 1 point for published reviews, meta-analyses, 1-1/2 points for no other treatments available, and 0 points for supportive randomized controlled or head-to-head studies. Consequently, for two different Evidence Based Evaluation systems, HBO meets the criteria on an Evidenced Based Indication for CROM.

TABLE 3. EVIDENCE BASED INDICATIONS; A SIMPLIFIED EVALUATION[34]

Criteria	Scoring (Use half points when the information is between the scoring points used for each criterion)
1. Outcomes **2. Mechanisms** (Appropriate for the pathophysiology of the condition) **3. Literature reviews/meta-analyses** **4. No other treatments available** (Failure with previous interventions, or outcomes poor with accepted management) **5. Randomized control trials and/or head-to-head studies**	**2 Points:** Overwhelming evidence **1 Point:** Evidence is consistent with the criterion **0 Points:** No information, no benefit or possible harm with the intervention

Interpretation: (Sum of scores for the five criteria)

    5 Points or greater: The intervention qualifies as an Evidence Based

    Less than 5 points: The intervention does not qualify as an Evidenced Based Indication

REFERENCES

1. Medicare Bulletin 424. May 11, 1999, Hyperbaric Oxygen (HBO) Therapy.

2. Hyperbaric oxygen therapy. 1999 Committee Report. Hampson NB, Chairman and Editor. Undersea and Hyperbaric Medical Society, Inc. Kensington, MD; pp. 51-56.

3. Fitzgerald RH Jr, Ruttle PE, Arnold PG, et al. Local muscle flaps in the treatment of chronic osteomyelitis. J Bone Joint Surg 1985;67A:175.

4. Mathes SJ. The muscle flap for management of osteomyelitis. N Engl J Med 1985; 306:294.

5. Weiland AJ, Moore JR, Daniel RK. The efficacy of free-tissue transfer in the treatment of osteomyelitis. J Bone Joint Surg 1984; 66A:181-193.

6. Ilizarov GA. The Principles of the Ilizarov Technique, Bulletin-Hospital for Joint Disease 1997; 56(1):49-53.

7. Waldvogel FA, Medoff G, Swartz MN. Osteomyelitis. Charles C. Thomas, Springfield, IL, 191: 4-12.

8. Hohn DC. Oxygen and lecocyte microbial killing. In: Davis JC, Hunt TK, eds. Hyperbaric Oxygen Therapy. Bethesda, MD: Undersea Medical Society, Inc; 1977; 101-110.

9. Hunt TK, Zederfeldt B, Goldstick TK. Oxygen and healing. Am J Surg. 1969; 118: 521-525.

10. Gottlieb SF. Oxygen under pressure and microorganisms in: Davis JC, Hunt TK, eds. Hyperbaric Oxygen Therapy. Bethesda, MD: Undersea Medical Society, Inc. 1977; 79-99.

11. Verklin RN Jr, Mandell GL. Alteration of effectiveness of antibiotics by anaerobosis. J Lab Clin Med. 1977; 89:65-71.

12. Bowersox, JC, Strauss MB, Hart, GB. Clinical experience with hyperbaric oxygen therapy in the salvage of ischemic skin flaps and grafts. J Hyperbar. Med 1986; 1:141.

13. Nemiroff PM, Lungu AL. The influence of hyperbaric oxygen and irradiation of vascularity in skin flaps: A controlled study. Surg Forum 1987; 38:565.

14. Perrins DJ. The effect of hyperbaric oxygen on ischemic skin flaps. In: Grabb WC, Myers MD, eds. Skin Flaps, Boston: Little Brown & Co, 1975; 53-63.

15. Zamboni WA, Roth AC, Russell RC, Smoot EC. The effect of hyperbaric oxygen on reperfusion of ischemic axial skin flaps: A laser Doppler analysis. Ann Plast Surg 1992; 28:339-341.

16. Strauss MB. Diabetic foot and leg wounds principles, management and prevention. Primary Care Reports, 2001; 7(22):187-198.

17. Cierny G II, Mader JT, Penninck JJ. A clinical staging system for adult osteomyeltiis. Contemp Orthop 1985; 10(5):17-37.

18. Mackey W, McCllough J, Conlon TP, et al. The costs of surgery for limb-threatening ischemia. Surgery 1986; 99:26-35.

19. Bingham EL, Hart GB. Hyperbaric Oxygen treatment of refractory osteomyelitis. Postgrad Med 1977; 61:70-76.

20. Davis JC, Heckman JD, DeLee JC, Buckwold FJ. Chronic non-hematogenous osteomyelitis treated with adjuvant hyperbaric oxygen. J Bone Jt Surg, 1986; 68A: 1210-1217.

21. Depenbusch FI, Thompson RE, Hart GB. Use of hyperbaric oxygen in the treatment of refractory osteomyelitis: A preliminary report. J Trauma, 1972; 12:807-812.

22. Perrins DJD, Maudsley RH, Colwill RR, et al. OHP in the management of chronic osteomyelitis. In: Brown IW, Cox BG, eds. Proceedings of the Third International Conference on Hyperbaric Medicine. Washington, DC: National Academy of Sciences-National Research Council, 1966; 578-584.

23. Strauss MB. Chronic refractory osteomyelitis: Review and role of hyperbaric oxygen. HBO Review, 1980; 1:231-255.

24. Nelson CL, Griffin FM, Harrison BH, Cooper RE. In vitro elution characteristics of commercially and noncommercially prepared antibiotic PMMA beads. Clin Orthop 1992; 284:303-309.

25. Papineau LJ, L'excision-greffe fermeture ret gardee delil berée dans l'osteomyelite chronique, Nouv. Presse Med 1973; 2:2753-2755.

26. Bouachour G, Cronier P, Gouello JP, et al. Hyperbaric oxygen therapy in the management of crush injuries: a randomized double-blind placebo-controlled clinical trial. J Trauma 1966; 41:333-330.

27. Johnson, L. Orthopedic Pathology in (Personal Communication), Armed Forces Institute of Pathology; Fall 1973.

28. Johansen K, Daines M, Howey T, Helfet D, Hansen ST Jr. Objective criteria accurately predict amputation following lower extremity trauma. J Trauma 1990; 30;568-573.

29. Renstra WR, Buras JA, Svoboda KS: Hyperbaric oxygen increases human dermal fibroblast proliferation, growth factor receptor number and in vitro wound closure. Undersea Hyperb Med 1998; 25(Suppl):53(#164).

30. Saulis AS, Davidson JD, Mustoe TA, Moford JE. Hyperbaric oxygen modulates PDGF receptor B expression and ERK1/2 activation in human dermal fibroblasts in vitro. Plastic Surgery Research Council, 45th Annual Meeting, Seattle, Washington. 2000:143

31. Hall BB, Fitzgerald RH Jr, Rosenblatt JE. Anaerobic osteomyelitis. J Bone Joint Surg 1983; 65(A):30-35.

32. Strauss MB.: Diabetic foot problems; keys to effective, aggressive prevention. Consultant 2001; 41(13):1693-1705.

33. Handbook of Emergency Cardiovascular Care for Health Care Providers. Hazinski ME, Cummins RD, eds. American Heart Association 1999; p. 3

34. Strauss MB. Evidence review of HBO for crush injury, compartment syndrome and other traumatic ischemia. Undersea and Hyperbaric Medicine 2001; 28(Suppl):35-36.

CHAPTER 4

PHYSIOLOGICAL AND PHARMACOLOGICAL BASIS OF HYPERBARIC OXYGEN THERAPY

P.J. Sheffield, A. PS Smith

Although pure dephlogisticated air might be useful as a medicine, it might not be so proper for us in the usual healthy state of the body. Who knows but that in a matter of time, this pure air might become an article of luxury...?

J Priestley (1775)

INTRODUCTION

Hyperbaric oxygen (HBO) therapy is high dose oxygen inhalation therapy that is achieved by having the patient breathe 100 percent oxygen inside a pressurized hyperbaric chamber. Since there is insufficient absorption of oxygen through the skin, delivery of oxygen to tissues is provided by way of the respiration. After hemoglobin is fully saturated, additional oxygen is carried to the tissues in physical solution in plasma. HBO elevates the capillary plasma oxygen content, which is proportional to the inspired oxygen pressure. The benefits of HBO are derived from both the physiological and pharmacological effects of high dose oxygen. In order to be effective as a treatment, the clinical status of the patient or the underlying pathology is altered pharmacologically. HBO is used as a drug, and as such, it has a specific dose, side effects, and contraindications.

Hyperbaric oxygenation is based on two physical factors related to the hyperbaric environment: mechanical effects of pressure and increased oxygenation of tissues. This chapter covers the physiological basis for hyperbaric therapy, the pharmacological effects of oxygen, some of the limitations of hyperbaric therapy, and the physiological basis of selected applications of HBO. More detailed information is provided in the references at the end of the chapter and in the chapters that follow.

PHYSIOLOGICAL EFFECTS

The physiological effects of HBO are based on physical chemistry laws that govern the effect of pressure up to 6 atmospheres absolute (ata) and oxygen breathing at pressures up to 3 ata (3.03 MPa). The pressure at 6 ata (6.06 MPa) is six times sea level pressure, or equivalent to the pressure attained by descending to 60 meters (165 feet) of seawater. The pressure at 3 ata (3.03 MPa) is equivalent to 30 meters (66 feet) of seawater, which is about the pressure level in most automobile tires. When the patient is pressurized inside the hyperbaric chamber, the total pressure increases and:

1. Gas volume in enclosed body areas (and bubbles) contracts according to Boyle's Law, which states that the volume is inversely proportional to the absolute pressure. The mathematical expression for Boyle's Law is: $P_1 / P_2 = V_2 / V_1$
2. The partial pressure of oxygen (PO_2) and each of the other component gases in the breathing media increases according to Dalton's Law, which states that the total pressure in a gas mixture is the sum of the partial pressures of each individual gas. The mathematical expression for Dalton's Law is: $P_{total} = PO_2 + PN_2 + P_{others}$
3. The amount of dissolved oxygen in plasma increases according to Henry's Law, which states that the amount of a gas in solution is directly proportional to the partial pressure of that gas above the solution. $P_1 / P_2 = A_1 / A_2$
4. As oxygen tension in the surrounding capillaries increases, tissue oxygenation is improved according to the Law of Gaseous Diffusion, which states that a gas will move from an area of higher pressure to an area of lower pressure.

The converse is true as the patient is depressurized and removed from the hyperbaric chamber. As total pressure decreases inside the chamber:

1. The volume of a gas in enclosed body areas (and bubbles) expands;
2. The PO_2 in the breathing media decreases;
3. Oxygen transport diminishes as the amount of dissolved oxygen taken up by plasma decreases;
4. Oxygenation of tissues diminishes as oxygen tension in surrounding capillaries decrease. Following a hyperbaric oxygen exposure for one hour, Wells et al. (1) reported that skin oxygen tension remained elevated >10 percent for up to three hours.

Gas Volume Effects

When the chamber is pressurized, the volume of gas in enclosed body areas such as the ears, sinuses, lungs, gastrointestinal tract, and gas-filled entities (such as intravascular bubbles) respond to the increased pressure by contracting in accordance with Boyle's Law. Figure 1 shows the expected decrease in bubble volume and diameter when the chamber is pressurized up to 6 ata (6.06 MPa). Doubling the pressure reduces gas volume to about one half and tripling the pressure reduces gas volume to about one third. This is significant to the patient because changes in chamber pressure may cause barotrauma and pain. For example, to avoid ear pain during pressurization air must be physically added to the ears by Valsalva or Frenzel technique, and during depressurization, the air must be allowed to escape through the Eustachian tube.

Air bubbles that occur in tissue also respond to pressure change. Elimination of the bubbles is accomplished by a combination of pressure and oxygen breathing. Figure 2 shows the effect of compression and oxygen breathing on establishing a gradient for nitrogen elimination from a bubble. Breathing pure oxygen while pressurized inside the chamber increases the pressure differential for nitrogen elimination and quickly resolves the bubbles. This is useful for treating decompression sickness, air or gas embolism, and gas gangrene. As gas volume is reduced, there is less tissue distension, better perfusion, and less pain. There are provisions for using HBO to treat air or gas embolism at pressures up to 6 ata (6.06 MPa), but 2.8 to 3 ata (3.03 MPa) is the usual treatment.

Oxygen in the Breathing Media

The patient's breathing media is contained within the chamber itself, or in a built-in-breathing system (BIBS) consisting of a mask or hood oxygen delivery system. Monoplace (single person) chambers may be pressurized with pure oxygen, enabling the patient to breathe oxygen from the chamber environment. Fire safety considerations require multiplace (large walk-in chambers that can treat more than one person) chambers to pressurize with air and administer oxygen to the patient via mask or hood. As hyperbaric chamber pressure increases, PO_2 in the breathing media also increases. Air at sea level pressure (1 ata, or 760 mm Hg) contains 21% oxygen at a PO_2 of 160 mm Hg. When the chamber is pressurized with air to 3 ata (3.03 MPa), PO_2 is 429 mm Hg which would be equivalent to breathing 56 percent oxygen at sea level. As chamber pressurization with air is increased to 5 ata (5.05 MPa) and beyond, PO_2 exceeds 798 mm Hg, which is greater oxygen pressure than can

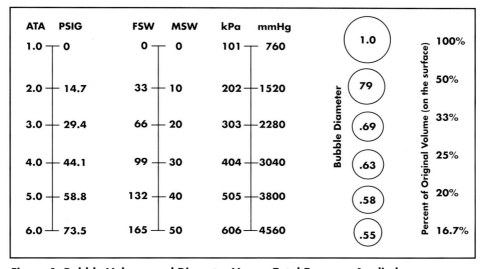

Figure 1. Bubble Volume and Diameter Versus Total Pressure Applied

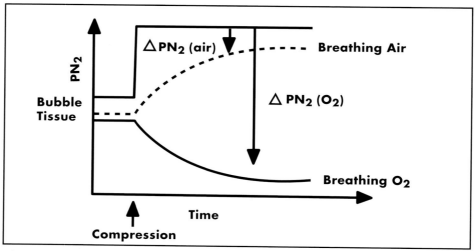

Figure 2. Effect of Compression and Oxygen on Establishing a Gradient for Nitrogen Elimination from a Bubble

be attained breathing pure oxygen at 1 ata. When the patient breathes pure oxygen from a mask, hood, or the chamber itself, PO_2 rises to 1520 mm Hg at 2 ata (2.02 MPa) and 2280 mm Hg at 3 ata (3.03 MPa).

Table 1 shows the partial pressure of oxygen in the breathing media, the alveolar oxygen tension, and the ideal dissolved oxygen in the plasma under various hyperbaric pressures as the subject breathes either air or oxygen. The ideal alveolar oxygen pressures (PAO_2) are calculated based on the alveolar gas equation:

$PAO_2 = (PB - PH_2O)FiO_2 - PACO_2 [FiO_2 + (1-FiO_2)/ R]$ where:

PB   - Barometric pressure
PH_2O - Water vapor at body temperature (47 mm Hg at 37°C)
FiO_2 - Percent of inspired oxygen, expressed as a fraction
$PACO_2$ - Mean alveolar PCO_2 measured in arterial blood (40 mm Hg)
R   - Respiratory exchange ratio (ml CO_2 excreted per ml O_2 absorbed)
          - 0.8 (when breathing air)
          - 1.0 (when breathing 100% O_2)

Oxygen Transport to Tissues

Oxygen is transported by blood from the lung to tissues by two methods: bound to hemoglobin, and physically dissolved in the plasma.

Oxygen Bound to Hemoglobin

The principal source of oxygen transport is the red blood cell in the form of oxyhemoglobin ($HbgO_2$). Normal concentration of hemoglobin is about 15 grams per dl. whole blood, and 1 gram of hemoglobin can combine with 1.36 ml of oxygen. When fully saturated ($SaO_2 = 100$), 1 dl. of whole blood will transport 20.4 ml O_2. At normal sea level pressure where alveolar oxygen pressure is about 100 mm Hg, hemoglobin is about 97% saturated

(SaO_2 = 97) and yields oxygen content of about 19.8 ml of oxygen per dl blood. When PAO_2 reaches about 200 mm Hg, hemoglobin becomes fully saturated with oxygen. Further increase in pressure will not increase the amount of oxyhemoglobin. Thus, oxygen transport by hemoglobin is not improved by hyperbaric oxygen therapy above oxygen administered at atmospheric conditions. Instead, additional oxygen is dissolved in the plasma and carried to the tissues in physical solution.

Oxygen Physically Dissolved in Plasma

When a person breathes air at sea level pressure, only 1.5 percent of the oxygen carried by the blood is transported physically dissolved in the plasma. However, oxygen transport by plasma is the key to hyperbaric oxygen therapy, for even poorly perfused wounded tissue can receive oxygen as the hyperoxygenated plasma seeps across it. Unlike hemoglobin saturation, which has an S-shaped curve, the amount of dissolved oxygen increases linearly as pO_2 increases. As shown in Table 1, by increasing the inspired oxygen pressure, one can significantly increase the amount of dissolved oxygen in the plasma. Thus, as the chamber is pressurized, the lung's elevated alveolar oxygen tension drives increasing quantities of oxygen into the

TABLE 1. OXYGEN VALUES ENCOUNTERED DURING HBO THERAPY

In The Breathing Media			In The Lung	In The Plasma
Total Pressure (ata)	Total Pressure (mm Hg)	PO_2 (mm Hg)	PAO_2 (mm Hg)	ml O_2/dl whole blood (vol%)
Breathing Air				
1	760	160	100	0.31
2	1520	319	269	0.83
2.36	1794	377	322	1.00
2.82	2143	450	400	1.24
3	2280	479	429	1.33
4	3040	638	588	1.82
5	3800	798	748	2.32
6	4560	958	908	2.81
Breathing 100% Oxygen				
1	760	760	673	2.08
2	1520	1520	1433	4.44
2.36	1794	1794	1707	5.29
2.82	2143	2143	2056	5.80
3	2280	2280	2193	6.80
4	3040			
5	3800	To minimize risk of oxygen toxicity, 100% oxygen is not used at pressures greater than 3 ata (3.03 MPa)		
6	4560			

plasma of the pulmonary circulation for its subsequent transport throughout the body. This is the principle on which hyperbaric oxygenation is based. Figure 3 graphically presents the combined oxygen carrying capacity of dissolved oxygen and the hemoglobin, assuming a normal hemoglobin level of 15 gm per dl of blood.

Oxygen Solubility

Henry's Law defines only the relative quantity of gas entering solution as related to the alveolar oxygen partial pressure (PAO$_2$), but does not define the absolute amount of gas in physical solution. The absolute amount varies with different fluids and is determined by the solubility coefficient of the gas in fluids, which is temperature dependent. Oxygen solubility in plasma at 37°C is 0.0028 ml of O$_2$ per dl plasma per mm Hg PAO$_2$. Oxygen is slightly more soluble in whole blood, and at 37°C is 0.0031 ml of O$_2$ per dl blood per mm Hg PAO$_2$. When air is breathed at sea level, arterial oxygen tension is about 100 mm Hg, so the blood transports about 0.31 ml of dissolved oxygen per dl whole blood. If 100 percent oxygen is breathed at sea level, the amount of dissolved oxygen can be increased to about 2.1 ml of O$_2$ per dl blood. Since alveolar water vapor and carbon dioxide pressures remain essentially constant during hyperbaric exposure, the PAO$_2$ increase with 100 percent oxygen administration under hyperbaric conditions is nearly 760 mm Hg per additional atmosphere of chamber pressure. Breathing 100 percent oxygen at 2 ATA (2.02 MPa) results in a PAO$_2$ of 1433 mm Hg or 4.4 ml of physically dissolved oxygen per dl blood. The maximum ambient pressure at which 100 percent oxygen can be safely breathed (for short periods) is 3 ata (3.03 MPa), which provides a PAO$_2$ of about 2200 mm Hg, and adds about 6.8 ml O$_2$ to each dl of blood. During the oxygen treatment, intermittent air breathing periods are programmed to prevent oxygen toxicity.

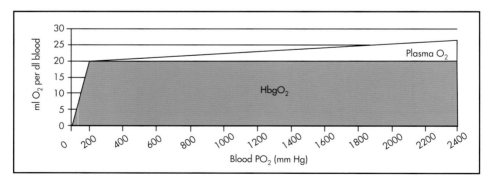

Figure 3. Combined Blood Oxygen Content Bound to Hemoglobin and Dissolved in Plasma at High Levels of Blood PO$_2$ (2)

Note: This figure is modified from C. J. Lambertsen. Physiological effects of oxygen inhalation at high partial pressures. In: Fundamentals of Hyperbaric Medicine, Washington DC: National Academy of Sciences, National Research Council, 1996, pp 12-20.

Carbon Dioxide Solubility

The solubility of carbon dioxide in plasma at $37\,^{\circ}C$ is 0.0697 ml CO_2/dl plasma/mm Hg $PACO_2$. Of the 493 ml of carbon dioxide in each liter of arterial blood, 27 ml (5%) is dissolved, 22 ml (5%) is in hemoglobin, and 444 ml (90%) is in carbonic acid or bicarbonate ion in the blood buffer system. In the tissues, 40 ml of CO_2 per liter of blood is added. Only 6 percent of the total venous content is carried as dissolved CO_2, even though carbon dioxide is about 20 times more soluble than oxygen. About 22 percent is combined with hemoglobin and 72 percent is transported in the blood buffer system. The pH of the blood drops from 7.40 to 7.37. In the lungs, the process is reversed, and the 40 ml of carbon dioxide is discharged into the alveoli for subsequent exhalation into the environment. Breathing hyperbaric oxygen fully saturates venous blood hemoglobin with oxygen and blocks carbon dioxide transport by hemoglobin. Some CO_2 retention occurs, but as long as blood flow is intact, the effects are minor because the carbon dioxide simply enters the plasma where it is buffered by bicarbonate with little change in pH. Because the person inside the chamber produces CO_2, continuous venting of the chamber or scrubbing with an absorbent is necessary to keep the CO_2 level within physiological ranges.

Gas Exchange between the Blood and Tissues

The usual oxygen transport to tissues is via hemoglobin. When the red blood cell arrives at the tissue capillary, it encounters an environment that encourages release of oxygen from the hemoglobin. Carbon dioxide leaves the tissue because its partial pressure is higher in the tissues than it is in the blood. As carbon dioxide diffuses from the tissues, oxygen diffuses into the tissues because its partial pressure is higher in the blood than in the tissues. Under hyperbaric conditions, the partial pressure of oxygen in the blood is significantly higher than normal. Although HBO treatment protocols vary by the type of disorder being treated, most require oxygen delivery at 2 to 3 ata (2.02 to 3.03 MPa), which results in an arterial oxygen tension of about 1200 to 2000 mm Hg. The increased oxygen tension causes the oxygen to diffuse further from functioning capillaries. One can relate this phenomenon to that seen in a garden hose where one can increase the water spray distance by increasing the pressure in the hose. Figure 4 is a comparison of healthy tissue response to air and oxygen breathing at 1 ata, 2 ata, and 2.4 ata as determined by invasive oxygen electrodes. Baseline subcutaneous oxygen tension of 30-50 mm Hg during air breathing at 1 ata (1.01 MPa) increases during oxygen breathing to 90-150 mm Hg at 1 ata, to 200-300 mm Hg at 2 ata, and up to 500 mm Hg at 2.4 ata. Table 2 is a comparison of tissue oxygen tension values for progressively increased inspired PO_2.

Cellular Respiration

The chemical energy produced from catabolism of food is stored in the energy-rich phosphate bonds of adenosine triphosphate (ATP), which exists in the cytoplasm of the cell. Because the supply of ATP in cellular cytoplasm is limited, new energy-rich bonds must be continually produced by oxidation of foodstuffs (protein, carbohydrates, and fat), making nutrition a very important component in tissue regeneration and repair. Figure 5 shows the

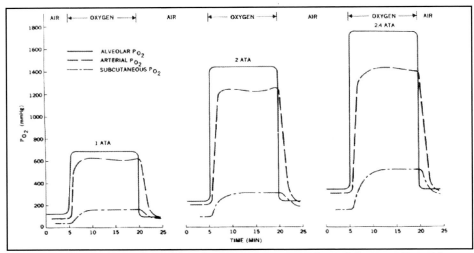

Figure 4. Comparison of Healthy Tissue Response to Air and Oxygen Breathing at 1 ATA, 2 ATA, and 2.4 ATA. (From Sheffield PJ, Heimbach RD, Respiratory Physiology. In: DeHart RL (ed) Fundamentals of Aerospace Medicine, Baltimore, MD: Williams & Wilkins, 1994; fig 5.8 p 84) (3).

TABLE 2: TISSUE OXYGEN TENSION VALUES FOR PROGRESSIVELY INCREASED INSPIRED PO_2

Ambient Pressure (ata) /Breathing Media	1.0 ata Air	1.0 ata O_2	2.0 ata O_2	2.4 ata O_2
	Representative Tissue Oxygen Tension in mm Hg			
Ambient PO_2	159	760	1,520	1,824
Alveolar PO_2 (Ideal)	104	673	1,433	1,737
Arterial PO_2 (Ideal)	100	660	1,400	1,700
Arterial PO_2 a	-	550±100	1,150±250	1,400 e
Venous PO_2 b	36±4	60±9	101±36	500 e
Muscle PO_2 b	29±3	59±13	221±72	-
Subcutaneous PO_2 c	30-50	90-150	200-300	250-500
Transcutaneous PO_2 –Chest d	67±12	450±54	-	1,312±112
Transcutaneous PO_2 –Calf Female d	63±13	367±59	-	1,174±127
Transcutaneous PO_2 –Calf Male d	49±4	281±78	-	1,027±164
Transcutaneous PO_2 –Midfoot d	63±13	280±82	-	919±214

a. Blood gas analyzer data from Lanphier et al. 1966 (4).
b. Mass spectrometer data from Wells et al., 1977 (1).
c. Invasive oxygen electrode from Sheffield 1985 (5).
d. Transcutaneous oxygen data from Dooley et al., 1997 (6).
e. Blood gas analyzer data from Sheffield (previously unpublished data).

process of cellular respiration, which starts with the foodstuffs being degraded in a series of enzymatic reactions to produce acetyl coenzyme A (CoA). Within the mitochondria of the cell, acetyl CoA is channeled into the Krebs tricarboxylic acid cycle, which is the final common pathway of oxidative catabolism. Hydrogen ions, or their equivalent electrons from this process, are then fed into the respiratory chain where energy-rich ATP is formed by oxidative phosphorylation of ADP as the electrons are transferred to molecular oxygen. This process requires a minimum oxygen tension of 0.5 to 3 mm Hg. The minimum tissue oxygen value required to achieve this level in the mitochondria is about 30 mm Hg. As tissue oxygen tension is increased above these minimum values in the mitochondria, oxidative phosphorylation is unaffected until levels above 250 to 300 mm Hg are reached. Above 300 mm Hg, the rate of oxygen consumption by the mitochondria falls sharply and oxygen toxicity occurs, presumably due to an interruption of the cytochrome oxidase enzyme system.

Tissue Oxygen Requirements

The respiratory chain in the mitochondria of the cell requires that molecular oxygen be present in abundance to meet the basic metabolic needs of the cell. About 90 percent of molecular oxygen is consumed in the process of oxidative phosphorylation that creates energy-rich ATP, about 9 percent is used to remove hydrogen during oxidation of amino acids and amines, and about 1 percent is incorporated into complex organic molecules during oxygenation of biogenic amines and hormones.

A healthy adult at rest uses about 6 ml of oxygen per dl of circulating blood. This can be determined from the mean tissue extraction, which is the difference between the oxygen content of arterial blood leaving the lung (20 ml oxygen/ dl blood) and mixed venous blood

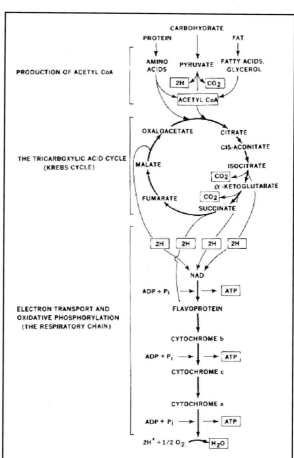

Figure 5. Cellular Respiration

Note: This figure is from Sheffield PJ, Heimbach RD. Respiratory Physiology. In: DeHart RL (ed) Fundamentals of Aerospace Medicine, Baltimore, MD: Williams & Wilkins, 1996, p 82 (3).

reaching the right atrium (14 ml oxygen/ dl blood), or 6 ml oxygen per dl of circulating blood. Thus, HBO at 3 ata (3.03 MPa) provides sufficient plasma oxygen to exceed the body's total metabolic requirement. In Boerema's 1960 classic "Life Without Blood" study at 3 ata (3.03 MPa), pigs that had their erythrocytes removed from their exsanguinated blood had sufficient oxygen in the plasma to sustain life (7). One of the applications of HBO is to overcome hemoglobin deficiency during massive blood loss. For example, the dissolved oxygen content of 6 ml oxygen per dl blood would be equivalent to the sea level oxygen carrying capacity of about 5 grams of hemoglobin. Thus, HBO at 3 ata (3.03 MPa) could be used to offset the loss of approximately one-third of the total blood volume that had been replaced by plasma expanders, buying time until the body could replenish the red blood cells.

The need for maintaining minimum tissue oxygen tension is demonstrated by measurements in chronic, non-healing hypoxic wounds (5). Wounds of HBO-treated patients were repeatedly measured at weekly intervals by inserting an invasive needle electrode into the wound to determine the wound oxygen tension (PwO_2). In a series of 20 patients, all wounds were hypoxic (PwO_2 = 5 to 20 mm Hg) before HBO treatment was initiated. Daily HBO treatments at 2.36 ata (2.4 MPa) elevated PwO_2 above 30 mm Hg in all patients in which healing occurred. Wounds that remained below 30 mm Hg failed to heal. Figure 6 shows the progressively improved wound response to oxygen breathing at 1 ata (1.01 MPa) for selected weeks of HBO treatment in a problem surgical wound of a high-thigh amputee.

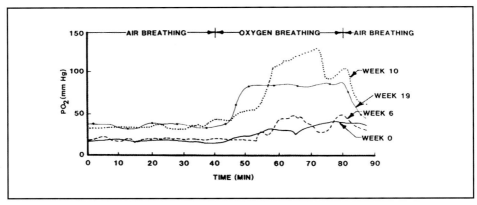

Figure 6.

Chronic wound response of a high-thigh amputee to oxygen breathing for selected weeks of HBO treatment (5). Measurements recorded by invasive oxygen electrodes over a course of 19 weeks in a long-term tissue oxygen study. Reprinted by permission from Sheffield PJ. Tissue oxygen measurements with respect to soft-tissue wound healing with normobaric and hyperbaric oxygen. In: Hyperbaric Oxygen Review. 1985 6(1): 18-46. Copyright by Plenum Publishing.

Note: This figure is from Sheffield PJ, Tissue oxygen measurements. In: Problem Wounds Role of Oxygen. Davis JC, Hunt TK, eds. New York: Elsevier Science Publishing. 1988; p 40.

Case 921 RC

The 46-year-old male presented with a non-healing high-thigh amputation site. The problem arose ten years previously when he received multiple shrapnel wounds to the right leg that subsequently healed. The patient had received a series of surgical procedures over the course of two years that included failed grafts and surgical procedures that serially progressed up the limb to this high-thigh amputation. There were four failed grafts attempted at this site. Rather than perform a hip disarticulation, HBO was chosen to prepare the site for grafting, and the patient was entered into a long-term tissue oxygen study. The wound was initially severely hypoxic, with baseline PwO_2 of 10-15 mm Hg. By the 10th week baseline PwO_2 values were above 30 mm Hg because of the presence of granulation tissue and improved capillary function, and the wound was determined to be ready for grafting. Because of the history of failed grafts, the surgeon requested that HBO be continued until the 19th week when successful grafting occurred. The patient was subsequently successfully fitted with prosthesis (5).

Oxygen Diffusion Limitations

Tissue oxygen content at any point depends on the distance from functioning capillaries, the oxygen demand of the tissue, and the oxygen tension in the capillary. During oxygen breathing at 3 ata (3.03 MPa), an arterial PO_2 of over 2000 mm Hg is achieved, compared to a normal sea-level value of 100 mm Hg. The Krogh Erlang mathematical model estimates that this 20-fold increase in PO_2 will cause oxygen diffusion distances to increase 4-fold at the arterial end of the capillary (8). Figure 7 shows the estimated oxygen diffusion from the capillaries to surrounding tissue under both normobaric and hyperbaric oxygenation. As shown in Figure 7, during air breathing at 1 ata (1.01 MPa), oxygen diffuses about 64 micrometers (less than the thickness of one sheet of typing paper) at the arterial end of the capillary. During oxygen breathing at 3 ata (3.03 MPa), oxygen diffuses about 250 micrometers (about the thickness of three sheets of typing paper).

Wound Oxygen Measurements

Data obtained with invasive oxygen electrodes have provided valuable information on wound oxygenation with normobaric and hyperbaric oxygen. The oxygen diffusion gradient in the healing wound was defined by Silver (9) in his classic microelectrode studies of rabbit granulation tissue as show at Figure 8. He recorded PwO_2 values less than 3 mm Hg at a distance of about 120-140 micrometers (about the thickness of two sheets of typing paper) from the nearest capillary. PwO_2 values were above 40 mm Hg at the capillary loops, and approached 100 mm Hg in areas of more densely populated capillaries.

Sheffield's tissue PO_2 measurements in human ischemic, indolent wounds revealed that initial PwO_2 were usually below 20 mm Hg, but responded to respired oxygen. Hyperbaric oxygen elevated PwO_2 on a single exposure and raised the baseline PwO_2 values over a course of HBO therapy. Finally, irradiated tissue had tissue PO_2 values similar to wounds. Studies of ischemic wounds revealed that many problem wounds were severely hypoxic, and that HBO corrected the severe hypoxia by daily

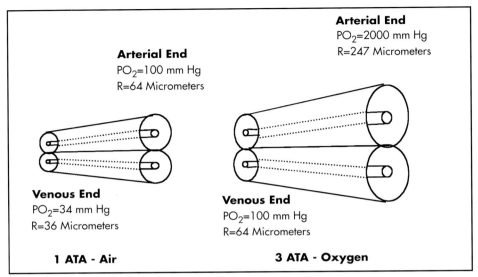

Arterial End
PO$_2$=100 mm Hg
R=64 Micrometers

Arterial End
PO$_2$=2000 mm Hg
R=247 Micrometers

Venous End
PO$_2$=34 mm Hg
R=36 Micrometers

Venous End
PO$_2$=100 mm Hg
R=64 Micrometers

1 ATA - Air

3 ATA - Oxygen

Figure 7.

Krogh Erlang oxygen diffusion model used to estimate oxygen diffusion from the capillaries to surrounding tissue and the potential increase in oxygen diffusion distances with hyperbaric oxygenation (8).

Note: This figure is from Sheffield PJ, Tissue oxygen measurements. In Problem Wounds Role of Oxygen. Davis JC, Hunt TK, eds. New York: Elsevier Science Publishing. 1988; p 38.

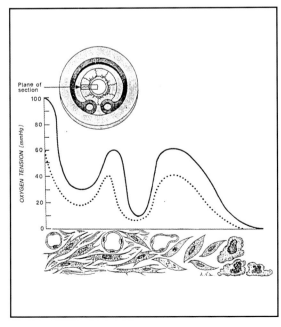

Figure 8.

Tissue oxygen tension profile of a rabbit ear wound as defined by the microelectrode studies of IA Silver (9). Wound PO2 shows the effects of systemic arterial hypoxia (lower line) as opposed to normal oxygen tension (upper line). (Hunt TK, van Winkle W Jr: Wound Healing: Disorders of Repair, in Dunphy JE (ed) Fundamentals of Wound Management in Surgery. South Plainfield; Chirurgecom, 1976. Redrawn with the gracious permission of IA Silver.

Note: This Figure is from Sheffield PJ, Tissue oxygen measurements. In: Problem Wounds Role of Oxygen. Davis JC, Hunt TK, eds. New York: Elsevier Science Publishing. 1988; p 35.

bringing the tissue oxygen tension up to normal level. About seven to ten days were required to see an appreciable change in the granulation base of the wound, and that change was reflected in the oxygen tracings.

Case 613 ES

A 51-year-old insulin-dependent diabetic female had a five-year history of neurotrophic ulcer with underlying osteomyelitis of the right foot. Multiple episodes of secondary cellulites required repeated antibiotic therapy and hospitalization. When the patient rejected amputation, her attending physician sought PwO_2 assessment in anticipation of HBO as a treatment option. The patient was enrolled in a long-term tissue oxygen study. Figure 9 shows PwO_2 values for three oxygen-breathing cycles at 1 ata (1.01 MPa) that were made initially (twenty-four weeks preHBO), one week preHBO, and three weeks after start of HBO. Baseline PwO_2 collected 24 weeks preHBO was 25 mm Hg compared to 40 mm Hg in healthy control tissue. During the six-month lapse before HBO treatments began, the wound continued to deteriorate and PwO_2 values decreased accordingly to a severely hypoxic condition of 10 mm Hg. After three weeks of HBO, baseline PwO_2 was above 30 mm Hg and response during oxygen breathing exceeded 400 mm Hg. HBO was continued until healing occurred (5).

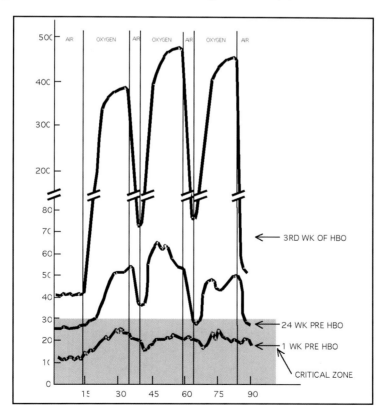

Figure 9. Wound Response to Oxygen Breathing at 1 ATA For Selected Weeks PreHBO and During a Course of HBO (original drawing)

When HBO restores the PO_2 to normal or slightly elevated values, it enhances epithelialization, collagen deposition, fibroplasia, angiogenesis, and bacterial killing. Human fibroblasts can survive in 3 mm Hg, but cannot undergo replication or migration with less than about 30 mm Hg oxygen tension. Balin (10) reported that if held continuously at 290-560 mm Hg (equivalent to 40-75% oxygen at sea level), fibroblastic replication was halted in early prophase, after DNA synthesis, but before metaphase of mitosis and at two specific stages during protein synthesis (Figure 10). When oxygen tension was

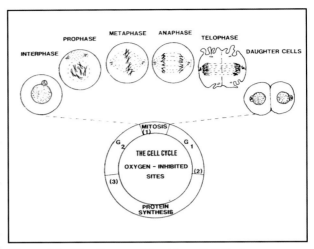

Figure 10. The Human Fibroblast Cell Cycle

The 24-hour cell cycle with markers (numbers in parentheses), indicating the sites of cellular accumulation of oxygen inhibited cells (11).

Note: This figure is redrawn from Sheffield PJ, Tissue oxygen measurements. In: Problem Wounds Role of Oxygen. Davis JC, Hunt TK, eds. New York: Elsevier Science Publishing. 1988; p 46.

returned to normal, the replication process continued. Thus, it would seem that a daily high dose of oxygen is needed to correct the hypoxic environment of fibroblasts in the problem wound, but oxygen must be delivered on an intermittent schedule to avoid possible toxic effects on the cells. Since the cell cycle for human fibroblasts is about 24 hours, and mitosis occurs in a period of about one hour, an oxygen dose of about one to two hours every 12 to 24 hours seems to be appropriate.

In general, capillary oxygen tension is more important than oxygen content for increasing the pressure differential and giving a greater diffusion distance from the functioning capillary. Hunt and associates reported only a one percent increase in arterial oxygen content when PaO_2 was increased from 82 mm Hg (air breathing) to 200 mm Hg (enriched O_2 breathing at sea level pressure), but the amount of hydroxyproline doubled (12) and the amount of collagen in granulation tissue increased by 50 percent (13). Conversely, animals breathing hypoxic gas mixtures (arterial PO_2 of 42 mm Hg) suffered a 50 percent reduction in collagen synthesis (13). Niinikoski (14) showed that twice as much hydroxyproline was produced in an environment of 70% oxygen than in an environment of 18% oxygen (Figure 11).

Transcutaneous Oximetry ($PtcO_2$)

Transcutaneous oximetry ($PtcO_2$) has become a standard technique for qualifying wounded patients for HBO treatment (15). $PtcO_2$ values indicate if the tissue is hypoxic and whether the tissue will respond to inspired oxygen. $PtcO_2$ measures the local tissue oxygen tension that is derived from

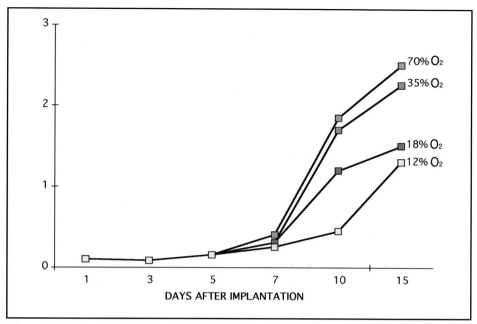

Figure 11.

Effect of different ambient oxygen tensions on production of collagen hydroxypro-line in subcutaneous cellulose sponge implants in rats. (Adapted from Niinikoski J.) Effect of oxygen supply on wound healing and formation of experimental granulation tissue. Acta Physiol Scand Suppl 1969; 334:1 (14).

Note: This figure is from Brakora MJ, Sheffield PJ, Hyperbaric oxygen therapy for diabetic wounds. In: Clinics in Podiatric Medicine and Surgery: The Diabetic Foot. LB Harkless, LA Lavery, KJ Dennis, eds. Philadelphia PA: WB Saunders; 1995. p 110.

capillary blood perfusion. Tissue oxygen values obtained with transcutaneous sensors are considerably greater than those attained with invasive electrodes because they are measuring different things. The invasive sensor measures what is in the tissues while the transcutaneous sensor measures what is in the capillary bed beneath the sensor. The transcutaneous sensor must be heated to aid oxygen migration to the skin surface where it is measured. In the absence of heat, diffusion of oxygen from tissue to skin surface contributes less than 3.5 mm Hg to the PO_2 at that location. When the sensor is heated to 44°C, normal healthy tissue has a baseline air $PtcO_2$ value that ranges from about 70 mm Hg at the chest to about 55 mm Hg at the foot (6).

Oxygen electrodes are attached to the periwound skin at a proposed surgical level to assess the oxygen released from the capillaries beneath the sensor. The electrodes are heated to create vasodilatation of the capillary bed. There is some local rebound vasoconstriction that is overcome by heating to temperatures between 42-44 degrees Celsius. The electrodes consume extremely low levels of oxygen, assuring the accuracy of measurements in poorly perfused tissue. Baseline air-breathing $PtcO_2$ values below 40 mm Hg are suggestive of local hypoxia and correlate with a reduced likelihood of healing. To assess whether the tissue will respond to oxygen administration, an "oxygen challenge" of 100% O_2 at 1.0 ata is provided via tight-fitting non-rebreather mask with at least 15 L per minute oxygen flow. Patients selected for HBO therapy usually have baseline air $PtcO_2$ values below 40 mm Hg (indicating presence of hypoxia) and a significant rise on oxygen breathing challenge. $PtcO_2$ values of 40 mm Hg or greater reached within ten to twenty minutes of breathing 100% oxygen indicate the tissue may respond to hyperbaric oxygen therapy. Observing the absolute value and the relative increase in $PtcO_2$ while breathing oxygen at sea level seems to increase the accuracy of the $PtcO_2$ predictive value in post amputation healing (16, 17, 18). Sheffield, Dietz, and Posey, et al. (19) reported that $PtcO_2$ in air >0 coupled with a $PtcO_2$ in O_2 >35 mmHg and an oxygen challenge increase of >50% was useful in predicting healing in 46 prospectively evaluated patients. Assessment of blood flow by laser Doppler with heat provocation also showed promise as a predictor of successful outcome (19).

In the event a patient has an inadequate response to a 100% oxygen challenge at 1.0 ata, an in-chamber oxygen challenge at 2.0-2.5 ata can be accomplished. To be considered an adequate response, $PtcO_2$ values taken while the patient is pressurized inside the chamber should rise to at least 100 mm Hg, and preferably 200 mm Hg. $PtcO_2$ values for transplanted flaps or grafts in which the vascular pedicle has been severed or severely compromised are expected to reach a value of 50 mm Hg. For the in-chamber oxygen challenge, 2.0 or 2.5 ata is usually selected based upon the treatment pressure anticipated in the chamber. It is important to note that the prescribed treatment pressure should be sufficient to achieve the desired tissue oxygen levels.

In a six-center outcome study of over 1,100 patients in which transcutaneous oximetry was used as a selection tool, Fife et al. (20) reported that 75% of the patients were improved after HBO therapy. When taken alone, baseline $PtcO_2$ while breathing air at sea level had no statistical relationship with outcome prediction, because some patients with very low $PtcO_2$ were improved after a course of treatment. However, in-chamber $PtcO_2$ had 74% reliability in predicting patients likely to benefit from HBO. Patients with an in-chamber $PtcO_2$ of 200 mm Hg or greater had a 76.6% benefit rate from treatment, with an accuracy of 74.7%. Fife's data support the use of in-chamber $PtcO_2$ as a screening tool as originally described by Wattel, Mathieu, et al. (21).

It is generally accepted that baseline air $PtcO_2$ values less than 20 mm Hg should undergo non-invasive vascular evaluation as part of a thorough assessment. Baseline air $PtcO_2$ values below 10 mm Hg are sometimes difficult to interpret, as it could be due to edema, inflammation, lack of blood perfusion, or capillary malfunction. Other etiologies for low $PtcO_2$ values include sclerotic/scar tissue, post-radiated tissue with vascular loss, transplanted flaps or grafts without adequate native vascular supply, cold room environment with resultant vasoconstriction, vasoconstrictive medications, placement over bone, palm or sole, and local inflammation or infection. Consumption of oxygen by the sensor will cause the $PtcO_2$ value to approach zero if placed on areas where the oxygen is not easily replenished.

PHARMACOLOGICAL EFFECTS OF OXYGEN

In order for hyperbaric therapy to be an effective treatment, it must pharmacologically alter the underlying disease pathology and thereby improve the clinical status of the patient. In this respect, hyperbaric oxygen (HBO) is used as a drug. It has a therapeutic index, a minimum effective concentration (MEC) under which oxygen is ineffective and a minimum toxic concentration (MTC) above which toxicity prevails. As with all drug dosing regimes, protocols for oxygen dosing for hyperbaric oxygen have to be designed with considerations of weight, age (physiologic maturity), body surface, genetics, diet, drug interactions, and disease states which all have profound effects on drug pharmacokinetics. The therapeutic window for oxygen is greatly influenced by the concentration of inspired oxygen (FiO_2) at a given pressure (ata) over a given time. Oxygen has a definable dose in available molecules/minute when ordered by the PO_2 (FiO_2 at a given pressure) and time, i.e., 100% O_2 at 2.0 ATA for 60 min or 100% O_2 at 2.4 ATA for 90 min. There is also a specific dose response to HBO. The oxygen dose provided in a hyperbaric treatment profile of 100% O_2 at 1.6 ATA x 60 minutes is not the same as the oxygen dose provided in a treatment profile of 100% O_2 at 2.4 ATA x 60 minutes.

Therapeutic Effects of HBO

The therapeutic effects of HBO are related to the ability of oxygen and/or pressure under hyperbaric conditions to:

1. Reverse hypoxia,
2. Alter ischemic effect,
3. Influence vascular reactivity,
4. Reduce edema,
5. Modulate nitric oxide production,
6. Modify growth factors and cytokine effect by regulating their levels and/or receptors,
7. Induce changes in membrane proteins affecting ion exchange and gating mechanisms,
8. Promote cellular proliferation,
9. Accelerate collagen deposition,
10. Stimulate capillary budding and arborization,
11. Accelerate microbial oxidative killing,
12. Improve select antibiotic exchange across membranes,
13. Interfere with bacterial disease propagation by denaturing toxins,
14. Modulate the immune system response, and
15. Enhance oxygen radical scavengers thereby decreasing ischemia-reperfusion injury.

HBO EFFECTS ON CEREBRAL VASCULATURE

Attention should be given to the effects of HBO upon the cerebral vasculature specifically focusing on blood flow, ischemia, and edema. Autoregulation is influenced by both cerebral arterial oxygen concentrations and cerebral arterial carbon dioxide concentrations. Carbon dioxide increases nitric oxide (NO) production and oxygen decreases NO production by the endothelial cells. An increase in NO leads to vasodilatation while a decrease in NO leads to vasoconstriction. The local endothelial NO effect does not explain the entire mechanism of cerebral autoregulatory responses. The human cerebral circulation is supplied with a fine network of nerve fibers containing vasoactive peptidergic and non-peptidergic transmitters. Neuronal NO has been noted to provide an autocrine effect with direct feedback upon vascular endothelial cells to influence cerebral vascular autoregulation. In addition to neuronal NO, several neurotransmitters appear to have a local effect upon cerebral vasoreactivity: 5-hydroxytryptamine (5-HT), noradrenaline (NA), and neuropeptide Y (NPY). Normal cerebral blood flow is 50-60 ml/100g/min and in healthy individuals cerebral blood flow is usually subjected to strong autoregulation rendering it independent of the systemic blood pressure (BP). HBO causes a significant increase in local oxygen. This section will review the affect of HBO on cerebral blood flow, cerebral hypoxia, cerebral edema, and cerebral hypoxia/reperfusion injury.

Cerebral Blood Flow (CBF)

HBO Mediates Vasoconstriction

HBO appears to influence cerebral vasoreactivity by modulating NO production. Initially, HBO exerts a cerebral vasoconstrictive effect. There is a measurable decrease in NO production, vasoconstriction ensues, and a measurable reduction in CBF (25% Vols) occurs. Hyperbaric oxygen at 2.0 ata for less than two hours has been shown to reduce CBF while concurrently increasing by tenfold the cerebral oxygen content. Thus, even though CBF is reduced, there is more oxygen delivered to the cerebral tissue.

HBO Mediates Vasodilatation

In response to prolonged hyperoxia and/or higher pressurization levels, continued hyperbaric oxygen exposure leads to cerebral vasodilatation and a subsequent increase in CBF. In animal studies, the increased CBF appears to be mediated by nitric oxide synthase (NOS). N-nitro-L-arginine, an NOS inhibitor, competes with the natural precursor L-arginine to bind NOS. Studies using N-nitro-L-arginine support a correlation between HBO induced CBF and NO production consistent with activation of nitric oxide synthetase (NOS).

CO_2 Effects on CBF

Cerebral vascular regulation is strongly influenced by cerebral carbon dioxide concentration ($PaCO_2$). The normal $PaCO_2$ value for cerebral blood is approximately 40 mm Hg. As cerebral plasma $PaCO_2$ increases, cerebral vessels vasodilate and results in increased CBF. Conversely, as $PaCO_2$ decreases, cerebral vessels vasoconstrict and results in decreased CBF. The vasoconstrictive properties of carbon dioxide have been attributed to local NO production. Oxygen and carbon dioxide appear to act in an opposing fashion to affect NO production. Severe hypocapnea leads to a critical reduction in cerebral perfusion as the $PaCO_2$ approaches 19 mm Hg. Recommendations limit the amount of iatrogenic hyperventilation to 24 mm Hg.

HBO Induces a Cerebral Ischemic Tolerance

Cerebral ischemia is the critical lack of blood flow to the brain, which presents in two forms: global ischemia and focal ischemia. Global ischemia results from a diffuse decrease in cerebral perfusion epitomized by cardiac arrest, and renders widespread necrosis in the neocortex, hippocampus, basal ganglia, and cerebellum. Focal ischemia results from a transient occlusion such as occurs with a stroke, and is more common than global ischemia.

Multiple occlusion studies of HBO administered prior to the ischemic insult have confirmed the neuroprotective properties of HBO in the cerebral cortex, hippocampus, and forebrain. Hyperbaric oxygen administered prior to, during, or immediately after a focal ischemic insult results in less neural tissue loss (stroke tissue volume). Hyperbaric oxygen does not induce vaso-constriction in the damaged area because chemical mediators generated during ischemia interact with local cerebral vasculature to override the local autoregulatory mechanisms.

Increases in neuroprotective enzymes and proteins such as superoxide dismutase (Mn-SOD) and heat shock protein 27 (HSP-27) also occur in cerebral ischemic areas. Superoxide dismutase scavenges free radicals thereby producing a neuroprotective effect. The level of neuroprotection depends upon the treatment profile. Single dose treatment regimes do not produce neuroprotection. Pretreatment with HBO prior to surgical vascular ligation and/or repetitive treatments improved the neuroprotection. Hyperbaric oxygen therapy at 3.0 ata for 60 minutes given immediately after a medial cerebral artery occlusion reduced the infarction volume, but only when the ischemic insult was less than two hours. Treatment profiles with 100% O_2 at pressures less than 2.0 ata are deemed more beneficial for treating neurologic post-ischemic insults. Minimizing the time between injury and treatment enhances the degree of neuroprotection (33).

Cerebral Edema

Clinically, HBO has been documented to produce a net reduction in cerebral edema. The reduction in CBF undoubtedly plays a major role in the reduction of cerebral edema but membrane ionic homeostasis and blood-brain barrier (BBB) permeability also have to be considered. Two primary types of brain edema that are categorized based upon the integrity of the BBB: 1) Intact-barrier edema (normal permeability) results from disturbances in ionic homeostasis. The increased brain fluid is located within the brain cells associated with a contraction of the extracellular space; and, 2) Open-barrier edema (increased permeability) results from an influx of serum proteins into the brain generating an oncotic force. Increased brain swelling is attributed to edema fluid accumulated primarily in the extracellular space. Typically both types of edema occur simultaneously; however, one form usually predominates.

The HBO influence upon the BBB permeability is variable. Intravenous ferritin treatments given concurrently with HBO at 1.6 ATA x 90 min increased the permeability of cerebral vessel walls in normal animals (31). In contrast to ferritin and protein enzyme studies, a 14C-sucrose study performed concurrently with HBO at 2.5 ATA x 90 min for 10 consecutive days did not show any difference when compared to controls treated with N_2-O_2

mixture (PO_2 = 0.3 ATA). These data confirm the finding that different HBO doses (FIO_2 and pressurization) have different effects. Additional studies are needed to further elucidate the full extent of influence HBO exerts over cerebral ionic exchange and permeability alterations to reduce cerebral edema.

HBO Affects CNS Response to Hemodilution

After a traumatic non-cerebral hemorrhagic event, resuscitation with normal saline or plasma expanders produces hemodilution which reduces cerebral blood viscosity. It also reduces cerebral blood oxygen content. Both of these effects alter cerebral blood flow (CBF). The reduced cerebral blood oxygen content is responsible for approximately 40-60% of the increased CBF. The contribution of blood viscosity toward changes in the CBF is more apparent prior to resuscitation when hemoconcentration is present. Tracking plasma viscosity is more accurate than tracking whole blood viscosity when monitoring the relationship between CBF and hemodilution. The type of fluid replacement (blood vs normal saline) does not influence CBF until the HCT falls below 19%, at which value blood is preferable. Adaptation occurs in response to long-term hemodilution. CBF normalizes more rapidly when HBO is administered during post-traumatic hemorrhagic resuscitation.

HBO Modulates Nitric Oxide (NO) Production

HBO appears to modulate a diverse variety of biological processes as a result of either elevating or reducing the level of oxidants produced through redox signaling. Oxidant production is applicable to infection control, proliferation, VEGF, collagen gene, and others. Oxidant generation in wounds is great and accounts for at least half of the oxygen that is consumed. Although there are many oxidants, NO production has received the most attention in hyperbaric oxygen studies. The process is quite complex and many pieces of the puzzle have yet to be assembled. Nonetheless, the biological significance of HBO-NO interaction mandates an in-depth review of nitric oxide to understand the many potent effects of hyperbaric oxygen treatment.

Nitric Oxide

NO is a free radical gas that can rapidly diffuse across membranes into cells and act as a biologic effector molecule. It was identified as the substrate that caused vascular relaxation, endothelial-derived relaxation factor, EDRF. It is frequently discussed in relation to its vasodilatory effects but NO plays a critical role in vast numbers and types of biological functions, including: neurotransmission; adhesion of platelets and leukocytes; promotion of the immune defense response; direction of various gastrointestinal, respiratory, and genitourinary tract functions; stimulation of penile erection; and regulation of cardiac contractility and cellular apoptosis. Overproduction or underproduction of NO has been implicated in the pathology of many disease processes. Low basal level or attenuated response has been noted in the blood vessels of patients with diabetes, hypertension, cardiovascular atherosclerotic disease, end-stage chronic lung disease, and chronic renal failure. High basal levels or excessive induced production has been identified in disease processes such as endotoxic shock, allograft rejection, cirrhosis, hepato-renal syndrome and ischemia/reperfusion injury. Overproduction of NO in neuroexitatory cells has been associated with epilepsy and cerebral ischemia.

Obviously close regulation of this potent molecule is necessary. NO is rapidly inactivated, t1/2 of 3-5 sec, in a reaction that converts oxyhemoglobin to methemoglobin. The affinity of hemoglobin for NO is about 3000 times that of oxygen. NO binds other metalloprotein heme sites such as myoglobin and iron-sulfur containing side chains. Albumin carries NO and renders it a slightly longer half-life. Endogenous metabolism produces plasma and urinary nitrate and nitrite, which is enhanced in patients exhibiting signs/symptoms of diarrhea, fever, and septic shock as well as during exercise. NO is rapidly oxidized to nitrosate molecules containing sulfhydryl groups, such as glutathione, cysteine, and albumin. The production, utilization, and metabolism of NO is very important because of the profound need for rapid yet tight control over local homeostasis.

L-arginine

L-arginine, the NO precursor, is a non-essential amino acid that becomes conditionally essential in stress situations such as starvation, injury, wound healing, growth, and development. It is "semi-essential" in childhood, since biological production does not usually generate enough L-arginine to meet the high levels needed for developmental growth. During adulthood, the amount of L-arginine produced predominately in the kidney is sufficient to meet demands except when significant injury or illness occurs. Dietary supplementation during stress may improve outcome. Absorption requires a specialized membrane receptor that also transports the amino acids L-lysine and L-histidine. L-arginine dietary supplementation following trauma decreases nitrogen loss and augments wound healing. In addition to being converted to NO, L-arginine performs a host of other biological functions. L-arginine stimulates pituitary growth hormone secretion without altering the innate physiological pulsatile pattern of steady state production. L-arginine is a secretogogue for prolactin hypothalamic corticotropin releasing factor (CRF), pancreatic insulin, pancreozymin, glucagons and polypeptide, aldosterone somatostatin, and adrenal catecholamines. Synthesized L-arginine is derived from L-citrulline in the proximal renal tubules where L-arginine is effective in converting ammonia to the non-toxic byproduct urea. Creatine is also a substantial byproduct of metabolized L-arginine with residual unchanged L-arginine released into the circulation. L-arginine synthesized in the liver is quickly and completely metabolized locally by the enzyme arginase. The majority of circulating L-arginine is absorbed through the jejunum and ileum from dietary intake. Figure 12 illustrates the production of NO from L-arginine.

Nitric Oxide Synthase

Human nitric oxide synthase has been described in three isoforms: nNOS (neural or I), iNOS (inducible-II), and eNOS (epithelial-III). Isoforms nNOS and eNOS are constitutive isoforms derived from brain and endothelial cells, respectively. They are present and continuously functioning. The iNOS is the inducible isoform derived predominately from activated macrophages.

$$L-Arginine + \begin{Bmatrix} FAD + FMD \\ nNADPH \\ BH4 \end{Bmatrix} \xrightarrow{\begin{array}{c} eNOS \\ nNOS \\ iNOS \end{array}} + O2 = L-Citrulline + NO + NADP^{+\cdot}$$

Figure 12. NO Production from L-Arginine

NO is derived from L-arginine in a two-step process, catalyzed by the membrane-bound enzyme nitric oxide synthetase (NOS). N-(omega)-Hydroxyarginine (not shown) is generated as an intermediate. The initial and final products of the reaction are shown in the diagram. L-arginine is a "semi-essential amino acid" that along with molecular oxygen is a precursor for the generation of NO and L-citrulline. The reaction requires reduced nicotinamide adenine dinucleotide phosphate (NADPH), flavin dinucleotide (FAD), fevin mononucleotide (FMD), tetrahydrobipterin (BH4), and heme. The NADPH, FAD, and FMD are high-energy molecules and BH4 is essential for NOS dimer formation.

NO is derived from L-arginine in a reaction catalyzed by NOS utilizing reduced nicotinamide adenine dinucleotide phosphate (NADPH), molecular oxygen (O_2), flavin dinucleotide (FAD), fevin mononucleotide (FMD), tetrahydrobipterin (BH4), and heme.

Figure 13 illustrates that NO is generated through a reversible enzymatic reaction catalyzed by nitric oxide synthase (NOS). Hyperbaric oxygen therapy (HBO) appears to influence this enzymatic reaction by preferably driving the reaction to the right. NO mediates several biological functions. It improves deamination of ammonia to produce urea. It elevates production of creatine which is essential for skeletal muscle to sustain contractions. It improves production of L-proline, which is a required precursor for collagen synthesis. It increases agmatine which binds the alpha-2 central adrenoreceptors (site of action of clonidine) with resultant centrally regulated blood pressure reduction. It also increases protein synthesis capability, which improves the rate of cellular and tissue growth.

Constitutive NOS is a membrane-bound protein, anchored to the cytoplasmic side of endoplasmatic reticulum, golgi, or plasma membrane of all human cells. The constitutive isoforms are typically found in cholesterol and glycolipid-rich membranes such as the vascular endothelial cells where it can quickly respond to local stimuli with the rapid production of NO. Initiating the NO effect begins with stimulation of the membrane receptors. A variety of stimuli have been identified, which include but are not limited to, local physiologic stress (pulsatile blood flow), cytokine receptor interaction (bradykinin), carbon dioxide elevation, or direct feedback by NO. Upon receptor activation a rapid influx of intracellular calcium occurs. Influxes of calcium (Ca^{2+}) evoke local potentials on the membrane and cause the migration of calmodulin (CaM). Intracellular calcium binds to calmodulin which activates constitutive NOS to produce NO. NO activates soluble (or cytosolic) guanyl cyclase (sGC), the enzyme that converts guanyl triphosphate (GTP) to cyclic-guanyl monophosphate (cGMP) and inorganic phosphate. Cyclic GMP

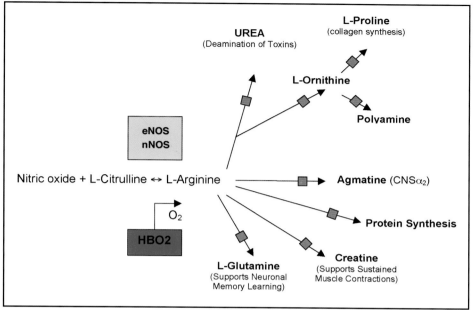

Figure 13. Constitutive NOS

Nitric oxide NO is generated through a reversible enzymatic reaction catalyzed by nitric oxide synthase (NOS). Hyperbaric oxygen therapy (HBO) appears to influence this enzymatic reaction by preferably driving the reaction to the right. Clinically, under HBO conditions, there is an improved deamination of ammonia to produce urea, elevated production of creatine which is essential for skeletal muscle to sustain contractions, improved L-proline production a required precursor for collagen synthesis, increased agmatine which binds the alpha-2 central adrenoreceptors (site of action of clonidine) with resultant centrally regulated blood pressure reduction, and increased protein synthesis capability to improve the rate of cellular and tissue growth. The symbol (⎯⎯■⎯▶) indicates downstream reactions catalyzed by other enzymes.

is a signaling molecule (similar to cAMP) secondary messenger for protein kinases. Most second messengers act by switching on a protein kinase that in turn regulates the activity of other proteins by covalently labeling them with phosphates at specific amino acid residues. Cyclic nucleotides cAMP and cGMP are second messengers that carry signals from the cell surface to proteins within the cell. Kinase signaling is normally terminated by a protein phosphatase that snips off the phosphate groups when energy is needed for the tagged protein to be activated.

    Inducible nitric oxide synthase, iNOS, is a calcium-independent endothelial and smooth-muscle cell enzyme that is usually induced by cytokine-receptor interaction. Inducible NOS is stimulated through a calcium-independent mechanism using cell receptors (Figure 14). Calmodulin is present and tightly bound to low levels of calcium present in the intracellular environment; therefore, additional calcium does not exert a significant effect. Instead, activated platelets and leukocytes secrete cytokines for a direct influence upon cellular receptors while endotoxin, cytotoxins, and lipopolysaccharides stimulate the production of cytokines (tumor necrosis

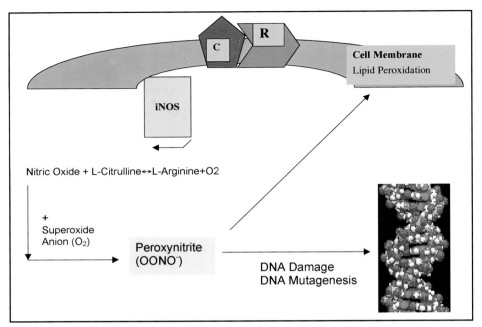

Figure 14. Inducible Nitric oxide (iNOS)

Inducible NOS is stimulated through a calcium-independent mechanism using cell receptors. Cytokines are the predominant stimuli and can be generated either directly by activated platelets, macrophages, or leukocytes or indirectly by lipopolysaccharides, endotoxins, and cytotoxins that stimulate these cells to produce cytokines. Initially at low levels of production the generated NO is cytoprotective. However, as the reaction progresses, such as occurs with septic shock, the excessive production of NO is cytotoxic as it combines with superoxide anion to produce peroxynitrite and leads to lipid peroxidation, DNA damage, and mutagenesis. (iNOS-inducible nitric oxide; C-cytokine; R-receptor; O_2-molecular oxygen.)

factor-alpha, [TNF-α] and gamma-interferon, [γ-IF]) to induce iNOS transcription through a receptor mechanism. Transcription of iNOS through this mechanism creates higher concentrations and more sustained production of NO than with the constitutive isoforms. Under clinical conditions where iNOS has been substantially induced, such as occurs following abdominal surgery or abdominal trauma complicated by bacterial infection, the profound NO production instigates a profound vascular relaxation that is resistant to conventional vasopressors, intravenous fluids, and antibiotic therapy. Early in the course, profound hypotension can be prevented with glucocorticoid therapy; however, glucocorticoids given late in the course may worsen the outcome.

Hypotension induced by cytokine therapy in cancer patients is thought to utilize this same mechanism. Induced NO production also occurs in response to other stresses, such as trauma, injury, pulmonary disease, and coronary artery disease. The induction of moderate levels of NO in these conditions may prove beneficial with NO acting in a cytoprotective fashion. Excessive induction of iNOS with resultant overproduction of NO can lead to cytotoxicity with increased morbidity and mortality. Treating patients with HBO in this clinical scenario may lead to a deleterious outcome.

Non-enzymatic NO synthesis has also been described experimentally using either D- or L-arginine and superoxide anion or hydrogen peroxide as precursors. This is important for hyperbaric therapy since HBO generates both reactive oxygen species. Through this mechanism the apparent inhibition of NO production is reversed as toxic reactive oxygen species (ROS) are converted to NO. Reactive oxygen species are the product of oxygen metabolism and include superoxide anion (O_2^-), hydrogen peroxide (H_2O_2), and hydroxyl radical (OH^-). Although high concentrations of NO have been associated with potential cytotoxic effects, NO is not as toxic as either hydrogen peroxide or superoxide anion. NO combines with superoxide to create cytotoxic peroxynitrite ($OONO^-$) which is also considered a reactive oxygen species. Peroxynitrite is responsible for lipid peroxidation, a process damaging proteins, nucleic acids, and the fatty acids in membrane lipids as well as DNA fragmentation and DNA mutations. The non-enzymatic pathway to synthesize NO may exist to decrease the local toxicity of very potent reactive oxygen species by local conversion to a less toxic entity, local destruction of bacterial/foreign agent that generated the oxidative stress, and local vasodilation to improve "washout" of an area. When HBO is administered at greater than 3.0 ata for two hours, NO production increases approximately four- to fivefold. Thus, hyperbaric therapy may at various concentrations produce opposing effects upon the production of NO, increasing NO in some conditions and decreasing NO in other conditions.

It is now recognized that although they were named to reflect characteristics of the activity or the original tissues in which they were first described the three isoforms described above all are expressed in a variety of tissues and cell types. Newer NOS enzymes have been discovered. Recent studies report a constitutively, expressed NOS in the paranasal sinuses that more closely resembles an inducible NOS with calcium-independent activation and glucocorticoid resistance. Sinus NO concentrations (1,000-30,000 parts per billion) exceed those needed for bacteriostatic function and may explain the sterility of the paranasal sinuses and suggest a role for host defense as large quantities of NO are generated in the paranasal sinuses and distributed throughout the lungs during nasal breathing. Documented increases in arterial oxygenation during nasal breathing as compared to oral breathing may be attributed to the increased local NO generated in the paranasal sinuses as well as effects of the inhaled NO. Undoubtedly, as the NO molecule undergoes further investigation, more isoforms of NOS with site-specific functions will be identified.

L-Arginine-NOS-HBO Oxygen Paradox
Reviewing the L-Arginine-NOS reaction in isolation presents an apparent paradox with regard to endothelial function (refer to Figure 12). Adding elevated levels of oxygen to this equation, as occurs with HBO, should drive the reaction towards the production of NO and result in vasodilation. However, under hyperbaric conditions producing "low levels" of hyperoxia suppression of NO generation is measured and vasoconstriction occurs. Intense investigation is ongoing to explain this apparent paradox. Nonetheless, several points present themselves for consideration and further investigation. NOS may act reversibly to synthesize and metabolize NO. The constitutive isoforms are activated under different circumstances than those

that activate the inducible isoform. When upregulated, the inducible form utilizes oxygen to synthesize NO. The constitutive forms when upregulated apparently result in a reduction of NO. It is difficult to determine if increased production to replace metabolized L-arginine is the culprit driving the reaction away from NO productions since L-arginine is quickly metabolized through other enzymatic systems and measured levels remain low. Other areas for investigation center on the cofactors NADPH, FAD, FMD, and BH4. Just as with the precursor (L-arginine) these cofactors are involved with other enzyme systems locally that may have a higher affinity, or higher kinetics (K_m) or maximal velocity reaction rate (V_{max}) that locally draws the reaction towards the production of more L-arginine inhibiting the metabolism of NO locally. At this time a mechanism proposing a direct inhibition of NO cannot be ruled out. And finally, a mechanism suggesting increased metabolism of generated NO may be plausible given the rapid rate at which NO is metabolized by oxyhemoglobin (t1/2=sec) and with O_2 in aqueous solutions to produce the relatively unreactive nitrate (NO_3^-) and nitrite (NO_2^-) ions. Hyperbaric oxygen treatment maximized both the levels of oxyhemoglobin and the levels of dissolved aqueous oxygen.

Nitric Oxide and cGMP and Glutamate

Glutamate is the main excitatory neurotransmitter in humans. However, excessive activation of glutamate receptors is neurotoxic, leading to neuronal degeneration and death. In many systems, including primary cultures of cerebellar neurons, glutamate neurotoxicity is mainly mediated by excessive activation of NMDA receptors, leading to increased intracellular calcium, which, after binding to calmodulin, activates neuronal NOS and increases NO which in turns activates guanylate cyclase and increases cGMP. Inhibition of NOS prevents glutamate neurotoxicity, indicating that NO mediates glutamate-induced neuronal death in this system.

Secondary Messenger cGMP

In addition to the above-described effects of cGMP in the central nervous system, cGMP regulates cardiovascular function and body fluid homeostasis. The secondary messenger mediates relaxation of cardiac muscle, vasodilation of vascular smooth muscle, increased excretion of sodium and water through the kidney, and decreased aggregation and adhesion of platelets. A cGMP-dependent protein kinase, protein kinase G, binds cGMP and then provides phosphorous groups (phosphorylation) to other enzymes, such as myosin light chain kinase in smooth muscle and platelets. Phosphorylation of myosin light chains in smooth muscle leads to vasodilation whereas phosphorylated light chains in platelets decreases platelet aggregation and adhesion.

Guanylate cyclase has two isoforms one is cytosolic (soluble), contains heme, and binds NO to generate cGMP. The other is membrane bound, does not contain heme, and binds atrial natriuretic factor (ANF) to regulate cardiovascular function and body fluid homeostasis. In cardiac tissue, activity of cytosolic guanylate cyclase requires ANF to be bound to the membrane isoform.

Immune System

NO plays a role in the immune system by contributing to host defense against bacteria, fungi, viruses, and parasites. It is toxic to tumor cells and combines with superoxide radicals as described above to form more toxic compounds (i.e., perioxynitrite).

HBO MECHANISMS THAT IMPROVE WOUND HEALING

Hyperbaric oxygen has been noted clinically to improve the rate of healing when used to treat wounds in patients suffering from chronic wound ischemia, chronic refractory osteomyelitis, mixed soft tissue infections, necrotizing fasciitis, myonecrosis, gas gangrene, post-radionecrosis injury in bone and soft tissue, diabetes microvascular arteriosclerosis, failing flaps and grafts, surgical re-anastomotic sites, crush injury, and acute arterial occlusive disorders. Clinical experience with HBO has shown that wound hyperoxia increases wound granulation tissue formation, accelerates wound contraction, and hastens secondary closure. The ability of HBO to improve wound healing traditionally has been attributed to increased availability of molecular oxygen at the wound site. However, new research tools and techniques have lead to a tremendous expansion in our understanding of the cellular and sub-cellular interactions that make up the "healing process." Some of these are: immuno-fluorescent staining, DNA and RNA sequence identification, DNA growth factor transfection techniques, Polymerase Chain Reactions (PCR), reverse transcriptase PCR (rt-PCR), Southern Blot tests, Fluorescent In-Situ Hybridization (FISH) and In-Situ Hybridization (ISH), electron microscopy, and recombinant gene therapy.

Wound Healing Events

Wound healing is classically described as occurring in four phases that include coagulation, inflammation, proliferation, and maturation. It is a complex series of events that are initiated instantly when tissue injury occurs.

As damaged blood vessels fill the wound space with erythrocytes and plasma, the body immediately recognizes the need to stop bleeding and initiates the clotting cascade at the wound site. During coagulation, fibrinogen from the plasma is activated in response to the injured, exposed epithelium and a mesh is formed. The mesh traps platelets that will adhere to each other and physically plug the injured vessels. The activated platelets release growth factors that are chemotactic for neutrophils and macrophages. Blood vessels contract and retract to aid in bleeding cessation.

Platelet activation initiates the first major escalation of the infammatory response to the injury. Within minutes, the platelets release a number of signaling molecules that attract macrophages, fibroblasts, polymorphonuclear cells (PMN), and vascular endothelial cells. The PMN membrane receptors are altered to allow neutrophil recognition and phagocytosis. The first neutrophils to arrive on the scene are those that are "marginated" along the blood vessel walls. Neutrophils remove necrotic tissue, foreign bodies, bacteria, and debris by secreting peroxidase and by engulfing the material, and then secreting peroxidase into the phagosomes. This process of oxidative killing is oxygen-dependent. The neutrophils secrete growth factors and chemotaxis factors that notify the T-cells (when necessary) and attract more macrophages to the area of injury. Macrophages ingest bacteria, further interact with white blood cells, self-regulate, and continue to orchestrate the wound healing process. Macrophages make H_2O_2 and respond to local accumulation of H_2O_2 by making vascular endothelial growth factor (VEGF), which develops the vascular network in the wound site. Vasodilation with resultant edema, warmth, and rubor are the result of factors secreted from the macrophage and other leukocytes present at the wound site as a component of the inflammatory process.

The combination of inflammatory growth factors released at the wound site is chemotactic for fibroblasts, the predominant cell type in granulation tissue. Cellular proliferation, mitosis, migration, and activation allow this cell to fill the void created by the injury. Fibroblasts secrete gel-matrix (glycosaminoglycans and fibronectin), collagen, elastin, and growth factors. Neoangiogenesis provides fibroblasts with the oxygen needed to function. Granulation tissue is the formation of collagen scaffolding for the vascular network supplying oxygen to the proliferating fibroblasts. Fibroblasts mature and differentiate into myofibroblasts with contractile function. As the wound contracts the wound edges move toward the center and the wound size decreases. Keratinocytes are activated by factors secreted from fibroblasts, macrophages, and other keratinocytes to multiply, migrate, and differentiate creating an epithelial layer that covers the wound. The cells migrate more effectively through moist tissue so it is important to keep the wound moist.

As the wound matures, collagen fibers rearrange into a triple-helix structure that is important for strength and function. Further wound contraction occurs and other cells migrate into the wound. Scar tissue is only 80% as strong as non-injured/healed tissue. The development of scar tissue with collagen deposit is the primary method of adult wound healing. Fetal tissue, on the other hand, heals by regeneration. The process of regeneration is similar to the process of scarring but in regeneration transforming growth factor β3 (TGF-β3) predominates instead of TGF-β1 as in adults. Under the guidance of TGF-β3, hyaluronic acid remains at the wound site for a longer duration, collagen deposition decreases, and the tissue more closely approximates non-injured tissue in composition and function. Maturity of the wound may continue for up to 1.5 years.

Effects of HBO on Growth Factors

Growth factors are soluble proteins that bind to receptors on the cell surface with the primary result of activating cellular proliferation and/or differentiation. Growth factors are either autocrine (acting on the cell that produced them), juxtocrine (acting on an adjacent cell), paracrine (acting on the local environment), or endocrine (acting on a distant cell). Cytokines are special growth factors secreted primarily from leukocytes to stimulate the humoral and cellular immune response and activate phagocytic cells. The term cytokine is generally used to include the insulin-like growth factors (IGFs), the transforming growth factors (TGF alpha and TGF beta), platelet-derived growth factor (PDGF), and fibroblast growth factors (FGFs). The cytokines released from monocyte/macrophage and lymphocyte cell lines are called monokines and lymphokines, respectively. Cytokines that are released from leukocytes and targeted for other leukocytes are called interleukins. More than 18 known interleukins have been identified. Growth factors are important in almost all cellular responses. Many diseases have been related to an over or under production of a variety of growth factors. HBO modifies a variety of growth factor and cytokine effects by regulating their levels and/or receptors.

Vascular Endothelial Growth Factor (VEGF)

The effect of HBO on vascular endothelial growth factor (VEGF) expression illustrates this point. Typically, after acute surgical wounding growth factors that exhibit an angiogenic response are released into the wound field. Angiogenesis is the name given to the development of new capillaries from preexisting blood vessels. Within the first three days an angiogenic factor, basic fibroblast growth factor-2 (bFGF-2), is released in large quantities from platelets. It subsequently decreases as VEGF released from macrophages begins to assume a predominant angiogenic role during the proliferative phase of wound healing. VEGF is important for the growth and survival of endothelial cells, and is found in plasma, serum, and wound exudates. There are four known members of the VEGF family (A, B, C, and D). Several splice variants also exist. Those that contain the heparin-binding domain have a higher potency and are better anchored to the extracellular matrix. This domain improves presentation to the VEGF receptors. Hypoxia stimulates the release of VEGF-A through hypoxia inducible factor-1α (HIF-1α) and hypoxia inducible factor-2α (HIF-2α). Transcription of mRNA must occur to activate the factor. Hypoxia specifically induces the production of VEGF-A differentially compared to other angiogenic factors or other variants of VEGF.

In normoxia, VEGF-A is activated by oncogenes including H-ras and several transmembrane tyrosine kinases such as epidermal growth factor (EGF) receptor and erbB2. There are three VEGF receptors (VEGF R1, VEGF R2, and VEGF R3). VEGF interacts with other receptors expressed by neuronal endothelial cells, Neurophilin-1, and Neurophilin-2. VEGF R1 is also found in a soluble form in the peripheral blood with antagonistic function. VEGF-A binds VEGF R1, VEGF R2, Neurophilin-1, and Neurophilin-2. VEGF-B binds VEGF R1 and Neurophilin-1. VEGF-C and VEGF-D bind VEGF R2 and VEGF R3. VEGF-C/VEGF R3 causes lymphatic proliferation. VEGF R3 is specifically expressed on lymphatic vessels. VEGF R1 and R VEGF R2 are upregulated in tumors and proliferating endothelium secondary to hypoxia and VEGF-A. VEGF R1 mediates motility and vascular permeability. VEGF R2 mediates proliferation.

Under normobaric conditions, VEGF production is stimulated by hypoxia, lactate, nicotinamide adenine dinucleotide (NAD), and NO. HBO induces the production of vascular endothelial growth factor (VEGF), thereby stimulating more rapid development of capillary budding, arborization, and granulation formation within the wound bed. HBO experiments at 2.1 ata for 90 minutes twice daily increased the level of VEGF by forty percent (40%) by five days of therapy. Levels of VEGF reverted to pretreatment range within three days of HBO discontinuation. Wound lactate levels remained unchanged (range, 2.0-10.5 mmol/L). The ability of HBO to generate NO may be the mechanism by which HBO upregulates VEGF expression (Figure 15). Once present in the wound base, VEGF induces the local synthesis of NO and prostacyclin which are thought to play a key role in vascular protection, defined as inhibition of vascular smooth muscle cell proliferation, enhanced endothelial cell survival, suppression of thrombosis, and anti-inflammatory effects. Since HBO works through the secondary messenger NO, it can initiate a positive feedback loop with long-term potentiation.

Chronic wounds differ biochemically from acute wounds. Chronic leg ulcer wound studies have shown a natural inhibition of VEGF function in chronic wounds unrelated to growth factor production. Although VEGF protein is expressed at elevated levels with a strong vascular endothelial growth factor mRNA signal, there are relatively low levels of VEGF detected in chronic wound fluid. Protease inhibitor studies utilizing recombinant vascular endothelial growth factor (rVEGF 165) indicate VEGF undergoes a significant level of degradation by serine proteases, such as plasmin. Degradative metalloproteinases have been identified in chronic wounds at greater amounts exhibiting different profiles than those found in acute wounds. There is also a reduction in the amount of available NO.

Platelet-derived Growth Factor (PDGF)

Although named for the cell type in which it was discovered, PDGF is now known to be produced by fibroblasts, macrophages, and keratinocytes. It is a mitogen for mesenchymally-derived cells, i.e., blood, muscle, bone/cartilage, and connective tissue cells. It is chemotaxic for macrophages and fibroblasts; activates macrophages; and stimulates fibroblasts to secrete extra-cellular matrix.

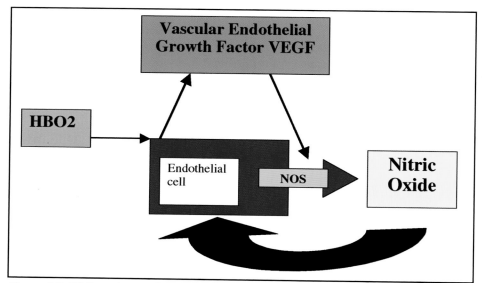

Figure 15. HBO and Vascular Growth

HBO potentiates vascular growth by stimulating the synthesis of NO.

Diabetes, chronic hypertension, and some cardiovascular disease states are well known for their reduced levels of NO. Boykin (54) conducted a retrospective study of chronic nonhealing wounds in diabetic patients treated with topical Becaplermin therapy (recombinant platelet derived growth factor, PDGF-ββ) showed that the addition of exogenous growth factor was effective in promoting granulation tissue growth only when wound NO production deficiency was corrected. HBO was thought to play a role in supplying the needed NO. Multiple studies and numerous reports supported the improved outcome in healing diabetic wounds when HBO was used in combination with exogenous PDGF-ββ.

Experimental investigations were conducted by Bonomo (55) in an ischemic rabbit ear wound model to evaluate the association between HBO and two growth factors, platelet derived growth factor (PDGF) and transforming growth factor beta (TGF-β). Acutely ischemic wounds treated with hyperbaric oxygen at 2 ata showed a significantly increased production of new granulation tissue without any significant new epithelial growth by seven days. HBO worked synergistically with PDGF-ββ to up-regulate mRNA for PDGF-beta receptor. In this experiment neither mRNA levels for PDGF-alpha receptor nor for PDGF-A were detected. Both growth factors alone were more effective than HBO in countering the ischemia induced impairment in wound healing. HBO alone was approximately 100% effective at seven days while both growth factors alone showed approximately a 200% increase in effectiveness at seven days. However, combination therapy of either growth factor with HBO produced a synergistic effect that totally reversed the deficit produced by ischemia.

Basic Fibroblast Growth Factor (bFGF)

FGF represents a family of approximately nineteen growth factors (FGF-8 mice only, all others are human) with four receptors. The FGFs are active in development, wound healing, cartilage and bone healing, hematopoiesis, and tumorigenesis. They are potent angiogenic factors but also act as potent mitogens for osteoblasts, chondrocytes, and endothelial cells, and stimulate proliferation of mesenchymal cells in the developing limb that leads to limb outgrowth. Basic FGF (bFGF) is also important at later stages of bone growth. Of note, bone FGFs are not secreted but are released after membrane disruption from degenerating chondrocytes, or they are located in the bone matrix. The FGF is then released during osteoclastic bone resorption. Cartilaginous angiogenesis and proliferation of osteoblastic precursor cells allow bFGF to play a significant role in bone regeneration. Experimental studies conducted by Wang (58) using HBO and bFGF either alone or in combination upon an irradiated hind leg model showed that a significant reduction in radiation effects on bone growth was achieved by HBO after 10 or 20 Gy, but not after 30 Gy. At 30 Gy bFGF still significantly reduced the degree of bone shortening, but HBO provided no added benefit to bFGF therapy.

Many chronic wounds have some measure of ischemia present. Zhao (57) conducted investigations in an ischemic model found bFGF/FGF-2 to be ineffective in stimulating healing under ischemic conditions even at high doses of 30 micrograms/wound. When HBO was administered with bFGF at low doses of 5 micrograms/wound, the rate of repair was similar to that found in non-ischemic wounds. In contrast, Wu (59) described a newly discovered variant Kaposi's fibroblast growth factor (K-FGF, FGF-4) stimulated repair in both non-ischemic and ischemic wounds demonstrating a differential responsiveness to bFGF based upon the oxygen content of the wound. Furthermore, the impediment to responsiveness can be resolved with the use of HBO in the ischemic wound model. Moreover, some growth factor variants are not oxygen dependent.

ANTIBACTERIAL EFFECTS OF HBO

White blood cells phagocytize bacteria in a variety of environments, ranging from oxygen rich to hypoxic. The energy needed for particle ingestion and degranulation are met primarily by anaerobic glycolysis. In hypoxic environments, ingestion occurs normally with glycogen consumption and lactic acid production, so leukocytes appear to be well equipped to function in low-oxygen states.

The main influence of HBO upon microbial oxidative killing is related to its ability to provide abundant oxygen to be used in the generation of reactive oxygen species. Neutrophils enter the wound site to remove necrotic material and kill bacteria in the wound space. They can kill organisms extracellularly by secreting peroxidases into the wound space or intracellularly by secreting peroxidases into phagosomes. Microbial oxidative killing occurs through both an oxygen-dependent and an oxygen-independent pathway. In oxygen-dependent microbial activity, stimulated neutrophils consume large amounts of oxygen in a respiratory burst. The products produced by oxygen include hydrogen peroxide (H_2O_2), superoxide anion (O^-), hydrochlorous acid (HOCl), and hydroxyl radical (OH^-). Neutrophils use NADPH (nicotinamide adenine dinucleotide), a high-energy electron donating reducing agent. NADPH oxidase enzyme causes NADPH to reduce oxygen and produce hydrogen peroxide (H_2O_2) and superoxide anion (O^-). Flavoproteins facilitate electron transport across membranes into the extracellular space or into phagosomes. In the presence of NADPH oxidase, the reaction is:

$$2\ O_2 + NADPH = NADP^+ + H^+ + 2\ O_2^-$$

Superoxide anions spontaneously combine with hydrogen cations to form oxygen and hydrogen peroxide. The reaction is most frequently catalyzed by superoxide dismutase (SOD).

$$2\ H^+ + 2\ O_2^- = H_2O_2 + O_2$$

Hydrogen peroxide is scavenged and degraded by catalase, glutathione peroxidase, or myeloperoxidase (MPO). Myeloperoxidase, released from neutrophil azurophilic granules into the phagosome in response to antibody-coated microorganisms, enhances the microbicidal activity by converting hydrogen peroxide (H_2O_2) to hydrochlorous acid (HOCl) and hydroxide anion (OH^-). Halides of chloride (Cl^-), bromide (Br^-), and iodine (I^-) can all be oxidized into strong acids but the chloride halide is the most common one utilized. Hydrochlorous acid attacks bacterial membrane transport function leading to non-viability and death of the organism.

$$H_2O_2 + Cl^- = OH^- + HOCl$$

Hydroxyl radical (OH) is another oxygen metabolite that is used in oxidative killing. It is formed from metal-catalyzed reactions between hydrogen peroxide (H_2O_2) and superoxide anion (O_2^-) in the Haber-Weiss reaction, a two-step process. Lactoferrin from neutrophil granules released into phagosomes or into the extracellular space donates the iron (Fe) used in this reaction. Hydroxyl radicals are very potent and prove toxic to bacteria, tissue, and other cells including neutrophils.

$$H_2O_2 + 2 \ O_2^- + Fe_3^+ = O_2 + Fe_2^+ + [\text{peroxide intermediate}] = Fe_3^+ + OH^- + OH$$

Mandell (64) showed that oxygen was essential for killing certain species of phagocytosed bacteria, such as *Escherichia coli*, *Klebsiella pneumoniae*, *Proteus vulgaris*, *Salmonella typhimurium*, and *Staphylococcus aureus*. Mader et al. (65) reported that *in vivo* leukocyte killing of *Staphylococcus aureus* was decreased markedly at an oxygen tension of 23 mm Hg, but improved at 45, 109, and 150 mm Hg, with greatest efficiency at 150 mm Hg (Figure 16).

In addition to its effect on leukocytes, oxygen also augments the bacterial killing action of certain antibiotics, such as tobramycin, vancomycin, and sulfonamides. Some aminoglycosides utilize an oxygen-dependent membrane transport system to enter the cell. Elevated oxygen tensions improve the transmembrane transport of the antibiotic. Moreover, HBO has direct lethal effects on anaerobic and microaerophilic aerobic organisms, based upon the intracellular formation of oxygen free radicals as noted above. These organisms do not possess superoxide radical dismutase or hydrogen peroxide catalase that would inhibit the oxygen radicals and afford the necessary protection. On the other hand, aerobic organisms do generate superoxide dismutase proportional to the amount of oxygen available that detoxifies the radicals. Therefore, aerobic organisms are protected in hyperoxic environments.

HBO has a role in denaturing toxins by forming oxygen free radicals in the relative absence of free radical degrading enzymes, such as superoxide dismutases, catalases, and peroxidases. In the study of toxin inhibition by HBO, Van Unnik reported that an oxygen tension of 250 mm Hg is needed to stop alpha toxin production by *Clostridium perfringens*, a commonly isolated pathogen in gas gangrene (83).

SPECIAL CONSIDERATIONS OF HYPERBARIC OXYGEN THERAPY

No medical procedure is absolutely free of risk. Thus, HBO therapy safety is the degree to which the risks are judged acceptable by the patient and the medical staff. The complications include side effects and contraindications.

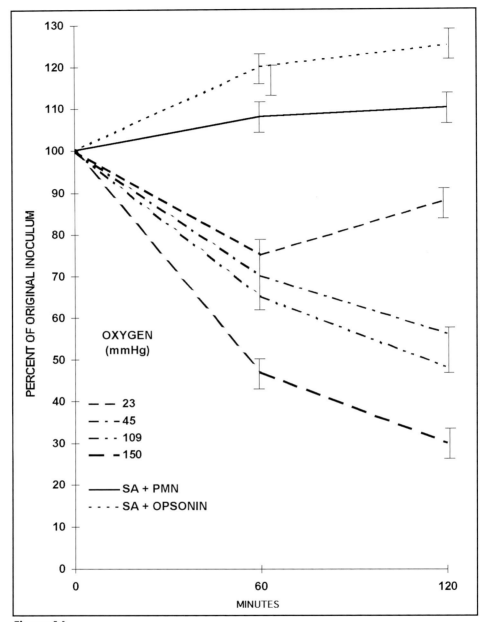

Figure 16.

Mean phagocytic killing of *Staphylococcus aureus* (SA) under different oxygen tensions. SA, rabbit peritoneal leukocytes (PMN), and opsonin were mixed at 37°C and removed after 60 and 120 minutes when the number of CFU of initial inoculum of SA was counted. (Adapted from Mader JT, Brown GL, Gockian JC, et al: A mechanism for amelioration of hyperbaric oxygen of experimental staphylococcal osteomyelitis in rabbits. J Infectious Disease 1980; 142:915-922.65.) (20)

Note: This figure is from Brakora MJ, Sheffield PJ, Hyperbaric oxygen therapy for diabetic wounds. In: Clinics in Podiatric Medicine and Surgery: The Diabetic Foot. LB Harkless, LA Lavery, KJ Dennis, eds. Philadelphia PA: WB Saunders; 1995: p 109.

TABLE 3. HBO COMPLICATION RATES AT SAN ANTONIO CIVILIAN MULTIPLACE HYPERBARIC FACILITIES DURING 21 YEARS (1979 THRU 2000)

No. Patients: 8,078
No. Exposures: 166,701

COMPLICATION	REMOVED FROM CHAMBER		REMOVED FROM OXYGEN	
	Total Occurences	Occurrences Per 10,000 Exposures	Total Occurrences	Occurrence Per 10,000 Exposures
Agitation, Combative	4	0.24	14	0.84
Barotrauma - Ear	729	43.65	0	0.00
Barotrauma - Sinus	129	7.72	0	0.00
Barotrauma - Teeth	5	0.30	0	0.00
Claustrophobia/anxiety	115	6.89	94	5.63
Clear Tracheal Secretions	0	0.00	2	0.12
Congestion/SOB/Diff Breathing	32	1.92	24	1.44
Contaminants in Chamber- Fumes	0	0.00	6	0.36
Coughing	0	0.00	10	0.60
Disorientation/ Hallucinations	7	0.42	0	0.00
Dizziness, Weakness	1	0.06	6	0.36
Doctors/ Other Appointments	25	1.50	0	0.00
Eyes Irritated	0	0.00	2	0.12
Equip Failure - Pacemaker, IV	3	0.18	8	0.48
High Blood Pressure	0	0.00	1	0.06
Hot Flashes, Overheated	0	0.00	11	0.66
Hyperventilation	7	0.42	3	0.18
Hypoglycemia	9	0.54	74	4.43
Nausea/ Vomiting	77	4.61	143	8.56
Nosebleed	0	0.00	2	0.12
Oxygen Toxicity/ Tingling	0	0.00	4	0.24
Pain- Abdomen/ Diarrhea	86	5.15	3	0.18
Pain-Chest	44	2.63	16	0.96
Pain-Headache	2	0.12	0	0.00
Pain-Other	6	0.36	2	0.12
PE Tubes-Unable to auto inflate	37	2.22	0	0.00
Pulmonary Edema	1	0.06	0	0.00
Refused to Continue Treatment	30	1.80	9	0.54
Seizure	29	1.74	7	0.42
Shakiness, Tremor	1	0.06	8	0.48
Social/ Family Problems	2	0.12	0	0.00
Unresponsive	1	0.06	0	0.00
Incidence per 10,000 exposures	1382	83.25	449	27.05

HBO Side Effects

Table 3 summarizes the results of a retrospective study conducted over 21 years of operation in three Texas wound care and hyperbaric medicine facilities in which over 8,000 patients received over 166,000 HBO treatments. There were 1,382 complications that resulted in removal from the chamber, for an incidence of 83 per 10,000 exposures. The ten top reasons for removal from treatment were: ear barotrauma (44/10,000 exposures), sinus barotrauma (8/10,000 exposures), claustrophobia/anxiety (7/10,000 exposures), abdominal pain/diarrhea (5/10,000 exposures), nausea/vomiting (5/10,000 exposures), chest pain (3/10,000 exposures), inability to autoinflate ears (2/10,000 exposures), refusal to continue treatment (2/10,000 exposures), seizure (2/10,000 exposures), and doctors/other appointments (2/10,000 exposures). There were 449 complications that resulted in temporary removal from oxygen during the treatment in the chamber, for an incidence of 27 per 10,000 exposures. The ten top reasons for removal from oxygen were: nausea/vomiting (9/10,000 exposures), claustrophobia/anxiety (6/10,000 exposures), hypoglycemic reaction (4/10,000 exposures), congestion/shortness of breath/trouble breathing (1/10,000 exposures), chest pain (1/10,000 exposures), agitation/combative (1/10,000 exposures), hot flashes/ overheated (1/10,000 exposures), coughing (1/10,000 exposures), refusal to continue treatment (1/10,000 exposures), and shakiness/tremor (1/10,000 exposures). There were occasional potentially life-threatening events (congestive heart failure, suspected heart attack, seizure, pacemaker failure, pulmonary edema, excessive tracheal secretions) but none resulted in fatality.

Barotrauma

Pain resulting from middle ear barotrauma is the most common side effect of receiving HBO therapy. Stone et al. (66) reported an incidence of approximately 2% among 1,446 military patients with 31,599 hyperbaric exposures. In a larger civilian patient series (67), 8,000 patients undergoing 166,000 exposures had a middle ear barotrauma incidence of 44 per 10,000 patient therapies or 0.4% (Table 3). This complication is usually prevented by teaching patients autoinflation techniques or by using tympanostomy tubes for those patients who cannot correctly autoinflate their middle ear. Sinus barotrauma is the second most common chamber complication. Both conditions usually occur in patients with allergic rhinitis or upper respiratory tract infections that are managed with decongestant nasal spray and/or antihistamines.

Oxygen Toxicity

Oxygen toxicity occurs in three major forms: pulmonary, central nervous system, and ocular. Pulmonary oxygen toxicity is rare and presents as chest pain and cough with symptoms resembling those of chronic obstructive pulmonary disease. Central nervous system oxygen toxicity most often manifests itself as a seizure that may be preceded by facial twitching and/or nausea and vomiting. The risk is exacerbated in patients who present with fever, who suffer from low glucose, or who take steroids or other "at risk medications." The incidence of oxygen convulsions during HBO exposures of 2.0 to

2.4 ata is approximately 1 per 10,000 patient therapies or 0.01%. Oxygen tolerance limits are well defined and safe but effective treatment regimes that avoid these potential complications have been published. Progressive myopia occurs in some patients after a prolonged series of HBO therapy. Difficulty with night vision and blurring of distant objects may impair driving. Most patients are instructed to not purchase new prescriptive lenses since these visual changes usually reverse within days to weeks of termination of HBO treatments.

Hypoglycemia in Diabetic Patients

Hypoglycemia in the hyperbaric environment presents with the same symptoms seen in a normobaric environment. Patients may become agitated, complain of palpitations, dizziness/lightheadedness, nausea, or sweating. Convulsions may occur if the patient's blood glucose level is not corrected. Patients are tested prior to HBO exposure and most conservative recommendations are not to treat a patient who is using antiglycemic therapy unless the pretreatment blood glucose is more than 100 g/dl. Three factors contribute to an HBO related hypoglycemic reaction: dietary intake, anti-diabetic medical regime, and a physiologic response to HBO environment in diabetic patients. In the 8,000 patient series at Table 3, 83 patients per 10,000 exposures (0.8%) had hypoglycemic reactions.

Confinement Anxiety

In the author's (Smith's) experience approximately one per twenty patients refused to be treated in the monoplace hyperbaric chamber. Of those patients accepting treatment approximately one in five request anti-anxiolytic medication during the initial portion of their treatment course. In the series of 8,000 patients treated in a multiplace chamber setting at Table 3, approximately 1-2% patients requested removal from oxygen or from the chamber because of confinement anxiety. In addition to anti-anxiolytic medications such as Ativan, patient anxiety can be tempered through familiarization with the treatment environment and reassurance training.

Decompression Sickness in Inside Attendants

Decompression sickness (DCS) can occur across the pressure continuum from deep sea to space. It can occur on ascent after a dive or a hyperbaric chamber exposure. In 1997, Baker (68) surveyed 33 North American hyperbaric treatment facilities and reported a total of 76 attendant DCS cases for an incidence of 0.01-0.6% for the estimated 29,000 exposures per year. Baker reported that breathing oxygen and rotating attendants to remain within no-decompression limits were better DCS avoidance techniques than using the standard air decompression methods.

During the 21 years from 1979 to 2000, 166,000 patient treatments were conducted at the Methodist Hospital and the Nix Medical Center in San Antonio. Two air-breathing inside medical attendants divided the 120-minute air-breathing time during each of the 40,000 2.4 ata elective treatments. There were no cases of decompression sickness in patients, but two attendants had suspected DCS episodes following 2.4 ata wound healing treatments.

Although classic signs and symptoms of DCS were absent, the decision was made to treat the vague complaints for the protection of the attendants. Two additional inside medical attendants had DCS on a single 6.0 ata air embolism treatment. Both attendants performed hard labor at 6 ata for a previously comatose patient who improved and went though a combative period. Despite oxygen decompression, both attendants required treatments for limb bends pain within six hours after the exposure (69). The incidence for attendant DCS in this series is 1 in 10,000 exposures (0.001%).

Contraindications

Absolute contraindications include untreated pneumothorax, untested pacemakers, and selected medications (70):

- **Untreated Pneumothorax**-The presence of untreated pneumothorax is an absolute contraindication for HBO treatment. Gas trapped between the chest wall and the pleural lining will expand upon ascent and develop into a tension pneumothorax. Mechanical inhibition to central venous return occurs and electromechanical dissociation leads to loss of consciousness. Treatment includes immediate placement of a needle thoracostomy followed by chest tube insertion. This condition is most commonly seen in patients with a prolonged smoking history, chronic obstructive pulmonary disease, and pulmonary blebs.
- **Pacemakers (Implanted)**-Early models of pacemakers malfunctioned under pressure. Newer models have been developed to withstand hyperbaric pressures. It is wise to check with the manufacturer before exposing a particular model to a pressurized environment.
- **Selected Medications**-Certain anticancer agents, alcohol abuse agents, and antibacterial drugs are contraindicated for HBO therapy (70).
  - **Doxorubicin** (Adriamycin)-Anticancer agent may cause myocardial toxicity. It may be inactivated and cleared from the tissues within 24 hours. It is wise to wait at least two days after the last dose before initiating HBO treatment (70).
  - **Bleomycin**-Anticancer agent has a side effect of pulmonary toxicity. If HBO is considered, it is recommendation to give an oxygen trial at 1 ata followed by pulmonary function testing to include a CO diffusion capacity (70).
  - **Disulfiram** (Antabuse)-Alcohol abuse agent that can block the production of superoxide dismutase, which is the body's major protection against oxygen toxicity. A single HBO treatment might be safe with little danger of convulsing, but subsequent exposures to HBO could have an increased risk due to lack of protection by the superoxide dismutase system (70).
  - **Cis-Platinum**-Anticancer agent that interferes with DNA synthesis that subsequently delays fibroblast proliferation and collagen production (70).
  - **Mafenide Acetate** (Sulfamylon)-Antibacterial drug used in burn wounds is a carbonic anhydrase inhibitor that promotes CO_2 build-up with a peripheral vasodilatation (70).

Relative Contraindications (70)

- Upper respiratory infections and chronic sinusitis
- Seizure disorders
- Emphysema with CO_2 retention
- High fevers
- History of spontaneous pneumothorax
- History of thoracic surgery
- History of surgery for otosclerosis
- Viral infections
- Congenital spherocytosis
- History of optic neuritis

PHYSIOLOGICAL BASIS OF SOME APPLICATIONS OF HBO

The physiological basis of HBO is provided for the following indications: decompression illness (decompression sickness, air or gas embolism), carbon monoxide poisoning, gas gangrene, and wound-healing enhancement applications, i.e., chronic osteomyelitis, osteoradionecrosis, maxillofacial osteomyelitis, and non-healing soft tissue wounds that require granulation tissue and epithelialization (26). This is not intended to be a complete list.

Rationale for HBO in Decompression Illness (DCS or AGE)

Decompression sickness (DCS) arises from bubbles that occur in tissues or blood following rapid decompression during ascent from diving, flying, or a hyperbaric/hypobaric chamber. Arterial gas embolism (AGE) occurs when gases enter or enucleate in arteries, veins, and/or capillaries, resulting in ischemia in the affected area. There is a current move to group both DCS and AGE into a single category of decompression illness. HBO is administered at 2.8 to 3.0 ata (2.85 to 3.03 MPa) to reduce bubble-size, create a positive nitrogen gradient to eliminate bubbles, oxygenate ischemic tissues, and correct local tissue hypoxia. During compression, bubbles deep within the body tissues respond to the pressure change. Pressurization to 3 ata (3.03 MPa) reduces bubble volume by one third. Breathing pure oxygen eliminates nitrogen from the body and creates a favorable nitrogen gradient for nitrogen to leave the bubble. As a bubble becomes very small, its own surface tension increases to the point that it is absorbed into solution. The first application of pressure might not eliminate all bubbles, but their size reduction should aid in partially restoring circulation in the case of intravascular bubbles and reducing the mechanical effects of extravascular bubbles. HBO increases the capillary oxygen tension that surrounds ischemic tissue, extends the oxygen diffusion distance from functioning capillaries, and corrects the local tissue hypoxia.

Rationale for HBO in Thermal Burns

In 1965, Wada and Ikeda reported an incidental observation that the use of HBO to treat coal miners exposed to carbon monoxide improved their rate of healing and the overall morbidity of associated burn injuries. HBO has subsequently been shown to produce a variety of effects including improved leukocyte bactericidal effect, inhibition and denaturing of toxins released by anaerobic organisms, increased flexibility of red cells, reduced tissue edema, preservation of intracellular adenosine triphosphate, and maintenance of tissue oxygenation in the absence of hemoglobin. Adjunctive HBO also appears to stimulate NO production ultimately affecting gene expression/suppression. Through these mechanisms HBO may be useful in treating both anaerobic and aerobic infections that are frequently associated with severe burns. Adjunctive HBO also promotes wound healing by facilitating the rapid spread and arborization of new capillaries, stimulating fibroblast growth, enhancing collagen formation, reducing lipid peroxidation, and subsequently improving epithelialization. Hyperbaric oxygen preserves ischemic tissues by relieving hypoxia, decreasing fluid loss, and limiting burn wound extension and conversion. All these factors are associated with better healing and improved morbidity.

Rationale for HBO in Carbon Monoxide Poisoning

Carbon monoxide poisoning results from exposure to products of incomplete combustion, as in automobile exhaust and smoke inhalation. Carbon monoxide binds with hemoglobin 200 times more readily than oxygen to form carboxyhemoglobin, thereby competing with oxygen for the same binding site. It also disrupts intracellular respiration by combining with the cytochrome oxidase system. In addition to the CO-induced hypoxic stress, neurologic injuries seem to be due to a complex cascade of biochemical events that involve several pathophysiologic processes. HBO administered at 2.4 to 3 ata (3.03 MPa) enhances tissue oxygenation and hastens dissociation of CO from hemoglobin. When the substrate O_2 is added on the left side of the chemical equation, $HbgCO + O_2 > HbgO_2 + CO$, the reaction is driven to the right by the Law of Mass Action, and CO is released from the hemoglobin. During 100 percent oxygen breathing, the half time for CO dissociation from hemoglobin is reduced to 23 minutes at 3 ata (3.03 MPa), compared to 80 minutes at 1 ata (1.01 MPa). Intracranial pressure caused by cerebral edema is reduced by as much as 50 percent shortly after commencing 100 percent oxygen breathing at 3 ata (3.03 MPa). HBO has been shown to be beneficial in animal studies by improving mitochondria oxidative processes, inhibiting lipid peroxidation, impairing leukocyte adhesion to injured microvasculature, and improving cardiovascular status.

Carbon monoxide and cyanide poisoning frequently occur simultaneously in victims of smoke inhalation. In addition to its effect on CO, HBO may have a direct effect on reducing the toxicity of cyanide and augmenting the benefit of antidote treatment. HBO is used to reduce mortality and possibly morbidity.

Rationale for HBO in Clostridial Myositis and Myonecrosis (Gas Gangrene)

Clostridial myositis and myonecrosis is an acute, rapidly progressive, invasive clostridial infection of the muscles, characterized by profound toxemia, extensive edema, massive death of tissue, and a variable degree of gas production. Gas gangrene (clostridial myonecrosis) is caused by an anaerobic, spore-forming, Gram-positive encapsulated bacilli of the genus Clostridium, most common of which is *C. perfringens*, which produces a tissue-necrotizing toxin. HBO is adjunctive to surgery and antibiotics in treating gas gangrene to halt the spread of infection and toxicity. On exposure to oxygen tensions of about 250 mm Hg, *C. perfringens* ceases alpha-toxin production and at 1500 mm Hg the dose is bactericidal. Adjunctive HBO treatments are given at 3 ata (3.03 MPa) with the patient breathing 100 percent oxygen for 90 minutes during each treatment. HBO, surgical, and antibiotic management is continued over five to seven treatments during the next three to five days. Using HBO for treating gas gangrene reduces morbidity and prevents or lowers the level of amputation necessitated by limb gas gangrene.

Rationale for HBO in Crush Injuries, Compartment Syndrome, and Other Acute Traumatic Peripheral Ischemias

Acute Traumatic Peripheral Ischemias (ATPI) include crush injuries, compartment syndromes, thermal burns, frostbite injuries, compromised skin grafts and flaps, and threatened replantations. The immediate threat to surviving injured tissue after an ATPI relates to the sufficiency of vascular perfusion. The primary rationale for using HBO at 2.0 to 2.5 ata (2.02 to 2.53 MPa) is to counteract trauma-related tissue hypoxia and edema, as well as their related consequences. Adjunctive HBO increases oxygen delivery in the blood, enhances oxygen availability to the injured tissue, and enhances post-traumatic edema reduction. HBO also protects tissue from reperfusion injury for which four actions have been identified. HBO antagonizes lipid peroxidation of the cell membrane that occurs after toxic oxygen radicals interact with membrane lipids. HBO interferes with initiation of reperfusion injury by blocking the sequestration of neutrophils on post-capillary venules, and antagonizing the beta2 integrin system which initiates the neutrophil adherence response to the post-capillary venule endothelium. It might also provide sufficient additional oxygen for reperfused tissues to generate oxygen radical scavengers. Using adjunctive HBO for ATPI reduces the number of surgeries and improves healing rates. Adjunctive HBO is widely accepted for use in limb salvage/reattachment to minimize an amputation site. The rationale for using HBO in frostbite is to prevent a foot or leg amputation and help with the reperfusion injury that is brought on after frostbite or other surgical procedures that reintroduce blood back into a hypoxic area of the body.

Rationale for HBO in Enhancement of Wound Healing

Problem wounds fail to respond to established medical and surgical management, and are usually compromised by tissue hypoperfusion, tissue hypoxia, and infection. They include diabetic feet, compromised amputation sites, nonhealing traumatic wounds, and vascular insufficiency ulcers. In the hypoxic environment of these wounds, healing is halted by decreased fibroblast proliferation, diminished collagen production, impaired capillary angiogenesis, and inability to control infection. The rationale for wound healing enhancement with adjunctive HBO at 2.0 to 2.5 ata (2.02 to 2.52 MPa) is to elevate oxygen tension in ischemic and infected wound tissue. HBO directly promotes wound healing by restoring the oxygen tension needed to enhance fibroblast replication, collagen synthesis, capillary budding, granulation tissue formation, epithelialization, and bacterial killing. Adjunctive HBO is used to enhance wound healing in problem wounds, salvage limbs, and reduce disability caused by amputation. HBO is also effective in establishing a healthy granulation base for skin grafting.

Rationale for HBO in Exceptional Blood Loss (Anemia)

Hyperbaric oxygen therapy has proven effectiveness in correcting the ion exchange disturbances in the heart and the kidney induced during the resuscitation of acute blood loss anemia. Adjunctive HBO at 3 ata provides dissolved oxygen content of 6 ml oxygen per dl blood which would be equivalent to the sea level oxygen carrying capacity of about 5 grams of hemoglobin. Thus, HBO at 3 ata (3.03 MPa) could be used to offset the loss of approximately one-third of the total blood volume that had been replaced by plasma expanders, buying time until the body could replenish the red blood cells.

Rationale for HBO in Osteomyelitis (Refractory)

The rationale for adjunctive HBO to aid the surgical and antibiotic management of chronic osteomyelitis is primarily to stimulate osteogenesis, improve fibroblastic activity, increase collagen production, and stimulate new capillary growth to fill dead space. Chronic, nonhealing wounds of bone and soft tissues are hypoxic, with oxygen tensions below 20 mm Hg compared to 30 to 40 mm Hg in healthy tissue. HBO elevates oxygen partial pressures in functioning capillaries and provides tissue tensions adequate to activate fibroblasts and osteoblasts. The effect of HBO on microorganisms in chronic osteomyelitis appears to be antibiotic enhancement and improved bacterial killing. HBO treatment at 2.0 to 2.5 ata (2.02 to 2.52 MPa) is combined with excision of sequestra and antibiotics.

Rationale for HBO in Delayed Radiation Injury (Soft Tissue and Bone Necrosis)

Delayed radiation injury may occur after a latent period of six months, and may occur many years after the radiation exposure. There is usually endarteritis with tissue hypoxia and secondary fibrosis. Dental extractions and other surgical procedures have high complication rates when done in irradiated tissue without the benefit of preoperative HBO therapy. Adjunctive HBO at 2.0 to 2.5 ata (2.02 to 2.52 MPa) is used to stimulate new capillary growth in irradiated tissue and to develop a rich granulation base for subsequent surgery in the irradiated field. Prophylactic preoperative HBO is used to reduce the risk of nonhealing when surgery is performed in the irradiated site.

Rationale for Skin Grafts and Flaps (Compromised)

Hyperbaric oxygen therapy improves survival of ischemic grafts and flaps—myocutaneous, rotated, free tissue transfers. In the process of generating a graft or flap the tissue will undergo periods of ischemia, reperfusion, and then secondary ischemia. Under hyperbaric conditions the rate of survival for grafts and flaps may improve partially or in "all or none" fashion depending upon the type of procedure being evaluated. Tissue oxygen tensions of 30 to 40 mm Hg are needed for the development of collagen matrix for capillary budding into avascular areas. Adjunctive HBO at 2.0 to 2.5 ata (2.02 to 2.52 MPa) can deliver the required levels of oxygen, thereby stimulating the fibroblasts and enhancing collagen synthesis. Controls treated with normobaric air or normobaric oxygen did not show the same level of improvement.

REFERENCES

Hyperbaric Physiology

1. Wells CH, Goodpasture JE, Horrigan DJ, et al. Tissue gas measurement during hyperbaric oxygen exposure, in Smith G (ed) Proceedings of the Sixth International Congress on Hyperbaric Medicine. Aberdeen, Scotland: Aberdeen University Press, 1977, pp 118-124.

2. Lambertsen CJ. Physiological effects of oxygen inhalation at high partial pressures. In: Fundamentals of Hyperbaric Medicine, Washington DC: National Academy of Sciences, National Research Council, 1966, pp 12-20.

3. Sheffield PJ, Heimbach RD. Respiratory Physiology. In: DeHart RL (ed) Fundamentals of Aerospace Medicine, Baltimore, MD: Williams & Wilkins, 1996, pp 69-108

4. Lanphier EH, Brown JW, Jr. The physiological basis of hyperbaric therapy, in National Research Council Committee on Hyperbaric Oxygenation (ed), Fundamentals of Hyperbaric Medicine. Washington DC: National Academy of Sciences, National Research Council, 1966, pp 33-55.

5. Sheffield PJ. Tissue oxygen measurements with respect to soft-tissue wound healing with normobaric and hyperbaric oxygen. Hyperbaric Oxygen Review 1985;6(1):18-46.

6. Dooley J, King G, Slade B. Establishment of reference pressure of transcutaneous oxygen for the comparative evaluation of problem wounds. Undersea Hyperb Med 1997; 24: 235-244.

7. Boerema I, Meyne NG, Brummelkamp WH, et al. Life without blood: A study of the influence of high atmospheric pressure and hypothermia on dilution of blood. J Cardiovascular Surgery 1960;1:133-146.

8. Krogh A. The number and distribution of capillaries in muscle with calculations of the oxygen pressure head necessary for supplying the tissue. J. Physiology 1919;52:409-415.

9. Silver IA. Measurement of Oxygen Tension in Healing Tissue. In Progress in Respiration Research, Herrog (Eq.) Vol III. Basel: S. Karger, 1969;124-135.

10. Balin AK, Goodman DG, Rassmussen H, et al. Oxygen sensitive stages of the cell cycle of human diploid cells. J Cell Biol 1978; 78: 390-400.

11. Sheffield PJ. Measuring Tissue Oxygen. In Davis JC, Hunt TK Problem Wounds: Role of Oxygen, New York: Elsevier, 1988; 17-51.

12. Hunt TK, MP Pai. Effect of Varying Ambient Oxygen Tensions on Wound Metabolism and Collagen Synthesis. Surgery, Gynecol. and Obstet. 1977;135: 561-567.

13. Hunt TK, J Niinikoski, BH Zederfeldt, IA Silver. Oxygen in Wound Healing Enhancement: Cellular Effects of Oxygen, In Hyperbaric Oxygen Therapy, JC Davis and TK Hunt (Eds.) Bethesda: The Undersea Medical Society, 1977; 111-122.

14. Niinikoski J. Effect of oxygen supply on wound healing and formation of experimental granulation tissue. Acta Physiol Scand Suppl 1969; 334:1.

15. Sheffield PJ, Measuring Tissue Oxygen: A Review. Undersea and Hyperbaric Medicine, 1998; 25(3):179-188.

16. Grolman RE, Wilkerson DK, Taylor J, Allinson P, Zatina MA. Transcutaneous oxygen tension measurements predict a beneficial response to hyperbaric oxygen therapy in patients with nonhealing wounds and critical limb ischemia. Am Surg 2001; 76(11): 1073-1079.

17. Harward TRS, Volny J, Golbranson F, Bernstein EF, Fronek A. Oxygen inhalation-induced transcutaneous PO2 changes as a predictor of amputation level. J Vasc Surg 1985; 2:220-227.

18. Smith BM, Desvigne LD, Slade JB, Dooley JW, Warren DC. Transcutaneous oxygen measurements predict healing of leg wounds with hyperbaric therapy. Wound Rep Reg 1996; 4:224-229.

19.   Sheffield PJ, Dietz D, Posey KI, Ziemba TA, Bakken B. Use of transcutaneous oximetry and laser Doppler with local heat provocation to assess patients with problem wounds. In: NM Petri, D Andric, D Ropac (eds), Book of Proceedings, 1st Congress of the Alps-Adria Working Community on Maritime, Undersea, and Hyperbaric Medicine. Split, Croatia: Croatian Maritime, Undersea and Hyperbaric Medical Society of Croatian Medical Association, 2001:341-344.

20.   Fife CE, Buyukcakir C, Otto GH, Sheffield PJ, Warriner RA III, Mader JT. The predictive value of transcutaneous oximetry in diabetic lower extremity ulcers treated with hyperbaric oxygen therapy: A retrospective analysis of 1000 patients. J Wound Repair, 2002 (In preparation)

21.   Wattel FE, Mathieu MD, Fossati P, et al. Hyperbaric oxygen in the treatment of diabetic foot lesions: search for healing predictive factors. J Hyperb Med 1991;6:263-268.

Pharmacology of Oxygen

22.   Hammarlund C. The physiologic effects of hyperbaric oxygen. In: Kindwall EP, Whelan HT (eds), Hyperbaric Medicine Practice, Flagstaff, AZ: Best Publishing, 1999;37-68.

23.   Knighton, DR (1994). The mechanisms of wound healing. In EP Kindwall (ed), Hyperbaric Medicine Practice. Flagstaff, AZ: Best Publishing. 1994;119-140.

Oxygen Effects on Cerebral Vasculature

24.   Ohta H. The effect of hyperoxemia on cerebral blood flow in normal humans. Brain Nerve. 1986;38:949–959.

25.   Lambertsen CJ, Kough RH, Cooper DY, Emmel GL, Loeschcke HH, Schmidt CF. Oxygen toxicity: effects in man of oxygen inhalation at 1 and 3.5 atmospheres upon blood gas transport, cerebral circulation and cerebral metabolism. J Appl Physiol. 1953;5:471–486.

26.   Franinovic-Markovic J, Kovacevic H, Franolic M. Transcranial doppler estimated cerebral blood flow velocity during hyperbaric oxygenation. pp.43-45 In: EUBS Diving and Hyperbaric Medicine, Collection of manuscripts for the XXIV Annual Scientific Meeting. Gennser M, ed. 1998 Aug 12-15, Stockholm, Sweden. 234 pages.

27.   Demchenko, I.T., Boso, A.E., O'Neill, T. J., Bennet, P.B, Piantadosi, C.A, Nitric oxide and cerebral blood flow responses to hyperbaric oxygen. J. Appl. Physiol. (2000) 88: 1381-1389.

28.   Ioroi T, Yonetani M, Nakamura H. Effects of hypoxia and reoxygenation on nitric oxide production and cerebral blood flow in developing rat striatum. Pediatr Res 1998 Jun;43(6):733-7.

29.   Buchanan JE, Phillis JW.) The role of nitric oxide in the regulation of cerebral blood flow. Increased carbon dioxide concentrations and cerebral vasculature vasodilation result in increased cerebral blood flow. Brain Res 1993 May 7;610(2):248-55.

30.   Betz AL, Iannotti F, Hoff JT. Brain edema: a classification based on blood-brain barrier integrity.

31.   Lanse SB, Lee JC, Jacobs EA, Brody H. Changes in the permeability of the blood-brain barrier under hyperbaric conditions. Aviat Space Environ Med 1978 Jul;49(7):890-4.

32.   Gruenau SP, Folker MT, Rapoport SI Lack of hyperbaric O2 effects on blood-brain barrier permeability in conscious rats. Aviat Space Environ Med 1981 Mar;52(3):162-5.

33.   Wada K, Miyazawa T, Nomura N, Yano A, Tsuzuki N, Nawashiro H, Shima K. Mn-SOD and Bcl-2 expression after repeated hyperbaric oxygenation. Acta Neurochir Suppl 2000;76:285-90.

34.   Xiong L, Zhu Z, Dong H, Hu W, Hou L, Chen S. Hyperbaric oxygen preconditioning induces neuroprotection against ischemia in transient not permanent middle cerebral artery occlusion rat model. Chin Med J (Engl) 2000 Sep;113(9):836-9.

35.   Wada K, Ito M, Miyazawa T, Katoh H, Nawashiro H, Shima K, Chigasaki H. Repeated hyperbaric oxygen induces ischemic tolerance in gerbil hippocampus. Brain Res 1996 Nov 18;740(1-2):15-20.

36.   Singhal AB, Dijkhuizen RM, Rosen BR, Lo EH.Normobaric hyperoxia reduces MRI diffusion abnormalities and infarct size in experimental stroke. Neurology 2002 Mar 26;58(6):945-52.

37.   Silbergleit R, Yeakley W. Narrow Window of Opportunity for Neuroprotective Effects of Hyperbaric Oxygen in Transient Focal Cerebral Ischemia. Academic Emergency Medicine Volume 7, Number 5 512, 2000.

38.   Tomiyama Y, Jansen K, Brian JE Jr., Todd MM. Hemodilution, cerebral O2 delivery, and cerebral blood flow: a study using hyperbaric oxygenation. AJP 1999; 276 (4): H1190-H1196.

39.   Tomiyama Y, Jansen K, Brian JE Jr., Todd MM. Plasma viscosity and cerebral blood flow, Am J Physiology, 2000; 279 (4): H1949-H1954.

40.   Rebel, A., Lenz, C., Krieter, H., Waschke, K. F., Van Ackern, K., Kuschinsky, W. Oxygen delivery at high blood viscosity and decreased arterial oxygen content to brains of conscious rats. Am. J. Physiol. 2001; 280: 2591H-2597.

41.   Ohta H. The effect of hyperoxemia on cerebral blood flow in normal humans. Brain Nerve. 1986;38:949–959.

42.   Oury TD, Ho Y, Piantadosi CA, Crapo JD. Extracellular Superoxide Dismutase, Nitric Oxide, and Central Nervous System O2 Toxicity. Proceedings of the National Academy of Sciences 1992; 89: 9715-9719.

43.   Ghabriel MN, Zhu C, Hermanis G, Allt G. Immunological targeting of the endothelial barrier antigen (EBA) in vivo leads to opening of the blood-brain barrier. Brain Res 2000 Sep 29;878(1-2):127-35.

44.   Kawamura S, Yasui N, Shirasawa M, Fukasawa H. Therapeutic effects of hyperbaric oxygenation on acute focal cerebral ischemia in rats. Surg Neurol 1990 Aug;34(2):101-6.

45.   Sukoff MH, Ragatz RE. Hyperbaric oxygenation for the treatment of acute cerebral edema. Neurosurgery 1982 Jan;10(1):29-38.

46.   Gross B, Bitterman N, Levanon D, Nir I, Harel D. Horseradish peroxidase as a cytochemical marker of blood-brain barrier integrity in oxygen toxicity in the central nervous system. Exp Neurol 1986 Sep;93(3):471-80.

47.   Elayan, Ikram M., Milton J. Axley, Paruchuri V. Prasad, Stephen T. Ahlers, and Charles R. Auker. Effect of Hyperbaric Oxygen Treatment on Nitric Oxide and Oxygen Free Radicals in Rat Brain. J. Neurophysiol. 2000; 83: 2022-2029.

48.   Kety SS, Schmidt CF. The effects of altered arterial tensions of carbon dioxide and oxygen on cerebral blood flow and cerebral oxygen consumption of normal young man. J Clin Invest. 1948;24:484-492.

Nitric Oxide

49.   Blair, E, Henning G, Esmond WG, Attar S, Cowley RA, and Michaelis M. The effect of hyperbaric oxygenation (OHP) on three forms of shock traumatic, hemorrhagic, and septic. J Trauma 4: 652-663, 1964.

50.   Inamoto Y, Okuno F, Saito K, Tanaka Y, Watanabe K, Morimoto I, Yamashita U, Eto S. Effect of hyperbaric oxygenation on macrophage function in mice. J Clin Invest 1987 Jun;79(6):1868-73.

51.   Masatomo Yamashita, Mamoru Yamashita. Hyperbaric oxygen treatment attenuates cytokine induction after massive hemorrhage. Am J Physiol-Endocrine and Metabolism2000; 278 (5), E811-816.

HBO in Wound Healing

52.   Lahat, N, Bitterman H, Yaniv N, Kinarty A, and Bitterman N. Exposure to hyperbaric oxygen induces tumor necrosis factor-alpha (TNF-α) secretion from rat macrophages. Clin Exp Immunol 102: 655-659, 1995.

53.   Frank S, Stallmeyer B, Kämpfer H, Kolb N, Pfeilschifter J. Nitric oxide triggers enhanced induction of vascular endothelial growth factor expression in cultured keratinocytes (HaCaT) and during cutaneous wound repair. Arterioscler Thromb Vasc Biol 2000 Jun;20(6):1512-20.

54.   Boykin JV Jr. The nitric oxide connection: hyperbaric oxygen therapy, becaplermin, and diabetic ulcer management. Undersea Hyperb Med 1998 Winter;25(4):211-6.

55.   Bonomo SR, Davidson JD, Yu Y, Xia Y, Lin X, Mustoe TA. Hyperbaric oxygen as a signal transducer: upregulation of platelet derived growth factor-beta receptor in the presence of HBO and PDGF. Arch Surg 1994 Oct;129(10):1043-9.

56.   Bonomo SR, Davidson JD, Tyrone JW, Lin X, Mustoe TA. Enhancement of wound healing by hyperbaric oxygen and transforming growth factor beta3 in a new chronic wound model in aged rabbits. Heart Lung Transplant 2002 Feb;21(2):244-50.

57.   Zhao LL, Davidson JD, Wee SC, Roth SI, Mustoe TA. Effect of hyperbaric oxygen and growth factors on rabbit ear ischemic ulcers. Int J Radiat Oncol Biol Phys 1998 Jan 1;40(1):189-96.

58.   Wang X, Ding I, Xie H, Wu T, Wersto N, Huang K, Okunieff P. Hyperbaric oxygen and basic fibroblast growth factor promote growth of irradiated bone. Growth Factors 1995;12(1):29-35.

59.   Wu L, Pierce GF, Ladin DA, Zhao LL, Rogers D, Mustoe TA. Effects of oxygen on wound responses to growth factors: Kaposi's FGF, but not basic FGF stimulates repair in ischemic wounds. Arch Surg 2000 Oct;135(10):1148-53.

60.   Ersson A, Linder C, Ohlsson K, Ekholm A. Cytokine response after acute hyperbaric exposure in the rat. Plast Reconstr Surg 1998 Apr;101(5):1290-5.

61.   Bayati S, Russell RC, Roth AC. Stimulation of angiogenesis to improve the viability of prefabricated flaps. J Clin Immunol 1997 Mar;17(2):154-9.

62.   Larsson A, Engstrom M, Uusijarvi J, Kihlstrom L, Lind F, Mathiesen T. Hyperbaric oxygen treatment of postoperative neurosurgical infections. Neurosurgery 2002 Feb;50(2):287-95; discussion 295-6.

63.   Bill TJ, Hoard MA, Gampper TJ. Applications of hyperbaric oxygen in otolaryngology head and neck surgery: facial cutaneous flaps. Otolaryngol Clin North Am 2001 Aug;34(4):753-66, vi.

64.   Mandell GL. Bacterial activity of aerobic and anaerobic polymorphonuclear neutrophils. Infect Immun 1974; 9:337-341.

65.   Mader JT, Brown GL, Guckian JC, et al. A mechanism for amelioration of hyperbaric oxygen of experimental staphylococcal osteomyelitis in rabbits. J Infectious Disease 1980; 142:915-922.

Complications of HBO

66.   Stone JA, Loar, H, Rudge, FW: An eleven year review of hyperbaric oxygenation in a military clinical setting. Undersea Biomed Res 1991; 18(Suppl):80.

67.   Sheffield, JC, Sheffield PJ, Ziemba AL, Posey KI. Complication rates for HBO treatments: a 21-year analysis. Proceedings of XIV International Congress on Hyperbaric Medicine, Flagstaff, AZ: Best Publishing, 2002 (In preparation)

68.   Baker PC. Decompression sickness incidence in inside attendants, Associates/BNA Precourse on Chamber Safety, Undersea and Hyperbaric Medical Society Annual Scientific Meeting, Cancun, Mexico, 1997.

69.   Davis JC, Dunn JM, Heimbach RD. Hyperbaric medicine: patient selection, treatment procedures and side effects. In: Davis JC, Hunt TK. Problem wounds: Role of oxygen, New York,NY: Elsevier 1988; 225-235.

70.   Kindwall EP. Contraindications and side effects to hyperbaric oxygen treatment. In Kindwall EP, Whelan HT, eds. Hyperbaric Medicine Practice, Falstaff, AZ: Best Publishing, 1999; 83-98.

71.   Balentine, JD. Pathology of Oxygen Toxicity. New York: Academic, 1982.

72.   Demchenko, I.T., Boso, A.E., O'Neill, T. J., Bennet, P.B, Piantadosi, C.A, Nitric oxide and cerebral blood flow responses to hyperbaric oxygen. J. Appl. Physiol. (2000) 88: 1381-1389.

73.   Demchenko IT, Boso AE, Bennett PB, Whorton AR, Piantadosi CA. Hyperbaric oxygen reduces cerebral blood flow by inactivating nitric oxide. Nitric Oxide 2000; 4(6):597-608.

74.   Sato T, Takeda Y, Hagioka S, Zhang S, Hirakawa M. Changes in nitric oxide production and cerebral blood flow before development of hyperbaric oxygen-induced seizures in rats. Brain Res 2001;918(1-2):131-40.

75.   Kurasako T, Takeda Y, Hirakawa M. Increase in cerebral blood flow as a predictor of hyperbaric oxygen-induced convulsion in artificially ventilated rats. Acta Med Okayama 2000; 54(1):15-20.

Rationale for HBO in Selected Indications

76.   Hampson NB. Hyperbaric Oxygen Therapy: 1999 Committee Report. Kensington Maryland: Undersea and Hyperbaric Medical Society, 1999; 1-75.

77.   Kindwall EP, Whelan HT, eds. Hyperbaric Medicine Practice, Falstaff, AZ: Best Publishing, 1999; 433-868.

78.   Zamboni WA, Roth AC, Russell RC, Graham B, Suchy H, Kucan JO. Morphologic analysis of the microcirculation during reperfusion of ischemic skeletal muscle and the effect of hyperbaric oxygen. Plast Reconstr Surg 1993 May;91(6):1110-23.

79.   Stevens DM, Weiss DD, Koller WA, Bianchi DA. Survival of normothermic microvascular flaps after prolonged secondary ischemia: effects of hyperbaric oxygen. Otolaryngol Head Neck Surg 1996 Oct;115(4):360-4.

80.   Nylander G, Lewis D, Nordstrom H, Larsson J. Reduction of postischemic edema with hyperbaric oxygen. Plast Reconstr Surg 1985 Oct;76(4):596-603.

81.   Nylander G, Nordstrom H, Eriksson E. Effects of hyperbaric oxygen on oedema formation after a scald burn. Burns Incl Therm Inj 1984 Feb;10(3):193-6.

82.   Kaiser W, Schnaidt U, von der Lieth H. [Effects of hyperbaric oxygen on fresh burn wounds]. Handchir Mikrochir Plast Chir 1989 May;21(3):158-63 [Article in German].

83.   Van Unnik AJM. Inhibition of toxin production in Clostridium perfringens in vitro by hyperbaric oxygen. Antonie Leeuwenhock Microbiol 1965; 31: 181-186.

NOTES

CHAPTER 5

WHEN HBO MEETS THE ICU: INTENSIVE CARE PATIENTS IN THE HYPERBARIC ENVIRONMENT

C.M. Muth, P. Radermacher, E.S. Shank

INTRODUCTION

There are well-recognized indications for treatment with hyperbaric oxygen (HBO) for which HBO therapy is either a first line therapy or a useful adjunct [1,2]. For some of these indications a need for intensive care is present between the hyperbaric sessions; for others the primary treatment is intensive care and HBO is the adjunct [2,3,4]. In either case, intensivists may be faced with HBO issues, and HBO therapists may be confronted with patients from the ICU. Quoting an editorial in Critical Care Medicine [5], to most physicians in the ICU "...HBO is not just a movie channel any more." Although interest in HBOT is growing, little is known about the advantages and the pitfalls of this therapy in intensive care patients. Only very few publications exist on how to perform HBO in ICU patients [3,4,6-10].

A Short Review on the Physiology of HBOT

Hyperbaric oxygen therapy is defined as the respiration of pure oxygen during a whole body exposure to ambient pressures exceeding the normal atmospheric pressure of 1 ata, usually values between 2 and 3 ata (Table 1). The following section briefly summarizes the essential physiologic effects associated with HBO.

Oxygen Uptake and Transport

While breathing air at normal atmospheric pressure, oxygen is predominantly transported hemoglobin-bound after diffusing through the alveolar capillary membrane. However, under these conditions a small amount is already physically dissolved in the plasma [11]. Under normobaric conditions and assuming an average hemoglobin content of 150 g per liter, blood carries approximately 200 ml O_2 per liter blood as can be derived from the following equation [11]:

$$(1) \ CAO_2 = (SAO_2 \ X \ [HB] \ X \ 1,34) + 3$$

In this formula CaO_2 represents the arterial content of oxygen in [ml/L blood], SaO_2 describes the arterial hemoglobin O_2 saturation (to be included as fraction of maximally 1.0 into the formula). [Hb] is the hemoglobin concentration of blood in [g/L]. 1.34 refers to the maximal amount of oxygen in [ml]

TABLE 1. PRESSURE CONVERSION

1 atm	= 1,013 bar
	= 101 kPa
	= 1,033 kg/cm²
	= 14,7 psi
	= 33 ft seawater
1 ata	≈ 1 bar abs

bound to 1 g hemoglobin. The finally added 3 ml O_2/L blood indicate the amount of oxygen physically dissolved in the plasma during normobaric air respiration. This calculation reveals that just a small fraction of approximately 1.5% of the entire blood oxygen transport capacity operates on physical dissolution under normal conditions. Hemoglobin, saturated by 97-98% in healthy humans breathing normobaric air, will already carry 100% of its maximum oxygen capacity while inhaling pure oxygen at atmospheric pressure. Consequently, any attempt to increase the amount physically dissolved remains the only possibility of enhancing the oxygen transport at a given hemoglobin content. In the hyperbaric environment, oxygen solution in the plasma increases proportionally to its partial pressure in the alveolar gas in accordance to Henry's and Dalton's law [12,13]. During routine HBO exposures the arterial pO_2 reaches values of approximately 1800-1900 mmHg increasing the amount of dissolved oxygen by a factor of 20.

Microcirculatory Oxygen Transport

The oxygen supply of tissues results from capillary convection and diffusion [14]. In this instance, the diffusion radius for oxygen is limited and essentially influenced by the partial pressure gradient between the capillaries and the dependent tissue. Already at the beginning of this century A. Krogh proposed a diffusion model to describe this interrelation [15]. In this model, a well-oxygenated tissue is characterized by a capillary density matching the oxygen demand of the dependent cells, so that a sufficient supply of all parts is guaranteed. With capillary rarefaction (i.e., by thermal or mechanical damage, microangiopathy, irradiation, edema, etc.) an adequate oxygen supply becomes impaired. Consequently, tissue hypoxia with anaerobic metabolism results.

The HBO-induced increase in oxygen partial pressure extends the oxygen diffusion radius into the extracapillary space up to four times as compared with the respiration of normobaric air. Anaerobia may be reversed as oxygenation of hypoxic cells becomes possible because of this enhanced diffusion radius compensating capillary rarefaction or swelling due to edema [16].

Circulatory Effects of HBO

Bradycardia is commonly seen during HBO treatment. The mechanisms which lead to bradycardia are still not fully understood; possibilities include direct influence on the pacemaker function of the heart, hyperoxia itself, increased work of breathing with dense gases, or the effects of dissolved inert gases [17]. Normally, over the course of a hyperbaric exposure the initial bradycardia will become less pronounced, but does not tend to return to baseline levels until the treatment is completed.

There are few human studies which examine the hemodynamic responses to HBO at clinically relevant pressures. In a study of volunteers [18] it was noted that cardiac output decreased significantly during continuous oxygen exposure, but this effect recovered during the latter part of the hyperbaric exposure. A standard hyperbaric treatment profile with intermittent air breaks was examined in another study [19]. Cardiac output, heart rate, and stroke volume were all significantly reduced, while mean arterial pressure increased compared with that at 1 ata. Cardiac output and stroke volume reduction rapidly reverted to control levels after cessation of HBO, but no change was noted during air breaks. Reduced cardiac output probably relates primarily to the combination of heart rate reduction as described above and increase in systemic vascular resistance.

A reduction of blood flow under hyperoxic conditions has been documented in various tissues and organs [20-23]. This effect is restricted to tissues with a preserved autoregulation and derives from a reactive vasoconstriction. This vasoconstriction results from a decreased release of nitric oxide from its binding to cystein in the heme molecule (S-nitroso-mehoglobin moiety) [24] which in turn is caused by the extremely elevated oxygen partial pressure. The latter prevents a decrease of tissue oxygenation as the oxygen diffusion radius remains enhanced despite the reduced blood flow. Nevertheless, in organs with preserved ability to autoregulation this effect favors the lymphatic drainage and contributes to the reduction of edema [16], and thereby a reduction of tissue pressure in organs unable to expand. Both mechanisms improve the microcirculatory blood flow, and in fact beneficial effects have been reported in patients suffering from crush injuries [25], compartment syndromes [26], or compromised transplants [27-29]. Hypoxic tissue does not react in the same way until hyperoxia as the crucial physiologic stimulus occurs. Several observations support this view and identify a dose-dependent reaction to oxygen. A redistribution of blood to improve the oxygenation of hypoxic tissues will result in the so called "inversed steal-effect" [23]. Finally, HBO has a potential of limiting reperfusion damage in previously ischemic areas. This is caused by the already mentioned reduction of edema as well as by reduced endothelial leukocyte adhesion in the venules [28]. To our current knowledge, these effects only occur if HBO is administered in the narrow therapeutic window directly previous to or within an hour after reperfusion [30].

Respiratory Effects

Hyperbaric oxygen therapy introduces several variables that can affect respiration (Table 2). These include hyperoxia, elevation of ambient pressure, elevation of ambient temperature, and an increase in patient anxiety. Autonomic respiratory control is under the influence of central and peripheral chemoreceptors. The peripheral chemoreceptors located in the carotid body consist of fast responding receptors sensitive to PaO_2, $PaCO_2$, and pH. As PaO_2 rises, the afferent impulse frequency from the carotid bodies decrease [31]. This response is normally small and insignificant, but in a patient dependent on hypoxic drive the introduction of hyperoxia can ablate their respiratory drive. Healthy patients have a reduced response to CO_2 during HBOT through this mechanism [32]. This reduced CO_2 reactivity

TABLE 2. RESPIRATORY EFFECTS OF HBO

Increased	Decreased
Tidal Volume	Et CO_2
Respiratory frequency	P_aCO_2
Minute ventilation	FVC
P 0.1 (central resp drive)	FEV 1
T ins, T exp, T total	CO_2 reactivity
Resistance	

Multiple studies investigating respiratory changes with HBOT suggest that the following respiratory alterations are likely. It is important to appreciate that in any given individual one or more of the above responses to HBOT may be dominant.

returns post HBOT [33]. Carbon dioxide is transported in the blood stream in three forms: bicarbonate ion, carbamino compounds, and dissolved in the plasma (in order of decreasing quantity). As oxygen content of the blood increases, carbon dioxide transport (as bicarbonate) is decreased (anti-Haldane effect) [34]. Thus, elevated PaO_2 depresses peripheral chemoreceptors, decreases CO_2 transport to the lungs, and decreases the CO_2 ventilatory response. This results in a transient decrease in respiration and elevation in Pa CO_2. By contrast, as Pa CO_2 rises, the P brain CO_2 also rises. This leads to a decrease in CSF pH ($CO_2 + H_2O \rightarrow H_2CO_3 \rightarrow H^+ + HCO_3^-$) and a stimulus to breathe. Ultimately a steady state arises with the brain CSF pH decreasing ~ 0.04 and an elevation in P brain $CO_2 \sim 5$ mm Hg.

The second influence of HBOT is related to the elevation in ambient pressure. As pressure increases, the density of a gas increases. In areas of the lung with turbulent flow, the density of the gas is proportional to the resistance. Thus as pressure increases, flow resistance and thereby work of breathing increases. Several studies [32,35-37] have demonstrated that as pressure increases, the body tends to optimize effort in breathing, i.e., respiratory rate decreases with an increase in tidal volume (preserving minute ventilation). Nevertheless spirometry shows a decline of FEV, FVC, and maximal ventilatory effort.

Effect of HBO on Angioneogenesis and Wound Healing

Uncomplicated healing of a wound requires a distinct microenvironment and the wound itself may be subdivided into two compartments: the wound space (hypoxic, acidotic, hypoglycemic, hypercapnic, hyperkalemic, and with high lactate concentration) and the wound edge, well vascularized and hyperemic due to inflammatory reactions [38,39]. Repair processes start from the latter and proceed towards the wound space, whereby concentration gradients essentially stimulate cell migration. In this context, hypoxia and high lactate concentrations are essential triggers for normal wound healing and capillary neoangiogenesis [40,41].

A proper initiation of wound healing also requires sufficient oxygen supply to maintain metabolism as well as proliferation and release of growth-factors or cytokines [42-44]. Therefore, mitoses are hardly recognized in marked hypoxic wound areas. Moreover, recent results demonstrate a dose-dependent stimulation of fibroblast proliferation by hyperbaric oxygen [45]. Fibroblastic collagen synthesis inevitably depends on molecular oxygen for the hydroxylation of the amino acid proline which is the limiting molecular step for extracellular collagen deposition [46,47]. In addition, not only the production, but also the stability of collagen essentially depends on oxygen. Cross-linking of collagen chains, crucial for the tensile strength of a wound, requires lysine hydroxylase which needs molecular oxygen as a substrate for the hydroxylation of the amino acid lysine [48]. Finally, a steep oxygen gradient between the edge and the space of a wound was identified as a mandatory prerequisite in the formation of granulation tissue [49]. As already mentioned above, a well-oxygenated wound edge with low lactate values induces neoangiogenesis and cell proliferation towards the hypoxic tissue of the wound center with its high lactate level [50]. Some angiogenic factors are stimulated in particular by low oxygen concentrations, although the most effective response to this proliferation stimulus occurs in the hyperoxic venules at the wound edge. This paradox is still unexplained and subject to further research. A physiological oxygen supply is also necessary to create a tissue matrix and to increase the capillary density. In fact an eight- to ninefold increase of the capillary density was demonstrated in animals previously irradiated and HBO-treated compared to irradiated and non-treated control animals [51].

Effects of HBO on Infection and Immunological Responses

Anaerobic or mixed aerobic-anaerobic infections respond to HBO, since a direct bactericidal effect is achieved against anaerobic organisms such as gas-forming clostridia (*Clostridium perfringens*, etc.) [52,53]. In addition, the production of the clostridial a-toxin is suppressed by HBO [54]. Finally, HBO exerts direct bacteriostatic effects on numerous bacteria, i.e., *Escherichia coli*, Staphylococci, and Pseudomonas [55,56,57].

A very important indirect effect is seen in aerobic infections, since the phagocytic killing by granulocytes requires oxygen and is impaired by hypoxia. A sufficient reoxygenation stimulates the oxidative burst and achieves a more effective killing and removal of the infectious source [58,59]. Additionally, hyperbaric oxygen enhances or at least restores the antimicrobial effect of several antibiotics, i.e., aminoglycosides [57,60].

The Dark Side of HBO: Unwanted Side Effects (Table 3)

Side effects and complications of HBO treatment are related to the three phases of its administration [61]: During compression barotrauma of the middle ear, inner ear, and the sinuses may occur, as described in detail later [62]. Therefore, in intubated or unconscious patients myringotomy should be performed prior to the HBO treatment [8-10].

Side effects at pressure are due to the toxicity of N_2 and O_2. The toxicity of N_2 is a dose-dependent, alcohol intoxication-like impairment of intellectual and neuromuscular performance, well known in diving [63]. The oxygen-breathing patient is not prone to this side effect, but the air-breathing attending medical staff in a multiplace chamber is particularly susceptible to N_2 toxicity. The full symptomatology of N_2 toxicity is generally limited to ambient pressures beyond 5 ata, but it may occur at lower pressures due to cold or respiratory acidosis. Most HBO treatments are limited to 3 ata, and in this range the effects are usually tolerable but can lead to a certain impairment.

The toxicity of O_2 is of particular practical importance; it affects the central nervous system (CNS), the lungs, and the eyes. In fact, O_2 toxicity is the limiting factor for the maximum PO_2 and the duration of HBO treatment [64,65,66].

Toxicity to the eyes is seen in about 30% of patients receiving HBO over several months duration and manifests as myopia. These changes of the refractory index of the lens usually resolve within a similar period of time as they occurred [67,68].

O_2 toxicity to the CNS in its most severe form manifests as seizures [65]. It is sometimes preceded by nausea, facial twitching, and/or unpleasant olfactory and gustatory sensations. Therapy is the immediate removal of 100% O_2 and switch to air breathing in the patient [69]. In contrast to generalized seizures of other origin (i.e., with arterial gas embolism, hypoglycemia, and more) barbiturate or benzodiazepine treatment is almost never indicated. Because of the special danger of an overinflation of the lungs, decompression must always be stopped when seizures occur! Several factors (most of which can be encountered in an ICU patient) influence CNS O_2 toxicity: While steroids, adrenergic drugs, thyroid hormones, respiratory acidosis, and fever or sepsis lower the seizure threshold, anesthetics and sedatives, ganglionic blocking drugs, and hypothermia are protective [70]. Recently, nitric oxide inhibition has also been shown to attenuate O_2-induced seizures in animal experiments [71,72] although this effect may be outweighed by the further reduction in cerebral blood flow [73].

In contrast to the acute CNS toxicity, pulmonary O_2 toxicity is cumulative [74]. It can be calculated in units of pulmonary toxic dose (UPTD) [75] as shown in Figure 1.

TABLE 3. IMPORTANT SIDE EFFECTS

Pressure induced:	others	iatrogenic
Barotrauma of • middle ear • Inner ear • sinuses	oxygen toxicity of the CNS	Mostly due to unawareness in combination with those to the left:
Pulmonary barotrauma	Pulmonary oxygen toxicity	ET-tube leakage
Pressure induced changes of other air/gas filled cavities and medical devices	Myopia	Overinflation of the lung
	Inert gas narcosis in attending staff	Gas embolism
	Risk of fire	

Pulmonary O_2 toxicity manifests as decreased functional residual capacity with subsequently impaired gas exchange (Figure 1) [76,77]. Therefore in most treatment protocols HBO is given intermixed with air-breathing periods ("air breaks") of 5-10 minutes every 20-30 minutes to lower toxicity [78]. Minimum inspired O_2 fractions for 5-10 minutes are likewise mandatory in ventilated patients. Whether or not the protective effect of antioxidants such as superoxide dismutase, N-aceytlcysteine [72], allopurinol, or vitamin E documented in experimental animals can be confirmed in humans remains to be elucidated.

Barotrauma is always a potential risk for patients for any closed air spaces while ambient pressures are altered [62]. Pulmonary barotrauma during decompression may result in cardiovascular instability secondary to a decrease in venous return [79], gas embolism, or pneumothorax [62]. Of course, barotraumas due to non-equilibration of pressure changes in air-filled cavities (middle ear, sinuses, lung) are a potential risk for attendant caregivers as well.

During decompression, first line attending nurses and physicians are susceptible to any decompression-induced complication. It is noteworthy that physical effort during or after the HBO treatment increases the risk of DCS for the attending personnel [8,80], and therefore nurses and physicians should decompress breathing 100% O_2 even if it is not formally required by the decompression schedule.

Although not a physiologic complication, the high risk of fire in a hyperbaric chamber has to be mentioned as well. In an atmosphere with elevated oxygen pressure or even pure oxygen almost any material easily can burn [81]. This has to be kept in mind with any device and any material

Units of Pulmonary Toxic Dose

$$UPTD = 1.78 \cdot t \, [min] \cdot (P \, O_2 \, [bar] - 0.5)^{0.8333}$$

$$\Delta\% \, VC = -0.011 \cdot (PO_2 \, [bar] - 0.5) \cdot t \, [min]$$

$\Rightarrow$ 600 Units $\approx$ 2 $\Delta\%$
$\Rightarrow$ 1000 Units $\approx$ 6 $\Delta\%$
$\Rightarrow$ 2000 Units $\approx$ 20 $\Delta\%$

Figure 1. Units of Pulmonary Toxic Dose: the UPTD Concept

The top part shows the equation were U is the number of units, t the time of exposure in minutes, and P the exposure pressure in bar. Pulmonary O_2 toxicity manifests as decreased functional residual capacity with subsequently impaired gas exchange. The bottom part shows the reduction in vital capacity (VC) induced by some standard HBO treatment schedules: about 2% after 90 min at 3 bar abs (approx 3 ata, Boerema table), 6% after 12 sessions of a common protocol for problem wounds (90 min O_2 at max. 2.4 bar abs/2.4 ata), and even 20% predicted after 3 sessions with the Boerema table used for gas gangrene.

which is brought into a chamber. Flammable materials and devices with a high risk of electrically produced sparks are to be banned from hyperbaric chambers, and patients should be dressed in clothing of pure cotton to limit likelihood of static electricity in the chamber. In addition, potential sources of electrical discharge, i.e., batteries, brush-motors, and lighters, are prohibited. Fires have been reported in both monoplace and, less commonly, multiplace facilities.

INDICATIONS THAT REQUIRE HBOT (TABLE 4)

Gas Embolism

Besides from diving medicine, gas embolism, the entry of gas into vascular structures, is a largely iatrogenic clinical entity responsible for serious morbidity, and even mortality, in many varied medical specialties [82,83].

Depending on the mechanism of gas entry and where the emboli ultimately lodge, two broad categories of gas embolism can be differentiated [82,83]. A venous embolism occurs by the entry of gas into the systemic venous system. This gas is then transported to the pulmonary vessels, where interference with gas exchange, arrhythmias, pulmonary hypertension, right ventricle strain, and finally cardiac failure, can occur [84]. In contrast to venous embolism, an arterial embolism arises through the entry and passage of air into the arterial system.

In this case, the gas bubbles are flow-directed to the distal endarteries occluding these vessels [82]. The occurrence is especially critical in brain-perfusing blood vessels because of the extremely short hypoxia tolerance of CNS, although this mechanism is possible in all arteries.

It should be noted, however, that any venous gas embolism can become an arterial one due to a paradoxical embolism [82]. This can result by passage of gas through the lung vessels, which normally filter gas-bubbles with good success; but after an overload of the lung with gas the passage of gas into the systemic circulation can happen [85]. Furthermore, a preexisting patent foramen ovale (PFO) may favor passage of gas into the systemic circulation under certain circumstances [86].

TABLE 4. IMPORTANT INDICATIONS FOR HBO IN ICU-PATIENTS

HBO as treatment of first choice	HBO as important adjunctive treatment	HBO as possible adjunctive treatment
decompression sickness	gas gangrene	exceptional blood loss and anemia
arterial gas embolism	necrotizing fasciitis	brain injury
CO intoxication (?)	crush injuries, reperfusion injuries	brain abscess
	impaired muskuloskeletal flaps	
	impaired wound healing	

From the hyperbaric point of view, the arterial gas embolism is clinically most important. Arterial gas embolism (AGE) occurs by the entry of gas into the pulmonary veins or directly into the arteries of the systemic circulation [82]. Mechanisms also include the overexpansion of the lung through decompression barotraumas [62], and paradox embolism. This entry of gas into the systemic circulation causes a distribution of gas bubbles into nearly all organs. Small emboli in the vessels of the muscular system or most of the visceral organs may stay silent. Embolization in the coronary arteries leads in most cases to changes in ECG typical of an infarction, while with larger quantities of gas myocardial suppression and dysrythmia may occur. With a small embolization these changes pass and are reversible; with an embolization of greater dimensions cardiac failure and cardiac arrest are possible [83]. Circulatory responses such as hypotension, arrhythmia, and cardiac arrest are possible as well by an embolization in the cerebral vessels [87].

When gas-bubbles disperse distally in the arteries of the brain until they cause an obstruction nutritive arteries the result is a reduction of the perfusion to the affected part of the brain with development of ischemia distal to the obstruction. From this initial local ischemia follow further functional/morphological failures, aggravated by a perifocal edema which further decreases cerebral blood-flow. Furthermore, development of edema and interference with brain perfusion as well as brain metabolism results with further impairment of the local tissues. But even areas not directly affected by the AGE are involved by disturbing cerebral autoregulation, and interrupting function of the blood-brain-barrier can arise. Besides the immediate effect of the obstruction of the vessel and the associated changes described above, more damages to structures emerge. Depending on the size of the gas bubbles, the complete disintegration or at least the reduction in the volume of the gas bubble is possible. But due to the mechanical irritation of the gas bubbles, on one hand, and due to their attribute as foreign body on the other, both mechanisms serve to generate a severe inflammatory response. The mechanical irritation of the vessel endothelium results in the adhesion of leukocytes and thrombocytes and triggers deposition of fibrin, which maintain the disturbance of perfusion. As the surface of the bubble represents a foreign surface in the vessel system, the activation of factors of the plasma clotting cascade, and activation of immunoglobulins and of the complement system occurs, resulting in a further decrease in perfusion and increase in tissue damage [82,83].

There are numerous mechanisms for the generation of gas emboli in the medical field, not limited to post-operative recovery of cardiac, neurosurgical, and vascular patients [82,83]. In patients requiring ventilatory support, pulmonary barotrauma may be induced and, analogous to barotrauma of the lung in diving medicine, gas embolism can develop [88,89]. Gas embolisms may also occur during mechanical circulatory interventions. These include hemodialysis, extracorporial membrane oxygenation (ECMO), or extracorporeal CO_2-elimination (ECCO$_2$-R) as well as cardiopulmonary bypass pumps [90,91]. Rare reports of catastrophic gas embolism have been reported from rupture of intra-aortic balloon pump balloons [92].

Decompression Illness

Decompression illness is a serious medical problem associated with a decrease in ambient pressure [62,83,93]. It encompasses both decompression sickness (DCS), which is caused by tissue bubble formation due to supersaturation of inert gases, and arterial gas embolism (AGE) caused by entry of gas into blood vessels during a rapid decompression due to pulmonary gas trapping and alveolar rupture [94]. As diving-associated AGE does not differ in pathophysiology from arterial gas embolism of any other etiology this section will focus on DCS. During diving the divers' tissues are loaded with increased quantities of nitrogen according to Henry's law, i.e., the nitrogen content of a tissue increases in proportion to the ambient pressure, the time under pressure, the tissue perfusion, and the tissue's nitrogen solubility [62,93]. When the diver returns to surface, the ambient pressure decreases and so do the partial pressures of the gases of the breathing gas (Dalton's law) and the additional nitrogen is eliminated from the tissues. When decompression is performed too fast, the pressure decrease can exceed the elimination rate and therefore the sum of the gas tensions in the tissue may exceed the absolute ambient pressure, which can result into a critical supersaturation in the tissues [62,83,93,94]. This mechanism assumes particular importance in tissues with shear stress due to movement of one tissue layer in relation to another which markedly enhances bubble formation, a phenomenon called tribonucelation [95,96]. As a consequence, the liberation of free gas from the tissue can occur with bubble formation and disturbance of organ function by blocking arteries, veins, and lymphatic vessels, or just tissue compression by expanding volume of the bubbles [97]. The volume of bubbles and their location in the body determine whether and how intense symptoms occur. Bubbles that form in the muscles and joints characteristically cause musculoskeletal pain (bends). Bubbles can also form in peripheral nerves and spinal cord, causing patchy hypesthesia and paraparesis. Girdle pain is often a sign for severe spinal cord involvement. Bubbles forming in the skin and lymphatics cause rash and lymphedema, and bubble formation in the inner ear causes vertigo and hearing loss. Tissue bubbles formed *in situ* can also migrate into the vasculature and produce venous gas embolism (VGE), which in most cases remain asymptomatic, but high levels of VGE can cause pulmonary hypertension, pulmonary edema, cough, and dyspnea, known collectively as chokes [98], VGE may also generate arterial gas embolisms as well when a right-to-left shunting occurs (patent foramen ovale and other mechanisms) [99].

DCS covers a continuum of signs and symptoms. In order to grade severity, decompression sickness has been subclassified into Type I, characterized as pain only and/or skin and lymphatic appearance, and into Type II with neurologic and/or respiratory disorders. Initial changes mainly are due to mechanical effects of the bubble. When gas bubbles form and expand they can obstruct the arterial and/or venous circulation, leading to tissue ischemia and tissue damage resulting in pain. Local edema and tissue ischemia, both of which have been observed after decompression, can reduce gas elimination by increasing diffusion distances and by reducing blood flow [100,101]. Therefore, besides the immediate effect of the obstruction of the vessel and the associated changes described above, more damages to structures may emerge.

EMERGENCY THERAPY IN BUBBLE-RELATED DISEASES

The protection and maintenance of vital functions is the primary goal. If necessary, cardiopulmonary resuscitation has to be performed. For somnolent or comatose patients endotracheal intubation should be performed to maintain adequate oxygenation and ventilation. Additionally oxygen should be administered in as high a concentration as available, if possible close to 100% oxygen [102]. This is important not only to treat hypoxia and hypoxemia but also for the elimination of the gas in the bubbles by the formation of a diffusion gradient and by this a diminution of the bubbles [103,104]. The next important step is the administration of fluids. In diving accidents, a dehydration with hypovolemia is very likely, due to fluid losses through airways and diver's diuresis during the dive [105,106]. Any kind of bubble injury with intravascular accumulation of bubbles leads to endothelial damage and capillary leakage, resulting in hemoconcentration and impaired microvascular flow [107-109]. Therefore, administration either orally or intravenously of one to two liters of fluid during the first hour is recommended. Further administration can be guided by clinical measurements [102]. The patient's positioning should be the flat supine position for comatose patients especially with CAGE. Head down positions are not sufficient to overcome the force of blood flow, propelling gas bubbles toward the head, but may aggravate the cerebral edema that develops in these patients.

Hyperbaric oxygen therapy is the treatment of choice in those emergencies since it causes a mechanical diminution of the gas bubble by both raising the ambient pressure and creating systemic hyperoxia. This hyperoxia produces an enormous diffusion gradient for oxygen into the gas bubble, as well as for egress of the inert gas from the bubble. Hyperoxia also enables significantly larger quantities of oxygen to be dissolved in the plasma and in addition increases the diffusion distance of oxygen in tissues. This improved oxygen carrying capacity and delivery is important to offset the embolic insult to the microvasculature [102].

Although immediate recompression demonstrates the best response, treatment in a hyperbaric chamber is still indicated after a longer period of time [110, 111]. As the treatment of decompression-related injuries as DCS and arterial gas embolism with hyperbaric oxygen is the first line treatment of choice, once the patient is stabilized from a cardiopulmonary standpoint, transfer to a hyperbaric oxygen facility should be accomplished without delay.

Carbon Monoxide Intoxication

Hyperbaric oxygen therapy has been considered the first line of therapy for severe acute carbon monoxide intoxication due to its ability to increase the speed of dissociation of carbon monoxide from the hemoglobin molecule [112,113], although recent randomized controlled clinical trials have raised some questions about that approach [114,115].

Carbon monoxide (CO), an odorless, colorless gas, is produced by the incomplete combustion of fossil fuels. Any device that runs on fossil fuels can be a hazard if inadequate ventilation is present; it is also found in tobacco smoke.

CO intoxication is a diagnosis determined largely by the history. Clinical signs may be non-specific and misleading [83]. Thus it is important that the diagnosis of CO poisoning be entertained early and a carboxy hemoglobin (COHb) level be obtained to confirm the intoxication. A COHb level greater than 10% establishes the diagnosis in all but the heaviest smokers. It is important to stress that the COHb level does not predict severity of the poisoning or possible outcome, but only that the patient has CO poisoning and should be treated. Some authors [116] suggest that presence of acidosis by arterial blood gas study may be a better measure of severity of poisoning.

The degree of CO poisoning is dependent on a number of factors. These include the concentration of CO inhaled, the duration of exposure, and the minute ventilation of the patient [117]. Additionally the severity is associated with the underlying health of the individual and how tolerant of hypoxia they may be. Thus elderly patients, patients with cardiopulmonary disease, and children and infants (higher oxygen consumption relative to body size) tend to be more affected. Pregnant patients are of special concern as not only the mother's history and physical state are important, but fetal hemoglobin has a higher affinity for the CO molecule than adult hemoglobin. hence CO concentration may occur in the fetus.

Historically, it was accepted that CO exerted its detrimental effects solely by aggravating oxygen delivery to the tissues. CO binds to hemoglobin with an affinity greater than 200 times that of oxygen. The binding of CO to hemoglobin causes an alteration in the structure of hemoglobin, making release of oxygen molecules to the tissues more difficult (i.e., a leftward shift of the oxygen hemoglobin dissociation curve occurs). Thus CO not only occupies binding sites normally carrying oxygen to the tissues, it also prevents the release of oxygen to the tissues [118,119]. Therefore, CO creates hypoxia both at the systemic and the cellular level. However, in a landmark study [120], carboxyhemoglobin was exchange transfused into non-CO exposed dogs, and survival, in spite of COHb levels as high as 60%, was demonstrated. It was concluded that binding of CO to hemoglobin was not enough; rather the CO must be dissolved in the plasma and delivered to tissues for CO to kill. CO also binds to other heme-containing molecules. These include myoglobin, interfering with oxygen transport to muscle, as well as intracellular heme moieties. These include the cytochrome c oxidase enzyme [121] interfering with cellular respiration and the cytochrome P 450 system responsible for hepatic metabolism, respectively [118]. Tissues with high cellular oxygen demand (i.e., brain and heart) are affected the greatest. CO induces the conversion of xanthine dehydrogenase to xanthine oxidase which enables the formation of multiple oxygen radicals including hydroxyl, singlet oxygen, and peroxyl species. These reactive molecules may interact with the membrane lipids of neurons, causing injury. Moreover, it was recently demonstrated that CO toxicity is at least partly caused by lipid peroxidation due to peroxynitrite formation which results from the CO-induced release of NO from the heme moiety and increased O_2 radical production because of the disrupted respiratory chain [121,122].

The signs and symptoms of CO poisoning, in order of most common presentation, are: headache, dizziness, weakness, nausea, difficulty concentrating, confusion, shortness of breath, visual changes, chest pain, loss of consciousness, abdominal pain, and muscle cramping [119]. The "classic" symptoms of cherry red pigmentation and retinal hemorrhages are both seen in less than 2% of patients and should not be relied upon to make the diagnosis. In addition to the acute and often dramatic symptomatology outlined above, there are more subtle manifestations of CNS neurotoxicity termed delayed neurologic sequelae (DNS), including aphasia, apraxia, apathy, disorientation, personality/mood changes, and more [124]. To better diagnose these neurological problems which can occur weeks post exposure, a thorough neurological examination and neuropsychological screening are important.

The therapy for CO treatment has been oxygen breathing. This therapy was first instituted under normobaric conditions, and then under hyperbaric conditions once it was demonstrated that the half life of carboxyhemoglobin was dramatically reduced employing this therapy [125,126]. Frequently quoted figures suggest the half life decreases from around five hours while breathing room air, to sixty minutes under normobaric 100% oxygen and as low as twenty-three minutes under hyperbaric oxygen at 3 ata [127]. Additional studies have suggested that HBOT also has other physiologic effects in CO poisoning: it accelerates the dissociation of CO from cytochromes, reduces brain lipid peroxidation, inhibits the adhesion of leukocytes to the compromised cerebral vascular endothelium, and prevents intracranial hypertension [127]. Although all these theoretical advantages of HBOT should help in CO poisoning, there are conflicting studies as to whether HBOT is advantageous, neutral, or actually deleterious to patients suffering from CO intoxication. Whether or not HBOT should be routinely used for patients with CO intoxication remains a matter of debate. There is still a powerful argument for HBOT in its ability to rapidly remove the CO molecule from intra- and extracellular heme molecules as well as the other theoretical benefits of HBOT mentioned above. At present it is recommended to treat all pregnant women with CO intoxication, and any patient with loss of consciousness, or evidence of cerebral or cardiac ischemia.

Clostridial Myonecrosis and Other Soft Tissue Infections

Clostridial myonecrosis is caused by anaerobic bacteria (*Clostridium perfringens*). Clostridial production of toxins, especially alpha toxin, leads to extensive tissue destruction and shock. The patients present with pain out of proportion to the apparent severity of their wounds and often have evidence of tissue gas (gas gangrene). The mainstay of treatment of clostridial myonecrosis has always been immediate surgical decompression and excision of all necrotic tissue together with administration of antibiotics. In addition, the available clinical and experimental evidence suggests that multiple early treatment sessions with hyperbaric oxygen at 3 atmospheres for 90 minutes, when administered in conjunction with antibiotics and surgery, confer the following benefits: the border between devitalized and healthy tissue is more clearly demarcated, permitting surgeons to be more conservative in their excisions; the extent of amputation required in clostridial myonecrosis involving the extremities is decreased; and systemically ill patients often improve substantially after a few treatments [53,54,128,129,130]. Somewhat similar in appearance, but totally different in origin is the necrotizing fasciitis [128,129], a rapidly progressive infection of the skin and underlying tissue. Because these infections have similarities to clostridial myonecrosis, hyperbaric oxygen in conjunction with surgery and antibiotic therapy has been used to treat them [128-131].

If hyperbaric oxygen can be safely administered, particularly in those with anaerobic infections, it is a reasonable adjunct to surgery and antibiotics in such severe soft tissue infections. Treatment regimens vary, but would commonly be once or twice daily treatments for 90 minutes at 3 atmospheres of pressure, only after and in conjunction with complete surgical debridement and antibiotic treatment. As with clostridial infections, the presumed benefits are from improved leukocyte function and bactericidal effects of hyperoxia previously discussed. The ICU physician should be prepared, however, for treatment of a suddenly occurring circulatory depression during HBO treatment of patients with gas gangrene: the bactericidal effect of the high O_2 tension on this microbe with resultant disruption of the cell membrane may lead to pronounced release of the α-toxin which per se has profound circulatory depressive effects.

OTHER INDICATIONS FOR HBO THERAPY THAT CAN BE ENCOUNTERED IN ICU PATIENTS

Anemia due to Exceptional Blood Loss

As described above, the amount of oxygen dissolved in the blood under hyperbaric conditions can be sufficient to meet cellular metabolic demands without any contribution from oxygen transported by hemoglobin. Hyperbaric oxygen has been used successfully to treat hemorrhagic shock in patients for whom suitable blood was not available or who refused transfusion for religious reasons [132].

Acute Traumatic Ischemic Injury and Compromised Skin Grafts and Flaps

Crush injury and other severe trauma to the extremities can result in tears of the major vessels and damage to the microcirculation, with resultant ischemia, edema, compartment syndromes, and tissue necrosis. Surgery remains the cornerstone of therapy for these injuries. Reduction of edema, protection from reperfusion injury, and enhanced wound healing are postulated benefits of adjunctive therapy with hyperbaric oxygen [25,26].

Skin grafts and reconstructive flaps may fail because of inadequate perfusion and hypoxia. Graft or flap failure is less frequent in animals receiving hyperbaric oxygen than in those receiving no treatment. Clinical studies have shown that adjunctive HBO treatment increased the rate of successful grafting in poorly vascularized tissue [28,133,134]. Hyperbaric oxygen treatments should therefore be considered when a graft or flap must be placed over a capillary bed with poor circulation, especially if previous reconstruction in the same area was unsuccessful [133,134].

Impaired Wound Healing

Impaired wound healing is a major problem in various localized and generalized diseases where blood and oxygen supply to the tissues and the oxygen demand of the tissues are imbalanced [134]. Therefore an important factor for impaired wound healing is a disturbance of tissue perfusion with resultant hypoxia [42,43,44]. Although acute hypoxia is an important trigger for healing mechanisms, a prolonged hypoxic state can impair wound healing as the presence of oxygen is known to be essential in a number of processes in the cascade of wound healing. Hyperbaric oxygen therapy (HBOT) is clinically used as a possible adjuvant therapeutical approach to treat such complicated wounds [135]. It should be underscored that experimental data suggest that HBOT even has beneficial effects when hypoxia is not present [136].

Hyperbaric Oxygen Treatment of Neurosurgical Infections

Larsson and coworkers evaluated the clinical usefulness of hyperbaric oxygen therapy for neurosurgical infections after craniotomy or laminectomy in a retrospective study [137]. They concluded that HBO treatment is an alternative to standard surgical removal of infected bone flaps and is particularly useful in complex situations. According to these findings they state that it can improve outcomes, reduce the need for reoperations, and allow infection control without mandatory removal of foreign material. The conclusions of these authors are that HBO therapy is a safe, powerful treatment for postoperative cranial and spinal wound infections, it seems cost-effective, and it should be included in the neurosurgical armamentarium. Others reported on beneficial effects of HBO therapy in patients with brain injuries [138-140]. Finally, intracranial abscesses have been accepted as an indication for HBO after successful treatment of 13 patients in different centers [141].

THE ICU PATIENT AND HYPERBARIC OXYGEN THERAPY: GENERAL CONSIDERATIONS

Hyperbaric oxygen therapy can be performed in monoplace or multiplace chambers, each with its own specific benefits and problems. In a monoplace chamber the patient is alone and no direct access is possible during the hyperbaric exposure. Points of criticism are also the lack of suitable equipment for optimal patient care, and the limitations of treatment pressures not exceeding 3 bar absolute pressure (approx. 3 ata). A clear advantage to monoplace chambers is avoidance of exposure of the healthcare team to hyperbaric pressures.

The chamber is pressurized with pure oxygen and air breaks have to be performed with built-in breathing systems (BIBS) and face masks in the cooperative patient or with manipulations of Fi O$_2$ in ventilated ones [10,142,143 (= recommended further reading)].

Multiplace chambers are designed to either treat several sitting patients simultaneously when the indications allow such procedure, or individual critically ill patients accompanied by attending staff. But even in multiplace, "walk-in" chambers physicians and nurses attending the patient are not able to freely move in or out of the chamber for obvious reasons, although modern chambers all are equipped with a small, separately locked front room, serving as a personal transfer lock. In addition, equipment, medications, etc. can only be moved into or out of the chamber via an additional small transfer lock [3,9]. Multiplace chambers are pressurized with air and patients breathe oxygen under pressure through face masks, head-tents, or T-tubes, when intubated or tracheostomized. In contrast, the attending staff breathes air from chamber atmosphere, but can also breathe oxygen via BIBS.

The particular consequences with respect to ICU patients will be discussed later. Some general considerations are of value for both ways of treatment (Table 5).

Critical care units provide specialized monitoring, organ-support systems, and intensive care to patients with severe or potential major organ dysfunction that could become rapidly life threatening. Successful optimal patient management depends on an integrated team of specialists with good experience. It is obvious that for the best treatment of the critically ill patient with HBO, the hyperbaric unit should also be staffed with personnel who are well and regularly trained in treating critically ill patients. The best way to meet this demand is by building the hyperbaric chamber as an extension of the ICU: in proximity, and in equipment and personnel. This allows for quick and safe transport and immediate consultation when needed.

Worldwide, only few hospitals have direct access to a hyperbaric chamber when needed, and even then the chamber may be in a distant

TABLE 5. CHECKLIST INTUBATED PATIENT

Prior to Therapy	During Therapy
Patient stabilized?	Patient stable?
All I.V.-lines working?	Both lungs ventilated? • At any time? • Control prior to any pressure reduction!
Myringotomy performed?	All I.V.-lines working?
Pneumothorax excluded? • chest roentgenogram! • when pneumothorax present: thorax drain first!	In case of CNS oxygen toxicity with convulsions: • switch to air breathing • **never** decompress during convulsions
Both lungs ventilated? • At any time?	Perform air breaks!
Breath sounds normal? • bronchospasm has to be treated prior to HBO • suctioning, when necessary	control ventilator, adjust if needed
ET tube: • Cuff filled with liquid (saline, distilled water)? • well positioned? • adequately fixed?	Check blood gases and TcpO$_2$
When patient is in the chamber: • monoplace: all wall penetrations work well? Ventilator tested? • multiplace: ventilator tested? Set for thorax drainage available inside the chamber? Emergency medication ? BIBS for attendants installed and working? Wound drains vented? Infusion containers vented?	Think of DCS risk for attending staff, when CPR had to be performed! Think of fire hazard with defibrillation and/or with ventilation with not optimized ventilation bag!

location in the hospital, so transportation of the critically ill patient is necessitated. It is well recognized that both inter- and intrahospital transfers may be an independent cause of patient morbidity [144,145]. Transportation as well as HBO treatment itself may result in the patient's absence from the ICU for 3-4 hours, which may even need to be repeated two to three times in a 24 hour period. This risk of increased morbidity can be reduced by minimizing patient transfers (i.e., using dedicated hyperbaric beds and/or barouches which do not require excessive patient movement during HBO sessions) and under ideal circumstances by maintaining similar ventilatory parameters to those carried out in the ICU. Unfortunately most ventilators which are in use under hyperbaric conditions do not meet the requirements for modern respiratory therapy. Minimum standards of monitoring are well recognized but not yet established in hyperbaric medicine. In addition, normal clinical observation can be difficult in HBO environments for technical reasons. These include limitation of patient access, noise, decreased ambient lighting, and altered sound transmission, making a simple technique such as chest auscultation difficult and unreliable [8,9].

    In most patients who require hyperbaric oxygen either as an emergency treatment or in an intensive care context, intravenous lines should be placed prior to the start of the HBO therapy since insertions within a hyperbaric chamber and especially under hyperbaric conditions is more difficult than under normobaric conditions [8]. Multiplace chambers can differ in a wide range with respect to inner diameter and space (Figure 2). Due to limited space and inadequate illumination, problems with access of peripheral veins can arise. This can be aggravated under hyperbaric conditions due to an oxygen-induced vasoconstriction and less distended peripheral veins or even due to a beginning nitrogen narcosis in the attending physician. In a monoplace chamber all preexisting intravenous lines should be checked prior to start of pressurization, as for obvious reasons there is no direct intervention possible once the treatment has started [10,142,143]. An I.V. line should be placed in all patients who will be treated in a monoplace chamber prior to treatment. When a central venous line is inserted via a subclavian or jugular vein in a patient prior to HBO therapy, a chest X-ray is strongly recommended to exclude any iatrogenic pneumothorax. Furthermore, the place of insertion should be sealed with a self-adhesive plastic drape. Nevertheless, a certain risk for occult pneumothorax during decompression still exists. Therefore, it is safer to place femoral central venous lines should central venous access be required.

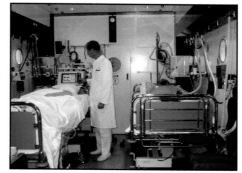

Figure 2. Multiplace Chamber

Very few chambers worldwide offer the opportunity to treat patients with hyperbaric oxygen in their normal clinical bed and with enough space for the attending staff as shown here (picture with kind permission of Dr. A Kemmer, Berufsgenossenschaftliche Unfallklinik (BGU) Murnau, Germany). In most multiplace chambers space is rather limited.

When HBO is performed as part of a surgical treatment protocol, wound drainage is not uncommon. Very often the draining containers are underpressurized to create a suctioning of blood and secretions. Under hyperbaric conditions the ambient overpressure adds to the already high forces which rest on the container walls. This can result in an implosion of the container which may not only injure the patient but can also lead to a widespread and difficult to clean contamination in the chamber [8]. Therefore, it is recommended to vent such containers prior to chamber pressurization and before and during decompression [8]. If from the surgical point of view it is necessary to maintain a vacuum in the wound area, the tubing from the patient to the container should be clamped off before venting and a fresh container with vacuum inside should be ready for a change immediately after the treatment. Using a monoplace chamber, suction can be continued through the chamber door if needed [142,143]. Chest tubes should be removed from drainage and a Heimlich valve inserted instead. Any untreated pneumothorax is a contraindication against HBO therapy.

Comatose patients or combative patients should be adequately sedated, and if indicated, intubated. Patients with altered mental status should be restrained carefully to prevent injuries or pulling out lines or tubes, and therefore sedation and intubation may be necessary as well [8,10,143]. With monoplace chambers, this has to be done before patients are brought into the chamber, but even with multiplace chambers adequate sedation and intubation should be performed before therapy starts and the chamber is pressurized.

Handling of endotracheal tubes in the hyperbaric field needs special emphasis (Figures 3a-3c):

According to Boyle's law the volume of the cuff changes during compression and decompression. Therefore, prior to HBO therapy, air has to be evacuated from the endotracheal cuff, which is then filled with the same amount of liquid to achieve an appropriate seal. In most cases, saline is used to block the cuff, but the use of distilled water has some advantages to saline: during the course of a HBO treatment schedule with intermittent stay on the ICU the cuff will be filled and emptied and refilled again several times, which can cause crystallization in the tubing between cuff and inlet-valve when saline is used. A blocking of this valve can possibly result [8]. Therefore equipment for emergency intubation should be readily available and checked periodically.

The endotracheal tube must be tightly secured and stabilized in place with documentation of its depth, cuff pressures, and bilateral breath sounds. In the multiplace chamber this has to be controlled carefully prior to every change of the chamber pressure, but especially during decompression. Unintended single lung ventilation not only will lead to atelactasis of the contralateral lung, but can also lead to overinflation of the ipsilateral lung with resultant barotraumas (Figure 4). There is heightened risk when the tube is displaced during the therapy. An early sign of overinflation of the lungs can be a sudden drop in blood pressure, because the expanding lung will lead to a decrease in venous return. This should be kept in mind if such an incident occurs, especially coinciding with chamber decompression. Barotrauma of the lung with lung rupture can lead to pneumothorax. An untreated pneumothorax in a hyperbaric atmosphere may easily result in an acute life-threatening tension pneumothorax just by decompression and expanding gases in the pleural space [8]. Therefore, tubing and instruments

Figures 3a-3c: Endotracheal Tubes Under Pressure

Air-filled cuffs of endotracheal tubes can cause problems under pressure, as described in the text. Figures 3a-3c show the behavior of three cuffs under varying conditions.

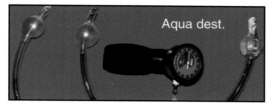

Figure 3a. The cuffs to the left and in the middle were filled with air; the cuff to the right was filled with water (distilled water). The cuff in the middle additionally was connected to a cuff pressure controlling device.

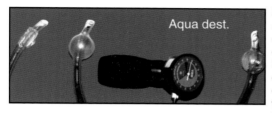

Figure 3b shows the effect of pressurization to 3 bar abs (approx 3 ata). The cuff to the left was compressed as predicted by Boyle's law, which would result in a significant tube leak. The cuff in the middle was continuously adjusted with the controlling device. The water-filled cuff to the right was unchanged.

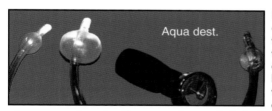

Figure 3c shows the effect of decompression. The air in the cuff to the left expanded again. The air in the cuff in the middle also expanded during decompression, but because of the additional filling due to adjustment at compression, air expanded dramatically. Therefore, close control and adjustment is needed during decompression as well. If this not performed adequately (i.e., due to unawareness or emergencies), rupture of the cuff or even the airways can result. This danger is eliminated when the cuff is filled with fluids as in the right cuff, which again remained unchanged during decompression. (Adopted from [8] with permission.)

for chest tube placement should be ready available inside the chamber, whenever an intubated patient has to be treated in the multiplace chamber.

Intubated patients with endotracheal or tracheostomy tubes are not able to perform a pressure equilibration to their middle ears by using the Valsalva manoeuvre, especially when they are sedated or even paralyzed. An increase in ambient pressure therefore will lead in most cases to barotrauma of the middle ear [8,10,143,146]. Therefore a myringotomy should be performed on all intubated or non-cooperative patients (comatose, altered mental status, intoxicated, children, mental retardation) to prevent middle ear or even inner ear barotraumas [147]. This applies especially to neurosurgical patients due to the pain-induced increase in intracranial pressure which may occur without prior myringotomy [138]. Other authors, however, do not routinely perform prophylactic myringotomies in intubated patients, but try to allow for a slow descent and passive inflation of the middle ear space during compression. When HBO therapy can be planned, the myringotomy should be performed by an ENT specialist in advance. As small incisions into the

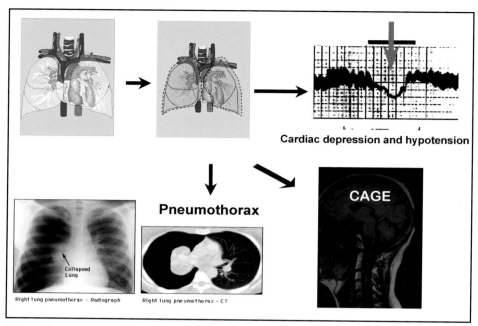

Figure 4.

Overinflation of the lungs during decompression can lead to serious problems. In intubated patients bilateral lung ventilation has to be controlled especially prior to any pressure reduction. Expanding breathing gases which cannot be exhaled due to air-trapping and/or dislocation of the ET-tube will lead to overinflation and pulmonary barotrauma. This may result in cardiac output depression (rapid fall of blood pressure due to impaired venous return), pneumothorax (rupture of alveoli near the pleural space), and/or arterial gas embolism.

tympanic membrane have a tendency to close rapidly, tympanostomy tubes should be placed prophylactically, when more than one HBO therapy is likely. In case of an emergency treatment where myringotomy is deemed necessary, the patient has to be sedated to facilitate the procedure. At most places an otolaryngologic operating microscope will not be accessible, but an otoscope with magnifying lens can be used to visualize the tympanic membrane (Figures 5a and 5b). Local anesthesia can be performed by filling the auditory canal with 2% lidocaine with epinephrine which vasoconstricts bleeding vessels after the myringotomy and offers some local pain relief. After a couple of minutes and removal of the local anesthetic by suctioning, a myringotomy knife is used to perforate the ear drum in the antero-inferior quadrant under direct vision. If a myringotomy knife is not available, a 21 gauge spinal needle can be used as well. Finally, patients after nasal intubation have the potential risk for a ipsilateral barotrauma of the sinuses when HBO therapy has to be performed [8].

Anesthesia and Sedation in the Hyperbaric Environment

General anesthesia with volatile anesthetics is not recommended in hyperbaric medicine [8]. Volatile anesthetics can contaminate the chamber

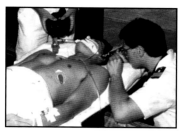 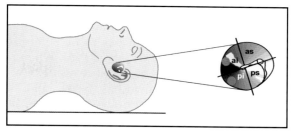

Figures 5a and 5b. Myringotomy

Emergency myringotomy can be performed with an otoscope and a 21 gauge spinal needle as described (5a). The myringotomy should be performed in the lateral anterior inferior (red dot) or posterior inferior quadrant (green dot). The posterior superior quadrant should never be used as in this area there is a serious danger for damage to the ossicles and oval or round window membrane (5b).

atmosphere, leading to impairment of attendants in the multiplace chamber [4,8]. Furthermore, vapors for volatile anesthetics change their characteristics with changes in ambient pressure, so the volume-percentage on the scale differs from that really given [4,148]. Ventilation with nitrous oxide can result in a potential risk of decompression sickness in the patient, and barotrauma may result from gas diffusion into hollow spaces [149-151]. Total intravenous anesthesia (TIVA) can be performed very safely with no unwanted side effects but possible malfunctions of infusion pumps. In hyperbaric medicine, every drug can be used for TIVA, which is in use for prolonged sedation on the ICU as well. Therefore, when deep sedation or general anesthesia is needed, TIVA is strongly recommended [8].

Miscellaneous

Patients with implanted internal pacemakers can undergo hyperbaric oxygen therapy without specific risks. Most manufacturers guarantee normal function up to 3 ata [152], whereas some data suggest no problems at even higher pressures up to 6 ata [153]. Automatic implanted cardiac defibrillators (AICD) can also tolerate pressures up to 6 ata [153]. In patients with external pacemakers, these devices suddenly can fail at 3 to 4 ata, but return to normal function during and after decompression [8,154]. As a pressure of 3 ata is used for the treatment of CO poisoning or necrotizing fasciitis, one should be aware of a potential for malfunction in those patients.

Flow-directed balloon-tipped pulmonary artery (PA) catheters can be used during HBO therapy. Of significant importance is, however, that the balloon at the tip of the catheter must not be inflated during decompression because of the potential risk of a decompression-induced rupture of an inflated balloon and consecutive rupture of the pulmonary artery. Therefore the balloon-port must be unlocked and open to air [8,9].

Monoplace Chamber

As discussed above, a monoplace chamber is pressurized with pure oxygen. Therefore, patients must be gowned in non-static 100% cotton or flame-proof material [10,142,143]. All cosmetics and especially hydrocarbon-based lotions and liquids have to be removed for fire safety reasons. Any item on the patient that can cause sparks such as metal clips or safety pins must be carefully searched for and removed. In chambers which are built in part from acrylic material all metal has to be removed from the patient to prevent scratches inside the acrylic glass [143]. When removal is impossible it has to be covered with cotton sheets and dressings. As there is no direct access to the patient once the treatment has started, all I.V. lines must have been checked. Some cooperative patients suffer from claustrophobia especially when brought into such a chamber for a longer period of time. In these patients, sedation may be required. In comatose or intubated patients, signs of oxygen toxicity, pneumothorax, seizure, or auditory or sinus pain may go unrecognized. It is critical that chamber personnel pay close attention in these patients to airway pressures, tidal volumes, hemodynamic changes, and evidence of auto-PEEP [10]. As with all patients, air breaks should be provided to reduce the risk of oxygen toxicity as outlined above.

Infusion Therapy

Intravenous infusions are provided to compressed patients in the monoplace chamber either by putting the infusion container inside the chamber or by passing the I.V. tubing through the chamber bulkhead via a special sterile I.V. pass-through (Figures 6a and 6b). As the first method has the problem of inadequate control of infusion, in most cases the infusion is pumped through the chamber wall with high-pressure I.V. pumps that permit the controlled delivery of I.V. fluids [142,143].

It should be mentioned, however, that monoplace chambers have a limited number of intravenous pass-through ports. Therefore careful planning of which drugs and solutions are really necessary during HBO therapy is required and eliminating unnecessary infusions that can be withheld during HBO or combining infusion lines should be considered. Weaver et al. [142,143] described specially constructed split-bolt path-throughs which allow up to four I.V. tubings to come out of one port.

The IVAC 530 and the Abbot Shaw Hyperbaric Pump for monoplace chambers can generate sufficient pressures to infuse I.V. solutions into patients compressed to 3 ata. These pumps both have inaccuracies at very low and high infusion rates, especially at chamber pressures exceeding 2 ata [10]. The IVAC pump is a pulsatile pump, so amount infused depends on the pump rate and the drip chamber type. The Abbot is a volumetric pump with certain inaccuracies under elevated pressure, which can be adjusted to the desired rate by the attending physician.

As there is no direct access possible it is critical to have a one-way or back-check valve to prevent retrograde blood return in case of I.V. line disconnect outside the chamber. In addition, only Luer-lock pressure tubing should be used inside the chamber [10,143].

Because of the large dead-space between the patient and the injection site outside the chamber, a certain risk for overshooting exists with bolus injections. Therefore, the I.V. lines should be carefully flushed.

Patient monitoring in the monoplace chamber

Most monoplace chambers allow for direct observation of the patients. ECG can be monitored by placing electrocardiographic leads on the

Figures 6a and 6b show the setup for Infusion therapy by passing the I.V. tubing through the chamber bulkhead via special pass-throughs.

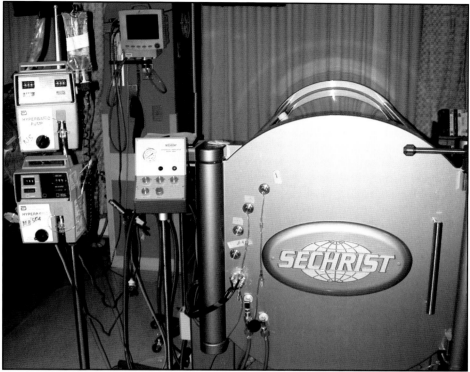

Figure 6a. On the left side two Abott Hyperbaric pumps can be seen, connected to the patient inside the chamber (right) with pass-throughs. In the middle the ventilator control panel of a Sechrist 500A ventilator can be seen.

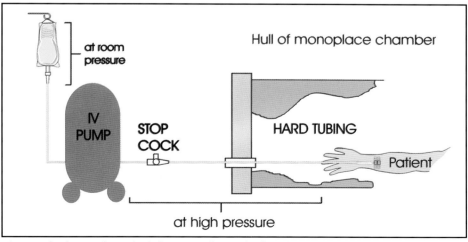

Figure 6b shows the principle as a schematic drawing.

patient, which pass out of the chamber via an electrical pass-through, and are connected to a standard monitor. In intensive care patients arterial blood pressure is generally measured by an indwelling arterial catheter connected to a pressure transducer through which an electrical signal is passed out of the chamber to a physiological monitor (Figure 7). The catheter and transducer are continually flushed with sterile saline at 3 ml per hour by a flush device. The pressure transducer should be zeroed prior to commencement of HBO therapy. The arterial line also permits arterial blood gas sampling during HBO therapy as described in detail by Weaver et al. [143,155]. The arterial waveform should be inspected for its dynamic response by ascertaining that there are no air bubbles or obstructions of the tubing that can alter the signal transduction. As an alternative to invasive blood pressure monitoring, non-invasive Doppler blood pressure monitoring in the monoplace chamber has been found to be adequate as well [156].

Intracranial pressure (ICP) monitoring has been performed under hyperbaric conditions on patients who suffered traumatic brain injury. The transducer used is analogous to invasive arterial pressure systems. Electroencephalogram monitoring can also be done in the chamber when needed and the signal can be passed out of the chamber via the 19-pin electrical pass-throughs [10].

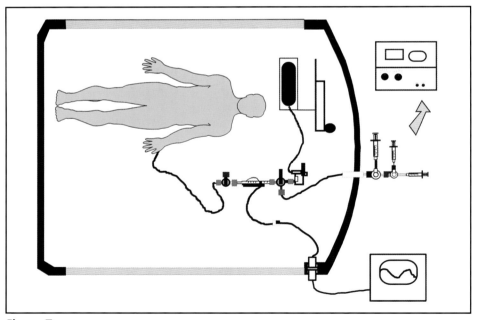

Figure 7.

Schematic representation of a system for invasive blood pressure monitoring and aspiration of arterial blood from a patient in a monoplace chamber. In this set-up both aspiration as well as the monitor screen are placed outside the chamber. Although designed for monoplace chambers, the system is suitable for multiplace chambers as well. (Redrawn and adopted from Dr. LK Weaver [143] with kind permission.)

In mechanically ventilated patients several respiratory variables are to be monitored during HBO. Ventilatory rate, expired volume, PEEP, and peak airway pressure are often displayed on the ventilator, but should nevertheless be continuously controlled by the attending physician. Alarms for pressure and rates should be calibrated and adjusted. End tidal carbon dioxide can be followed during HBO and may provide useful information regarding the adequacy of alveolar ventilation. $EtCO_2$ can be used to adjust the mechanical ventilator but it must be kept in mind that a substantial arterial-end tidal PCO_2 gradient may arise when acute lung injury is present. Arterial blood gases of patients treated with HBO can be monitored but require a set-up permitting aspiration of arterial blood in the pressurized chamber (Figure 7) [155,157]. It is important to use luer-lock connections and hard-pressure tubing. In addition, minimizing the dead-space volume in the lines and the transducer is important, as at least five times the system dead-space has to be drawn before the blood sample is obtained [143]. When flushing the system, it is important to ensure that air is not entrained, as this not only dampens the wave form but can also cause gas embolism. The ABL 330 (Radiometer) has been proven to operate with oxygen partial pressures up to 2200 mmHg [155].

The use of transcutaneous PO_2 ($PtcO_2$) sensors, which are frequently used in hyperbaric medicine for other reasons, can give rough information on adequate oxygenation as well. It has been performed mainly on lower extremity vascular diseases, diabetic feet, and in mechanical trauma to vessels where it may help to predict the response to HBO in problem wounds [158].

Suctioning

As outlined above, wound drainage and redon drains are not uncommon in surgical patients for suctioning of blood and secretion. Whenever possible, handling of drainage should be performed as described earlier. Whenever necessary suctioning should be performed as described by Weaver et al. [142,143]: an Ohmeda vacuum regulator and suction canister are mounted on an aluminum plate that hangs within the chamber on the hatch ventilator bracket. The Sechrist 500A ventilator can be used concurrently with the suction system. The vacuum hose that drives the regulator is passed out of the chamber via a specially constructed pass-through port. Intravenous passports can be used as well. The pressure gradient necessary to operate the vacuum regulator is provided by the pressurized chamber, but caution must be used to make sure that the regulator should never be turned to "full" but rather to the "regulate" position. The pass-through outside the chamber is connected to a three-way stopcock or to an adjustable flow control valve. The degree of vacuum can be adjusted by the attendant outside the chamber. The authors emphasize that a 20-gauge blunt needle should be inserted between the regulator and the suction canister to vent the degree of vacuum [142,143].

This suction system allows nasogastric, oral, wound, or pleural suction during HBO therapy but should not be used for endotracheal suction because there is a potential for complications including negative pressure pulmonary edema, negative pressure barotraumas of the lungs, and airway bleeding.

Ventilation

Intensivists need to know that the mechanical ventilators in use with HBO in a monoplace chamber do not meet the requirements demanded of modern ventilators in intensive care units, as they are rather simply designed and unable to offer most of the features used in modern ventilatory therapy. In most cases, just controlled ventilation is possible (IPPV mode), similar to those simple ventilators used for transportation purposes. Because of the very limited options in ventilation modes and the very special situation especially in monoplace chambers with little opportunity to interfere, most ventilated patients will require deep sedation or even muscle relaxation. This is in clear contrast to modern respiratory care strategies where, under optimized circumstances, relaxation of the ventilated patient should be avoided.

There are two types of ventilators in the U.S. for monoplace chambers: the Sechrist 500A hyperbaric ventilator and the Omni-Vent. The 500A circuit is located inside the chamber hatch (Figure 8) while the ventilator controls are located outside the chamber (Figure 9). The 500A is a pneumatic, time-cycled ventilator that permits adjustments for flow, inspiratory time, and expiratory time. When the ventilator cycles, O_2 moves through the ventilator control unit into the ventilator block supply hose and into the ventilator block, simultaneously closing the exhalation valve to augment tidal volume. Tidal volume is measured with a spirometer also located inside the chamber (Figure 8) and connected to the expiratory limb of the ventilator circuit. Some of the oxygen is routed through a water-filled nebulizer to provide humidity to the inspiratory circuit. PEEP is provided by placing PEEP valves into the expiratory circuit, but "occult" PEEP with chamber pressurization has been reported [159]. The peak pressure pop-off valve of the 500A ventilator should be adjusted prior to use for each patient. A one-way valve permits the patient to inspire. In a modified version the 500A ventilator can deliver air breaks as well. The 500A ventilator operates in a controlled mode only, so in order to reduce patient-ventilator asynchrony resulting in auto-PEEP and gas trapping, patients have to be sedated. For optimal ventilator performance, the ventilator driving pressure exceeds the wall pressure for oxygen of most hospitals, so an auxiliary gas source by, for example, gas cylinders is recommended [10,142]. With very high ventilatory volumes (>10 l/min), the 500A uses an inverted expiratory ratio, with the inspiratory time exceeding the expiratory time. This may cause auto-PEEP and air-trapping, leading to hypotension. In this case, the I:E ratio has to be reduced by increasing expiratory time [10].

The other ventilator in use with monoplace chambers is

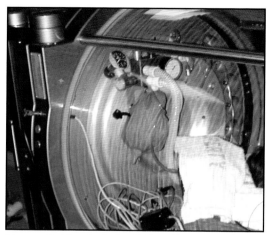

Figure 8. The Sechrist 500A Circuit Inside the Chamber

the Omni-Vent, a pneumatic ventilator with controls for

inspiratory time, expiratory time, and flow [142]. The airway port of the Omni-Vent can be passed through the chamber hatch. Inside the chamber, a peak pressure pop-off valve needs to be adjusted to 10 to 15 cm H_2O above the patient's peak airway pressure. A manometer located inside the chamber measures airway pressures. The exhalation valve tubing needs to be passed through another hatch penetrator. According to Weaver it is crucial that there is no disruption of the high-pressure circuit between the chamber hatch and the ventilator while a patient is compressed in the chamber and mechanically ventilated with the Omni-Vent [142,160]. A one-way valve needs to be installed inside the chamber or at the hatch connection to prevent gas backflow in the event of a disruption of the airway circuit external to the chamber. Weaver explicitly points out that without these safeguards, potential serious harm could ensue. The Omni-Vent also requires operation pressures which are generally in excess of the hospital supply. Air breaks can easily be accomplished by switching the ventilator's driving gas to air.

Cardiopulmonary Resuscitation (CPR)

CPR can only be performed outside the chamber. In case of an emergency with immediate need for CPR, the monoplace chamber can be decompressed at any time without the risk for decompression sickness as the patient breathes pure oxygen with minimal saturation of nitrogen during air breaks and quick wash-out when oxygen breathing is resumed.

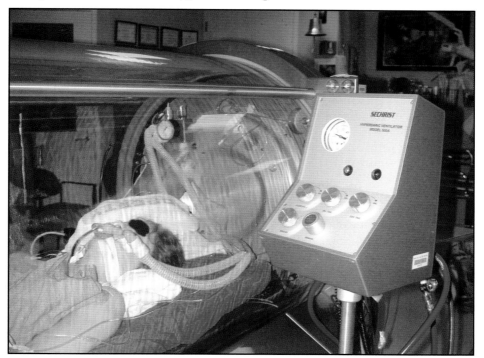

Figure 9. Ventilated Patient in a Monoplace Chamber with the Sechrist 500A Ventilator

The 500A circuit is located inside the chamber hatch (left) while the ventilator controls are located outside the chamber (right).

A potential risk remains for pulmonary barotrauma, especially when the emergency coincides with an oxygen-induced seizure or with displaced endotracheal tubes.

As soon as the chamber is totally decompressed, the patient can be taken out and CPR performed. When external defibrillation is needed as well, the patient has to be removed from the chamber. It is not enough to just remove him partially, as oxygen flowing out of the chamber increases the risk of fire (Figure 10).

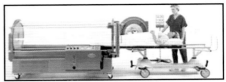

Figure 10. Evacuation of Patients from a Monoplace Chamber

In case of emergencies, especially when a cardiac defibrillation has to be performed, an evacuation of the patient to the extent shown in this figure is insufficient with still a high risk of fire. Due to out-flow of oxygen from the chamber the patient is surrounded by oxygen-enriched air, causing a remaining explosion hazard. Therefore, patients have to be removed completely from the chamber. (Figure with kind permission of Sechrist Industries.)

Multiplace Chambers

A number of practical aspects have to be considered when critically ill patients are treated with HBO in a multiplace chamber. First of all, even in multiplace "walk-in" chambers physicians and nurses attending the patient are not able to freely move because of limited space. For obvious reasons, simply going in or out of the chamber is impossible, and therefore equipment, medications, etc. can only be moved into or out of the chamber via a transfer lock, which requires careful planning of what is really needed. In addition, even experienced personnel may exhibit impaired physical or psychologic performance, as already mentioned.

Multiplace chambers are pressurized with air and patients breathe oxygen under pressure through special devices. Therefore the fire hazard in a multiplace chamber is reduced when compared to monoplace chambers, but nevertheless is still present. Contamination of the multiplace chamber's atmosphere with oxygen must be avoided as this dramatically increases the risk for fire (Figure 11).

Practical Considerations

Only few multiplace chambers are big enough to allow the patient to stay in a normal hospital bed (Figure 2). In most cases, special stretchers are used which are designed to fit perfectly into the chamber. When a patient is transferred from his bed to such a stretcher, special attention has to be paid to any drainage or tubing. Endotracheal tubes must be inspected after such transfers. Even when the chamber itself and/or the opening allow the use of the normal bed, high-tech beds commonly used in ICU units may not be suitable for hyperbaric conditions. Especially those which inflate or create vacuum can present with severe malfunction, and any electronic device not encapsulated or specially adapted for high ambient pressures can be a problem source. Furthermore, only equipment specifically designed for use in the hyperbaric environment, or tested for that specific purpose, should be used. As only very few devices meet that criterion, the following precautions should be made: All equipment used in the chamber should have a power supply

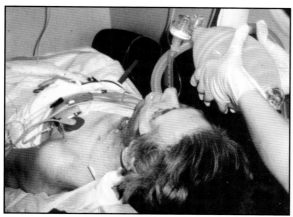

Figure 11. Bag-to-Tube Ventilation

Intubated patients may be ventilated by bag-to-tube ventilation during transportation, or in rare occasions even during therapy. In this case it is crucial that the bag is equipped with a device which ensures that the exhaled gas is vented out of the chamber and cannot contaminate the chamber atmosphere, as the exhaled gas is still oxygen-rich and increases the risk of fire. The situation shown in Figure 11 is only allowed prior or post treatment with the chamber door wide open.

independent from the main power supply. Therefore it should run on battery or accumulator or on direct current, which in the best case is a dual power supply. In addition, all are required to be waterproof, explosion proof, and protected from the sprinkler system of the chamber. Finally, monitors must work effectively with the electrical module on the outside, connected to the patient through dedicated penetrations in the chamber wall [8,9].

Venous Lines

In the hyperbaric chamber special emphasis must be paid to I.V. lines as disconnected lines can be the source of severe gas embolization [161]. Although this is especially relevant for central venous lines [162] it has importance for lines in peripheral veins as well [163]. According to Boyle's law entrance of even small amounts of gas into the vessels under hyperbaric conditions can cause severe injury during decompression just by expansion of the gas bubbles. For the same reasons the fittings of two- or three-way stopcocks should be evacuated by suctioning fluid when I.V. medications are to be injected to avoid iatrogenic entry of gas bubbles.

Fluid Management and Infusion Therapy

During HBO therapy the fluid management per se does not differ from that outside a chamber. However, the technique of fluid administration itself can raise certain problems.

Fluid administration by gravity

The use of glass bottles with intravenous fluids should be avoided and fluids contained in plastic bags or bottles should be used instead [8] (Figures 12a-12c). The major problem with gravity-driven systems is that massive gas embolism can result during decompression: for every volume of fluid an equal amount of atmospheric gas will enter the bottle through a little outlet in the drip chamber. Under hyperbaric conditions this gas will expand during decompression and increase its volume depending on the treatment schedule up to 3-fold. This will result in an overpressurization of the fluid container. This overpressurization can lead to a forced infusion of the remaining fluids and, when the container emptied but still under pressure, the remaining gas will be infused as well (Figures 12a-12c). Therefore all containers for intravenous fluids must be vented. Especially nonvented glass containers can be potentially dangerous for additional reasons: implosion during compression or explosion during decompression are the possible risks. The easiest way to avoid such problems is to ban glass containers for intravenous fluids from hyperbaric chambers, and to vent plastic bags and bottles with a syringe needle on the upper side, so a pressure equilibration between inside the bottle and surrounding atmosphere is guaranteed.

The use of flow-controlled automatic infusion pumps for accurate fluid administration is possible as well, when the device is equipped with a battery as a power supply for minimized risk of fire (Figure 13). Nevertheless, technical problems can arise since not all commercially available devices function well during hyperbaric conditions and some pumps are unable to operate under hyperbaric conditions at all [164-169]. Several factors affect the accurate performance of infusion pumps under high ambient pressure, such as possible depression of electronic components and the control buttons (especially with soft touch buttons) whenever an air pocket is present. Such air pockets will respond to pressure changes and can lead to malfunction [8,165]. Lavon and co-workers [165] reported that the Graseby 3100 syringe pump did not meet the performance criterion, since at chamber pressures of 2.5 ata and higher (treatment pressures, frequently met in emergency treatment schedules) the infusion rate could not be changed, and no response could be elicited to any other control panel key. The same study reports that the Easy-pump MZ-257 failed to function completely beyond a chamber pressure of 1.4 ata, making it unsuitable for use inside the hyperbaric chamber, while the Imed 965 exhibited an acceptable volume deviation during most hyperbaric conditions. During the compression phase of the profiles used and for low infusion rates only, exceptional volume deviations of 20-40% were monitored with this device. The Infutec 520 demonstrated an acceptable deviation (within 10%) throughout all the hyperbaric profiles used which was unaffected by changes in ambient pressure or infusion rate. In addition, Ray and co-workers [166] reported that the Baxter Flo-Gard 6201 infusion pump demonstrated acceptable performance for infusing saline, enteral formula, and PRBC at low and high infusion rates into the pressurized monoplace hyperbaric chamber up to 3 ata, with the exception of low flow rates during compression and decompression.

It was also reported by Sanchez-Guijo et al. [169] that patient controlled analgesia pumps (PCA) can fail under hyperbaric conditions, which in a best case scenario can result in malfunction, and in a worst case can result in a severe drug overdose. Analgesia therefore should be performed by bolus dose as required or by continuous infusion with a suitable and tested device.

Monitoring the Patient

Non-invasive blood pressure monitoring is certainly more difficult during HBO treatment because of noise within the chamber as well as altered acoustic properties of compressed air, but it is possible with the limitation that sphygmomanometers still using mercury should be banned [4,8,9]. By using pressure transducer cables plumbed through the chamber wall to preamplifiers kept outside, any invasive pressure as well as ECG-monitoring is possible [9,170]. The display should be visible from inside through a porthole.

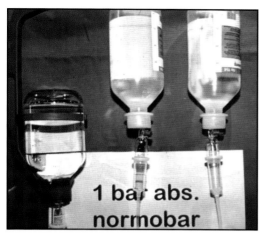

Figures 12a–12c demonstrate fluid administration by gravity. Shown is the effect of pressurization and decompression on a fluid container made from glass (to the left) and a vented (middle) and unvented (right) plastic container.

Figure 12a shows the normobaric situation at 1 bar abs (approx 1 ata). All containers were equipped with a flow-controlling device and adjusted to the same outlet flow. The plastic container in the middle was vented with a syringe needle.

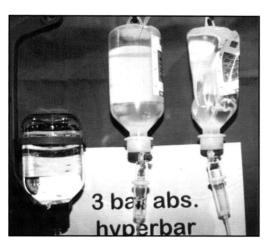

Figure 12b. Containers after compression to 3 bar abs (3 ata, Boerema table). The glass container to the left seems to be unchanged. The container in the middle was enabled to perform a pressure equilibration via the syringe needle (clearly seen now). The container to the left shows pressure induced deformation.

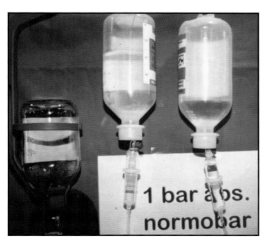

Figure 12c. After decompression, the glass bottle was empty. The fluid was forced out of the bottle by expanding air with enormous power not only through the regular tubing but also through the equilibration valve. The dark spot in the background is wet cotton. With this glass bottle a venous gas embolism would have resulted in a patient. The vented plastic container in the middle shows the amount of fluid which had really been used. The plastic canister to the right is almost empty with high pressure inside. Due to expanding deformation some of the driving force could be equalized. A potential risk for venous gas embolism is obvious as well. (From [8] with permission.)

For invasive blood pressure monitoring, rezeroing of the transducers after compression is recommended because of potential temperature-induced offset [9]. The indwelling arterial catheter is continuously flushed as described in the monoplace section. In the multiplace the plastic bag with saline used for flushing can be taken into the chamber. As in this setup the bag is compressible, air is evacuated from the bag anyway, and no venting mechanism exists in the tubing, venting of this system as described for venous infusion is not needed. Continuous flushing is performed by a pressure bag, which surrounds the saline container and is pumped to approx. 300 mmHg with air. Due to compression in the chamber this pressure bag has to be refilled under pressure. It has to be kept in mind, however, that this additional portion of air needed while under pressure will expand massively during decompression. Therefore, the manometer of the pressure bag has to be controlled carefully during decompression, and the bag pressure has to be adjusted to prevent the bag from overinflation or even explosion.

Blood sampling requires meticulous attention to avoid bubbles, but it must be remembered that sample decompression in a transfer lock produces bubbles and may thereby render analysis impossible [9]. With very slow decompression rates in the transfer lock, bubbling can be minimized, but any bubbling will lead to false low values of oxygen partial pressure.

In contrast, pH and PCO_2 values are interpretable, as minimal changes will occur [143].

Accurate measurement of PO_2 requires a blood gas machine operated and calibrated at ambient pressure of the chamber. Furthermore, blood gas measurements require blood sampling with aspiration from outside of the pressurized chamber as described for monoplace chambers [142,143,155]. As this is limited to very few centers, the already mentioned very slow decompression has to be performed. Weaver and co-authors have shown that PO_2 values can be measured reasonably accurately if the sample is processed immediately after decompression [155]. At least for clinical purposes it may not be necessary to have more than 10% to 20% accuracy under hyperbaric conditions. Whether commercially available blood gas analyzers allow to measure blood PO_2 values as high as 2.000 mmHg has up to now only been demonstrated for the radiometer ABL 330 [155].

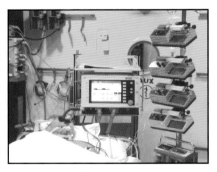

Figure 13. Flow-Controlled Automatic Infusion Pumps for Accurate Fluid Administration under Hyperbaric Conditions in a Multiplace Chamber

Accurate fluid administration with automatic infusion pumps inside the chamber (left side). The devices are equipped with batteries as power supplies for minimized risk of fire and do not have any soft-touch control buttons. Note the Dräger Evita 4 ventilator in the background. Although this ventilator meets all requirements for modern respiratory care strategies and obviously seems to work even under hyperbaric conditions, it has to be stated, however, that there only exists this single prototype for hyperbaric use. The Evita 4 designed for clinical use only are NOT suitable for use in the hyperbaric field. (Picture with kind permission of Dr. Kemmer, BGU Murnau, Germany.)

While SaO_2 monitoring with pulse oximetry is only of limited value in the hyperbaric field, the use of transcutaneous PO_2 and PCO_2 ($TCPO_2$ and $TCPCO_2$) sensors, which are frequently used in hyperbaric medicine for other reasons, can give rough information on adequate oxygenation as already described in the monoplace section.

Advanced Cardiac Life Support and Cardiopulmonary Resuscitation (CPR)

CPR requires the consideration of some practical aspects. To perform chest compressions adequately and over longer periods of time, excessive physical exercise is done. This physical effort may be of concern since the density-induced expiratory flow limitation will reduce the maximal physical effort sustainable by the personnel. In any case, since the attending physicians and nursing staff will normally breathe air, physical exercise under hyperbaric conditions will lead to substantially increased upload of the body tissues with nitrogen (like in scuba divers) [80]. This must be kept in mind in decompression: either the attending staff inside the chamber starts to breathe oxygen via the built-in-breathing systems at a very early time, or decompression stops are necessary to prevent the staff from suffering decompression injury. An early start of oxygen breathing while still under therapeutical pressure implicates a certain risk of central nervous oxygen toxicity with generalized convulsions [65], but decompression stops will lead to a longer time until the patient can be brought outside the chamber. The best way is to stop the hyperbaric treatment when CPR is necessary and to decompress slowly with attendants breathing oxygen from 1.9 ata until reaching surface pressure. When CPR has to be performed, in most cases ventilation of the patient will be by bag-to-mouth or, when intubated, with bag-to-tube. As stated earlier, in this case a specially equipped resuscitation bag is strongly recommended, because exhaled gas should not be released into the chamber atmosphere but led into the scavenging system of the chamber (Figure 11). Otherwise a contamination of the chamber with high oxygen levels is very likely, thereby increasing the risk of fire.

Drug therapy can be performed as usual, although due to vasoconstriction a physiologic response can be delayed [171].

Defibrillation

Some hyperbaric physicians reported anecdotally that cardiac defibrillation inside a multiplace chamber is possible. Although multiplace chambers with an upper oxygen limit of 23% have a certain safety margin, problems associated with defibrillation inside a chamber include the risk of fire and explosion along with equipment malfunction, i.e., cathode ray screen implosion. Therefore, the defibrillator itself should be placed outside the chamber, and the leads with the defibrillation pads should be lead through an electrical porthole inside the chamber. In a CPR situation the risk of fire is even increased, as contamination of the atmosphere in the chamber with oxygen is not completely avoidable. Some authorities therefore recommend that during defibrillation, one inside attendant wears an emergency breathing apparatus and readies the fire hose while defibrillation is proceeding. With the defibrillator outside the chamber and leads extending through the chamber wall via dedicated penetrations to specially designed gelled monitoring defibrillation pads, the fire hazard is minimized. Nevertheless, the safest approach is to decompress while performing conventional CPR and to defibrillate in the unpressurized chamber with the door wide open.

Mechanical Ventilation

Breathing is more difficult at higher pressures because gas density is increased in direct proportion to absolute pressure and this movement of denser air requires more effort (work) to move [35,36,37,172]. Consequently, increased respiratory resistance at depth leads to increased energy cost of breathing which may result in increased oxygen demand, carbon dioxide retention, dyspnoea, and in some cases adverse cardiovascular reactions. Critically ill patients may exhibit increased metabolic demand, and the work of breathing in these patients may be further increased due to reduced lung compliance [173]. Therefore spontaneous breathing under hyperbaric conditions can lead to respiratory muscle fatigue in ICU patients. The hypoventilation with a consecutive increase in arterial PCO_2 that may occur in this situation can create additional excessive work of breathing. In clinical practice it is therefore recommended to always use an inspiratory pressure support or increase the level of a preexisting pressure support in intubated, spontaneously breathing patients.

The higher density of the inspiratory gas in the hyperbaric environment raises the demands on the function of mechanical ventilators [174]. According to Boyle's Law the volume of a given mass of a gas varies inversely with the absolute pressure at constant temperature. In monoplace chambers the function of any ventilator placed outside the chamber is limited by this law: as the pressure within the chamber increases the tidal volume delivered diminishes. Gas flow rates are proportional to the gas density so that in the hyperbaric chamber the flow rate will fall as the ambient pressure increases. Hence, since ventilators are designed for use in a normal atmospheric environment, their normal function is disturbed at increased ambient pressure in most cases. For this reason expiratory volumes should be measured (Figure 14) and $ETCO_2$ monitoring should be performed under hyperbaric conditions. Performing this standard monitoring of the operating room and the ICU may present fundamental problems in the hyperbaric environment. Mainstream capnometry (with the detector placed at the ISO connector of the endotracheal tube) becomes grossly erroneous since the infrared absorption characteristics of CO_2 are modified with increased gas density [8]. In contrast side stream capnometry is reliable as it can be performed outside the chamber. Unfortunately a rather complex passing of the sampling tubes through the chamber wall is mandatory [8].

Ventilators Under Pressure

A number of artificial respirators can be used in the hyperbaric chamber, but it is important to know that pressure-cycled ones have to be continuously adjusted in rate and cycling pressure with the varying ambient pressure [3,8,9]. Volume-cycled respirators therefore are superior, and several devices have been tested under hyperbaric conditions [9]. ICU respirator therapy is highly sophisticated and so are modern ventilators. Most of the respirators used in the hyperbaric field do not meet the standards set in the

ICU, but are comparable to those used for transportation of ventilated patients. During the last three decades several respirators have been tested.

In 1982 Saywood and co-workers [175] reported on the function of the Oxford Ventilator at high pressure. The ventilator functioned well to 6 atmospheres absolute in an air environment and even to 31 atmospheres absolute in an oxyhelium environment, as assessed remotely utilizing a lung ventilator performance analyzer. In the opinion of the authors it features easily comprehensible controls and functions, and its use in prolonged ventilatory support could be taught to non-anaesthetists with relative ease. In addition to its relative simplicity, it is reported as reliable, readily available, and requires only fitting with a male Schrader valve for use at high pressures. The authors recommend the ventilator therefore for ventilatory support under extreme hyperbaric conditions.

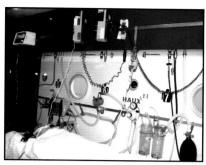

Figure 14. Ventilated Patient in a Multiplace Chamber

The patient is ventilated by a Dräger Oxylog 2000 Ventilator. Because of pressure-induced shift of the tidal volume a volumeter inserted in the exhalation tubing, so the ventilator can be adjusted to deliver controlled tidal volumes. Suctioning is possible with an adapted suctioning device. (With kind permission of Dr. A. Kemmer, BGU Murnau, Germany.)

In 1986 Moon et al. [176] tested the Monaghan 225 ventilator at ambient pressures of up to 6 atmospheres absolute (ata). The tidal volume delivered was independent of ambient pressure. At 6 ata, the ventilatory rate was 45 percent of the preset rate at 1 ata. By decreasing the circuit resistance and increasing the inspiratory flow rate, the 6 ata rate could be increased to 72 percent of the 1 ata value. The maximum minute ventilation of the ventilator at 1 ata was approximately 48 L/min; at 6 ata, its maximum was 18 L/min. Synchronized intermittent mandatory ventilation, assist/control, and PEEP functions were satisfactory at 6 ata. While using 100 percent O_2 to power the ventilator at 2.82 ata, the oxygen leakage was 57.7 L/min (converted to 1 ata pressure, 20 degrees C), of which 33.7 L/min was successfully scavenged using simple techniques. A minor modification was made to the ventilator, allowing it to be driven by compressed air while maintaining complete flexibility in setting the FIO_2. The ventilator has proven stable and reliable in clinical use at ambient pressures up to 6 ata.

In 1991, Lewis et al. [177] reported on the use of the Penlon Nuffield 200 which was modified for use in a monoplace hyperbaric oxygen chamber by feeding back the chamber pressure to the reducing valve. As reported, this provides a compensating mechanism, allowing the ventilator to deliver adequate tidal volumes at pressures of up to 3 atmospheres. Although compensation is not complete the authors conclude that modification is adequate for short-term clinical use in patients in whom the airway is compromised but who need hyperbaric oxygen therapy.

Spittal et al. in 1991 [178] gave a short report on the performance of the pneuPAC Hyperbaric variant HB, a ventilator designed for use in a monoplace hyperbaric chamber. In this report the ventilator delivered minute volumes of 11-23 liters at 1 ata. These volumes decreased due to compression to 7.6-16 liters at 2.5 ata. The authors described that the delivered minute volume can be adjusted from outside the chamber by manipulation of the ventilator rate.

Finally, Stahl and co-workers recently evaluated the function of four currently available [179], not specifically modified time-cycled ICU ventilators (EVITA 4, Oxylog 2000 HBO and Microvent from Drägerwerk, Germany, and Servo 900C, Siemens-Elema, Sweden) under hyperbaric conditions using volume-controlled ventilation (VCV) and, if available, pressure-controlled ventilation (PCV). All ventilators were studied on an electromechanical lung simulator consisting of a motor driven bellows (LS 1500, Drägerwerk, Germany) at normobaric (1 ata) and hyperbaric ambient pressures (1.3, 1.6, 1.9, 2.8 ata). Servo 900C and Microvent were additionally tested at 6 ata. During VCV the tidal volume (VT) was set at 750 ml at normobaric conditions prior to starting hyperbaric exposure. During PCV the same VT setting was achieved by adjusting the inspiratory pressure level. Ambient pressure airway pressure (measured inside the bellows) and flow (derived from the linear displacement of the bellows) were registered. From these data off-line VT, inspiratory airway peak and plateau pressure (Ppeak and Pplateau) and, during PCV only, peak inspiratory flow (Vmax) and the time delay between onset of and peak inspiratory flow (Vdelay) were calculated. During VCV inspiratory flow VT consequently consistently decreased with increasing ambient pressure. In contrast, during PCV VT remained stable at each chamber pressure despite a slight decrease in Vmax. The authors conclude that, whenever available, PCV should be preferentially used during hyperbaric oxygen therapy due to the stability of ventilator function. Based on the specific ventilator properties at increasing ambient pressures, appropriate correction tables are mandatory allow the safe use of ICU ventilators during VCV, but limitations for these corrections are to be expected with increasing respiratory rates at ambient pressures beyond 3 ata.

More ventilators for hyperbaric use:

- *Dräger Hyperlog (Drägerwerke, Lübbeck, Germany)* (Figure 15)
  The Dräger Hyperlog which basically is an adaptation of the Oxylog for the use in the hyperbaric chamber was the first artificial ventilator to be especially designed for this purpose. As an emergency respirator it is suitable only for mechanical ventilation in adults and children < 5kg. This pneumatically driven, time-cycled device has no alarms and only provides volume-controlled ventilation at ambient pressures of up to 6 ata. Ventilator settings are minute volume and respiratory rate, PEEP ventilation is possible with an additional valve hooked onto the expiratory limb.

- *The Oxylog 2000 Hyperbar (Drägerwerke, Lübeck, Germany)* is an adaptation of the time-volume cycled emergency and transport ventilator Oxylog 2000 for use under increased ambient pressures. It provides IPPV, SIMV and spontaneous breathing with CPAP as ventilatory modes, the inspiration/expiration time ratio as well as the PEEP level can be freely set, and airway pressures and expiratory minute volume are displayed. It can be distinguished from the Oxylog 2000 because of a correction table on the device which allows for ambient pressure-dependent correction of the tidal volume.

- *EKU MAV3-H (Hyperbar) Ventilator* (Figure 16)
  This device (EKU Elektronik GmbH, Leiningen, Germany) was specially designed for use under hyperbaric conditions. Therefore emphasis was made on high flow rates and automatic correction of the pressure-dependent decrease in tidal volume, and in fact, the respirator automatically adapts to varying ambient pressure. Ventilator settings are volume- as well as pressure-controlled ventilation, PEEP, and inspiratory pressure support during spontaneous ventilation.

- *The Servo 900C (Siemens-Elema, Sweden)* (Figure 17) is well known in intensive care medicine and is certainly the device for which most experience under hyperbaric conditions is available. The Servo 900C is well adapted to any requirement for ventilator therapy of ICU patients undergoing HBO treatment. For use in hyperbaric chambers the pneumatic and electronic parts are separated from each other so that all ventilator settings are made outside the chamber. Therefore well-trained attending personnel both within and outside the chamber is required if this ventilator is used.

In conclusion, hyperbaric oxygen may be an important therapeutic modality for the intensive care patient. However, the hyperbaric environment presents many unique challenges in the care of the critically ill patient. To administer HBOT safely to these patients, a thorough understanding of the physical and physiologic changes is essential.

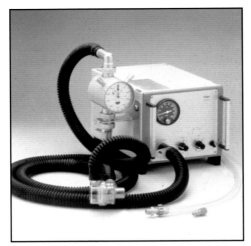

Figure 15. Dräger Hyperlog – Ventilator

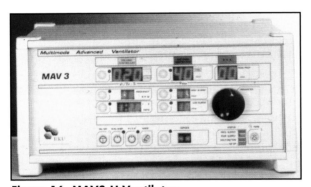

Figure 16. MAV3-H Ventilator

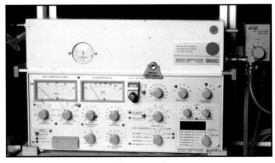

Figure 17. Servo 900C Ventilator

REFERENCES

1. Tibbles PM, Edelsberg JS. Hyperbaric oxygen therapy. N Engl J Med 1996;334:1642-1648

2. UHMS Hyperbaric Oxygen Therapy 1999- Committee report. Undersea & Hyperbaric Medical Society, Kensington, 1999

3. Frey G, Lampl L, Radermacher P, Bock KH. Hyperbare Oxygenation - Ein Betätigungsfeld für Anästhesisten? Anaesthesist 1998;47:269-289

4. Moon RE, Camporesi EM. Clinical care in the hyperbaric environment. In: Miller RD (Ed.) Anesthesia third edition, Vol. 2. Churchill Livingstone 1990; pp. 2089-2111

5. Slotman GJ. Hyperbaric oxygen in systemic inflammation ... HBO is not just a movie channel anymore. Crit Care Med 1998;26:1932-3

6. Holcomb JR, Matos-Navarro AY, Goldmann RW. Critical Care in the hyperbaric chamber. In: Davis JC, Hunt TK(eds): Problem Wounds: The role of oxygen. Elsevier 1988 pp.187-209

7. Kluger M. Implications of hyperbaric medicine for Anaesthesia and Intensive Care. SPUMS Journal 1997;27:62-73

8. Muth CM. Intensivmedizin unter hyperbaren Bedingungen. In: Almeling M, Böhm F, Welslau W (Eds): Handbuch Tauch- und Hyperbarmedizin. Ecomed Landsberg, Germany, 1998 IV-4.3, pp 1-26

9. Radermacher P, Frey G, Berger R. Hyperbaric oxygen therapy - intensive care in a hostile environment? In: Vincent JL (Ed) Yearbook of Intensive Care and Emergency Medicine 1997. Springer 1997, 821-835

10. Barach P. Management of the critically ill patient in the hyperbaric chamber. Int Anesthesiol Clin. 2000; 38:153-66

11. Nunn JF. Oxygen. In: Nunn JF: Nunn's Applied Respiratory Physiology. Butterworth-Heinemann, London, 1993; pp 255-287

12. Oriani G, Michael M, Marroni A, Longoni C. Physiology and physiopathology of hyperbaric oxygen. In: Oriani G, Marroni A, Wattel F (Eds.): Handbook on Hyperbaric Medicine. Springer, Berlin, 1996; pp 1-34

13. Camporesi EM, Mascia MF, Thom SR. Physiological principles of hyperbaric oxygenation. In: Oriani G, Marroni A, Wattel F (Eds.): Handbook on Hyperbaric Medicine. Springer, Berlin, 1996; pp 35-58

14. Ellsworth ML, Pittman RN. Arterioles supply oxygen to capillaries by diffusion as well as by convection. Am Physiol Soc 1990;258 (Heart Circ. Physiol 27):H1240-H1243

15. Krogh A. The Anatomy and Physiology of Capillaries. New Haven;CT: Yale University Press 1929

16. Nylander G, Lewis D, Nordström H, Larsson J. Reduction of postischemic edema with hyperbaric oxygen. Plast Reconstruct Surg 1985;76:596-601

17. Ornhagen HC, Hogan PM. Hydrostatic pressure and mammalian cardiac-pacemaker function. Undersea Biomed Res. 1977;4:347-58

18. Whalen RE, Saltzman HA, Holloway DH, et al. Cardiovascular and blood gas responses to hyperbaric oxygenation. Am J Cardiol 1965;15:638

19. Pelaia P, Rocco M, Conti G, et al. Hemodynamic modifications durino hyperbaric oxygen therapy. J Hyperbaric Med 1992;7:229-237

20. Muhvich KH, Piano MR, Myers RAM, Ferguson JL, Marzella L. Hyperbaric oxygenation decreases blood flows in normal and septic rats. Undersea Biomed Res 1992;19:31-40

21. Bergö GW, Tyssebotn I. Cerebral blood flow distribution during exposure to 5 bar oxygen in awake rats. Undersea Biomed Res 1992;19:339-354

22. Norman JN, Shearer JR, Napper AJ, Robertson IM, Smith G. Action of oxygen on the renal circulation. Am J Physiol 1974;227:740-741

23. Cason BA, Wisneski JA, Neese RA, Stanley WC, Hickey RF, Shnier CB, Gertz EW. Effects of high arterial oxygen tension on function, blood flow distribution, and metabolism in ischemic myocardium. Circulation 1992;85:828-838

24. Stamler JS, Jia L, Eu JP, MacMahon TJ, Demchenko IT, Bonaventura J, Gernert K, Piantadosi CA. Blood flow regulation by S-nitrososhemoglobin in the physiological oxygen gradient. Science 1997;276:2034-7

25. Bouachour G, Cronier P, Gouello JP, Toulemonde JL, Talha A, Alquier P. Hyperbaric oxygen therapy in the management of crush injuries: A randomized double-blind placebo-controlled clinical trial. J Trauma 1996;41:333-339

26. Strauss MB, Hargens AR, Gershuni DH. Reduction of skeletal muscle necrosis using intermittent hyperbaric oxygen in a model compartment syndrome. J Bone Joint Surg 1983;65A:656-662

27. Zamboni WA, Wong HP, Stephenson LL. Effect of hyperbaric oxygen on neutrophil concentration and pulmonary sequestration in reperfusion injury. Arch Surg 1996;131:756-760

28. Zamboni WA, Roth AC, Russel RC, Graham B, Suchy H, Kucan JO. Morphologic analysis of the microcirculation during reperfusion of ischemic skeletal muscle and the effect of hyperbaric oxygen. Plas Reconstruct Surg 1993;91:1110-23

29. Buras J. Basic mechanisms of hyperbaric oxygen in the treatment of ischemia-reperfusion injuries. Int Anesthesiol Clin 2000;38:91-109

30. van der Kleij AJ. Which role for HBO-Therapy in the prevention of reperfusion injury? In: Marroni A, Oriani G, Wattel F (Eds.): Proceedings of the XXII. International Joint Meeting on Hyperbaric and Underwater Medicine. Milano, Italy 1996 Sept. 4.-8.; pp 677-681

31. Nunn JF. Control of Breathing. In: Nunn's Applied Respiratory Physiology, 4th Edition, Butterworth-Heinemann, London 1993:90-116, 537-555

32. Rocco M. Pelaia P, et al. Effects of Hyperbarism on Central Respiratory Drive and Respiratory Pattern in Humans, Undersea & Hyperbaric Medicine, 1994;21:315-319

33. Gelfand R, Lambertsen CJ, et al. Hypoxic Ventilatory Sensitivity in Men is Not Reduced by Prolonged Hyperoxia (Predictive Studies V and VI), Journal of Applied Physiology 1998;84:292-302.

34. Nunn JF. Carbon Dioxide. In: Nunn JF: Nunn's Applied Respiratory Physiology, 4th Edition. Butterworth-Heinemann, London, 1993; pp 219-246

35. Dragonat P, Drenckhahn D. Spirographische Untersuchung der Ventilatorischen Lungfunktion unter Überdruckbedingungen, European Journal of Physiology 1974;32:341-348.

36. Hrncir E. Forced Expiration and Inspiration under Hyperbaric Conditions, Physiology Research 1996;45:471-473

37. Clarke JR, Flook V. Respiratory function at depth. In: Lundgren CEG, Miller JN (eds): The lung at depth. Marcel Dekker, New York, 1999; pp.1-72

38. Hunt TK. The physiology of wound healing. Ann Emerg Med 1988;17:1265-1273

39. Silver IA. The physiology of wound healing. In: Hunt TK (Ed.). Wound Healing and Wound Infection: Theory and Surgical Practice. Appleton-Century-Crofts, New York 1980, pp11-31

40. Hunt TK, Pai MP. The effect of varying ambient oxygen tensions on wound metabolism and collagen synthesis. Surg Gynecol Obstet 1979;135:561-567

41. Siddiqui A, Galiano RD, Connors D, Grunskin E, Wu L, Mustoe TA. Differential effects of oxygen on human dermal fibroblasts: acute versus chronic hypoxia. Wound Rep Reg 1996;4:211-218

42. Niinikoski J. The effect of oxygen supply on wound healing and formation of experimental granulation tissue. Acta Physiol Scand 1969;334 (Suppl):1-72

43. Niinikoski J, Gottrup F, Hunt TK. The role of oxygen in wound repair. In: Janssen H, Raaman R, Robertson JIS (Eds.): Wound healing. Wrightson Biomedical Publishing 1991, pp 165-174

44. Vihersaan T, Kivisaari J, Niinikoski J. Effect of changes in inspired oxygen tension on wound metabolism. Ann Surg 1974;179:889-895

45. Herenberger K, Brismar K, Lind F, Kratz G. Dose-dependent hyperbaric oxygen stimulation of human fibroblast proliferation. Wound Rep Reg 1997;5:147-150

46. Prockop DJ, Kivirikko KI, Tuderman L, Guzman NA. The biosynthesis of collagen and its disorders. N Engl J Med 1979;301(1):13-23 and 1979;301(2):77-85

47. Hutton JJ, Tappel AL, Udenfriend S. Cofactor and substrate requirements of collagen proline hydroxylase. Arch Biochem 1967;118:231-240

48. Stephens FO, Hunt TK. Effect of changes in inspired oxygen and carbon dioxide tensions on wound tensile strength. Ann Surg 1971;173:515-519

49. Silver IA. The measurement of oxygen tension in healing tissue. In: Herzog, H. (Eds.): Progress in Respiration Research. Karger, Basel 1969, pp 124-135

50. Knighton DR, Silver IA, Hunt TK. Regulation of wound-healing angiogenesis - effect of oxygen gradients and inspired oxygen concentration. Surgery 1981;90:262-270

51. Marx RE, Ehler WJ, Tayapongsak P, Pierce LW. Relationship of oxygen dose to angiogenesis introduction in irradiated tissue. Am J Surg 1990;160: 519-524

52. Hill GB, Osterhout S. Experimental effects of hyperbaric oxygen on selected clostridial species. I. In-vitro studies. J Infect Dis 1972;125:17-25

53. Kaye D. Effect of hyperbaric oxygen on clostridia in vitro and in vivo. Proc Soc Exp Biol. Med 1967;124:360-366

54. van Unnik AJM. Inhibition of toxin production in clostridium perfringens in vitro by hyperbaric oxygen. Antonie Van Leeuwenhoek 1965;31:181-186

55. Mader JT, Brown GL, Guckian JC, Wells CH, Reinarz JA. A mechanism for amelioration by hyperbaric oxygen of experimental staphylococcal osteomylitis in rabbits. J Infect Dis 1980;142:915-922

56. Bertoye A, Bolot JF, Roussel-Argenson C, Rousset C, Vincent P. Action inhibitrice de l´oxygène hyperbare (O.H.B.) sur le développement des bactéries aérobies. I. Comparaison des effets de l´O.H.B. à 2 atmosphères absolues, sur 3 espèces bactériennes de type métabolique différent. C. R. Séances Soc Biol. Fil 1970;164:2309-2312

57. Park MK, Muhvich KH, Myers RAM, Marzella L. Hyperoxia prolongs the aminoglyco-side-induced postantibiotic effect in pseudomonas aeruginosa. Antimicrob. Agents Chemother 1991;35:691-695

58. Allen DB, Maguire JJ, Mahdavian M, Wicke C, Marcocci L, Scheuenstuhl H, Chang M, Le AX, Hopf HW, Hunt TK. Wound hypoxia and acidosis limit neutrophil bacterial killing mechanisms. Arch Surg 1997;132:991-6

59. Hopf HW, Hunt TK, West JM, et al. Wound tissue oxygen tension predicts the risk of wound infection in surgical patients. Arch Surg 1997;132:997-1004

60. Knighton DR, Halliday B, Hunt TK. Oxygen as an antibiotic - the effect of inspired oxygen on infection. Arch. Surg 1984;19:199-204

61. Kindwall EP. Contraindications and side effects to hyperbaric oxygen treatment. In: Kindwall EP, Whelan HT (Eds): Hyperbaric Medicine Practice, 2nd Ed. Best Publishing Comp, Flagstaff, 1999, pp.83-98

62. Edmonds E, Lowry C, Pennefather J. Dysbaric Diving Diseases. In: Edmonds E, Lowry C, Pennefather J (Eds). Diving and subaquatic medicine, 3rd Ed, Butterworth-Heinemann, Oxford, UK, 1992, pp. 95- 139

63. Edmonds E, Lowry C, Pennefather J. Inert gas narcosis. In : Edmonds E, Lowry C, Pennefather J (Eds). Diving and subaquatic medicine, 3rd Ed, Butterworth-Heinemann, Oxford, UK, 1992, pp. 215-226

64. Donald KW. Oxygen poisoning in man I and II. Br Med J. 1947, I:667-672, II: 712-717

65. Clark JM. Oxygen toxicity. In: Bennett P, Elliott D (Eds.), The Physiology and Medicine of Diving, 4th Ed. Saunders, London, UK, 1993, pp121-169

66. Nunn JF. Hyperoxia and oxygen toxicity. In: Nunn's Applied Respiratory Physiology, 4th Edition, Butterworth-Heinemann, London 1993, 537-555

67. Anderson B Jr, Farmer CJ Jr. Hyperoxic myopia. Trans Am Ophtalmol. Soc. 1978, 76:116-124

68. Palmquist BM, Philipson B, Barr PO. Nuclear cataract and myopia during hyperbaric oxygen therapy. Br J Ophtalmol 1984, 68:113-117

69. Kindwall EP. Management of complications in hyperbaric treatment. In: Kindwall EP, Whelan HT (Eds): Hyperbaric Medicine Practice, 2nd Ed. Best Publishing Comp, Flagstaff, 1999, pp. 365-376

70. Clark JM, Whelan HT. Oxygen toxicity In: Kindwall EP, Whelan HT (Eds): Hyperbaric Medicine Practice, 2nd Ed. Best Publishing Comp, Flagstaff, 1999, pp. 69-82

71. Oury TD, Ho Ys, Piantadosi CA, Crapo JD. Extracellular superoxide dismutase, nitric oxide, and central nervous system O_2 toxicity. Proc Natl Acad Sci USA 1992;89:9715-9

72. Bernareggi M, Radice S, Rossoni G, Oriani G, Chiesara E, Berti F. Hyperbaric oxygen increases plasma exsudation in rat trachea: involvement of nitric oxide. Br J Pharmacol 1999;126:794-800

73. Chavko M, Braisted JC, Outsa NJ, Harabin AL. Role of cerebral blood flow in seizures from hyperbaric oxygen. Brain Res 1998;791:75-82

74. Clark JM, Lambertsen CJ. Pulmonary oxygen toxicity: A review. Pharmacol Rev 71, 23:37-133

75. Bardin H, Lambertsen CJ. A quantitative method for calculating pulmonary oxygen toxicity.Use of the 'Unit pulmonary toxic dose' (UPTD).Institute for Environmental Medicine Report. Philadelphia, University of Pennsylvania 1970

76. Caldwell PRB, Lee WL Jr, Schildkraut HS, Archibald ER. Changes in lung volume, diffusing capacity, and blood gases in men breathing oxygen. J Appl. Physiol 66, 21: 1477-1483

77. Clark JM. Pulmonary limits of oxygen tolerance in man. Experimental Lung Research 1988, 14:897-910

78. Hendricks PL, Hall DA, Hunter WL Jr, Haley PJ. Extension of pulmonary oxygen tolerance in man at 2 ata by intermittent oxygen exposure. J Appl. Physiol. 1977, 42:593-599

79. Radermacher P, Muth CM, Santak B, Wenzel J. A case of breath holding and ascent-induced circulatory hypotension. Undersea Hyperb Med 1993;20:159-161

80. Radermacher P, Santak B, Muth CM, Wenzel J, Hampe P, Vogt L, Hahn M, Falke KJ. Nitrogen partial pressures in man after decompression from simulated scuba dives at rest and during exercise.Undersea Biomed Res 1990;17:495-501

81. Sheffield PJ, Desautels DA. Hyperbaric and hypobaric chamber fires: a 73-year analysis.Undersea Hyperb Med. 1997;24:153-64

82. Muth CM, Shank ES. Gas embolism. N Engl J Med. 2000;342:476-482

83. Shank ES, Muth CM. Decompression illness, iatrogenic gas embolism, and carbon monoxide poisoning: The role of hyperbaric oxygen therapy. Int Anesthesiol Clinic 2000;38:111-138

84. Palmon SC, Moore LE, Lundberg J, Toung T. Venous air embolism: a review. J Clin Anesth 1997;9:251-257

85. Vik A, Brubakk AO, Hennessy TR, Jenssen BM, Ekker M, Slørdahl SA. Venous air embolism in swine: transport of gas bubbles through the pulmonary circulation. J Appl Physiol 1990;69:237-244

86. Gronert GA, Messick JM, Cucchiara RF, Michenfelder JD. Paradoxical air embolism from a patent foramen ovale. Anesthesiology 1979;50:548-549

87. Evans DE, Kobrine A, Weathersby PK, Bradley ME. Cardiovascular effects of cerebral air embolism. Stroke 1981;122:338-344

88. Cullen DJ, Caldere DL. The incidence of ventilator-induced pulmonary barotrauma in critically ill patients. Anesthesiology 1979;50:185-189

89. Powner DJ. Pulmonary Barotrauma in the intensive care unit. J Intensive Care Med 1988;3:224-232

90. Baskin SE, Wozniak RF. Hyperbaric oxygenation in the treatment of hemodialysis associated air embolism. N Engl J Med 1975; July 24:184-185

91. Pelaia P, Rocco M, Volturo P, Conti G. Arterial air embolism during cardiopulmonary bypass: twelve years experience. J Hyperbaric Med 1992;7:115-121

92. Frederiksen JW, Smith J, Brown P, Zinetti C. Arterial helium embolism from a ruptured intraaortic ballon. Ann Thorac Surg 1988; 46:690-692

93. Melamed Y, Shupak A, Bitterman H. Medical problems associated with underwater diving. N Engl J Med 1992;326:30-34

94. Moon RE, Dear GL, Stolp, BW. Treatment of decompression illness and iatrogenic gas embolism. Respir Clin N Am 1999;5:93-135

95. Gorman D. Problems in the modelling of inert gas kinetics. Anaesth Intensive Care 1995;23:187-90

96. McDonough PM, Hemmingsen EA. Bubble formation in crabs induced by limb motions after decompression. J Appl Physiol 1984;57:117-22

97. Vann RD, Thalmann ED. Decompression physiology and practice. In: Bennett P, Elliott D (eds.). The physiology and medicine of diving, 4th edition. Saunders, London 1993, pp. 376-432

98. Zwirewich CV, Mueller NL, Abboud RT, Lepawsky M. Noncardiogenic pulmonary edema caused by decompression sickness: rapid resolution following hyperbaric therapy. Radiology. 1987;163:81-82

99. Moon RE, Camporesi EM, Kisslo JA. Patent foramen ovale and decompression sickness in divers. Lancet 1989; 1(8637): 513-514

100. Francis TJR, Gorman DF. Pathogenesis of decompression disorders. In: Bennett P, Elliott D (eds.). The physiology and medicine of diving, 4th edition. Saunders, London 1993, pp. 455-480

101. Brubakk AO. The effect of bubbles on the organism. Proceedings of the 25th annual meeting of the EUBS, Haifa and Eilat, Israel 1999, 143-153

102. Moon RE, Sheffield PJ. Guidelines for treatment of decompression illness. Aviat Space Environ Med 1997; 68:234-43

103. Annane D, Trouché G, Delisle F, Devauchelle P, Paraire F, Raphael JC, Gajdos P. Effects of mechanical ventilation with normobaric oxygen therapy on the rate of air removal from cerebral arteries Critical Care Medicine 1994;22: 851-857

104. Van Liew HD, Conkin J, Burkhard ME. The oxygen window and decompression bubbles: estimates and significance. Aviat Space Environ Med 1993;64:859-865

105. Flook V. Physics and Physiology in the hyperbaric environment. Clin Phys Physiol Meas 1987;8:197-230

106. Lin YC. Applied physiology of diving. Sports Med 1988;5:41-56.

107. Brunner FP, Frick PG, Buehlmann AA. Post-decompression shock due to extravasation of plasma. Lancet 1964;1:1071-1073

108. Smith RM, Van Hoesen KB, Neuman TS. Arterial gas embolism and hemoconcentration. J Emerg Med 1994;12:147-153

109. Boussuges A, Blanc P, Molenat F, Bergmann E, Sainty JM. Haemoconcentration in neurological decompression illness. Int J Sports Med 1996;17:351-355

110. Ball R. Effect of severity, time to recompression with oxygen, and re-treatment on out come in forty-nine cases of spinal cord decompression sickness. Undersea Hyperb Med 1993;20:133-145

111. Myers RA, Bray P. Delayed treatment of serious decompression sickness. Ann Emerg Med 1985;14:254-257

112. Hardy KR, Thom SR. Pathophysiology and treatment of carbon monoxide poisoning. J Toxicol Clin Toxicol 1994;32:613-629

113. Weaver LK, Hopkins RO, Larson-Lohr V. Carbon monoxide poisoning: a review of human outcome studies comparing normobaric oxygen with hyperbaric oxygen. Ann Emerg Med. 1995 Feb;25:271-2.

114. Scheinkestel CD, Bailey M, Myles PS, Jones K, Cooper DJ, Millar IL, Tuxen DV. Hyperbaric or normobaric oxygen for acute carbon monoxide poisoning: a randomised controlled clinical trial.Med J Aust. 1999 Mar 1;170:203-210

115. Tibbles PM, Perrotta PL. Treatment of carbon monoxide poisoning: a critical review of human outcome studies comparing normobaric oxygen with hyperbaric oxygen. Ann Emerg Med 1994;24:269-276

116. Turner M, Esaw M, Clark RJ. Carbon monoxide poisoning treated with hyperbaric oxygen: metabolic acidosis as a predictor of treatment requirements. J Accid Emerg Med. 1999;16:96-98

117. Weaver LK, Hopkins RO, Larson-Lohr V. Neuropsychologic and functional recovery from severe carbon monoxide poisoning without hyperbaric oxygen therapy. Ann Emerg Med. 1996;27:736-740

118. Weaver LK. Carbon Monoxide Poisoning, Crit Care Clin 1999;15: 297-317

119. Ernst A, Zibrak J. Carbon Monoxide Poisoning. N Engl J Med 1998;339:1603-1608

120. Goldbaum LR, Orellano T, Dergal E. Mechanism of the toxic action of carbon monoxide. Ann Clin Lab Sci 1976 ;6: 372-376

121. Miró O, Casademont J, Barrientos A, Urbano-Marquez A, Cardellach F. Mitochondrial cytochrome c oxidase inhibition during acute carbon monoxide poisoning. Pharmacol Toxicol 1998;82:199-202

122. Stamler JS, Piantadosi CA. O = O NO: It's CO. J Clin Invest 1996;97:2165-2166

123. Ischiropoulos H, Beers MF, Ohnishi ST, Fisher D, Garner SE, Thom SR. Nitric oxide production and perivascular nitration in brain after carbon monoxide poisoning in the rat. J Clin Invest 1996;97:2260-2267

124. Thom SR, Taber RL, Mendiguren II, Clark JM, et al. Delayed neuropsychologic sequel-lae after carbon monoxide poisoning: prevention by treatment with hyperbaric oxygen. Ann Emerg Med. 1995;25:474-480.

125.   Pace N, Strajman E, Walker EL. Acceleration of carbon monoxide elimination in man by high pressure oxygen. Science 1950;111:652-654

126. Weaver LK, Howe S, Hopkins R, Chan KJ. Carboxyhemoglobin half-life in carbon monoxide-poisoned patients treated with 100% oxygen at atmospheric pressure. Chest 2000;117:801-808

127. Myers RA, Thom SR. Carbon monoxide poisoning, in Hyperbaric Medicine Practice, 2nd Edition, Kindwall EP, Whelan HT, (Eds), Flagstaff: Best publishing, 1999, pp. 509-548

128. Bakker DJ, van der Kleij AJ. Soft tissue infections including clostridial myonecrosis: Diagnosis and treatment. In: Oriani G, Marroni A, Wattel F(Eds) Handbook on hyper-baric medicine. Springer. Berlin Heidelberg New York, 1996, pp 343-386

129. Clark LA, Moon RE. Hyperbaric oxygen in the treatment of life-threatening soft-tissue infections. Respir Care Clin N Am 1999;5: 208-219

130. Korhonen K, Klossner J, Hirn M, Niinikoski J.Management of clostridial gas gangrene and the role of hyperbaric oxygen. Ann Chir Gynaecol. 1999;88:139-142.

131. Korhonen K. Hyperbaric oxygen therapy in acute necrotizing infections with a special reference to the effects on tissue gas tensions. Ann Chir Gynaecol Suppl. 2000;214:7-36

132. Hart GB. Exceptional blood loss anemia. Treatment with hyperbaric oxygen.JAMA. 1974 ;228:1028-1029

133. Lozano DD, Stephenson LL, Zamboni WA. Effect of hyperbaric oxygen and medicinal leeching on survival of axial skin flaps subjected to total venous occlusion. Plast Reconstr Surg. 1999 Sep;104(4):1029-32.

134. Mutschler W, Muth CM. Hyperbaric oxygen therapy in trauma surgery. Unfallchirurg. 2001;104:102-114

135. Wattel F, Mathieu D, Coget JM, Billard V. Hyperbaric oxygen therapy in chronic vascular wound management. Angiology 1990;41:59-65

136. Muth CM, Toss A, Born K, Koschnick M, Mutschler W, Frank J. Hyperbaric oxygen therapy improves wound healing in normal and impaired wounds in a mouse wound model. Proceedings XXV. Ann. Meeting EUBS, Israel, Aug 27-Sept 3, 1999

137. Larsson A, Engstrom M, Uusijarvi J, Kihlstrom L, Lind F, Mathiesen T. Hyperbaric oxygen treatment of postoperative neurosurgical infections. Neurosurgery. 2002;50: 287-295

138. Rockswold GL, Ford SE, Anderson DC, Bergman TA, Sherman RE. Results of a prospective randomised trial for treatment of severely brain-injured patients with hyperbaric oxygen. J Neurosurg 1992;76:929-934

139. Neubauer RA, Gottlieb SF. Hyperbaric oxygen for brain injury. J Neurosurg 1993;78:687-688

140. Neubauer RA, James P. Cerebral oxygenation and the recoverable brain. Neurol Res 1998;20 Suppl 1 :S33-36

141. Lampl LA, Frey G, Dietze T, et al. Hyperbaric oxygen in intracranial abscesses. J Hyperbaric Med 1989 ;4 :111-126

142. Weaver LK. Operational use and patient care in the monoplace hyperbaric chamber. Respir Care Clin N Am. 1999;5:51-92

143. Weaver LK. Management of critically ill patients in the monoplace hyperbaric chamber. In: Kindwall EP, Whelan HT (Eds): Hyperbaric Medicine Practice, 2nd Ed. Best Publishing Comp, Flagstaff, 1999, pp. 245-322

144. Braman SS, Dunn SM, Amico CA, Millman RP. Complications of intrahospital transport in critically ill patients. Ann Intern Med. 1987;107:469-473

145. Link J, Krause H, Wagner W, Papadopoulos G. Intrahospital transport of critically ill patients. Crit Care Med. 1990;18:1427-1429.

146. Presswood G, Zamboni WA, Stephenson LL, Santos PM. Effect of artificial airway on ear complications from hyperbaric oxygen. Laryngoscope. 1994;104:1383-1384

147. Kidder TM. Myringotomy. In: Kindwall EP, Whelan HT (Eds): Hyperbaric Medicine Practice, 2nd Ed. Best Publishing Comp, Flagstaff, 1999, pp. 355-364

148. Camporesi EM. Anesthesia in the hyperbaric Environment. In: Jain KK (ed). Textbook of hyperbaric medicine, 3rd ed. Hogrefe&Huber Publishers, Seattle 1999, pp. 549-555

149. Acott CJ, Gorman DF. Decompression illness and nitrous oxide anaesthesia in a sports diver .Anaesth Intensive Care. 1992 ;20:249-250

150. Bailie R, Restall J.Otic barotrauma due to nitrous oxide. Anaesthesia 1988;43:888-889.

151. Eagle C, Tang T.Anaesthetic management of a patient with a descending thoracic aortic aneurysm and severe bilateral bullous pulmonary parenchymal disease. Can J Anaesth. 1995;42:168-172

152. Medtronic. Personal communication. January 1997

153. Moon RE. Answer in "Ask the expert." Pressure 1999, 28:16-17

154. Kratz JM, Blackburn JG, Leman RB, Crawford FA. Cardiac pacing under hyperbaric conditions. Ann Thorac Surg. 1983;36:66-88

155. Weaver LK, Howe S. Normobaric measurement of arterial oxygen tension in subjects exposed to hyperbaric oxygen. Chest 1992;102:1175-1181

156. Weaver LK Howe S. Management of critically ill patients in the monoplace hyperbaric chamber. Appendix III- Noninvasive Doppler blood pressure monitoring in the monoplace hyperbaric chamber. In: Kindwall EP, Whelan HT (Eds): Hyperbaric Medicine Practice, 2nd Ed. Best Publishing Comp, Flagstaff, 1999, pp. 295-301

157. Rogatsky GG, Shifrin EG, Mayevsky A. Physiologic and biochemical monitoring during hyperbaric oxygenation: a review. Undersea Hyperb Med. 1999;26:111-122

158. Sheffield PJ. Tissue oxygen measurements. In: Davis JC, Hunt TK(eds): Problem Wounds: The role of oxygen. Elsevier 1988 pp. 17-52

159. Weaver LK, Larson-Lohr V. Hypoxemia during hyperbaric oxygen therapy. Chest 1994;105:1270-1271

160. Layton W, Weaver L, Haberstock D. Modifications to the Omni-Vent ventilator for use within the monoplace hyperbaric chamber. Undersea Hyperb Med 1998, 25(Suppl):56

161. Colquhoun BP. Air embolism and intravenous catheters. Br. J. Med.1979;1:1489

162. Schlotterbeck K, Tanzer H, Alber G, Muller P. Cerebral air embolism after central venous catheter. Anasthesiol Intensivmed Notfallmed Schmerzther. 1997;32:458-462

163. Groell R, Schaffler GJ, Riesenmueller R. The peripheral intravenous cannula: a cause of venous air embolism. Am J Med Sci 1997;314:300-302

164. Levecque JP, Vincenti-Rouquette I, Rousseau JM. Electric pumps and hyperbaric treatment. Anesthesiology 2000;93:586

165. Lavon, H; Shupak, A.; Tal, D.; et al. Performance of Infusion Pumps during Hyperbaric Conditions. Anesthesiology 2002;96: 849-854

166. Ray D, Weaver LK, Churchill S, Haberstock D. Performance of the Baxter Flo-Gard 6201 volumetric infusion pump for monoplace chamber applications.Undersea Hyperb Med 2000;27:107-12

167. Dohgomori H, Arikawa K, Kubo H. The accuracy and reliability of an infusion pump (STC-3121; Terumo Inst., Japan) during hyperbaric oxygenation. Anaesth Intensive Care 2000;281:68-71

168. Story DA, Houston JJ, Millar IL. Performance of the Atom 235 syringe infusion pump under hyperbaric conditions. Anaesth Intensive Care 1998;26:193-195

169. Sanchez-Guijo JJ, Benavente MA, Crespo A. Failure of a patient-controlled analgesia pump in a hyperbaric environment. Anesthesiology 1999;91:1540-1542

170. Poulton TJ. Monitoring critically ill patients in the hyperbaric environment. Med Instrum 1981;15:81-84

171. Kindwall EP. The use of drugs under pressure. In: Kindwall EP (Ed.):Hyperbaric Medicine Practice. Best Publishing, Flagstaff 1995, pp.247-260

172. Calzia E, Stahl W, Radermacher P. Work of breathing imposed by different ventilators under pressure. Undersea Hyperbaric Med 1998;25(Suppl):21

173. Skinner M. Ventilatory function under hyperbaric pressure. SPUMS J 1998;28:62-71

174. Blanch PB, Desaultes DA, Gallagher TJ. Deviations in function of mechanical ventilators during hyperbaric compression. Respir Care 1991;36:808-814

175. Saywood AM, Howard R, Goad RF, Scott C. Function of the Oxford Ventilator at high pressure. Anaesthesia 1982;37:740-744

176. Moon RE, Bergquist LV, Conklin B, Miller JN. Monaghan 225 ventilator use under hyperbaric conditions. Chest 1986;89:846-851

177. Lewis RP, Szafranski J, Bradford RH, Smith HS, Crabbe GG. The use of the Penlon Nuffield 200 in a monoplace hyperbaric oxygen chamber. An evaluation of its use and a clinical report in two patients requiring ventilation for carbon monoxide poisoning. Anaesthesia 1991;46:767-770

178. Spittal MJ, Hunter SJ, Jones L. The pneuPAC hyperbaric variant HB: a ventilator suit able for use within a one-man hyperbaric chamber. Br J Anaesth 1991;67:488-491

179. Stahl W, Radermacher P, Calzia E. Functioning of ICU ventilators under hyperbaric conditions--comparison of volume- and pressure-controlled modes. Intensive Care Med 2000;26:442-448

NOTES

CHAPTER **6**

HYPERBARIC CHAMBER DESIGN AND FACILITY SAFETY

W.T. Workman

INTRODUCTION

Two key components of successful clinical hyperbaric medicine programs are an understanding of hyperbaric chamber design and a strong facility safety program. Appreciating these components results in a multi-faceted program that incorporates a variety of complementing elements: carefully controlled operational procedures, attention to detail, practice, preventive maintenance, vigilance, training, equipment knowledge, etc. It is not sufficient to simply have a well-crafted program; staff members must fully understand their responsibilities in maintaining the highest level of safety. Maintaining a safe environment for patients and staff is not automatic; it results, in part, from a focused mindset. Creation of this mindset generally begins by learning the fundamentals that any hyperbaric safety program should embrace. Clinical hyperbaric facility accreditation programs can assess this mindset against other parameters such as quality of patient care.

TYPES OF HYPERBARIC CHAMBERS

In the United States, hyperbaric chambers used for clinical application are classified by the National Fire Protection Association (NFPA) as either Class A-multiple patient occupancy or Class B-single patient occupancy. Though the specific designation of a Class A or Class B hyperbaric chamber is only applied in the United States, the commonly accepted nomenclature for hyperbaric chambers worldwide is multiplace (multiple patient) and mono-place (single patient).

Monoplace Hyperbaric Chambers

Though there are a few exceptions throughout the world, monoplace chambers generally are of two basic types: those that are primarily constructed of metal and those constructed mostly of an acrylic cylinder with metal ends.

The most common type is a single acrylic cylinder held in place by steel tie rods that connect the two metal end caps. One of the end caps has a door opening/closing mechanism to allow patient entry and egress. The design of this mechanism can range from an interrupted breech rotating lock to a simple cam action lever closure. All closures should be designed to meet fundamental safety requirements while under pressure yet maintaining the ability for rapid opening and patient access.

Acrylic cylinders are mostly produced with outside diameters ranging from 25 to 40 inches and lengths up to eight feet. Larger diameter monoplace chambers are becoming more popular as they increase patient comfort by providing a less confining space. Larger diameter monoplace chambers however do have drawbacks such as increased oxygen consumption, extra weight and additional installation considerations.

Acrylic monoplace chambers are generally designed for a maximum pressure of 3 atmospheres absolute (3 ATA) or an operational treatment pressure equivalent to 66 feet of seawater (66 fsw). Though there are some monoplace chambers designed to be pressurized with compressed air and deliver oxygen by mask, most are designed to operate off of oxygen pressurization thus eliminating the need for additional oxygen delivery equipment for the patient.

Variations of the acrylic cylinder now include chambers with up to a half-length acrylic cylinder balanced by the remainder of the chamber being metal. There is one monoplace chamber that has two acrylic cylinders with a central metal cylinder section where connections are made for controls and monitoring.

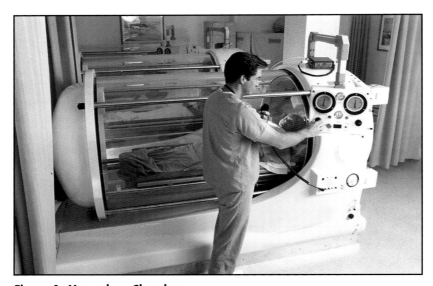

Figure 1. Monoplace Chamber

Monoplace chambers constructed mostly of steel, stainless steel or aluminum cylinders will usually contain acrylic viewports for patient viewing. It is not unusual to find these types of monoplace chambers used in harsher environments than encountered in a hospital setting such as offshore commercial diving locations.

Multiplace Hyperbaric Chambers

As the name implies, a multiplace chamber is designed to provide treatment to several persons at a time and may be better suited to larger hospitals and clinics with higher patient treatment demands. Multiplace chambers are designed to be pressurized with compressed air and deliver oxygen to the patient either through a breathing mask or oxygen hood with their exhaled gases being dumped to the outside of the chamber. Provisions for medical attendants inside the chamber allow for traditional hands-on patient care while accommodating more sophisticated treatments with difficult to manage medical conditions. Multiplace hyperbaric chambers can even be used as operating suites when special precautions are followed to comply with mandatory fire safety requirements of the NFPA.

Multiplace chambers are made of metal with acrylic viewports and are typically designed for operation at higher pressures than monoplace chambers. Multiplace chambers designed for pressures to 6 atmospheres absolute (6 ATA) or 165 feet of seawater (165 fsw) make them more suitable to treat deep water diving accidents and to conduct research into the physiological effects of depth and pressure.

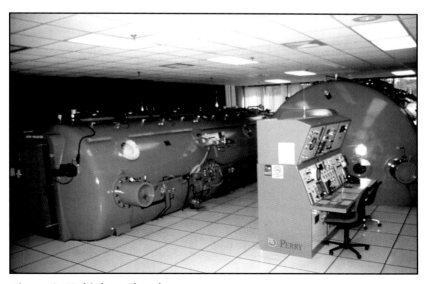

Figure 2. Multiplace Chamber

The size and variety of multiplace chambers is virtually unlimited. Multiplace chambers can be purchased for the treatment of as few as two patients or up to 20 or more. Sizes range from 40 inches in diameter to more than 20 feet and can be found in configurations ranging from upright cylinders to more traditional horizontal cylinders with multiple compartments to spherical shapes with interconnecting chambers. Rectangular chambers, which provide the advantage of the chamber being more "room-like," are now available. It is reported that rectangular chambers also lessen patient confinement anxiety and fears of being in a capsule or tube structure.

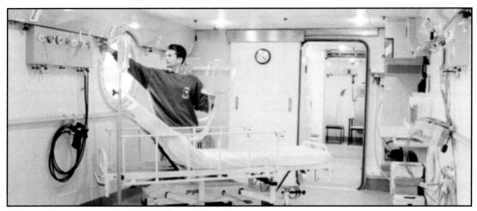

Figure 3. Rectangular Multiplace Chamber

MULTIFACETED PROGRAM

As mentioned above, a properly developed safety program is multifaceted. Although there can be a variety of program elements depending on the specific setting and need, there are common aspects that are elementary in program development, management and execution. These basic elements are:

- **Operational procedures** – managers should develop a comprehensive set of operational procedures that cover the complete spectrum of issues based upon the type of equipment employed by a given facility. Not only should these procedures cover all items of medical equipment to include the chamber or chamber system, they should address patient care activities as well. Written operating instructions form the foundation of any proper safety program.

- **Attention to detail** – procedures should address every aspect, no matter how mundane, of operating and maintaining a given type of chamber system, medical device or patient treatment process. The level of detail should be sufficient to ensure that no critical process or procedure has been omitted. Being thorough is a time-consuming process and one that some can easily justify not completing; however, thoroughness is absolutely necessary.

- **Vigilance** – an organization may have the most comprehensive safety plan possible; but, if the staff is not constantly aware of their surroundings and the consequence of their actions or the actions of others, it means little. As noted in the chapter titled "How Accidents Happen" (in *Hyperbaric Facility Safety: A Practical Guide*, Best Publishing) mishaps are rarely the result of a single event but usually result from a chain of events that lead to an accident. Maintaining constant awareness of one's situation may help break a link in this chain.

- **Preventive maintenance** – keeping all equipment in peak working order depends directly on a comprehensive preventive maintenance program. In general, hyperbaric equipment is well designed and highly reliable, requiring relatively little maintenance (except perhaps for large multiplace hyperbaric complexes). As a result, in times of fiscal restraint, preventive maintenance often is relegated to a lower priority. Such management decisions usually prove to be very costly. Senior management must fully support routine maintenance expenditures since it is generally cheaper to keep equipment in good working order than to face the higher cost of repairing a component after a major failure.

- **Proper training** – the importance of this element cannot be overly stressed. Safety awareness begins in the classroom and is applied in the facility. Mishap data clearly points to the dominance of operator errors in recent hyperbaric accidents. Proper initial instruction and timely continuing education can help mitigate these tragic findings in the future. Minimum training standards must be developed, adopted and enforced throughout the international hyperbaric community. Training outcomes should be focused at providing all staff members with sufficient information for them to know when to question a particular action or situation. It is neither practical nor desired to educate every staff member to be an expert on every aspect of hyperbaric operations. However, if a person notes that something does not seem right, stops and investigates the situation, then a major training objective has been met. This person may have broken the chain of events leading to an accident. The ones that should cause concern are those staff members whose knowledge level is not high enough to recognize that something is not right, continues to allow the situation to exist, perhaps ending in a tragic mishap.

- **Practice, practice, practice** – the proper response to an emergency situation should be calculated and immediate. Although it is not practical for each staff member to memorize every emergency procedure, it is important for them to routinely practice planned reactions to a range of emergency situations. Each should be familiar enough with all department or equipment emergency procedures to allow them, with the aide of emergency checklists, to deal with any quick response situation. Being aware of others' responsibilities is crucial in that anyone may find themselves in a position of having to respond to an incident when the staff member normally responsible for that particular function is not immediately available. Practicing as a group helps the staff to better appreciate the responsibilities of others and fosters development of the hyperbaric team. As difficult as it is, time should be set aside on a recurring basis for focused unit safety training. Although monthly staff safety training is recommended, the minimal interval should be no less than quarterly.

- **Safety mindset** – attention to the above elements helps cultivate a safety mindset for the entire hyperbaric facility staff. This obvious attitude then becomes very evident to the patient, helping to instill confidence and easing any fear they may have. Safety must be an overriding philosophy that guides the attitudes and actions of the entire staff.

PRECEDING SAFETY ELEMENTS (EQUIPMENT)

Thanks to the extremely hard work done over the years by many people representing a variety of engineering and safety disciplines, there are codes and standards working behind the scenes to ensure the safety of the equipment installed in hyperbaric facilities. These various groups exert their influence before the doors of the hyperbaric facility are open for business.

The first group coming into contact with the basic equipment for a hyperbaric facility is the American Society of Mechanical Engineers (ASME) and the standards developed by the Pressure Vessel for Human Occupancy Committee (PVHO). In summary, the ASME-PVHO establishes the design and fabrication rules for hyperbaric chambers. Although not recognized throughout the world as the internationally accepted standard, it is considered by many as the premier guidance governing this issue. Unfortunately, compliance with ASME-PVHO is not yet mandatory in all 50 American states. Of primary importance, however, is that a pressure vessel intended for human occupancy be designed and fabricated in accordance with some sort of recognized safety standard.

A second group having tremendous influence on the safe design of a hyperbaric system is the National Fire Protection Association and their fire safety standard for hyperbaric facilities. NFPA 99, Safety Standard for Health Care Facilities, Chapter 20-Hyperbaric Facilities establishes minimum performance criteria for ancillary hyperbaric support equipment and systems such as the fire suppression system, intercommunications system, air quality monitoring, electrical requirements, etc. Though ASME-PVHO is not yet mandatory in all 50 American states, NFPA 99 is. It requires that any hyperbaric chamber intended for clinical treatment installed in a healthcare facility or business occupancy be in compliance with ASME-PVHO.

A third group which, in this author's opinion, is underestimated and certainly not well understood for the role it plays is the Food and Drug Administration. The FDA classifies hyperbaric chambers as Class II medical devices and requires that manufacturers comply with 510(k) Pre-market Notification Requirements before a specific chamber design can be legally placed into commercial sales. Unfortunately, not all U.S. hyperbaric chamber manufacturers are in compliance with these requirements. Any healthcare organization considering purchase of a hyperbaric chamber or hyperbaric system should require the manufacturer to produce evidence of pre-market clearance. Such documentation verifies that the manufacturer surpassed a rigorous third party review of design and fabrication adequacy and that the system complied with recognized industry standards. If a hyperbaric system under consideration for purchase does not have a cleared 510(k), or is not "grandfathered" (few are), it is suggested that other equipment alternatives be considered. Similar requirements, such as CE Marking in Europe, are being established in other world regions that will ultimately raise the level of quality of hyperbaric systems. Improved quality leads directly to improved safety.

Guidelines developed by the American Society for Testing and Materials (ASTM) are used extensively to direct designers of oxygen equipment and oxygen system components to proper material selection, design and maintenance. These guidelines help ensure that consideration is given to these elements to minimize the risk of fire due to improper materials, inadequate design or sub optimal maintenance. More information on ASTM interests is found in the chapters titled "The Role of Oxygen in Hyperbaric Chamber Fire Safety" and "Hyperbaric Fire Risk Assessments and Forensics" (in *Hyperbaric Facility Safety: A Practical Guide*, Best Publishing).

The Compressed Gas Association (CGA) sets guides for the installation of primary and secondary gas delivery systems and gas purity. Compliance with these industry guidelines gives the new operator assurance that the necessary steps have been taken to ensure delivery of high quality gas supplies to either the patient or the chamber.

Additionally, the Undersea & Hyperbaric Medical Society (UHMS) produced companion safety guidelines for both monoplace and multiplace hyperbaric chamber systems. Originally intended to provide a potential purchaser with a better understanding of the issues that needed to be understood when contemplating installation of a hyperbaric system, they have now become valuable source documents for users and engineers alike. Referring to these documents in the early stages of facility planning has proven to be a valuable effort by many.

Though hyperbaric medicine is poised for rapid expansion into developing areas of the world, comprehensive safety standards like those mentioned above are not in place in most of these countries to help establish and support the growth of the specialty. Aggressive efforts are underway to promote adoption of comprehensive safety standards throughout the world.

PRECEDING SAFETY ELEMENTS (FACILITIES)

Not only are there codes and standards that govern the design and fabrication of hyperbaric chambers and their affiliated component systems, there are also standards in the United States and a few other countries, that establish minimum facility requirements that must be met before the hyperbaric chamber can be installed. These building requirements as set forth in NFPA 99, Safety Standard for Health Care Facilities, Chapter 20-Hyperbaric Facilities were developed for facilities in operation in designated healthcare facilities. However, NFPA 101, Life Safety Code, 2000 Edition requires compliance to NFPA 99, Chapter 20 for any hyperbaric chamber conducting medical treatment in business-classed occupancies governed by the Life Safety Code. The UHMS monoplace and multiplace safety guidelines previously mentioned also address general facility issues that should be considered. In reality, the type of building into which a hyperbaric chamber is installed is immaterial—there are basic facility standards that should be met to ensure continued safe operation regardless of arbitrary classification.

PRECEDING SAFETY ELEMENTS (STAFF TRAINING)

The previous elements that frame equipment and facility requirements generally work quite well, and for the most part, are conducted behind the operational scene. Most hyperbaric staff personnel are not even aware of many of the details of the above requirements. However, it all comes together with the initial training the staff receives before beginning hyperbaric chamber operations. Although these aspects of a viable hyperbaric safety program are all important in their own right, training is, in this author's opinion, the most critical element.

As in any discipline, training is central to successful outcomes. The operator must acquire the knowledge to understand the what, why, when, where and how. Raising the knowledge level of each hyperbaric operator high enough to know when to ask a question when something does not seem right has already been stressed. Experience also contributes to this higher order awareness. I encourage the reader's support in adopting the philosophy to obtain a thorough hyperbaric knowledge and to expand it through experience. More basic, however, is the need to have a minimum skill and knowledge level in place before hyperbaric operations even begin. Training after the fact, although better than no training at all, leaves an organization open to all sorts of potential legal pitfalls should an accident occur involving a person who has not been properly trained.

More directly, training is one of the links in the accident chain of events over which the management of any hyperbaric facility has direct control of. At present, there are no mandatory requirements in the United States for minimum training standards for all hyperbaric staff. Though there are efforts underway to establish these minimums, there is much work that needs to be done. This is a universal need recognized by the international hyperbaric medicine community and movement in this direction among our peers encourages the author.

CORE PROGRAM ELEMENTS

The basic elements of any comprehensive hyperbaric facility safety program should include at least the following:
- Defined responsibilities
- Documented safety procedures based on the type and size of the facility
- Documented in-service training
- Documented maintenance
- Documented measurement and validation

Responsibilities

Borrowing from the preceding discussion on training, one of the first individual responsibilities is to ensure that each person directly involved in hyperbaric operations is knowledgeable of all potential hazard sources.

If there is ever doubt about a particular situation or procedure, then stop and ask for clarification. Do not continue blindly down what may be the beginning of the accident chain of events. Once again, each individual has direct control over his or her level of hyperbaric knowledge and understanding.

Broadly speaking, each organization should develop a program that includes four major checkpoints. Unfortunately, this is generally not the case. The development, execution and management of the safety program is usually left entirely up to the hyperbaric facility. It is important to do all that is practically possible to indoctrinate everyone from the most senior hospital executive to the most junior technician on the hyperbaric program. The more they understand about what hyperbaric medicine is, what its limitations are, and what the requirements are to provide high quality care safely, the better they can serve as an advocate for the program. The four checks are:

- The governing body (Hospital Board of Directors, etc.) should set a firm hyperbaric safety policy
- The hyperbaric facility management should develop comprehensive safety procedures
- The technical staff of the hyperbaric facility should implement the procedures
- Accrediting agencies should survey for compliance

As mentioned above, the governing body should establish a firm hyperbaric safety policy. Within a given institution, the ultimate responsibility resides with this senior management group. They must work closely with the safety director (SD) to ensure that these policies are developed and rigidly adhered to. Adherence implies there is an ongoing dialog between the governing body and the hyperbaric facility. This should be encouraged. Developing a close working relationship between the governing body and the SD is extremely important in that it helps establish the credibility of the SD with senior institutional management. Again, the more institutional management understands your program, the better they can serve as you spokesman.

Continuing down the hierarchy, the administrator of the host institution plays an important role as well. Specifically, the institution's administration should adopt and correlate regulations and standard operating procedures to ensure that both the physical qualities and operating maintenance methods pertaining to the hyperbaric facility meet the standards required of other departments of the institution. In particular, administration must have an appreciation of the unique compliance issues cited by various codes and standards pertaining to hyperbaric facilities. The more administration understands the requirements, they better they can offer support and funding for major department expenditures such as periodic maintenance, etc.

As this hierarchy becomes more functional, the hyperbaric medical staff is not exempt from responsibility. The department medical director should work closely with the safety director to develop department-specific regulations and procedures. Other medical personnel should also make themselves available to the SD to assist in this effort. Finally, the medical director should adopt and ensure that all staff adhere to the procedures developed.

Perhaps the most visible position of a comprehensive hyperbaric safety program is that of the designated safety director. This is the only position directed by NFPA 99, Chapter 20. Every facility, regardless of size, or the type or number of chambers employed, shall have a safety director. This individual has a tremendous responsibility to ensure the safe order and discipline among the staff and patients. Specific responsibilities of the SD are covered later in this chapter.

Documented Safety Procedures

There are a variety of issues that should be documented in your safety program. It is not the intent of this text to provide a specific list for your use. Instead, you are encouraged to think through each process, procedure, concern, activity, etc., and conduct a step-by-step analysis of each. From that detailed assessment, then construct a set of guidelines for each action that is appropriate for your facility. There will be many procedures that you will have in common with all other hyperbaric facilities, but there will also be those that are unique to your department.

There are a few general and specific areas identified in NFPA 99, Chapter 20 that are recommended for inclusion in your documentation.

General Facility Safety

- **Conduct of personnel** – this area should address such issues as staff performance and evaluation, conduct around patients, etc.
- **Apparel and footwear** – based on documented mishap data, this is also an area of great concern. It was mentioned earlier that training is one aspect over which any hyperbaric department has direct control; this is another. The Sheffield and Desautel analysis of recent mishaps indicates a high percentage of accidents where contraband or unauthorized items and synthetic materials were allowed into the chamber interior. Research is very clear on the benefits of fire resistant or fire retardant materials in minimizing the fuel available to help propagate a fire. Garments made of 100% cotton are used widely because of their ability to reduce the buildup of static electricity. Unfortunately, many hyperbaric facilities throughout the world allow patients to enter the chamber in regular street clothes, shoes, etc. **This practice is highly discouraged**. Garments made from anything other than natural fibers are a potential source of increased fuel. Many argue that it takes too much time to have the patient change from their regular clothing into prescribed garments provided by the facility and that the staff is too limited to assist those patients unable to change clothes on their own. *It is this author's opinion that you CANNOT AFFORD NOT TO!* As long as the process of assisting patients in the change of clothing is planned, any well-managed program can afford the few extra minutes and effort to perform this vital function.

  Contraband can also more easily be managed by having the patient wear only garments provided by the facility. Personal clothing may have numerous pockets where items such as cigarette lighters, matches, fuel or chemical warmers, etc., may go unnoticed. If the patient is given a garment to wear that has had the pockets sewn closed, or better yet, no pockets at all, then the likelihood that contraband could be brought into the chamber is greatly minimized. Once again, this is an action that you can control!

- **Posting of procedures** – although it is not recommended to post all emergency procedures throughout the facility for the patients and others to see, there are key procedures that should be posted in public view. Procedures such as building evacuation routes, etc. fall into this category. For multiplace hyperbaric chambers with auxiliary control stations, the chamber operator should post emergency procedures at each control station in a quick-reading flip chart folder for ready access. Any chamber operator, whether monoplace or multiplace, should have immediate access to a complete series of emergency procedures for use in any emergency situation.

- **Staff familiarity with procedures** – the operative words here are practice, practice, practice! Though each person has his or her specific responsibility within the unit, each should be aware enough of the duties of others to be able to respond to any emergency that might happen when they may be the only one around. Frequent practicing, playing the role of other staff members, etc., will help develop an *esprit de corps* and a sense of being a member of the hyperbaric team that will be advantageous in the event of an accident. During mishaps, things may happen very quickly, possibly leaving little time to contemplate your next action. Practice helps minimize this hesitation and facilitates one's confidence in dealing with the adverse situation regardless of how drastic.

  In many organizations, it is difficult to set aside sufficient time to conduct in-service safety training. If an organization, from the very beginning, weaves recurring in-service safety training into the fabric of their organizational structure, then it becomes second nature, part of the routine. For those organizations that seldom or never devote the time necessary to hone staff safety skills, there is, in this author's opinion, higher risk for a mishap.

Specific Facility Safety

- There should be specific procedures developed, based on the unique characteristics of your hyperbaric chamber or system, that cover situations such as fire in the chamber, patient egress, contaminated air, equipment component failure, fire in the building, etc. Failure to develop these specific response actions will add to the confusion that generally accompanies a mishap situation and will certainly increase one's response time necessary to interrupt the accident chain of events. As noted earlier, these procedures should also be posted at auxiliary control stations for multiplace hyperbaric chamber systems.

- In addition to developing a comprehensive response posture to mechanical or operational emergency situations, a companion list should also be developed to address physiological emergencies such as ear/sinus pain, confinement anxiety, oxygen toxicity, etc. The reader is referred to the chapter on emergency procedures in the textbook*Hyperbaric Facility Safety: A Practical Guide* for a more detailed discussion on developing these crucial operational safety aides.

Documented In-Service Training

The familiar theme of practice, practice, and more practice cannot be stressed too strongly. Having said that, it is realized that it may be easier said than done. Time must be routinely set aside; otherwise, in-service training will often take the back seat to other important activities. Ideally, an organization should devote time to monthly safety training. However, if this is not feasible, it is recommended to establish the frequency best suited to your needs, but no less than quarterly. The important thing is that training be routinely done. Safety must be given priority in the ongoing business of a hyperbaric facility.

Examples of training topics are as varied as the mind is creative. Several suggestions are offered to stimulate thinking:

- **Fire drills** – not only should your fire suppression system (FSS) be exercised periodically (for multiplace chambers so equipped), the local fire department should be frequently involved.

  All too often, the FSS is ignored, sitting idle for months and then expected to perform flawlessly when needed. They must be routinely activated to maintain peak efficiency. There have been several mishaps in which a faulty FSS has been implicated in the accident chain of events. Activating the FSS every six months (preferably) or annually (at minimum) will help instill operator confidence in the system and better assure proper function when needed.

  Some organizations are reluctant to invite local fire department personnel into their facility. This attitude is foolish. The patient egress requirements for a hyperbaric environment are different from those of a regular healthcare facility setting. This is especially true in multiplace hyperbaric chamber facilities, where both patients and chamber operators may be required to stay with the chamber longer than usual in order to decompress the chamber safely. Fire department personnel need to understand these unique requirements and be given the opportunity to practice them. Otherwise, they will be unable to provide the quality support necessary during any mishap situation. The needs are different; they need to be able to practice their response to that difference.

- **Mock patient emergencies** – the staff must be capable of responding to the complete spectrum of patient emergencies such as confinement anxiety, ear/sinus pain, oxygen toxicity reactions, etc. Practice helps the staff develop those reflexive actions necessary to deal with a patient emergency in a timely fashion.

- **Simulated equipment failure** – although hyperbaric equipment is generally reliable, they are mechanical devices which are subject to failure. A good example for multiplace chamber operations is to practice the steps necessary to deal with a failed viewport. A good example for monoplace chamber operations is the operator's response to loss of pressure control. There are numerous other equipment failures for any type of chamber that can be simulated for practice.

- **Contaminated air** – usually, the quality of the air produced for hyperbaric chamber operations depends on the quality of the air ingested for compression and proper function of the compressor. Fortunately for the human, one of the most sophisticated alarms for air contamination is the nose. Hydrocarbon-based contaminates can easily be detected. Of concern, of course, is carbon monoxide, which is odorless. Regardless, dealing with contaminated air should be routinely practiced.

- **Updates on codes and standards** – fortunately for the in-service trainer, change in this area is very slow making it easy for the trainer to stay current. Changes do occur, however, and hyperbaric personnel are encouraged to be aware of them. The advantage here is that emphasizing these issues in your training program helps broaden your staff's knowledge base for factors that influence the everyday world of hyperbaric medicine.

Vital to an effective ongoing hyperbaric training program are those sessions for which continuing education credits are offered. This is especially crucial for technical personnel. Generally, there is no problem with professional medical staff personnel in satisfying continuing medical educational credits. Unfortunately, technical staff do not often have the administrative support to routinely participate in these ongoing educational activities. They can rarely afford to attend these functions at their own expense, and as a result, they usually do not attend. This situation needs to change. As an alternative, larger clinical hyperbaric medicine programs are encouraged to apply to organizations such as the National Board of Diving and Hyperbaric Medical Technology for continuing education credits for their ongoing in-service training program. This approach will help ensure staff members have the opportunity to maintain currency for minimal cost and less time away from the facility. Further, it is highly recommended that technical personnel attend courses such as the ASTM course Fire Hazards in Oxygen Delivery Systems, or International ATMO's Advanced Course in Hyperbaric Safety and the Hyperbaric Safety Director Training Course. There are others. If a good working relationship has been established with the institution's administrative management, it is easier for the director of hyperbaric medicine to advocate on the technician's behalf to help justify funding the educational need.

Continuing to grow in importance is certification in hyperbaric technology. Suffice it to say this is a valuable tool to recognize staff competence and should be a priority for every hyperbaric facility. Developing a comprehensive in-service training program assists those technicians not yet certified to achieve the background preparation necessary to successfully complete the certification exam.

Finally, there is an old military saying that goes something like, "If you did not write it down, you did not do it!" That speaks for itself. It is very important for you to document what you do. This is the one thing surveyors have to review to determine department activity in this area. Additionally, one tends to be more organized in program development and execution when documentation is required.

Documented Maintenance

Preventive and responsive maintenance on any component of a hyperbaric chamber or system is required. Considering the total number of hyperbaric facilities in the United States, few are fortunate enough to maintain sufficient technical expertise on staff to handle the majority of maintenance needs in-house. Generally, third-party contractors or the chamber manufacturer is relied upon. Regardless of your particular situation, all aspects of maintenance ranging from daily inspections to major component overhauls should be documented in detail. Failure to maintain detailed maintenance records often makes future repairs more costly since historical system actions cannot be validated.

Documented Measurement and Validation

In setting up any program for which outcomes are important, the processes developed to achieve those outcomes must be measurable. If not, there is no mechanism for feedback to determine if the process is actually needed, if it is achieving the desired result, or if it is as efficient as it can be. It is relatively easy to measure outcomes in an industrial setting where a product is produced. You can measure machining tolerances, component rejection rates, etc. It is more difficult to measure management outcomes, yet this is still attainable. If organizations have no tool by which they can assess performance, regardless of the measurement area, then they are omitting an important tool that management can use to ascertain the success of a given program. This is equally true with the need to assess outcomes of a hyperbaric safety program. Compliance organizations such as the Joint Commission on Accreditation of Healthcare Organizations traditionally review such interdepartmental documentation to assist with their survey of a particular department or patient service. Good documentation cannot be stressed too strongly.

SAFETY DIRECTOR

As previously mentioned, one of the key positions of every hyperbaric facility is that of the Safety Director. Every hyperbaric facility, regardless of type, shall have a designated Safety Director. Due to the extensive nature of responsibilities of the Safety Director, no attempt will be made to provide a detailed discussion of each. Instead, these responsibilities are provided in list form.

Knowledge and Experience

- Completion of a recognized course in hyperbaric medicine (Undersea and Hyperbaric Medical Society, The American College of Hyperbaric Medicine, The National Board of Diving and Hyperbaric Medical Technology, etc., or similar nation-specific requirement)
- Training or experience in hyperbaric chamber maintenance and operations (primarily for multiplace hyperbaric facilities)
- Working knowledge of safety codes and decompression requirements
- Certification in hyperbaric technology (highly desired)

General Responsibilities

- In charge of all hyperbaric equipment in the absence of a Technical Director. (Note: there is no requirement in NFPA 99, Chapter 20 for a designated Technical Director as it is for the Safety Director. Generally, monoplace hyperbaric facilities do not have a Technical Director whereas multiplace hyperbaric facilities do. This is due, in part, to the increased complexity of multiplace systems.)
- Responsible for the safe/effective operation and maintenance of the hyperbaric chamber and related support systems and ancillary components
- Works closely with facility management and hyperbaric physician(s)
- Recommends and implements safety procedures as appropriate
- Serves on institutional safety committee (recommended)
- Has authority to restrict or remove potentially hazardous items or supplies from inside the chamber
- Provides training and leadership
- Maintains all safety related codes and standards as required by various licensing and regulatory agencies

Specific Responsibilities

- Ensures compliance with NFPA 99, Chapter 20, Hyperbaric Facilities (or other country equivalent as appropriate) and unit safety policies and procedures
- Reviews safety incidents, collects information on equipment/patient safety, reports relevant incidents, and provides periodic in-service training on accident prevention
- Works closely with the medical, nurse and technical directors to develop and annually review and revise documents pertaining to policies, procedures, operations and maintenance
- Fosters positive relationships between department personnel and local regulators such as the local fire marshal, director of emergency services, pressure vessel inspector, etc.
- Works with the Technical Director to coordinate/approve all upgrades, modifications and repairs to the hyperbaric chamber or hyperbaric system
- Interacts with hospital maintenance personnel and outside contractors to ensure all maintenance is performed in accordance with applicable codes and standards
- Ensures that all system modifications are tested prior to manned chamber operations
- Evaluates equipment and supplies before they are used inside the chamber
- Maintains a safe environment for the staff and patients alike
- Monitors to ensure that appropriate decompression procedures are used for all persons with hyperbaric exposure to inert gases
- Informs personnel of any special work condition such as infection control, hazard control, etc.
- Serves as technical trainer for full-time and part-time staff

- Provides in-service training on aspects of hyperbaric physiology, equipment operations, safety, decompression requirements and treatment protocols
- Validates in-chamber safety training of new staff before their initial entry into the hyperbaric chamber (multiplace)
- Generates and supervises safety drills which are tailored to the special needs of the facility
- Conducts annual review of safety-related events in order to identify trends and monitor improvements
- Sets up procedures to assist the medial director in reviewing, documenting, and reporting safety-related events to the staff to facilitate learning

HYPERBARIC FACILITY ACCREDITATION

With over 500 clinical hyperbaric facilities in the United States alone, the specialty of hyperbaric medicine has matured sufficiently to warrant a third-party quality assessment program. Though there are many organizations and agencies with an interest in hyperbaric medicine, there is no single agency with ultimate responsibility to assure that the highest quality of care is provided to the hyperbaric patient. With the ever-changing reimbursement climate there is a demonstrated need to implement a national quality assessment program to improve the quality of care across the continuum of clinical hyperbaric facilities.

As the primary professional hyperbaric medicine society in the United States, the Undersea & Hyperbaric Medical Society has developed a clinical hyperbaric medicine facility accreditation program. The program is intended to assure that clinical hyperbaric facilities are:
- Staffed with specialists who are well trained
- Using quality equipment that is properly installed, maintained and operated to the highest possible safety standards
- Providing high quality care
- Maintaining proper documentation of informed consent, treatment procedures, physician involvement, etc.

SUMMARY

A well-structured safety plan consists of a variety of components, each with its relative importance. Not to diminish the other elements, proper training serves as the foundation for continued safety.

In order to maintain a safe operational hyperbaric environment, everyone must realize it is a team effort. Although a particular aspect of daily operation may not be a specific person's responsibility, each must appreciate the role of another. Each person must do his or her part by developing a safety mindset to strengthen the chain of mishap avoidance.

The safety director is a key figure in any hyperbaric medicine department's safety program and has wide-ranging responsibilities to ensure that the functions of hyperbaric safety are properly planned, executed, documented and validated.

Hyperbaric facility accreditation provides a mechanism to provide a high level of assurance that the quality of care being provided the hyperbaric patient is as high as possible.

REFERENCES

1. ANSI/ASME PVHO-1-1997, Safety Standard for Pressure Vessels for Human Occupancy, American Society of Mechanical Engineers, New York, 1997.

2. GCA Pamphlet G-7.1-1989, Commodity Specification for Air, Compressed Gas Association, Inc., Arlington, Virginia, 1989.

3. Guidelines for Clinical Multiplace Hyperbaric Facilities. Undersea & Hyperbaric Medical Society, Kensington, MD. 1994.

4. Health Care Facilities Handbook, 5th Edition, Burton R. Klein, Ed., National Fire Protection Association, Quincy, Massachusetts, 1999.

5. Hyperbaric Facility Safety: A Practical Guide, W.T. Workman, Ed., Best Publishing Company, Flagstaff, AZ, 1999.

6. Hyperbaric Facility Accreditation Manual, Undersea & Hyperbaric Medical Society, Kensington, MD. 2002.

7. Monoplace Hyperbaric Chamber Safety Guidelines. Undersea & Hyperbaric Medical Society, Kensington, MD. 1997.

8. Safe Use of Oxygen and Oxygen Delivery Systems. Guidelines for Oxygen System Design, Materials Selection, Operations, Storage, and Transportation. Harold D. Beeson, Walter F. Stewart, and Stephen S. Woods, Editors. ASTM, 100 Barr Harbor Drive, West Conshohocken, PA. 2000.

9. Sheffield PJ, Desautels, DA. Hyperbaric and hypobaric chamber fires: a 73-year analysis. Undersea Hyper Med 1997; 24(3): 153-164.

10. Standard for Health Care Facilities, NFPA 99, 2002 Edition, National Fire Protection Association, Quincy, Massachusetts, pp. 102-112.

CHAPTER 7

CLINICAL ASPECTS OF DECOMPRESSION DISORDERS

A. Marroni

INTRODUCTION

Decompression illness (DCI) is a complex condition which can appear with a wide variety of signs and symptoms.

Any organic or functional decrements in individuals who have been exposed to a reduction in environmental pressure must be considered as a decompression illness case and treated as such until the contrary is proven. This applies to acute, sub-acute and chronic changes related to decompression and may be related to acute clinical symptoms or to situations which may develop sub-clinically and deceptively. It is in fact generally accepted that sub-clinical forms of decompression illness, with little or no reported symptoms, may cause changes in the bones, the central nervous system, and in the lungs.

Generally speaking a disorder is a physical derangement, frequently slight and transitory in nature; a disease is instead a condition of an organ, part, structure or system of the body in which there is incorrect function resulting from the effect of heredity, diet or environment. A disease is a serious, active, prolonged and deep-rooted condition (*Webster's Dictionary*).(114) Decompression illness should be considered a disorder due to a physical primary cause that can transform into a disease if adequate and timely action is not undertaken to abort or to minimize the pathophysiological effects of bubbles on the body tissues.

The primary physical cause of decompression illness is the separation of gas in the body tissues, due to inadequate decompression and determining an excessive degree of gas supersaturation in the body tissues. Inadequately rapid speed of ascent after an exposure to increased environmental pressure, as much as the omission of the prescribed decompression stops, are the origin and the cause of gas separation in body tissues. The best prevention of decompression illness is therefore achieved by calculating and observing appropriate ascent and decompression procedures.

Unfortunately the current knowledge as to which ascent or decompression procedures are the most appropriate is largely empirical and not yet reliable. The incidence of "unexplainable" cases of DCI is very significant and about 50% of the recreational diving DCI cases reported by DAN internationally are apparently "undeserved."

In fact the role of other contributing factors of DCI, such as a patent foramen ovale, the wide variation in individual susceptibility to DCI, the role of complement activation in the presence of gas bubbles and the relationship between gas bubbles, blood cells, the capillary endothelial lining and DCI, are still undefined and obscure.

It is apparent that DCI can manifest itself with minor and very subtle changes and is likely to be ignored or denied if adequate information is not provided to individual divers as well as to diving training organizations and to the examining non-specialized physicians. There is growing evidence that underreported, underestimated and undertreated signs and symptoms of DCI can result in permanent organic or functional damage.

Although the presence of doppler-detectable gas bubbles in the blood is not always predictive of clinically evident DCI, it has been observed during many field and experimental human studies that no individual without detectable pulmonary artery and venous bubbles developed signs and symptoms of DCI. On the contrary, there is growing experimental and clinical evidence that asymptomatic "silent" bubbles present in the body tissues can cause cellular and biological reactions and the release of potentially damaging biochemical substances in the blood.

Definition

The previously adopted classification criteria—i.e., Type I or Type II decompression illness and arterial gas embolism—are generic and presume that the underlying diagnostic criteria are of common and uniform knowledge. Indeed a great variation and a significant level of disagreement has been observed between different experienced specialists called to define the same cases of decompression disorders using the traditional classification. A descriptive form of classification, using the common term "decompression illness," followed by a description of the clinical signs and symptoms and of their onset and development characteristics, has been considered both more universally understandable and simpler to explain, and it showed a much higher degree of concordance between the specialists who were asked to define the same cases of decompression disorders using this kind of classification criteria.

Epidemiology

Epidemiologically, there is universal consensus among the diving medicine international community, that the incidence of DCI is generally very low and that there is no gender-related significant difference. There is equally uniform consensus on the fact that neurological manifestations of DCI are by far the most common form of the condition among recreational divers. Universal data, based on wide epidemiological information, are unfortunately still lacking.

Many yet unknown aspects of DCI are currently the object of ongoing international studies such as: the relationship between gas separation and DCI injury, the relationship between clinical symptoms and the severity of the disease, the relationship between initial clinical onset, treatment results and permanent sequelae, the reason for the large variation in individual susceptibility to DCI, the lifetime of gas bubbles and the real incidence of DCI.

Treatment

One hundred percent oxygen should be administered immediately as the single most important first aid treatment of any DCI case related to surface-oriented diving; appropriate rehydration is an important adjunct during field first aid.

Hyperbaric treatment started with the shortest possible delay, using 100% oxygen at pressures not exceeding 2.8 bar, showed to assure very good results in more than 80% of the treated cases. There is no significant evidence that any other therapeutical scheme may provide better results and be therefore preferable as the hyperbaric treatment of first choice.

The administration of adjunctive fluid therapy is generally recommended by the diving-hyperbaric medicine specialists in Europe; the role of other drugs, such as steroids and anticoagulants, is still controversial.

HISTORY

In 1670, Robert Boyle demonstrated that decompression illness could be produced in the reptile by sudden lowering of atmospheric pressure.

The first case of decompression illness (DCI) recorded in writing was in a compressed air worker. In 1845, Triger reported that two men had suffered "very sharp pain" in the left arm and another had pain in the knees and left shoulder 30 minutes after emerging from a seven-hour exposure at pressure (the pressure could have ranged between 2.4 atmospheres and 4.25 atmospheres).(104)

The first reported form of treatment for DCI in man, as reported by Triger, was "rubbing with spirits of wine soon relieved this pain in both men and they kept working on the following days."

Two years later, Pol and Watelle (93) wrote to feel "justified in hoping that a sure and prompt means of relief would be to recompress immediately, then decompress very carefully."

In 1878, Paul Bert (7) demonstrated that the cause of DCI was nitrogen going into gas phase in the tissue and that this bubble formation was responsible for symptoms. Bert also highlighted the existence of "silent bubbles" in the venous blood. He understood that prompt recompression was the key to effective treatment. He also used oxygen at one atmosphere following very rapid decompression and observed that cardiopulmonary symptoms, but not spinal cord paralysis, were relieved by normobaric oxygen breathing.

The *Journal of the Society of Art* of May 15, 1896 describes the work of E.W. Moir during the digging of the Hudson River tunnel in 1889. (85)

Facing a decompression illness fatality rate of over 25% of the employed workers, he installed a recompression chamber at the worksite, with the result that only two deaths occurred out of 120 workers during the next 15 months. He wrote:

With a view to remedying the state of things an air compartment like a boiler was made in which the men could be treated homeopathically, or reimmersed in compressed air. It was erected near the top of the shaft, and when a man was overcome or paralyzed, as I have seen them often, completely unconscious and unable to use their limbs, they were carried into the compartment and the air pressure raised to about 1/2 or 2/3 of that in which they had been working, with immediate improvement. The pressure was then lowered at the very slow rate of one pound per minute or even less. The time allowed for equalization being from 25 to 30 minutes, and even in severe cases the men went away quite cured.

Prompt recompression followed by slow decompression has since been universally considered the key for treatment even if there have been and still are different opinions about the best treatment schedule to use.

ETIOLOGY AND PATHOPHYSIOLOGY OF DECOMPRESSION ILLNESS

Decompression illness is a disease of protean clinical manifestations which is produced by excessively rapid lowering ambient pressure. This reduction causes inert gas dissolved in tissue to come out of physical solution and enter the gas phase. The result is the formation of gas bubbles in tissues, and in arterial and venous blood.

Synonyms for all or portions of the clinical syndrome of decompression illness include decompression sickness, decompression injury, caisson disease, bends, staggers, chokes, aeroembolism, and arterial gas embolism.

Clinical settings of decompression illness:
- Diving
- Aviation
- Hyperbaric oxygen therapy (nurses, chamber assistants, medical personnel)

Predisposing Factors

Exercise during exposure to increased ambient pressure (during the bottom phase of the dive) appears to increase the incidence of decompression illness. The probable explanation of this is that the increased perfusion during exercise leads to an increased uptake of inert gas which must be subsequently eliminated during decompression.

Exercise during decompression may at first sight appear to lower the incidence of decompression illness by an opposite mechanism. The reverse is true; exercise during decompression seems associated with increased incidence of DCI.

Two mechanisms may explain this:

1. The formation of gas micronuclei. Rapidly flowing blood, especially in the area of bifurcation of vessels, may create foci of relative negative pressure through a Venturi effect. Small numbers of molecules of gas from the surrounding supersaturated blood may then diffuse into these foci down a partial pressure gradient. The resulting localized collections of small numbers of gas molecules are known as gas micronuclei and are thought to act as a nidus for bubble formation.
2. Increased local CO_2 production in exercising muscle may play a role since CO_2 is a highly diffusible gas and might contribute to the formation of gas micronuclei.

Recent local injury seems to lead to an increased incidence of decompression illness manifested by pain at or near the site of the injury. The mechanism responsible for this phenomenon is unclear. Changes in local perfusion and increased gas micronuclei formation in injured tissue are postulated mechanisms.

Diving in cold water tends to increase the incidence of decompression illness. Inert gas uptake is generally not affected since the exercising diver is usually warm and has increased tissue perfusion because of exercise. However, when the diver leaves the bottom and reaches his decompression stop where he remains at rest he is likely to become cold. The resulting peripheral vasoconstriction may then impair inert gas elimination.

Even small increases in $FICO_2$ seem to increase the incidence of DCI. The mechanism of this effect is not clearly understood; the increased availability of this highly diffusible gas for diffusion into gas micronuclei is one possible mechanism. This may play a role in the reported higher incidence of DCI after stressful dives with high levels of physical exercise.

Advancing age is thought to increase the incidence of decompression illness for reasons which are not yet clearly known.

Dehydration was reported as a factor which increases the risk of decompression illness during studies on aviators during World War II, and it is still considered a significant risk factor by the international flying and diving medical communities. The mechanism is, however, again unclear and reliable scientific evidence is missing. Changes in the surface tension in serum favoring bubble formation have been postulated.

Anecdotal reports and well as epidemiological studies from Divers Alert Network (DAN) suggest that prior alcohol ingestion increases the incidence of decompression illness. As with alcohol, there are anecdotal as well as epidemiological reports suggesting that significant fatigue preceding a dive increases the incidence of DCI.

Pathogenesis of Decompression Illness

Vascular obstruction by bubbles or bubble-formed complexes occurs in the periphery and in the lung and is considered as the most important element in the pathogenesis of decompression illness. Vascular obstruction may occur in peripheral arteries and/or veins by either bubble formation *in situ* or by embolization of bubbles formed elsewhere. Malfunction and impairment of critical organs and tissues, such as the central nervous system, may have considerable impact on the patient.

Diffuse peripheral vascular obstruction and stasis with resultant tissue hypoxia or anoxia may lead to metabolic acidosis and hypovelemia due to increased capillary permeability. Acidosis and hypovolemia may considerably impair cardiovascular function.

Vascular obstruction of pulmonary capillaries secondary to embolization of bubbles or bubble-formed complexes in venous blood results in increased pulmonary vascular resistance, bronchiolar constriction and peribronchiolar edema. These changes may lead to alterations in ventilation-perfusion ratios with resultant arterial hypoxemia.

Blood-Bubble Interactions

Currently much attention is given to the possible consequences of blood-bubble interaction. Bubbles are a foreign element in the blood. One of the consequences of the blood bubble interaction is thought to be the "denaturization" of lipoproteins with release of lipids.

Electron-micrographic studies in animals have shown vascular obstruction by a complex which appears to be composed of a gas bubble surrounded by a layer of lipid, to which platelets are agglutinated. This and similar observations have given rise to a variety of experimental work investigating the possible usefulness of anticoagulants in decompression illness.

Bubbles are thought to be capable of activating Hageman Factor (Factor XII) with activation of coagulation, contributing to vascular obstruction.

To date there is no experimental evidence to indicate that disseminated intravascular coagulation occurs in decompression illness. Enhanced coagulation at local sites in tissue, however, may contribute to the pathogenesis of DCI.

Coagulation Factor XIIa is capable of triggering the reaction of the complement system. The sequence of reactions of this system produce factors which increase capillary permeability and factors which are chemotaxic for leukocytes.

Factor XIIa is also capable of activating the Kinin system with liberation of bradykinin and histamine. Bradykinin may cause local pain. Both are capable of increasing capillary permeability.

Relationship between Vascular Bubbles and DCI

There is little reason to doubt that the localized pain in a joint is mainly caused by local gas formation. Webb, Ferris and Engels (113) showed that gas could be seen in periarticular and perivascular tissue spaces, and demonstrated a correlation between the presence of gas and the occurrence of pain and that strain was correlated with pain at the site where the strain had been applied. This seems also supported by the common clinical knowledge that local compression often relieves the pain.

However, vascular gas bubbles are a common finding in divers after almost any dive. If a diver reports only a limb or joint pain, he is also and very likely subject to gas invasion in the vascular system and in the pulmonary circulation.

Gas bubbles, detected by precordial doppler monitoring in the pulmonary artery, have been claimed not to be a very reliable predictor of DCI, as they are frequently observed in the absence of any clinical sign or symptom.

On the other hand, there seems to be agreement about the fact that DCI risk increases with the increase of circulating gas bubbles.

In my own experience, as well as the experience of many other colleagues, based on the monitoring of several hundreds of air, heliox, trimix and saturation dives, I have never seen DCI symptoms in individuals without doppler-detectable circulating venous gas bubbles.

Similar observations have been made by Brubakk and Davis, (9, 13, 14) who claim that clinical symptoms were never observed when gas bubbles could not be detected in the pulmonary artery and in muscles of the thigh, respectively, and by Nishi (90, 91) who reported that decompression illness was always accompanied by bubbles if all monitoring sites are considered. Table 1 provides an overview of the results of some related studies.

Surprisingly, DCI incidence is above what is normally accepted in all groups with bubbles shown in Table 1. As it is sometimes very difficult to distinguish between occasional bubble signals and the absence of bubbles, with precordial doppler monitoring, it has been argued by Brubakk (9) that the few DCI cases that did not show any gas bubbles may actually have had "undetected" bubbles.

Effect of Bubbles

Gas bubbles have an effect upon cells and biochemical processes. Thorsen showed, *in vitro*, that gas bubbles are associated with aggregation of thrombocytes, and the degree of aggregation seems to be independent from the gas content of the bubble, but related its surface properties.

Ward and Bergh (6, 110-112) separately reported that gas bubbles activate complement *in vitro*, the response being similar irrespective of the content of the bubble, indicating that activating factor is on the surface of the bubble. Ward (111) also noted a difference between sensitive and non-sensitive individuals, according to the degree of complement activation, which was itself related to the clinical manifestations of decompression illness.

TABLE 1. DOPPLER BUBBLE DETECTION (PRECORDIAL) AND INCIDENCE OF DCI (MODIFIED FROM BRUBAKK)

		Bubble grade	
		0	**I-IV**
Spencer & Johansen 1974 (98)	n	110	64
	DCI inc (%)	1.0	22
Nashimoto & Gotho 1977 (89)	n	64	88
	DCI inc (%)	0	19
Marroni 1981 (61)	n	64	33
	DCI inc (%)	0	9
Nishi 1993 (90)	n	1265	331
	DCI inc (%)	0.6	8
Brubakk 1994 (9)	n	68	40
	DCI inc (%)	1.5	7.5

Individuals with low C5a levels before the dive produced many gas bubbles, and a single air dive seemed to reduce C5a levels, apparently indicating that diving and gas bubbles may activate both C5a and C5a receptors. This has been shown by Stevens in divers up to 14 hours after treatment for DCI. (99)

Complement activation (Kilgore) (53) triggers the activation of neutrophils and the formation of multiple membrane attack complexes (MAC) that eventually lead to cellular destruction. This also causes the leukocytes to adhere to the endothelium and to eventually pass through it. Neutrophil activation has been demonstrated to occur during decompression (Benestad). (4)

C5a activation may be related to erythema, edema and infiltration of inflammatory cells in the skin (Swerlick). (100) Another important effect of C5a is vasoconstriction and blood flow reduction (Martin). (83) If circulation of blood is reduced during decompression, gas elimination is reduced with considerable local bubble formation. After circulation is restored, flow to the affected area does not show the expected "overflow" reaction. This may be due to both vascular bubbles and C5a activation (Brubakk). (9)

Brubakk also observed that pulmonary alterations in pigs after decompression are similar to those observed after complement activation, with considerable leukocyte invasion of the lungs in a pig exposed to significant amounts of bubbles for about 100 minutes after decompression. Complement activation was considered to be the most important mechanism for acute lung injury (Ward). (112)

Certain pulmonary function changes observed in divers, with a reduction in carbon monoxide diffusion capacity and compliance (Thorsen) (101-103), have been considered as evidence that inflammatory processes in the lungs may represent a result of the decompression process. In fact the reduction in carbon monoxide diffusion capacity is rapid and appears related to the development of bubbles (Dujic). (17)

Brubakk (9) considers the lungs to be a primary target organ for gas bubbles. They are probably exposed to gas bubbles effects in each and every decompression. This interpretation is in apparent contrast, when dealing with minimal gas loads, with the concept of the lungs' role as a filter, eliminating the bubbles before they can pass to the arterial side, where the damage can be more significant.

If the gas load on the lungs is large, the filtering capabilities of the lungs will be exceeded and gas will enter the arterial circulation (Vik). (109) An increase in pulmonary artery pressure of only about 30% is considered sufficient to cause arterialization of venous gas bubbles.

Central nervous alterations in DCI are caused by multiple mechanisms, where both vascular and tissuetal bubbles play a role (Francis). (32-37)

Exposure to vascular bubbles does not seem to have a pathologically detectable effect on the spinal cord. In a group of ten amateur and ten professional divers, five of whom had neurological DCI, no changes could be seen (Morild). (27)

However, other authors reported changes in the endothelial layer of the brain ventricles in a group of divers (Mørk). (88) Brubakk (9) considered this as probably not an effect of intravascular gas bubbles in the brain, but possibly related to circulatory changes in venous pressure, such as in pulmonary embolism.

Another possible explanation he gives is that this damage is caused by gas bubbles in the spinal fluid, where bubbles may adhere to the lining of the ventricles.

Chryssantou (10) had indeed shown that animals exposed to decompression show alterations of the blood-brain barrier and Broman (8) had demonstrated that even a short contact between gas bubbles and endothelium (1-2 minutes) would lead to such changes.

Further studies in rabbits showed that bubble-endothelium contact causes endothelial damage and progressive reduction in cerebral blood flow and function (Helps). (44)

CLINICAL MANIFESTATIONS OF DCI

The clinical presentation of DCI used to be divided into two broad categories based on the severity of symptoms.

TYPE I (also called "pain only" decompression illness)
This category used to include the following mild forms of DCI:
*   Limb pain
*   Lymphatic manifestations
*   Cutaneous manifestations

TYPE II (this included more serious manifestations)
*   Pulmonary DCI
*   Central nervous system DCI (brain, spinal cord, inner ear)
*   Shock
*   Abdominal, thoracic, or back pain
*   Extreme fatigue

TYPE I DCI

Pain

The upper extremities are involved three times more often than the lower limbs. This applies to recreational and compressed air diving, while the situation is reversed for both caisson workers and in commercial saturation diving.

The pain can range from slight discomfort to dull, deep, boring and unbearable pain. It is usually not affected by movement and there can rarely be some degree of local pitting edema.

Lymphatic Manifestations

The lymphatic manifestations of decompression illness presumably result from obstruction of lymphatics by bubbles. The manifestations can include pain and swelling of lymph nodes, with lymphedema of the tissues drained by the obstructed lymph nodes.

Cutaneous Manifestations
*   Itching is commonly reported during decompression from dry chamber dives where the skin is surrounded by chamber atmosphere

rather than water. It is thought to depend upon the diffusion of gas from the chamber atmosphere into the skin, followed by expansion during decompression and a consequent itching sensation. This symptom is not a form of decompression illness and should not be treated with recompression. Itching after a regular wet dive is different and very likely related to a form of cutaneous DCI. However, this is usually accompanied by some degree of skin rash or visible skin change.

- Cutis Marmorata is a form of DCI which is thought to result from bubble-generated cutaneous venous obstruction. It usually presents as an area of erythema, frequently affecting the upper back and chest. Prominent linear purple markings are frequent. These manifestations are to be considered a clear form of DCI and should be promptly treated. Recompression often, although not always, leads to immediate resolution. This sign is frequently a herald of more serious forms of DCI.

TYPE II DCI

Pulmonary Decompression Illness

This is a syndrome usually presenting with a triad of evolving symptoms:

a) Substernal pain, usually burning and progressively increasing. Initially the pain may be noted only when coughing. Over time the pain may become constant.

b) Cough, initially intermittent and easily provoked by cigarette smoking. Paroxysms of coughing may become uncontrollable.

c) Progressive respiratory failure and dyspnea.

The manifestations of pulmonary decompression illness are believed to result from the combined effects of gas emboli in the pulmonary artery and obstruction of the vascular supply to the bronchial mucosa. Untreated pulmonary DCI may be fatal.

Neurological Decompression Illness

Decompression illness causes vascular obstruction secondary to random bubble formation within the vascular system. The neurological manifestations of DCI are, therefore, unpredictable. Any focal neurological symptom or sign may be the presenting problem. All neurological symptoms and signs occurring in the course of decompression illness should be assumed to represent central nervous system involvement and be treated accordingly.

Cerebral Decompression Illness

Brain involvement in DCI appears to be especially common in aviators. In this group a migraine-like headache accompanied by visual disturbances is a common manifestation of Decompression Illness. Brain involvement also occurs in divers as in the form of hemiparesis.

Collapse with unconsciousness is a rare presentation of decompression illness and presumably represents brain involvement in a hyperacute form of DCI.

Spinal Cord Decompression Illness

Paraplegia is a "classic" symptom of decompression illness in divers and clearly represents spinal cord involvement. Bladder paralysis with urinary retention and fecal incontinence frequently accompany paraplegia.

In the last few years, cases of serious paralysis in recreational divers dropped from 13.4 percent in 1987 to only 2.9 percent in 1997, and the number of cases of divers losing consciousness dropped from 7.4 percent to 3.9 percent of total injuries during the same period. The incidence of loss of bladder function, another sign of neurological DCI, dropped from 2.2 percent to 0.4 percent during this period (DAN Diving Accident Reports). (16, 77, 79, 80)

However, this has not been balanced by an equivalent rise in the frequency of pain only or skin DCI; on the contrary there seems to be a clear trend towards an increased incidence of milder neurological manifestations, such as paresthesia, with more or less undefined subjective symptoms, such as numbness and/or tingling, when not vague, ambiguous and ill-defined symptoms, which, however, normally respond well to oxygen administration and therapeutical recompression.

Inner Ear Decompression Illness

Cochleo-vestibular decompression illness is a not an uncommon manifestation of CNS involvement. Usually both the cochlea and vestibular apparatus are involved and the presenting symptoms include tinnitus, deafness, vertigo, nausea, vomiting, and ataxia. Nystagmus may be present on physical examination.

It is not clear whether the situation depends predominantly on bubble formation in the perilymph or is due to embolization of the auditory vestibular areas of the brain. Inner ear decompression illness is a serious medical emergency and must be treated immediately to avoid permanent damage. Since the nutrient arteries of the inner ear are very small, rapid reduction in bubble diameter, with immediate 100% oxygen administration and prompt recompression, is essential.

Shock

Shock occasionally occurs in decompression illness; it is usually associated with serious pulmonary manifestations, and indicates a hyperacute form of DCI. Multiple mechanisms may contribute to the pathogenesis of shock in DCI, including loss of vascular tone from spinal cord involvement, myocordial depression from hypoxemia and acidosis, pulmonary embolization and hypovolemia due to increased capillary permeability, loss of plasma water and hemocencentration.

Back, Abdominal, or Chest Pain

Pain in these areas, in contrast to limb pain, should be given great attention, as it frequently heralds spinal cord involvement.

Extreme Fatigue

Fatigue out of proportion from that normally occurring after a dive has long been regarded as a serious manifestation of decompression illness. However, the biochemical and pathophysiological mechanisms of this symptom are unknown.

Time to Onset of Symptoms (general)

- 50% occur within 30 minutes of surfacing
- 85% occur within one hour of surfacing
- 95% occur within three hours of surfacing
- 1% delayed more than 12 hours

However, symptoms have been reported to begin as late as 24 hours and more after surfacing.

NEW DCI CLASSIFICATION

The simple classification into Type I DCI and Type II DCI implies that the different categories are well-defined disease entities and that there is reasonable agreement about the classification (Brubakk).

Smith and Kemper (51, 96, 97), however, in two separate studies, showed considerable uncertainty between experts using the classical classification system. For instance, cerebral DCI could not, in many cases, be distinguished from arterial gas embolism or vestibular barotrauma. Other studies have shown that solely articular symptoms are rare, as they are usually accompanied by central nervous symptoms (Denoble, (15)Kelleher(50)). Extreme fatigue can be classified as a minor symptom, but could also be a sign of subclinical pulmonary embolism (Hallenbeck). (43)

Francis (32-37) therefore suggested the currently widely adopted term "decompression illness," to include the two previously used definitions of decompression sickness and arterial gas embolism. He also suggested not using the classification (Type I and Type II), while adopting instead a descriptive classification method according to the clinical manifestations (signs and/or symptoms) and their evolution in time. Using this classification scheme, a very high degree of concordance between different specialists was possible (Smith). (96, 97)

Dutka (18-20) proposed the following Classification Table for Decompression Injuries, which is a useful guideline to correctly describe the various possible manifestations of a decompression disorder (Table 2).

THE TREATMENT OF DCI

Air was nearly always used as the breathing gas in the treatment of DCI for many years, and oxygen treatment was not really explored until Yarbrough and Behnke's preliminary experiments in 1939. (115)

The early treatment theory was conceptually homeopathic, in trying to decide how deep to take the injured diver. The original depth of the dive was used as a guide. For example, if decompression from a depth of 40 meters caused the symptoms, recompression to the same pressure should alleviate them.

However, there were controversies, as others thought that the situation of the diver should lead the decision and that the depth of relief should mark the beginning treatment pressure, while still others argued that bubbles may be compressed, but never disappear and should always be assumed as being present.

For these reasons the recommendation was to compress the patient to the depth of relief plus at least one atmosphere. The rationale was that if a bubble became extremely small, surface tension may cause it to collapse and disappear. It was generally realized that bubbles remaining in the tissues and circulation would continue to take up inert gas, as more nitrogen was absorbed during the recompression treatment.

TABLE 2. CLASSIFICATION TABLE FOR DECOMPRESSION INJURIES

		DEFINITION ➤	ABRUPT	EVOLVING	STATIC
		ONSET TIME ➤	IMMEDIATE	FIRST DAY	DAYS TO YEARS
L O C A L I Z A T I O N	**S O M A T I C**	PAINFUL	Limb bend: Periarticular pain	Limb bend: fluctuating pain after dive	Osteonecrosis
		PARESTHETIC	Tingling or numbness, may herald spinal DCI	Tingling or numbness, may be combined with pain	Recurrent or episodic after treatment; probably benign
		ASYMPTOMATIC	Skin changes or painless swelling	Skin changes or painless swelling	Asymptomatic osteonecrosis
		CEREBRAL	Loss of consciousness, hemiplegia, "air embolism"	Hemiparesis, delirium, brainstem signs, vertigo	Chronic neuropyschologic changes
		SPINAL	Girdle pain, loss of leg movement and bladder control	Waxing and waning weakness, bladder dysfunction, sensory levels	Chronic gait and bladder disturbances
		CEREBRO-SPINAL	Unconscious diver with spinal findings	Combined spinal and cerebral signs, varying	Combined cerebral and spinal disability; spinal predominates
		SYSTEMATIC	Chokes; acute systematic respiratory collapse	Fatigue, rare visceral DCI	Rare cases of ARDS and lung damage

In the 1924 edition of the U.S. Navy Diving Manual, a suggested recompression treatment procedure was first published, but more than 50% of the treatments were unsuccessful. The U.S. Navy published treatment tables again in 1942 without much improvement in the results. In 1945, Van Der Aue and Behnke (107) experimented with better treatment methods which resulted in the publication of the U.S. Navy air recompression Tables I to IV. They became the standard of the world for the next 20 years. (105) The outcome improvement over the previous approach was dramatic and over 90%.

The principles of these tables were:

- Recompression to depth of relief plus at least one atmosphere. In practice, this meant going to a minimal depth of 30 meters.
- A maximum treatment depth of 50 meters. This depth was considered a good compromise between optimal recompression of any bubble while minimizing nitrogen narcosis risk and subsequent decompression.
- The use of a 12-hour stop at 9 meters before surfacing. Theoretically, this "overnight soak" was intended to allow all the tissues to saturate or desaturate to the 9 meter level, from where, according to Haldane, direct decompression to the surface would be safe.
- The use of intermittent oxygen breathing during the last hours of treatment.

These tables were at first very successful, with a failure rate on the initial recompression of only 6% in 1946. Despite their great length—from six hours 20 minutes for Table I to 38 hours 11 minutes for Table IV, they represented the only available therapeutical solution at the time.

In 1963, however, the observed failure rate for serious symptom cases was 46% on the initial recompression. The reason for the failure of these tables, which had initially been so successful, was that more and more civilian recreational scuba diving cases were being treated. The civilians often dove in total ignorance of decompression requirements, to say nothing of the pretreatment intervals, which were significantly longer than with the military divers.

Goodman and Workman (40) started investigating the use of oxygen at moderate depths (2.8 ATA) for the treatment of decompression illness. Oxygen treatment had first been suggested by Behnke in 1937.(2) At that time, however, the U.S. Navy Bureau of Medicine and Surgery was concerned that oxygen breathing in the chamber may be dangerous. The risks of oxygen toxicity and fire were too great (Kindwall). (54) For this reason Behnke's excellent results were ignored. (24)

Edgar End, (24) in Milwaukee, had also noted in 1947 that treating with compressed air was ineffective. He introduced oxygen breathing with excellent results in over 250 cases of DCI in compressed air workers (Kindwall). (54)

The first 52 cases treated with the "new" Goodman and Workman (40) oxygen tables demonstrated that a 30-minute stay—at least—at the maximum depth of 18 meters and a total oxygen breathing treatment time of 90 minutes could be considered "adequate" treatment, allowing for a 3.6% failure rate.

Treatment schedules were lengthened to two hours and four hours of oxygen breathing, with air breathing intervals of 5 to 15 minutes, to avoid oxygen toxicity. The two- and four-hour schemes were called U.S. Navy Tables 5 and 6 respectively and officially published in 1967. (106)

The most significant conceptual difference, with respect to the previous approach, was the importance given to the time of relief, instead of the depth of relief (Kindwall). (54)

Compression ceased to be limited to the scope of reducing the bubbles, hopefully until they could disappear, and then decompress the diver along a safe profile. The concept of a real "therapeutical" treatment scheme was introduced. Compression is also the vehicle for a therapeutical drug (oxygen) that exerts its treating action during the time of the treatment schedule, while also offering a (now twofold) tool for the reduction of the offending gas bubbles, both by pressure and by a favorable diffusion gradient.

Serial treatment of decompression illness had been advocated by many. At a meeting of the North Sea off-shore diving groups (Royal Society of Medicine in London in 1976), a consensus was reached that if the diver had residual symptoms after the initial treatment, daily hyperbaric oxygen treatment should be continued for at least two weeks or until the patient's signs and symptoms had plateaued (Elliott). (21)

Several modification treatment schemes were then introduced, such as the Comex table 30. This used mixed gas at a maximum pressure of four, and the concept of saturation treatment. This was first introduced by Miller (84) in 1978, with saturation treatment to start at four atmospheres while the patient breathed oxygen at 0.35 to 0.5 bar.

Currently many different treatment protocols are in use, while the U.S. Navy Table 6 is probably the most commonly used internationally. Available evidence indicates that this table is adequate in the majority of cases where treatment is initiated without delay (DAN Diving Accident Reports). (16) Unfortunately, there is often considerable delay in initiating treatment, and many of the secondary effects of the bubbles on blood and tissues become important.

Kelleher (50) has shown that initial treatment is effective in only about 66% of the cases. Other studies have demonstrated that none of the alternative proposed protocols, including saturation decompression, are superior to U.S. Navy Table 6 (Leitch). (56-57)

The severity of symptoms should not be the only variable to be considered. Heliox and trimix dives may differ from air dives, due to the differences in partition coefficients of helium and nitrogen in the tissues (Brubakk, James). (9, 49)

The use of different gas mixes (particularly heliox) for the treatment of DCI, following compressed air diving, remains controversial. Some reports seem to indicate that helium is beneficial; air bubbles in tissue have been observed to disappear faster from the spinal cord, if heliox is used instead of pure oxygen at 1 ATA. However, the reverse is true at the pressure of 2.8 ATA (Hyldegaard). (46-48)

Brubakk believes, having showed an increased shunt in the lung and a reduction of gas elimination at increased oxygen tensions, that there is actually little benefit in using high oxygen tensions and that lower tensions may be more advantageous.

Ancillary pharmacological treatment to recompression began to be emphasized in the late 1960s and 1970s.

In 1979 the Undersea Medical Society organized a workshop on the management of severe and complicated cases of decompression illness, where the importance of hydration, steroids, heparin, aspirin, and other agents were discussed. (13)

Over the years, many attempts have been made to improve the treatment of decompression illness with other drugs, generally with little success.

Some of these possibilities have not been sufficiently studied and may deserve further attention, such as the use of fluorocarbons, which have a higher solubility for nitrogen than plasma. Lutz and Herrmann were able to substantially reduce the mortality of rats undergoing rapid decompression from 8 ATA when fluorocarbon was infused after decompression. (58)

A further point which deserves attention and study is complement activation and its effect on the leukocyte-endothelium adhesion. This appears to have a certain role in DCI, and for which drugs could have a role.

In 1994, the European Committee for Hyperbaric Medicine organized its first European Consensus Conference, where decompression illness was one of the topics. (26)

In 1996 a second, more specific Consensus Conference was organized, the theme of which was "The Treatment of Decompression Accidents in Recreational Diving." Following both conferences, and after extensive presentations by leading international experts, the two International Juries formulated recommendations. They have since been adopted in Europe as the current standards for the definition and treatment of DCI in Europe and are reproduced in Appendix 1. (27)

CONCLUSION

DCI is generally considered a benign condition, if adequate treatment is promptly started, with a success rate in excess of 80-90%.

There is a consensus that 100% oxygen should be administered immediately as the single most important first aid treatment of any DCI case related to surface-oriented diving. Rehydration is also a very valuable adjunct during field first aid of such DCI cases.

Hyperbaric treatment should be started with the shortest possible delay from surfacing or from the onset of the first DCI signs and symptoms. Hyperbaric treatment tables using 100% oxygen at environmental pressures not exceeding 2.8 bars, with various depth/time profiles, demonstrated to assure excellent results in more than 80% of the treated cases. There is no evidence that other therapeutical schemes provide better results.

It is accepted by many specialists that the use of high pressure (generally 4 bars maximum) treatment tables using a gas mixture of 50% helium and 50% oxygen may prove highly effective and provide good results in the cases that do not quickly and satisfactorily respond to the standard low pressure hyperbaric oxygen treatment tables.

Although conclusive scientific evidence suggesting the use of any pharmacological treatment other than oxygen is missing, the administration of adjunctive fluid therapy is considered very important. Hydration is generally recommended by diving-hyperbaric medicine specialists, whereas the role of other drugs, such as steroids and anticoagulants, is still controversial.

The continuation of hyperbaric oxygen therapy, combined with a specific rehabilitation protocol in neurological cases, when the initial DCI treatment tables are not totally successful is considered important. There is growing scientific evidence that physical therapy can significantly contribute to achieve an eventually better functional recovery. (69, 78)

APPENDIX 1

Extract from the final recommendations of the Jury of the First European Consensus Conference on Hyperbaric Medicine. European Committee for Hyperbaric Medicine. Lille, September 1994. (26)

QUESTION N°1: Which treatment for diving decompression accidents?

- The primary cause of DCI is the separation of gas in the body tissues (bubbles).
- The best prophylaxis is achieved by adequate ascent/ decompression procedures.
- DCI is best classified descriptively.
- On-site 100% oxygen first aid treatment is strongly recommended (Type 1 recommendation).
- On-site fluid administration for the first aid of decompression accidents is recommended (Type 2 recommendation).
- Therapeutical recompression must be initiated as soon as possible (Type 1 recommendation).
- Aside immediate recompression treatment tables which may be used on the site of the accident, the "low pressure oxygen treatment tables" are recommended as the treatment tables of first choice (Type 1 recommendation). High pressure oxygen/inert gas tables can be used in selected and/or recalcitrant cases (Type 3 recommendation). Deep, not surface-oriented, mixed gas or saturation diving accidents require special treatment protocols.
- Adjunctive pharmacological treatment is controversial but:
  - I.V. fluid therapy is recommended (Type 2 recommendation).
  - The use of steroids and anticoagulants, although widely adopted without any apparent adverse effect, is considered optional (Type 3 recommendation).
- The continuation of a combined hyperbaric oxygen therapy and rehabilitation treatment is recommended until clinical stabilization or no further amelioration is achieved (Type 2 recommendation).

Final recommendations of the Jury of the Second European Consensus Conference of the European Committee for Hyperbaric Medicine on "The Treatment of Decompression Accidents in Recreational Diving." Marseilles, May 1996. (27)

After listening to the presentations by the experts and the following floor discussion, the jury met to answer the six questions posed by the Conference Scientific Committee. The recommendations of the jury were based on the analysis of the clinical and experimental studies, according to the current scientific standards, although considering the limited data provided by the—otherwise scientifically correct—clinical studies presented. The jury evaluated the data on the basis of their general concordance and of the fact that the studies refer to several years of observations by many independent international groups. The jury also considered that its recommendations are intended as aimed at recreational diving performed in

European waters and that, regarding logistical conditions of other diving sites that may not allow for the full respect of the jury's recommendations, rather than downgrading the jury's conclusions, its recommendations should be taken as a stimulus towards optimal diving safety worldwide.

QUESTION N°2: Is there a difference between recreational and commercial diving decompression accidents?

Whatever the reasons and the methods for diving, they all share similar risk (the same decompression profile after the same dive will bring about the same decompression risk), similar physiopathology (a decompression accident will generate similar disorders in both circumstances) and similar results (if the delay to treatment is similar). The observed differences between decompression accidents in the two types of diving essentially regard the degree of risk (fitness to dive, training, work load, depth, environment, safety standards) and the delay before treatment (symptom recognition, hyperbaric chamber availability).

The recommendations of the jury (Type 1 recommendation) are the following:
- Implementing fitness-to-dive standards, both for recreational and commercial diving
- Implementing an adequate classification of decompression accidents
- Implementing a coordinated network for the collection and the retrospective analysis of data concerning decompression accidents
- Improving the recreational diving safety standards to approach the current
- Standards applied in commercial diving, with special regard to:
  - availability of oxygen on every dive site
  - availability of a recompression chamber within a delay of four hours
  - preparation of an emergency plan before any dive
- Recreational divers should be trained, like commercial divers are, to recognize signs and symptoms of decompression accidents

QUESTION N°3: How to classify decompression accidents?

Depending on the intended utilization objective, there are three possible ways to classify decompression accidents:
- Immediate clinical use, need for rapid and efficient communication between divers and emergency services, on-site first aid and medical evacuation of injured divers, data selection and availability for clinical studies
- Epidemiological use for the retrospective analysis of data and of treatment results
- Description of lesions based on anatomo-pathological observations

The recommendations of the jury (Type 1 recommendation) are the following:
- Immediate use classification should be simple and objective.
  The jury recommends that it is based on that adopted by the UHMS (Smith and Francis). (96-97)

- Epidemiological use classification for retrospective analysis should allow for the institution of a data bank collecting the observations from a great numbers of countries. To this purpose, harmonization between national classifications should be established in order to allow transcodification.
- This classification should:
  - be multithematic in its conception
  - include the type of diving, chronological data, clinical manifestations and a two-year follow-up

QUESTION N°4: Which experimental model for decompression studies?

Considering the complexity of the question and the difficulty in conducting rigorous clinical studies with sufficient numbers of experimental subjects, the jury agreed that animal studies are still needed.

The recommendations of the jury (Type 1 recommendation) are the following:

- Experimental studies are necessary for more information on decompression accidents.
- The variables to study are many and include:
  - the bubble phenomenon
  - central neurological manifestations
  - bone and skin manifestations
  - pulmonary disorders
  - cardiovascular disorders
- As a general principle *in vitro* studies should precede *in vivo* studies, and *ex vivo* studies should be done before *in vivo* ones.
- Among the animal models so far used, small animals (rodents) do not seem to adequately reproduce the human observations. Among the larger animals, the dog is less and less used, sheep and ewes are mainly used for pulmonary studies, while the pig seems to be the animal that better reflects human reactions to decompression.

Concerning methodology, the jury recommends that studies:
- Consider clinically significant parameters
- Consider experimental conditions, particularly when anesthesia
- Modalities may interfere with the observations, include a detailed description of the animal model in each published paper

QUESTION N°5: Which initial recompression modality?

Decompression accidents are true medical emergencies that must benefit from treatment in specialized centers as soon as possible. A specialized center is considered as a hospital-based facility, having not only a hyperbaric chamber but also a permanent and adequately trained medical and paramedical staff.

- The victims of a decompression accident should be immediately directed from the site of the diving accident to the closest specialized center (Type 1 recommendation).
- Minor decompression accidents (pain only) should be treated

with oxygen recompression tables at 18 meters depth maximum
(Type 1 recommendation).
- Regarding more serious decompression accidents (neurological
  and vestibular accidents), the jury observed that there are
  presently two acceptable protocols, as neither one has been
  proved better by any scientifically valid study to date:
  - oxygen recompression tables at 2.8 ATA (with possible
    extensions)
  - hyperoxygenated breathing mixtures at 4.0 ATA

The choice between the two may depend on personal experience
and on local logistics. However, under no circumstance should the
unavailability of one of the two accepted modalities delay the
treatment (Type 1 recommendation).

The jury also considered the following optional treatment modalities
(Type 3 recommendation):
- Compression to 6 ATA in case of cerebral arterial gas embolism, with
  the condition that this compression is performed using hyperoxygenated mixtures and not compressed air and that the delay to treatment is not more than a few hours.
- Saturation treatment tables in case of persistent symptoms.

Finally the jury recommends that:
- In-water recompression should never be undertaken as the
  initial recompression modality for a decompression accident
  (Type 1 recommendation).
- All decompression accidents should be the object of a
  standardized recording method aimed at the creation of a
  database for epidemiological studies (Type 1 recommendation).

QUESTION N°6: Which fluid replacement protocol and which role for drugs in the treatment of decompression accidents?

1 - Fluid treatment

Victims of decompression accidents generally suffer from a
certain degree of dehydration, depending on decreased fluid input, increased
urinary output, capillary fluid leakage and disorder-related relative hypovolemia.
The degree of dehydration should be evaluated:

On site:
- history, dive conditions, thirst, clinical evaluation of neurological conditions, hemodynamics, temperature, vasoconstriction, dryness of
  mucosae, urinary output

At hospital:
- urinary output, hemodynamics to include CVP, hematocrit, plasma
  proteins and electrolytes

Recommended hydration protocol:

On site:

- Oral hydration is recommended only if the patient is conscious (Type 1 recommendation)
- Contraindications to oral rehydration are stringent and include:
  - any consciousness abnormality
  - nausea and vomiting
  - suspected lesions of the gastro-intestinal tract.
- Oral rehydration should be done with plain water, possibly with the addition of electrolytes but with no gas. The administered fluid should be cold if the patient is hyperthermic. Sugar is not recommended. The amount of fluids administered should be adapted to the patient's thirst and acceptance.
- Venous rehydration should be preferred if a physician is present. Recommended procedures are as follows:
  - Use a peripheral venous catheter (18 gauge) and preferably Ringer Lactate as infusion fluid. Glucose-containing solutions are not recommended.
  - The addition of colloids can be considered if large quantities of fluids are needed. Recommended colloids, in order of preference, are starch-containing solutions, gelatines, haptene added dextranes (Type 3 recommendation).

At the hospital:

- Intravenous rehydration is recommended while controlling the routine physiological parameters: urinary output, hemodynamics, CVP, standard laboratory tests.

2 - Drug treatment

Strongly recommended (Type 1 recommendation):

- Normobaric Oxygen. The administration of normobaric oxygen allows for the treatment of hypoxemia and favours the elimination of inert gas bubbles. Oxygen should be administered with an oro-nasal mask with reservoir bag, at a minimal flow rate of 15 l/min, or with CPAP mask circuit, using either a free flow regulator or a demand valve, in such a way to obtain a F_iO_2 close to 1. In case of respiratory distress, shock or coma, the patient should be intubated and ventilated with a $F_iO_2 = 1$ and setting the ventilator to avoid pressure and volume trauma. Normobaric oxygen should be continued until hyperbaric recompression is started (with a maximum of six hours when the F_iO_2 is 1).

Recommended (Type 2 recommendation):

- Any necessary drug for the support treatment of an intensive care patient (adequate first aid kit)

Optional (Type 3 recommendation):
On site:
- Any way to prevent hyperthermia
- Aspirin: 500 mg orally in the adult patient (contraindications similar to oral rehydration)

At the hospital:
- Use drugs having no significant collateral effects, such as:
  - aspirin: 500 mg if not already administered or contraindicated
  - lidocaine
  - low dose heparin (avoid complete decoagulation)
  - steroids, calcium channel blockers, antioxydants

QUESTION N°7: Which treatment protocol for persistent symptoms after the initial recompression?

The jury concluded that there are no scientifically valid data to allow for a recommended approach to this issue. More studies are necessary as well as the adoption of standardized evaluation methods. Concerning spinal cord injuries, a specific scoring system (such as the ASIA scale) is recommended for pre and post treatment evaluation and during the two-year follow-up.
- Randomized prospective studies are needed to better evaluate the efficacy of hyperbaric oxygen therapy and of rehabilitation before any protocol can be proposed or recommended. However, in analogy with any other neurological injury, rehabilitation should be started as soon as possible (Type 1 recommendation).
- Hyperbaric oxygen treatment is recommended to a maximum of 10 treatment sessions after the initial recompression, in combination and during rehabilitation therapy. The continuation of HBO therapy can be accepted if objective improvement is observed under pressure during the hyperbaric treatment sessions (Type 3 recommendation).

REFERENCES

1. Balestra C, Germonpré P, Marroni A. Intrathoracic pressure changes after Valsalva strain and other maneuvers: implications for divers with patent foramen ovale. Undersea Hyper Med 1998; 25(3): 171

2. Behnke AR, Shaw LA. The use of oxygen in the treatment of compressed air illness. Nav med Bull 1937;35:61.

3. Behnke AR. Decompression sickness following exposure to high pressures. In: Fulton JF. Decompression sickness. WB Saunders Company, London 1951: 53. 1993:293.

4. Benestad HB, Hersleth IB, Hardersen H, Molvær OI. Functional capacity of neutrophil granulocytes in deep-sea divers. Scand J Clin Lab Invest 1990;50:9.

5. Bennett PB, Dovenbarger J, Corson K. Etiology and Treatment of Air Diving Accidents. In Diving Accident Management. Forty-first Workshop of the Undersea and Hyperbaric Medical Society. PB Bennett, RE Moon Eds. 1990:12

6. Bergh K, Hjelde A, Iversen O-J, Brubakk AO. Variability over time of complement activation induced by air bubbles in human and rabbit sera. J Appl Physiol 1993, 74:1811

7. Bert P. Barometric Pressure (1878) page 894, Translation by MA Hitchcock and FA Hitchcock—College Book Company, Columbus, Ohio, 1943. Republished by Undersea and Hyperbaric Medical Society, Bethesda, 1978.

8. Broman T, Branemark PI, Johansson B, Steinwall O. Intravital and post-mortem studies on air embolism damage of the blood-brain-barrier. Acta Neur Scand 1966;42:146

9. Brubakk A. Decompression Illness. What we do know, what we don't know?. In: F. Wattel, D. Mathieu eds) First European Consensus Conference on Hyperbaric Medicine European Committee for Hyperbaric Medicine, University of Lille., C.R.A.M. Nord-Picardie, Sécurité Social 1994:2. ISBN 3-908229-05-7

10. Chrysantou C., Springer M, Lipschitz S. Blood-brain and blood-lung barrier alterations by dysbaric exposure. Undersea Biomed Res 1977;4:111.

11. Curley MD, Schwartz HJ, Zwingelberg K~. Neuropsychologic assessment of cerebral decompression sickness and gas embolism. Undersea Biomed Res. 1988; 15:223.

12. Daniels S, Bowser-Riley F, Vlachonikolis IG. The relationship between gas bubbles and symptoms of decompression sickness. In: In Brubakk AO, Hemingsen BB, Sundnes G.(eds), Supersaturation and bubble formation in fluids and organisms. Tapir Publishers Trondheim 1989:pp 387.

13. Davis JC, (Chairman). Treatment of serious decompression sickness and arterial gas embolism. UMS Workshop #20, Publication No. 34WS(SDS), Nov. 30, 1979.

14. Davis JC, Piantadosi CA, Moon RE.. Saturation Treatment of Decompression Illness in a hospital based hyperbaric facility. In Treatment of Decompression Illness. Forty-fifth Workshop of the Undersea and Hyperbaric Medical Society. RE Moon, PJ Sheffield Eds. 1996:267

15. Denoble P, Vann RD, Dear GL. Describing decompression illness in recreational divers. Undersea & Hyperbaric Medicine 1993;20(suppl):18.

16. Divers Alert Network. 2002 Report on Decompression Illness, Diving Fatalities and Project Dive Exploration (Based on 2000 Data). Divers Alert Network, Durham, N.C, USA. 2002. www.diversalertnetwork.org

17. Dujic Z, Eterovic D, Denoble P, Krstacic G, Tocilj J, Gosovic S. Effect of single air dive on pulmonary diffusing capacity in professional divers. J Appl Physiol 1993;74:55.

18. Dutka AJ, Mink R and Hallenbeck JM. Dexamethasone prevents secondary deterioration only when given 3 hours prior to cerebral air emboflsm. (Abstract), Undersea Biomedical Research (SuppL), 1988; 15:14.

19. Dutka AJ, Overlock R, Farra F, Okamoto G, Suzuki D. The Neurologic Residua of Decompression Sickness. Neurology 1990; 40(Suppl 1):744.

20. Dutka AJ. Clinical Findings in Decompression Illness. A proposed Terminology. In Treatment of Decompression Illness. Forty-fifth Workshop of the Undersea and Hyperbaric Medical Society. RE Moon, PJ Sheffield Eds. 1996:1

21. Elliott DH (Ed). Treatment offshore of decompression sickness, EUBS Workshop— Reported on behalf of the UMS—Supported by the U.K. Off-Shore Operators Assoc. London, Feb. 17, 1976. UMS Report No. 4-9-76.

22. Elliott D, Moon RE. Manifestations of the decompression disorders. In Bennett PB, Elliott DH (eds). The Physiology and Medicine of Diving, 4th ed. WB Saunders Company, London 1993:481.

23. Elliott DH, Hallenbeck JM, Bove AA. Acute Decompression Sickness. Lancet, 1974; 16: 1193

24. End, Edgar. Personal Communication, 1956. In Kindwall EP, Management of Diving Accidents: Historical Review. In Diving Accident Management. Forty-first Workshop of the Undersea and Hyperbaric Medical Society. PB Bennett, RE Moon Eds. 1990:1

25. Erde, A, Edmonds, O. Decompression sickness: a clinical series. Journal of Occup Med 1975; 17: 324.

26. European Committee for Hyperbaric Medicine. First European Consensus Conference on Hyperbaric Medicine European Committee for Hyperbaric Medicine, F. Wattel, D. Mathieu eds. University of Lille., C.R.A.M. Nord-Picardie, Sécurité Social 1994 ISBN 3-908229-05-7

27. European Committee for Hyperbaric Medicine. Second European Consensus Conference on the Treatment of Decompression Accidents in Recreational Diving. European Committee for Hyperbaric Medicine, F. Wattel, D. Mathieu eds . Conseil Général des Bouches du Rhone. 1996

28. Evans DE, McDermott JJ, Kobrine AL and Flynn ET. Effects of intra-venous Lidocaine in experimental cerebral air embolism (Abstract). Undersea Biomedical Research (Suppl.), 1988; 15:17.

29. Farmer JC. Inner Ear Decompression Sickness versus Inner Ear Barotrauma: differential diagnosis and treatment of diving related Inner Ear dysfunction. In Treatment of Decompression Illness. Forty-fifth Workshop of the Undersea and Hyperbaric Medical Society. RE Moon, PJ Sheffield Eds. 1996:163

30. Ferris EB, Engel GE. The clinical nature of high altitude decompression sickness. In: Fulton JF. Decompression sickness. WB Saunders Company, London 1951: 4.

31. Flynn ET, Catron PW. Recognition and Treatment of Diving Casualties. Publications A-4N-0018, US Naval School, Diving and Salvage, Washington D.C..

32. Francis TJR, Gorman DF. Pathogenesis of the decompression disorders. In: Bennett PB, Elliott DH (eds). The physiology and medicine of diving, 4th ed. WB Saunders Company, London 1993:454.

33. Francis TJR, Pezeshkepour GH, Dutka AJ, Hallenbeck JM, Flynn ET. Is there a role for the autochthonous bubble in the pathogenesis of spinal cord decompression sickness? J. Neuropath and Exp Neurol 1988; 47:475.

34. Francis TJR, Smith DJ, Sykes JJW. The prevention and management of diving accidents. INM Report No. R93002, Institute of Naval Medicine, Alverstoke, 1993.

35. Francis TJR, Smith, DH; eds. Describing Decompression Illness 42nd UMHS. Forty-second Workshop. Bethesda, MD: Undersea and Hyperbaric Medical Society, 1991.

36. Francis, TJR, Dutka, AJ, Flynn, ET. Experimental determination of latency, severity and outcome in CNS decompression sickness. Undersea Biomedical Res 1988; 15:419.

37. Francis TJR. The Pathophysiology of Decompression Sickness. In Diving Accident Management. Forty-first Workshop of the Undersea and Hyperbaric Medical Society. PB Bennett, RE Moon Eds. 1990:38

38. Frankel HL. Paraplegia due to decompression sickness Paraplegia 1977; 14:306.

39. Germonpre P, Dendale, P, Unger P, Balestra C. Patent Foramen Ovale and decompression sickness in sport divers. J. Appl. Physiol. 1998; 84(5): 1622

40. Goodman MW and RD Workman. Research Report 5-65. Minimal recompression, oxygen-breathing approach to treatment of decompression sickness in divers and aviators. BuShips Project SF011 06 05, Task 1151 3-2, November 15, 1965.

41. Gorman DF, 0W Edmonds, DW Parsons, et al. Neurologic sequelae of decompression sickness: a clinical report. Proceedings of the Ninth International Symposium on Underwater Hyperbaric Physiology, Undersea and Hyperbaric Medical Society, Bethesda, Maryland, 1987: 993

42. Gregg PJ, Walder DN. Caisson Disease of Bone. Clin Orthopedics and Related Res. 1986; 210:43.

43. Hallenbeck JM, Elliott DH, Bove AA. Decompression sickness studies in the dog. In Lambertsen CJ (ed). Underwater Physiology V, Fed Am Soc Exp Biol, Bethesda 1975

44. Helps SC, Parsons DW, Reilly PL, Gorman DF. The effect of gas emboli on rabbit cerebral blood flow. Stroke 1990;21:94.

45. Hjelde A, Brubakk AO, Bergh K, Iversen O-J. Complement activation in divers following repeated air/heliox dives and its possible relevance to decompression sickness. Submitted J Appl Physiol 1994.

46. Hyldegaard O, Madsen J, Kerem D, Melamed Y. Effect of combined recompression and air, heliox or oxygen breathing on air bubbles in rat spinal white matter. In: Eidsmo Reinertsen R, Brubakk AO, Bolstad G (eds). Proc XIX EUBS, Trondheim1993: 292

47. Hyldegaard O, Møller M, Madsen J. Effect of He-O2, O2 and N2-O2 breathing on injected bubbles in spinal white matter. Undersea Biomed Res 1991;18:361.

48. Hyldegaard O, Madsen J. Effect of different breathing gas on bubble resolution in lipid and aqueous tissues. Animal experiments. In Treatment of Decompression Illness. Forty-fifth Workshop of the Undersea and Hyperbaric Medical Society. RE Moon, PJ Sheffield Eds. 1996:313

49. James PB. Recompression Therapy in Commercial Diving. In Diving Accident Management. Forty-first Workshop of the Undersea and Hyperbaric Medical Society. PB Bennett, RE Moon Eds. 1990:314

50. Kelleher PC, Francis TJR. INM diving accident database analysis of 225 cases of decompression illness. INM Report No. R93048, Institute of Naval Medicine, Alverstoke 1994.

51. Kemper GB, Stegman BJ and Pilmanis AA. Inconsistent classification and treatment of Type I / Type II decompression sickness. Aviat Space Environ Med 1992;63:386.

52. Kidd DJ, Elliott DH. Decompression disorders in divers. In Bennett PB, Elliott DH (eds). The Physiology and Medicine of Diving. 2nd ed, Bailliere Tindall, London 1969: 471.

53. Kilgore KS, Friedrichs GS, Homeister JW, Lucchesi BR. The complement system in myocardial ischemia/reperfusion injury. Cardiovascular Res 1994;28:437.

54. Kindwall EP. Management of Diving Accidents: Historical Review. In Diving Accident Management. Forty-first Workshop of the Undersea and Hyperbaric Medical Society. PB Bennett, RE Moon Eds. 1990:1

55. Imbert JP. Evolution and performances of Comex treatment tables. In Treatment of Decompression Illness. Forty-fifth Workshop of the Undersea and Hyperbaric Medical Society. RE Moon, PJ Sheffield Eds. 1996:389

56. Leitch DR, Green RD. Additional pressurization for treating non responding cases of serious air decompression sickness. Aviat Space Environ Med 1985;56:1139.

57. Leitch DR, LA Greenbaum, Jr and JM Hallenbeck. Cerebral arterial air embolism I-IV. Undersea Biomedical Research, 1984; 11(3):221.

58. Lutz J, Herrman G. Perfluorochemicals as a treatment of decompression sickness in rats. Pflugers Archiv 1984;401:174.

59. Marroni A, La saturazione terapeutica in aria per la terapia dei casi gravi e refrattari di MDD. Med.Sub.Ip. 1980; 6:19

60. Marroni A, Bianchi P. Rilevazione di bolle gassose circolanti dopo immersione in aria compressa. Med Sub Ip 1980;6:27

61. Marroni A, Zannini D, Effetti della variazione della velocità di risalita sulla produzione di bolle gassose circolanti dopo immersione ad aria compressa. Med.Sub.Ip.(Min.:Med.)1981;1:83

62. Marroni A, Catalucci G et al. Alcune considerazioni su 209 casi di MDD trattati nei centri iperbarici italiani nel 1978 e 1979. Med.Sub.Ip.(Min.Med.)1981;1:55

63. Marroni A, Catalucci G et al. Alcune considerazioni su 169 casi di malattia da decompressione trattati nei centri iperbarici italiani nel biennio 1980-1981 Med.Sub.Ip.(Min.Med.)1983; 3:9

64. Marroni A, The critical care of patients involved in severe diving accidents. Program and Abstracts: International Symposium on Hyperbaric Oxygen in Critical Care Medicine, Eilat, Israel 1985

65. Marroni A et al. Critical care and HBO treatment at depth of a saturation diving traumatic injury. In: Diving and Hyperbaric Medicine:Proceedings of the XII Congress of the EUBS, Rotterdam 1986

66. Marroni A et al. Some observations on 548 cases of sport diving decompression sickness treated in Italy in the last seven years. In: Diving and Hyperbaric Medicine: Proceedings of the XIII Congress of the EUBS, Palermo 1987

67. Marroni A, Il Trattamento delle Sequele della Malattia da Decompressione. Corsi di Aggiornamento sull'Ossigenoterapia Iperbarica. Lega Navale Italiana, Assessorato Sanità Regione Puglia, Bari 6-7 April 1989

68. Marroni A. La MDD nel subacqueo sportivo: dati sulla incidenza e standardizzazione dei protocolli di intervento. Atti del Secondo Convegno di Medicina Subacquea, USL 21, Castiglioncello 2 Giugno 1990

69. Marroni A., Lo Pardo D., Helzel V., Guarino U. Neurological Decompression Sickness treated with early recompression, HBO and under-water rehabilitation with oxygen underwater breathing apparatus. In: Proceedings of the tenth International Congress on Hyperbaric Medicine. DJ Bakker, FS Cramer Eds. Best Publishing Company 1992:84. And In: Program and Abstracts Joint Meeting on Diving and Hyperbaric Medicine, Amsterdam August 1990. Undersea Biomed Res 1990;17(suppl):141

70. Marroni A. Recreational Diving today, risk evaluation and problem management. In: Proceedings of the XXth Annual Meeting of the EUBS. Cimsit M. Ed. Istanbul 1994: 121 ISBN 975.7958.00.X

71. Marroni A., Lo Pardo D., Guarino U., Helzel V., L'uso dell' Autorespiratore ad Ossigeno nella riabilitazione dei postumi neurologici della M.D.D. In: Atti IX Congresso S.I.M.S.I. Lerici 29-30 settembre 1990

72. Marroni A. - Recreational Diving Safety. In Elliott DH Ed. Medical Assessment of Fitness to Dive Biomedical Seminars, Ewell, England, 1995: 41 - ISBN 0-9525162-0-9

73. Marroni A. Decompression Illness, Final Report. In: F. Wattel, D. Mathieu eds) First European Consensus Conference on Hyperbaric Medicine European Committee for Hyperbaric Medicine, University of Lille., C.R.A.M. Nord-Picardie, Sécurité Social 1994:28. ISBN 3-908229-05-7

74. Marroni A., Patologia Da Decompressione. Una valutazione alla luce delle più recenti acquisizioni. In: EM Camporesi, GC Caroli, A. Pizzola, G. Vezzani (eds), Proceedings of the International Symposium "Update on Hyperbaric Oxygen Therapy", Tipografia La Commerciale, Fidenza, Italy, 1995:195

75. Marroni A., La plongée moderne de loisir; la gestion des accidents de décompression. Le protocole d'intervention del l'International Divers Alert Network. Bull Medsubhyp 1994;4(2):41

76. Marroni A. (Clinical Indications) Decompression Illness- Final Report. In: Oriani G, Marroni A, Wattel F, (eds). Handbook on Hyperbaric Medicine. Springer-Verlag Berlin Heidelberg New York, 1996: 96. ISBN 3-540-75016-9

77. Marroni A. (The Divers Alert Network: Epidemiology of Diving Accidents) The Divers Alert Network in Europe: Risk Evaluation and Problem Management in a European Recreational Divers Population. In: Oriani G, Marroni A, Wattel F, (eds). Handbook on Hyperbaric Medicine. Springer-Verlag Berlin Heidelberg New York, 1996: 265. ISBN 3-540-75016-9

78. Marroni A. New Frontiers: Use of Combined Hyperbaric Oxygenation and In-Water Rehabilitation for Neurological Conditions due to Stroke and to Spinal Decompression Sickness. In: Oriani G, Marroni A, Wattel F, (eds). Handbook on Hyperbaric Medicine. Springer-Verlag Berlin Heidelberg New York, 1996: 809. ISBN 3-540-75016-9

79. Marroni A. Cali Corleo R. Fontaneto C. DAN Europe Diving Incident Report 1996. Proceedings of the 25th EUBS Annual Meeting. Israel Aug 28 - Sept 2, 1999

80. Marroni A, Cali Corleo R, Balestra C, Voellm E, Pieri M. Incidence of asymptomatic circulating venous gas emboli in unrestricted uneventful recreational diving DAN Europe's Project Safe Dive first results Proceedings of the XXVI Annual Scientific Meeting of the EUBS, Malta 14-17 September 2000:9

81. Marroni A, Cali Corleo R, Balestra C, Longobardi P, Voellm E, Pieri M, Pepoli R Effects of the variation of ascent speed profile on the production of venous gas emboli and the incidence of DCI in compressed air diving. Proceedings of the XXVI Annual Scientific Meeting of the EUBS, Malta 14-17 September 2000: 1

82. Marroni A. Acute management of Decompression Accidents in normal and remote locations. Proceedings of the XXVI Annual Scientific Meeting of the EUBS, Malta 14-17 September 2000: 127

83. Martin SE, Chenoweth DE, Engler RL, Roth DM, Longhurst JC. C5a decreased regional coronary blood flow and myocardial function in pigs; implications for a granulocyte mechanism. Circ Res 1988;63:483.

84. Miller JN, L Fagreus, PB Bennett, DH Elliott, TG Shields and J Grimstad. Nitrogen-oxygen saturation therapy in serious case of compressed air decompression sickness. The Lancet, 1978; July 22:169.

85. Moir, E.W., Tunelling by Compressed Air, Journal of the Society of Arts, 44:567, May 15, 1896.

86. Moon RE, Camporesi EM, Kisslo JA. Patent foramen ovale and decompression sickness in divers. Lancet 1989; 1:513.

87. Morild I, Mørk SJ. A neuropathologic study of the ependimorentricular surface in divers brains. Undersea & Hyperbaric Medicine 1994;21:43.

88. Mørk S, Morild I, Eidsvik S, Nyland H, Brubakk AO, Giertsen JC. Does diving really damage the spinal cord? A neuropathological study of 20 professional and amateur divers. Undersea Biomed Res 1992;19(suppl):111.

89. Nashimoto I, Gotoh Y, Relationship between precordial Doppler ultrasound records and decompression sickness. In Shilling CW, Beckett MW (eds). Underwater Physiology VI. Undersea Medical Society, Bethesda 1978:497.

90. Nishi RY. Doppler and ultrasonic bubble detection. In Bennett PB, Elliott DH (eds). The physiology and medicine of diving. 4th ed, WB Saunders Company London 1993: pp433-453.

91. Nishi RY. Doppler evaluation of decompression tables. In Lin YC, Shida KK (eds). Man in the sea. Best Publishing Company San Pedro 1990

92. Peters BH, Levin HS, Kelly PJ. Neurologic and psychologic manifestations of decompression illness in divers. Neurology 1977; 27: 125.

93. Pol M and M Wattelle. Memoire Sur Les Effets De La Compression De L'Air Applique Au Creusement Des Puits A Houille: Ann. D'Hygiene Publique Et De Medicine Legale. Second Series, 1854; 1:241.

94. Rivera JC. Decompression sickness among divers; an analysis of 935 cases. Milit Med 1964;129:314.

95. Shupak A. He-O2 treatment for severe air diving-induced neurological decompression illness. Treatment of Decompression Illness. Forty-fifth Workshop of the Undersea and Hyperbaric Medical Society. RE Moon, PJ Sheffield Eds. 1996:329

96. Smith DJ, Francis TJR, Tehybridge RJ, Wright JM, Sykes JJW. Concordance: A problem with the current classification of diving disorders. Undersea Biomed Res 1992;19(suppl):40.

97. Smith DJ, Francis TJR, Tehybridge RJ, Wright JM, Sykes JJW. An evaluation of the classification of decompression disorders. Undersea & Hyperbaric Medicine 1993;20(suppl):17

98. Spencer MP, Johanson DC. Investigation of new principles for human decompression schedules using the Doppler ultrasonic blood bubble detector. Tech Report, Inst. Environ Med and Physiol, Seattle 1974.

99. Stevens DM, Gartner SL, Pearson RR. Complement activation during saturation diving. Undersea & Hyperbaric Med 1993;20:279.

100. Swerlick RA, Yancey KB, Lawlwy TJ. A direct in vivo comparison of the inflammatory properties of human C5a and C5a des arg in human skin. J Immunol 1988;140:2376.

101. Thorsen E. Segadal K, Kambestad B, Gulsvik A. Divers' lung function: small airways disease. Brit J Industr Med 1990;47:519.

102. Thorsen T, Brubakk A, Øvstedal T, Farstad M, Holmsen H. A method for production of N2 microbubbles in platelet-rich plasma in an aggregometer-like apparatus, and effect of platelet density in vitro. Undersea Biomed Res 1986;13:271.

103. Thorsen T, Klausen H, Lie RT, Holmsen H. Bubble-induced, aggregation of platelets: effects of gas species, proteins and decompression. Undersea & Hyperbaric Med 1993;20:101.

104. Triger M. Letter to Monsieur Arago, Comptes rendus de l'academie des sciences, 1845; 20:445-449 (Paris).

105. U.S. Navy Diving Manual, Navsea 00994-LP-001-9010. Revision 1, 1 June 1985, Navy Department, Washington, D.C. 20362.

106. U.S. Navy, BuMed Instruction 6420.2, BuMed 74, Oxygen breathing treatment for decompression sickness and air embolism, 22 August 1967, Bureau of Medicine and Surgery, Washington, DC., 1967.

107. Van Der Aue OE, WA White, R Hayter, ES Brinton, JR Kellar and AR Behnke. Physiologic factors underlying the prevention and treatment al decompression sickness (1945), report number 1, U.S. Navy Experimentai Diving Unit, Washington, DC.

108. Vann RD. Exercise and circulation in the formation and growth of bubbles. In Brubakk AO, Hemingsen BB, Sundnes G.(eds), Supersaturation and bubble formation in fluids and organisms. Tapir Publishers Trondheim 1989:235.

109. Vik A, Brubakk AO, Hennessy, Jenssen BM, Ekker M, Slørdahl SA. Venous air embolism in swine: transport of gas bubbles through the pulmonary circulation. J Appl Physiol 1990;69:237.

110. Ward CA, Koheil A, McCullough D, Johnson WR, Fraser WD. Activation of complement at plasma-air or serum air interface of rabbits. J Appl Physiol 1986;60:1651.

111. Ward CA, McCullough D, Fraser WD. Relation between complement activation and susceptibility to decompression sickness. J Appl Physiol 1987;62:1160.

112. Ward CA, Till GO, Kunkel R et al. Evidence for the role of hydroxyl radical in complement and neutrophil-dependent tissue injury. J Clin Invest 1983;72:789.

113. Webb JP, Engel GL, Romano J, Ryder HW, Stevens CD, Blankenhorn MA, Ferris EB. The mechanism of pain in aviators bends. J Clin Invest 1944;23:934.

114. Webster's Encyclopedic unabridged Dictionary of the English Language. Gramercy Books, New York 1989.

115. Yarbrough OD and AR Behnke. The treatment of compressed air illness utilizing oxygen. J Md Hyg Toxicol, 1939; 21 :213.

116. Yount DE. Growth of bubbles from nuclei. In Brubakk AO, Kanwisher J, Sundnes G (eds). Diving in animals and man. Tapir Publishers, Trondheim 1986: 131

CHAPTER **8**

ADJUNCTIVE HYPERBARIC OXYGEN THERAPY IN THE TREATMENT OF THERMAL BURNS AND FROSTBITE

P. Cianci

INTRODUCTION

The use of hyperbaric oxygen therapy as an adjunct in the treatment of thermal injury remains a subject of considerable controversy. It is frequently condemned as being too dangerous and/or too expensive for routine use. A comprehensive review of the world literature fails to support these conclusions. Indeed, a significant body of data suggests it is of great benefit. Any therapy should pass scrutiny based on its merits; that is, can it favorably affect the pathology? Will it improve currently accepted results? Is it safe? Is it cost effective? This chapter will explore the specific application of hyperbaric oxygen therapy in the treatment of thermal injury, its relation to the pathophysiology, how it can favorably affect outcome, discuss relevant side effects and complications, and demonstrate its cost effectiveness when utilized as part of a comprehensive program of burn care.

The use of hyperbaric oxygen therapy in the treatment of thermal burns began in 1965 when Ikeda and Wada noted more rapid healing of second-degree burns in a group of coal miners being treated for carbon monoxide poisoning.(51) They followed this serendipitous observation with a series of experiments that demonstrated a reduction of edema and improved healing in animal studies.(26) The Japanese experience (25-27,50,51) stimulated interest in other countries, and there followed a series of reports of uncontrolled clinical experience with favorable results.(32,48) In 1970 Gruber, (18) (Figure 1) working at the U.S. Army biophysics laboratory at the Edgewood Arsenal in Maryland, devised a series of experiments placing rats in a hyperbaric chamber breathing 100% oxygen at sea level and at 2 and 3 atmospheres, respectively. He demonstrated that the area subjacent to a third-degree burn was hypoxic when compared to normal skin and that the tissue oxygen tension could only be raised by oxygen administered at pressure. This important study suggested that hyperbaric oxygen therapy could have a direct effect on the pathophysiology of the burn wound.

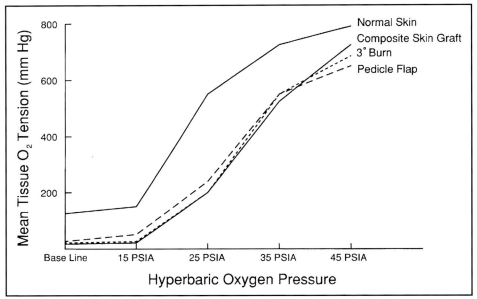

Figure 1. Tissue Oxygen Tension

Mean oxygen tension of normal skin and various hypoxic tissues as a function of hyperbaric oxygen pressure. Note: Oxygen tension rises in burned skin only with increasing pressure.

PATHOPHYSIOLOGY

In order to understand the rationale for therapy, it is necessary to review the physiology of the thermal injury. The burn wound is a complex and dynamic injury characterized by a central zone of coagulation surrounded by an area of stasis and bordered by an area of erythema. The zone of coagulation or complete capillary occlusion may progress by a factor of 10 during the first 48 hours after injury. Ischemic necrosis quickly follows. Hematologic changes, including platelet microthrombi and hemoconcentration, occur in the postcapillary venules. Edema formation is rapid in the area of the injury but also develops in distant, uninjured tissue. There are also changes occurring in the distal microvasculature where red cell aggregation, white cell adhesion to venular walls, and platelet thrombo-emboli occur.(6) "This progressive ischemic process, when set in motion, may extend damage dramatically during the early days after injury."(22) The ongoing tissue damage seen in thermal injury is due to the failure of surrounding tissue to supply borderline cells with oxygen and nutrients necessary to sustain viability.(4) The impediment of circulation below the injury leads to desiccation of the wound as fluid cannot be supplied via the thrombosed or obstructed capillaries. Topical agents and dressings may reduce but cannot prevent desiccation of the burn wound and the inexorable progression to deeper layers.

INFECTION

Susceptibility to infection is greatly increased due to the loss of the integumentary barrier to bacterial invasion, the ideal substrate present in the burn wound, and the compromised or obstructed microvasculature which prevents humoral and cellular elements from reaching the injured tissue. Additionally, the immune system is seriously affected, demonstrating decreased levels of immunoglobulins and serious perturbations of polymorphonuclear leukocyte (PMNL) function, (1,2,15,50) including disorders of chemotaxis, phagocytosis, and diminished killing ability. These functions greatly increase morbidity and mortality; infection remains the leading cause of death from burns.

Regeneration cannot take place until equilibrium is reached; hence, healing is retarded. Prolongation of the healing process may lead to excessive scarring. Hypertrophic scars are seen in about 4% of cases taking 10 days to heal, in 14% of cases taking 14 days or less, in 28% of cases taking 21 days, and up to 40% of cases taking longer than 21 days to heal.(12) Therapy of burns, then, is directed towards minimizing edema, preserving marginally viable tissue, protecting the microvasculature, enhancing host defenses, and providing the essential substrate necessary to sustain viability.

EXPERIMENTAL EVIDENCE

A significant body of animal data support the efficacy of hyperbaric oxygen in the treatment of thermal injury. Ikeda noted a reduction of edema in burned rabbits.(26) Ketchum in 1967 reported an improvement in healing time and reduced infection in an animal model.(30) He later demonstrated dramatic improvement in the microvasculature of burned rats treated with hyperbaric oxygen therapy.(29) In 1974 Hartwig (21) working in Germany reported similar findings and additionally noted less inflammatory response in those animals that had been treated with hyperbaric oxygen. He suggested at that time that hyperbaric oxygen might be a useful adjunct to the technique of early debridement. Wells and Hilton, (53) in a carefully designed and controlled experiment, reported a marked decrease in extravasation of fluid in a series of dogs with 40% flame burns. The effect was clearly related to oxygen and not simply increased pressure (Figure 2). They additionally reported a reduction in hemoconcentration and improved cardiac output in oxygen-treated dogs. Nylander (39) in a well-accepted animal model showed that hyperbaric oxygen therapy reduced the generalized edema associated with burn injury (Figure 3).

Kaiser (28) showed that hyperbaric oxygen treatment resulted in shrinkage of third-degree (full thickness) injury in a rabbit model. Untreated animals demonstrated the expected increase in wound size during the first 48 hours. Treated animals showed shrinkage of their wounds. At all times treated animal wounds remained smaller than those of the controls (Figure 4).

Korn and colleagues (31) in 1977 showed an early return of capillary patency in the hyperbaric-treated animals using an India ink technique. He also demonstrated survival of the dermal elements and more rapid epithelialization from these regenerative sites. He suggested the decreased desiccation of the wound he observed was a function of subjacent capillary integrity

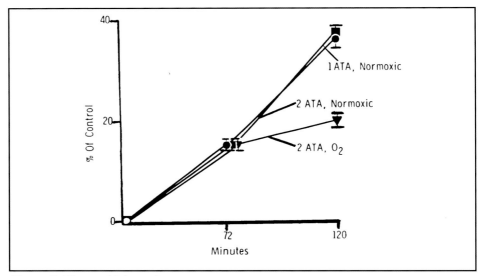

Figure 2. Plasma Volume Losses

Plasma volume losses after burn in untreated animals (1 ATA, normoxic), animals exposed to hyperbaric oxygen (2 ATA O$_2$) and to pressure alone (2 ATA, normoxic).

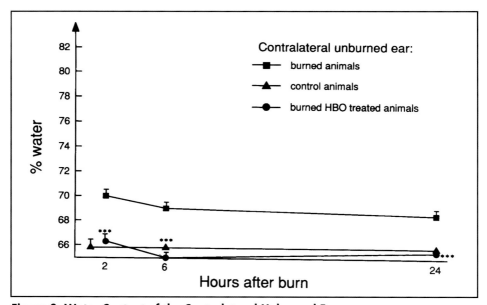

Figure 3. Water Content of the Contralateral Unburned Ear

Water content (± SEM) of the contralateral unburned ear in burned animals with and without HBO treatment.

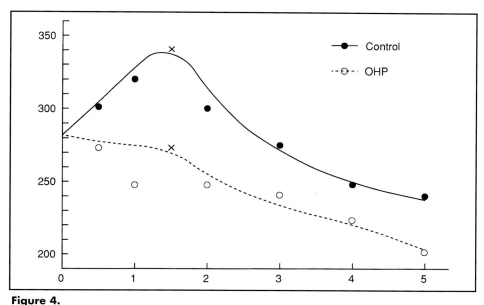

Figure 4.

Kaiser demonstrated in a full thickness animal model a significant reduction of wound size in the hyperbaric-treated animals vs. an increase in the control group, which remained larger at all times measured. (28)

noted in the HBO-treated animals. Saunders (44) and colleagues have shown similar results. They have also reported an improvement in collagen synthesis in HBO-treated animals. Perrins failed to show a beneficial effect in a small scald wound in a pig model treated with HBO.(41) Niccole (36) in 1977 reported that HBO offered no advantage over topical agents in controlling wound bacterial counts. He proposed that HBO acted as a mild antiseptic. His data, however, supported the observation of improved healing of partial thickness injury noted by earlier investigators. Stewart (46,47) and colleagues subjected rats to a controlled burn wound resulting in a deep partial thickness injury. Both experimental groups were treated with topical agents. The hyperbaric oxygen treated group showed preservation of dermal elements, no conversion of partial to full thickness injury, and preservation of adenosine triphosphate (ATP) levels; whereas, the untreated animals demonstrated marked diminution in ATP levels and conversion of partial to full thickness injury (Figures 5, 6).

These studies may relate directly to the preservation of energy sources for the sodium pump. Failure of the sodium pump is felt to be a major factor in the ballooning of the endothelial cells that occurs after burn injury and subsequent massive fluid losses.(3) Bleser (5) in 1973 in a very large controlled series reported reduction of burn shock and a fourfold increased survival in 30% burned animals vs. controls. Reduction of PMNL killing ability in hypoxic tissue has been well documented by Hohn et al.(23) The ability of hyperbaric oxygen to elevate tissue oxygen tension and the

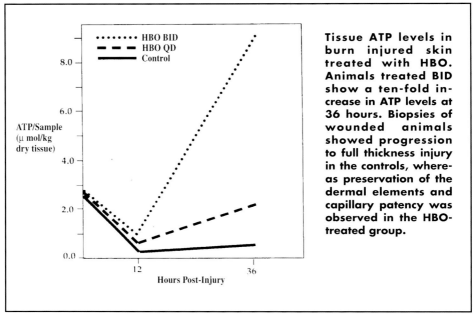

Tissue ATP levels in burn injured skin treated with HBO. Animals treated BID show a ten-fold increase in ATP levels at 36 hours. Biopsies of wounded animals showed progression to full thickness injury in the controls, whereas preservation of the dermal elements and capillary patency was observed in the HBO-treated group.

Figure 5. Rats: Burn with Silvadene Dressing

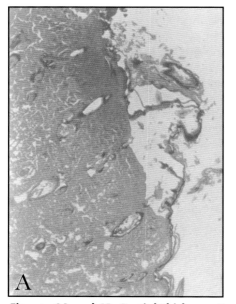
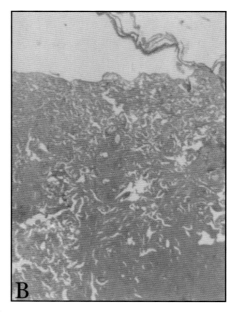

Figures 6A and 6B. Partial Thickness Burns

Biopsy of experimental partial thickness burns at five days.
(A) HBO-treated animals show preservation of the dermal elements.
(B) Nontreated animals show coagulation necrosis.

enhancement of PMNL killing in an O_2 enriched animal model as demonstrated by Mader (33) suggests that this may be an additional benefit of HBO. Recent data from Zamboni (55) suggest that hyperbaric oxygen is a potent blocker of white cell adherence to endothelial cell walls, interrupting the cascade which causes vascular damage. The mechanism is felt to be an inhibitory effect on the CD18 locus.(56) Germonpre's data tends to bear out this observation and may explain the beneficial effect of hyperbaric oxygen therapy on the microcirculation previously observed. (13,21,44,46,47) Shoshani reported no benefit of HBO in a rat model where all animals received standard sulfadiazene treatment.(45) There was no improvement reported in Doppler studies of blood flow, epithelialization, or wound contraction. All groups were treated with topical agents. The authors postulated that hyperbaric oxygen added little to the topical therapy. These data are not in agreement with the report by Stewart, who also treated all animals with topical burn therapy. Hussman et al. have shown no evidence of immunosuppression in a carefully controlled animal model.(24) Tenenhaus and colleagues showed reduction in mesenteric bacterial colonization in a hyperbaric oxygen treated mouse model.(49) Intestinal villus damage was also minimized in the hyperbaric oxygen group. Bacterial translocation the gut is felt to be a major source of infection in burn sepsis. Thus, the overwhelming evidence in a large number of controlled animal studies suggests that hyperbaric oxygen reduces edema, prevents conversion of partial to full thickness injury, preserves the microcirculation, preserves ATP, and perhaps secondarily the sodium pump, improves survival, and, though not yet proven, may enhance PMNL killing.

CLINICAL EXPERIENCE

Beginning with the reports of Wada in 1965 and continuing with Ikeda, (25-27,50,51) Lamy, (32) and Tabor, (48) reports of clinical series began to accumulate. In 1974 Hart (20) reported a controlled, randomized series showing a reduction of fluid requirements, faster healing, and reduced mortality when his patients were compared to controls and to U.S. National Burn Information Exchange standards. Waisbren (52) in 1982 reported a reduction in renal function, a decrease in circulating WBCs, and an increase in positive blood cultures in a retrospective series of patients who had received hyperbaric oxygen therapy. He stated he could demonstrate neither a salutory nor deleterious effect; however, his data showed a 75% decrease in the need for grafting in the hyperbaric treated group. Grossman and colleagues (16,17,54) have reported a very large clinical series showing improved healing, reduced hospital stay, and reduced mortality. Merola (35) in 1978 in a randomized study reported faster healing of partial thickness burns in 37 patients treated with HBO vs. 37 untreated controls. Niu and his associates (38) from the naval burn center in Taiwan have reported a very large clinical series showing a statistically significant reduction in mortality in 266 seriously burned patients who received adjunctive hyperbaric oxygen when compared to 609 control patients who did not receive this additional modality of therapy. Hammarlund and colleagues (19) have reported a reduction of edema and wound exudation in a carefully controlled series of human volunteers with ultraviolet irradiated blister wounds (Figure 7).

The author has shown a significant reduction in length of hospital stay in burns of up to 39% total body surface area (Table 1).(9) Additionally, a reduction in the need for surgery, including grafting, in a series of patients with up to 80% burns was noted when they were compared to non-HBO treated controls (Table 2).

HBO-treated patients in this study experienced an average savings of $95,000 per case.(7) In a series of patients with burns of up to 50% TBSA averaging 28% total body surface area injury, similar results were obtained.(11) In a retrospective, blinded review, this same group examined resuscitative fluid requirements in a group of severely burned patients. A 25% reduction in resuscitative fluid administration and a statistically significant reduction in maximum weight gain and percent weight gain was noted in the hyperbaric oxygen-treated group vs. the controls.(8) Maxwell and colleagues in 1991 reported a small controlled series showing a reduction of surgery, resuscitative weight gain, intensive care days, total hospitalization time, wound sepsis, and cost of hospitalization in the hyperbaric oxygen-treated group.(34) Data from our facility demonstrate continuing improvement in outcome of large burns with a reduction of surgeries of 86% (p<0.03).(10) Niezgoda and colleagues have demonstrated a similar reduction of wound exudate and wound size in a randomized, blinded human study utilizing normoxic controls (Figure 8).(37)

Considerable attention has been given to the use of hyperbaric oxygen in inhalation injury. There is fear that it may cause worsening of pulmonary damage, particularly in those patients maintained on high levels of

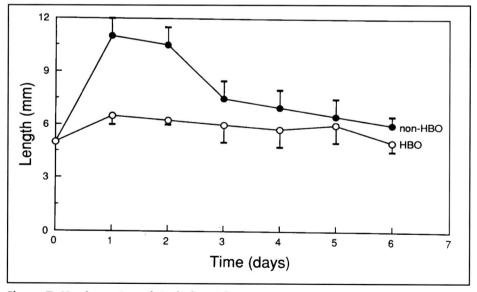

Figure 7. Maximum Length Including Edema

Maximum length (including edema adjacent to the wound) (mean ± s.d.) of u.v.-irradiated (•) and HBO-treated U.V.-irradiated (ọ) blister wounds as a function of time. The value on day 0 is approximately the diameter of the suction cup used to create the blister. (p<0.05)

inspired O_2. Grim et al., (14) have studied products of lipid peroxidation in the exhaled gases in HBO-treated burn patients and found no indication of oxidative stress. Ray et al., (42) have analyzed serious burns being treated for concurrent inhalation injury, thermal injury, and adult respiratory distress syndrome. She noted no deleterious effect, even in those patients on continuously high inspired oxygen. More rapid weaning from mechanical ventilation was possible in the HBO-treated group (5.3 days vs. 26 days, $p < 0.05$). A significant saving in cost of care per case ($60,000) was effected in the HBO-treated patients ($p < 0.05$). There is presently no evidence to controvert these studies.

TABLE 1. COMPARISON OF FACTORS IN HBO AND NON-HBO GROUPS IN PATIENTS WITH 18-39% TBSA

VARIABLE	HBO (N=8)	CONTROL (N=12)	
Age			
Average	29.5	30.9	
Range	16-47	18-42	p<0.57NS
Standard Deviation	9.6	8.5	
Total Body Surface Burn (%)			
Average	24.0	25.8	
Range	20-33	18-39	p<0.91NS
Standard Deviation	4.3	7.6	
Full Thickness Injury			
Average	5.2	5.6	
Range	0-18	0.20	p<0.96NS
Standard Deviation	6.1	6.2	
Surgeries			
Average	1.3	1.7	
Range	0-2	0.3	p<0.42NS
Standard Deviation	0.88	1.2	
Days Hospitalized			
Average	20.8	33.0	
Range	16-33	16.58	p<0.012*
Standard Deviation	6.7	13.1	
Cost of Burn Care			
Average	$44,838	$55,650	
Range	$27,600-$75,500	$21,500 $98,700	p,0.47NS
Standard Deviation	$9,200	$11,300	

NS, Not Significant
*p<.012, significant (Mann-Whitney U test)

TABLE 2. COMPARISON OF CONTROLS AND HBO TREATED PATIENTS WITH 40-80% TBSA BURNS

Variable	Control (n=7)	HBO (n=11)	HBO Since '87 (n=6)
Age			
Average	26	31.3	35
Range	14-24	20-60	24-60
Total Body Surface Burn (%)			
Average	48%	61.8%	60%
Range	40-60%	45-80%	40-80%
Days Hospitalized			
Average	108	51.8	44.6
Range	47-184	22-95	22-80
Cost of Burn Care			
Average	$391,000	$215,000	$200,000
Range	$151,000-801,000	$72,000-350,000	$76,000-394,000
Surgeries			
Average	7.8	2.1	1.1
Range	3-12*	0-6*	0-6*
Average HBO Tx			
Average	0	40	32
Range		13-77	13-64
HBO Cost*			
Average	0	$16,600	$17,000
Range		$5,000-$23,000	$5,000-$27,000
% Reduction			
Days Hospitalized		53	86
Surgeries		73	59
Care cost		46	49

*p<0.03

Brannan et al. (7a) failed to show any reduction in length of stay or the number of surgical procedures in a recent study. The failure to demonstrate any reduction in surgical procedures is not surprising as both groups underwent very early and aggressive excision, thus invalidating an important study parameter. There was, however, a reduction in overall cost of care in the group treated with hyperbaric oxygen.

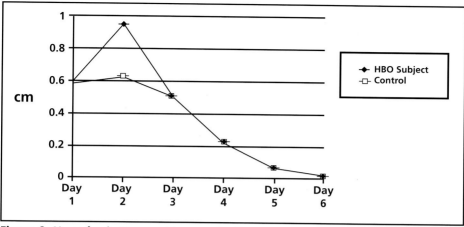

Figure 8. Hyperbaric Oxygen Therapy for Burns

Wound size measurements (cm) of ultraviolet-irradiated suction blister wounds in control group (□) and hyperbaric oxygen group (♦).

SURGICAL PERSPECTIVES

Over the past 30 years, the pendulum has rapidly swung to an aggressive surgical management of the burn wound, i.e., early tangential or sequential excision and grafting of the deep second-degree and third-degree burns, especially to functionally important parts of the body.(24a,44a) Hyperbaric oxygen, as adjunctive therapy, has allowed the surgeon another modality of treatment for these deep second-degree or so-called "indeterminant burns" of the hands and fingers, face and ears, and other areas where the surgical technique of excision and coverage is often difficult and imprecise. These wounds, not obvious third degree, are then best treated with topical antimicrobial agents, bedside and enzymatic debridement, and adjunctive hyperbaric oxygen therapy, allowing the surgeon more time for healing to take place and definition of the extent and depth of injury (Illustrations 1, 2). (9) Adjunctive hyperbaric oxygen therapy has drastically reduced the healing time in the major burn injury, especially if the wounds are deep second degree (Illustration 3).(7,9,10,34) There is some theoretical benefit of hyperbaric oxygen therapy for obviously less well defined third-degree burns. (28) Fourth-degree burns, most commonly seen in high voltage electrical injuries, are benefited by reduction in fascial compartmental pressures and need for fasciotomies as injured muscle swelling is lessened by preservation of aerobic glycolysis and, later, by a significant reduction of anaerobic infection.

Finally, reconstruction utilizing flaps, full thickness skin, and composite grafts, i.e., ear to nose grafts, has been greatly facilitated using this technique. Often the decision to use hyperbaric oxygen has been made intraoperatively as the surgeon is concerned about a compromised cutaneous or musculocutaneous flap. Patients are, in many instances, prepared preoperatively about the possibility of receiving this form of adjunctive therapy immediately after surgery.

PATIENT SELECTION

Hyperbaric oxygen therapy is presently utilized to treat serious burns, i.e., greater than 20% total body surface area, deep partial or full thickness injury, or with involvement of the hands, face, feet, or perineum. Patients with superficial burns or those not expected to survive are not accepted for therapy.

TREATMENT PROTOCOLS

We utilize a twice-a-day regimen of 90 minutes at 2 atmospheres plus descent and ascent time. Treatments typically take 105 minutes. Treatment is rendered as soon as possible after injury, often during initial resuscitation.

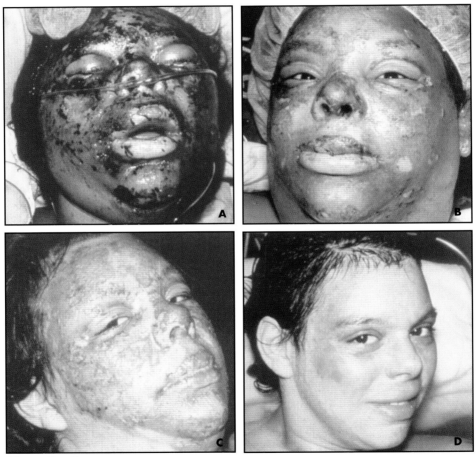

Illustration 1

A. 23-year-old white female with facial burns from flaming gasoline and tar 12 hours after injury.
B. 24 hours later (36 hours after injury) after two HBO treatments. Note resolution of edema.
C. 72 hours later (84 hours after injury) after six HBO treatments.
D. Shortly before discharge.

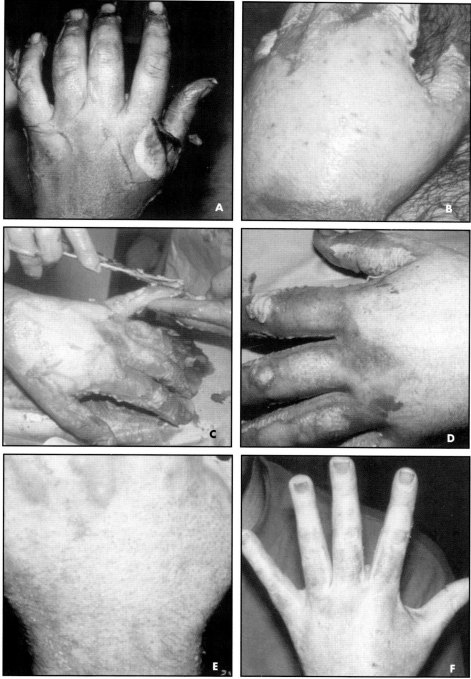

Illustration 2

A. A deep partial thickness of hand in 30-year-old male with 60% total body surface burn and inhalation injury, on admission.

B. Six days later.

C. At surgery, light debridement.

D. Immediately afer surgery. Note preservation of dermal appendages.

E. Two weeks after admission. Note re-epithelialization.

F. Appearance on discharge 25 days post-injury. Healed without grafting.

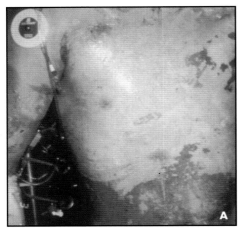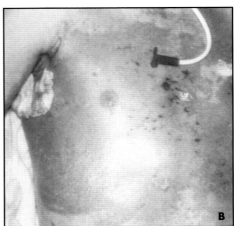

Illustration 3

A. 19-year-old white male with flame burn of chest from burning clothing
estimated to be deep partial-to-full-thickness burn.
B. One month later with no grafting required. Patient received adjunctive HBO
therapy twice daily.

Patients are carefully monitored during initial treatments until stable and as necessary thereafter. Children are treated for 45 minutes twice a day.(16) In the monoplace configuration, we are now able to monitor blood pressure non-invasively using a special cuff. We attempt to treat three times in the first 24 hours and BID thereafter. Treatments are rendered twice during a normal workday, that is, a normal 8-10 hour period. Careful attention to fluid management is mandatory. Initial requirements of burn patients may be several liters per hour, and pumps capable of this delivery at pressure must be utilized in order to maintain appropriate fluid replacement. Patients can be maintained on ventilatory support during treatment. This is frequently the case in larger burns. Maintenance of a comfortable ambient temperature must be accomplished, and treating patients within two hours of tubbing or dressing changes is not recommended as temperature control may be difficult. Febrile patients must be closely monitored and fever controlled as O_2 toxicity is reported to be more common in this group. We have not observed evidence of O_2 toxicity in the patients we have treated.

Patients may be treated in a multiplace or monoplace hyperbaric chamber. Monoplace chamber treatment appears to be easier in terms of maintaining the patient environment, especially in head and neck burns. A multiplace chamber is obviously preferable, if available, for those patients who are hemodynamically unstable. Movement over long distances is not recommended. Patients should not be transported to a hyperbaric chamber that is not within the burn center facility. Careful attention to infection control is mandatory. In large burns of 40% Total Body Surface Area (TBSA) or greater, treatment is rendered for 10-14 days in close consultation with the burn surgeon. Many partial thickness burns will heal without surgery during this time frame and obviate the need for grafting. Treatment beyond 30 sessions is usually utilized to ensure graft take. While there is no absolute limit to the number of hyperbaric treatments rendered, it is rare to exceed 40-50 except in very unusual circumstances.

SIDE EFFECTS

Barotrauma to the ears is common, particularly in burns of the head and neck.(43) Routine ear, nose, and throat (ENT) evaluation and early myringotomy is recommended in this subset of patients. We have established capabilities for myringotomy in our hyperbaric unit as this will often facilitate more rapid and more comfortable treatment.

In larger burn injuries, adequate fluid and electrolyte resuscitation during the first 24 hours can be problematic. Certain patients have developed hypotension shortly after exiting the chamber. We feel this represents hypovolemia that was masked during hyperbaric oxygen treatments. Careful volume replacement and assessment is mandatory prior to, during, and immediately after hyperbaric treatment. We have elected to increase fluids during ascent to compensate for any masked hypovolemia. We have not seen O_2 seizures or pulmonary toxicity in our patients.

RECOMMENDATIONS

We recommend that units planning treatment of burn patients be thoroughly versed in the management of critical care patients in the hyperbaric setting and to the peculiar problems of burn patients prior to initiation of a therapy program. Patients with severe burns are among the most challenging encountered in medicine. The hyperbaric team must be experienced in the management and monitoring of central lines, ventilators, and all aspects of critical care in the hyperbaric chamber. HBO treatment must be carefully coordinated to work around the busy schedule of the burn center. Our hyperbaric department is an extension of the burn center. Our personnel are trained in burn care and hyperbaric medicine and are an integral part in the "team approach" to burn care.

SUMMARY

Current data show that hyperbaric oxygen therapy, when used as an adjunct in a comprehensive program of burn care, can significantly improve morbidity and mortality, reduce length of hospital stay, and lessen the need for surgery. It has been demonstrated to be safe in the hands of those thoroughly trained in rendering hyperbaric oxygen therapy in the critical care setting and with appropriate monitoring precautions. Careful patient selection and screening is mandatory.

FROSTBITE

Much has been said about frostbite injuries through the ages. Napolean's problems are well known and often quoted in the literature, (13f) but the basic mechanism has remained little understood. As burns were once thought merely to represent direct thermal injury to cells, the mechanism of frostbite injury has been thought to be a direct effect of freezing on the tissue cells. At various times, ice crystals, either intracellular or extracellular, were thought to be the main cause of cellular damage.(19f) The outcome of frost-bite injury was inevitable; and the basic treatment has been to thaw the tissue, cover it with a sheet, wait, and debride or amputate everything that turns black.(11f) Even in recent years, much effort has been made to speed up the amputation process by the use of nuclear imaging techniques to predict the level of needed amputation so the "wait" phase can be eliminated.(8f,15f) This has done little to provide insight into the mechanism of frostbite injury much less provide needed treatment options to prevent rather than to predict amputation.

The mechanism of frostbite injury on a cellular level is much more complex than previously believed. When a frozen limb is initially thawed, it appears viable; and various studies have shown that blood flow is reinstituted after thawing.(12f,22f) Over the next few days, however, there is a process of progressive ischemia which can result in tissue necrosis depending on the severity of the injury. It is this progressive tissue ischemia which is most interesting. The pathophysiology of

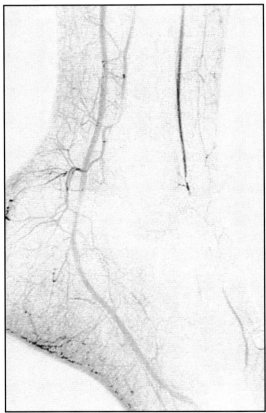

Illustration 4

Arteriogram of young, active-duty army soli-er with a severe frostbite injury. Note occlu-sion of dorsalis pedia artery.

Photo courtesy of Dr. Bill Clem of the Hyperbaric Medicine Center, Presbyterian/ St. Luke's Medical Center, Denver, Colorado.

ischemia-reperfusion injury is well studied and well described. (5f,7f,21f) Several studies have shown that many of the characteristics of frostbite pathophysiology are similar to ischemia-reperfusion injury, although they may be seen at different times in the injury process.(22f) These include neutrophil adhesion to the endothelial wall, breakdown of the endothelial cell membrane, erythrocyte extravasation, production of potent vasoconstrictors such as thromboxane A2 and prosta-glandin F2a, free radical generation, and the amelioration of some tissue damage with free radical scavengers such as deferoxamine and superoxide dismutase (SOD). (1f,10f,14f) Additionally, several studies have found that thrombus formation may play a significant role in the later stages of the ischemic injury process.

Although better understood than frostbite, it has been difficult to clinically intervene in the process of ischemia-reperfusion injury. This is partially due to the inability to stage the process in any individual patient. Likewise in frostbite injury, each patient may be in a different stage of injury and the degree of tissue injury varies from virtually uninjured to severely affected. The successful use of deferoxamine, SOD (at least experimentally), selective prostaglandin inhibitors, and thromboxane A2 inhibitors in frostbite treatment is encouraging.(10f,14f) One very interesting study by Salimi et al. (17f) as well as other studies (20f) have demonstrated extensive vascular thrombosis and subsequent tissue salvage using thrombolytic agents. Other clinical evidence, including emergent arteriography in recently thawed frostbite patients, has shown significant vascular thrombus formation, even in larger arteries such as the dorsal pedis artery (Illustration 4).(1f,4f,6f,18f) Unlike cardiac thrombolytic therapy where a guide wire can be used to first cannulate a thrombus, thrombolytic therapy in small and microvascular structures is more difficult due to the limited "face" that the clot presents to the thrombolytic agent. It may be that anticoagulation therapy, if given early in the process, can prevent the formation of microvascular thrombus. At present, there is sufficient clinical and experimental evidence to support the use of selective prostaglandi inhibitors (ibuprofen), deferoxamine, thromboxane A2 inhibitors (topical aloe vera), and anticoagulation in certain patients. Selective thrombolytic therapy may be beneficial if there is arteriography documented occlusion and the agent can be infused over many hours. Hyperbaric oxygen therapy, if used early and aggressively, may be beneficial when added to a regimen designed to minimize the production of vasoconstrictive agents and free radicals, limit endothelial damage, and prevent thrombosis. Hyperbaric oxygen therapy has been shown to increase capillary diffusion distance in ischemic tissue, helping to salvage marginal tissue until recannalization occurs. It also has been proven to reduce free radical production, stabilize and reverse lipid peroxidation of the cell wall, and prevent neutrophil adhesion to the endothelium, a major contributor to ischemia-reperfusion injury.(2f,3f,9f,55) Objections to its use have been made when it has been erroneously said to cause vasoconstriction and reduction of blood flow.(16f) This only occurs in healthy tissue. HBO actually reverses vasoconstriction in ischemic tissue.(20f) In all cases the hyperoxia induced by HBO overwhelms any potential reduction in blood flow. The benefits of hyperbaric oxygen therapy greatly outweigh any potential deleterious effects.

While it would be satisfying to recommend a single treatment for frostbite, it is clear that the mechanism is a cascade of causative factors. As different portions of the injured tissue are likely to be at different stages of injury, it is likely to be necessary to use a combination of agents, each intervening at a different stage of the injury. What is clear is that amputation should be considered an outcome, not an intervention.

The similarities of frostbite to thermal burns and reperfusion injury suggest that application of adjunctive hyperbaric oxygen in the treatment of frostbite, particularly if utilized in the early stages of injury, may prove an area of fruitful investigation.

THANKS FROM THE AUTHOR

The author is indebted to Ronald Sato, M.D., Director, Burn/ Wound Care Center, Doctors Medical Center, San Pablo, CA, for his contribution to the chapter on thermal burns and to William B. Clem, M.D., F.A.C.E.P., from the Hyperbaric Medicine Center, Presbyterian/St. Luke's Medical Center, Denver, CO, for his contribution to the chapter on the subject of frostbite.

REFERENCES

1. Alexander JW, Mekins JL. "A physiological basis for the development of opportunistic infections in man." Annals of Surgery. 1972;176:273.

2. Alexander JW, Wilson D. "Neutrophil dysfunction and sepsis in burn injury." Surg Gynec Obstet. 1970;130:431.

3. Arturson G. "The pathophysiology of severe thermal injury." J Burn Care Rehabil. 1985;6(2):129-146.

4. Arturson G. "Pathophysiology of the burn wound." Ann Chir Gynaecol. 1980;66:178-190.

5. Bleser F, Benichoux R. "Experimental surgery: The treatment of severe burns with hyperbaric oxygen." J Chir. (Paris). 1973;106:281-290.

6. Boykin JV, Eriksson E, Pittman RN. "In vivo microcirculation of a scald burn and the progression of postburn ischemia." Plast and Recon Surg. 1980;66:191-198.

7a. Brannen AL, Still J, Haynes M, Orlet H, Rosenblum F, Law E, Thompson WO. "A randomized prospective trial of hyperbaric oxygen in a referral burn center population." Am Surg 1997;63(3):205-208.

7. Cianci P, Lueders H, Lee H, Shapiro R, Sexton J, Williams C, Green B. "Adjunctive hyperbaric oxygen reduces the need for surgery in 40-80% burns." J Hyper Med. 1988;3:97-101.

8. Cianci P, Lueders H, Lee H, Shapiro R, Sexton J, Williams C, Green B. "Hyperbaric oxygen and burn fluid requirements: Observations in 16 patients with 40-80% TBSA burns." Undersea Biomed Research Suppl. 1988;15:14.

9. Cianci P, Lueders HW, Lee H, Shapiro RL, Sexton J, Williams C, Sato R. "Adjunctive hyperbaric oxygen therapy reduces length of hospitalization in thermal burns." J Burn Care Rehab. 1989;10:432-435.

10. Cianci P, Sato R, Green B. "Adjunctive hyperbaric oxygen reduces length of hospital stay, surgery, and the cost of care in severe burns." Undersea Biomed Research Suppl. 1991;18:108.

11. Cianci P, Williams C, Lueders H, Lee H, Shapiro R, Sexton J, Sato R. "Adjunctive hyperbaric oxygen in the treatment of thermal burns: An economic analysis." J Burn Care Rehab. 1990;11:140-143.

12. Deitch E, Wheelahan T, Rose M, Clothier J, Cotter J. "Hypertrophic burn scars: Analysis of variables." J Trauma. 1983;23:895-898.

13. Germonpre P, Reper P, Vanderkelen A. "Hyperbaric oxygen therapy and piracetam decrease the early extension of deep partial-thickness burns." Burns 1996;22(6):468-473.

14. Grim PS, Nahum A, Gottlieb L, Wilbert C, Hawe E, Sznajder J. "Lack of measurable oxidative stress during HBO therapy in burn patients." Undersea Biomed Research Suppl. 1989;16:22.

15. Grogan JB. "Altered neutrophil phagocytic function in burn patients." J Trauma. 1976;16:734.

16. Grossman AR. "Hyperbaric oxygen in the treatment of burns." Ann Plast Surg. 1978;1:163-171.

17. Grossman AR, Grossman AJ. "Update on hyperbaric oxygen and treatment of burns." HBO Review 1982;3:51-59.

18. Gruber RP, Brinkley B, Amato JJ, Mendelson JA. "Hyperbaric oxygen and pedicle flaps, skin grafts, and burns." Plast and Recon Surg. 1970;45:24-30.

19. Hammarlund C, Svedman C, Svedman P. "Hyperbaric oxygen treatment of healthy volunteers with u.v.-irradiated blister wounds." Burns. 1991;17(4):296-301.

20. Hart GB, O'Reilly RR, Broussard ND, Cave RH, Goodman DB, Yanda RL. "Treatment of burns with hyperbaric oxygen." Surg Gynecol Obstet. 1974;139:693-696.

21. Hartwig VJ, Kirste G. "Experimentelle Untersuchungen Über die Revaskularisierung von Verbrennungswunden unter Hyperbarer Sauerstofftherapie." Zbl Chir. 1974;99:1112-1117.

22. Heggers JP, Robson MC, Zachary LS. "Thromboxane inhibitors for the prevention of progressive dermal ischemia due to the thermal injury." J Burn Care Rehab. 1980;6:466-468.

23. Hohn DC, McKay RD, Halliday B, Hunt TK. "Effect of oxygen tension on the microbicidal function of leukocytes in wounds and in vitro." Surg Forum 1976;27:18-20.

24a. Hunt JL, Sato RM, Baxter CR. "Early tangential excision and immediate mesh autografting of deep dermal hand burns." Annals Surg 1979;189(2):147-151.

24. Hussman J, Hebebrand D, Erdmann D, Roth A, Kucan JO, Moticka J. "Lymphocyte sub populations in spleen and blood after early wound debridement and acute/chronic treatment with hyperbaric oxygen." Hanchir Mikrochir Plast Chir 1996;28(2):103-107.

25. Ikeda K, Ajiki H, Kamiyama I, Wada J. "Clinical application of hyperbaric oxygen treatment." Geka (Japan) 1967;29:1279.

26. Ikeda K., Ajiki H, Nagao H, Karino K, Sugh S, Iwa T, Wada J. "Experimental and clinical use of hyperbaric oxygen in burns." Proceedings of the Fourth International Congress on Hyperbaric Med. J Wada and T Iwa, (Eds.) Tokyo: Igaku Shoin, Ltd., 1970;370-380.

27. Iwa T. Discussion. In: JW Brown and BG Cox, (Eds.) Proceedings of the Third International Conference on Hyperbaric Medicine. Washington, DC; National Academy of Science - National Research Council Publication No. 4, 1966;611-612.

28. Kaiser VW, Schnaidt U, Von der Lieth H. "Auswirkungen Hyperbaren Suerstoffes auf die frische Brandwunde." Handchir Mikrochir Plast Chir. 1989;21:158-163.

29. Ketchum SA, Thomas AN, Hall AD. "Angiographic studies of the effect of hyperbaric oxygen on burn wound revascularization." Proceedings of the Fourth International Congress on Hyperbaric Med. J Wada and T Iwa, (Eds.) Tokyo: Igaku Shoin, Ltd., 1970;388-394.

30. Ketchum SA, Zubrin JR, Thomas AN, Hall AD. "Effect of hyperbaric oxygen on small first, second and third degree burns." Surg Forum. 1967;18:65-67.

31. Korn HN, Wheeler ES, Miller TA. "Effect of hyperbaric oxygen on second-degree burn wound healing." Arch Surg. 1977;112:732-737.

32. Lamy ML, Hanquet MM. "Application opportunity for OHP in a general hospital - a two years experience with a monoplace hyperbaric oxygen chamber." Proceedings of the Fourth International Congress on Hyperbaric Med. J Wada and T Iwa, (Eds.) Tokyo: Igaku Shoin, Ltd., 1970;517-522.

33. Mader JT, Brown GL, Guckian JC, Wells CH, Reinarz JA. "A mechanism for the amelioration of hyperbaric oxygen of experimental staphylococcal osteomyelitis in rabbits." J Inf Disease. 1980;142:915-922.

34. Maxwell G, Meites H, Silverstein P. "Cost effectiveness of hyperbaric oxygen therapy in burn care." Winter Symp on Baromedicine. 1991.

35. Merola L, Piscitelli F. "Considerations on the use of HBO in the treatment of burns." Ann Med Nav. 1978;83:515-526.

36. Niccole MW, Thornton JW, Danet RT, Bartlett RH, Tavis MJ. "Hyperbaric oxygen in burn management: A controlled study." Surgery. 1977;82:727-733.

37. Niezgoda JA, Cianci P, Folden BW, Ortega RL, Slade JB, Storrow AB. "The effect of hyperbaric oxygen therapy on a burn wound model in human volunteers." Plast Reconstr Surg 1997;99(6):1620-1625.

38. Niu AKC, Yang C, Lee HC, Chen SH, Chang LP. "Burns treated with adjunctive hyperbaric oxygen therapy: A comparative study in humans." J Hyper Med. 1987;2:75-86.

39. Nylander G, Nordstrîm H, Eriksson E. "Effects of hyperbaric oxygen on oedema formation after a scald burn." Burns. 1984; 10:193-196.

40. Ogle CK, Alexander JW, Nagy H, Wood S, Palkert D, Carey M, Ogle JD, Warden GD. "A long-term study and correlation of lymphocyte and neutrophil function in the patient with burns." J Burn Care Rehab. 1990;11(2):105-111.

41. Perrins DJD. "Failed attempt to limit tissue destruction in scalds of pig's skin with hyperbaric oxygen. Proceedings of the Fourth International Congress on Hyperbaric Med. J Wada and T Iwa, (Eds.) Tokyo: Igaku Shoin, Ltd., 1970;381-387.

42. Ray CS, Green B, Cianci P. "Hyperbaric oxygen therapy in burn patients: Cost effective adjuvant therapy (poster presentation). Undersea Biomed Res Suppl. 1991;18:77.

43. Ross JC, Cianci PE. "Barotitis media resulting from hyperbaric oxygen therapy. A retrospective study of 395 consecutive cases." Undersea Biomed Res Suppl. 1990;17:102.

44a. Sato RM, Beesinger DE, Hunt JL, Baxter CR. "Early excision and closure of the burn wound." Current Topics in Burn Care. TL Wachtel et al. (eds). Rockville, Aspen Publication, 1983, pp 65-76.

44. Saunders J, Fritz E, Ko F, Bi C, Gottlieb L, Krizek T. "The effects of hyperbaric oxygen on dermal ischemia following thermal injury." Proc of Am Burn Assoc. 1989;58.

45. Shoshani O, Shupak A, Barak A, Ullman Y, Ramon Y, Lindenbaum E, Peled Y. "Hyperbaric oxygen therapy for deep second degree burns: an experimental study in the guinea pig." Brit J Plast Surg 1998;51:67-73.

46. Stewart RJ, Yamaguchi KT, Cianci PE, Knost PM, Samadani BA, Mason SW, Roshdieh BB. "Effects of hyperbaric oxygen on adenosine triphosphate in thermally injured skin." Surg Forum. 1988;39:87-90.

47. Stewart RJ, Yamaguchi KT, Cianci PE, Mason SW, Roshdieh BB, Dabbass N. "Burn wound levels of ATP after exposure to elevated levels of oxygen." Proc of the Am Burn Assoc. 1989;67.

48. Tabor CG. "Hyperbaric oxygenation in the treatment of burns of less than forty percent." Korean J Int Med. 1967.

49. Tenenhaus M, Hansbrough JF, Zapata-Sirvent R, Neumann T. "Treatment of burned mice with hyperbaric oxygen reduces mesenteric bacteria but not pulmonary neutrophil deposition." Arch Surg 1994;129(12):1338-1342.

50. Wada J, Ikeda K, Kegaya H, Ajiki H. "Oxygen hyperbaric treatment and severe burn." Jap Med J. 1966;13:2203.

51. Wada J, Ikeda T, Kamata K, Ebuoka M. "Oxygen hyperbaric treatment for carbon monoxide poisoning and severe burn in coal mine (Hokutanyubari) gas explosion." Igakunoaymi (Japan) 1965;54:68.

52. Waisbren BA, Schultz D, Collentine G, Banaszak E, Stern M. "Hyperbaric oxygen in severe burns." Burns. 1982;8:176-179.

53. Wells CH, Hilton JG. "Effects of hyperbaric oxygen on post-burn plasma extravasation." Hyperbaric Oxygen Therapy. JC Davis and TK Hunt, (Eds). Undersea Medical Society, Inc., 1977;p259-265.

54. Wiseman DH, Grossman AR. "Hyperbaric oxygen in the treatment of burns." Crit Care Clin. 1985;2:129-145.

55. Zamboni WA, Roth AC, Russell RC, Graham B, Suchy H, Kucan JO. "Morphologic analysis of the microcirculation during reperfusion of ischemic skeletal muscle and the effect of hyperbaric oxygen." Plast Reconstr Surg 1993;91(6):1110-1123.

56. Zamboni WA, Stephenson LL, Roth AC, Suchy H, Russell RC. "Ischemia-reperfusion injury in skeletal muscle: CD18 dependent neutrophil-endothelial adhesion." Undersea & Hyperbar Med 1994;suppl 21:53.

FROSTBITE REFERENCES

1f. Bourne MH, Piepkorn MD, Clayton F, Leonard LG. "Analysis of microvascular changes in frostbite injury." J Surg Res 1986;40:26-35.

2f. Buras J. "Basic mechanisms of hyperbaric oxygen in the treatment of ischemia-reperfusion injury." Int Anes Clinics 2000;38:91-109.

3f. Buras JA, Stahl GL, Svoboda KKH, Reenstra WR. "Hyperbaric oxygen downregulates ICAM-1 expression induced by hypoxia and hypoglycemia." Am J Phys 2000;278: 292-302.

4f. Clem B. Personal communication. 2002.

5f. Grace PA. "Ischaemia-reperfusion injury." Brit J Surg 1994;81:637-647.

6f. Gralino BJ, Porter JM, Rosch J. "Angiography in the diagnosis and therapy of frostbite." Radiology 1976;119:301-305.

7f. Granger DN, Korthuis RJ. "Physiologic mechanisms of postischemic tissue injury," Anual Rev Phys 1995;57:311-332.

8f. Greenwald D, Cooper B, Gottlieb L. "An algorithm for early aggressive treatment of frostbite with limb salvage directed by triple-phase scanning." Plast Reconstr Surg 1998;102:1069-1074.

9f. Haapaniemi T, Nylander G, Sirsjo A, Larsson J. "Hyperbaric oxygen reduces ischemia-induced skeletal muscle injury." Plast Reconstr Surg 1996;97:602-607.

10f. Heggers JP, Robson MC, Manavalen K, Weingarten MD, Carethers JM, Boertman JA, Smith DJ, Sachs RJ. "Experimental and clinical observations on frostbite." Ann Emerg Med 1987;16:1056-1062.

11f. Kyosola K. "Clinical experiences in the management of cold injuries: a study of 110 cases." J Trauma 1974;14:32-36.

12f. Lange K, Boyd L. "The functional pathology of experimental frostbite and the prevention of subsequent gangrene." Surg Gynecol Obstet 1945;80:346-350.

13f. Larrey DJ. "Memoirs of military surgery and campaigns of the French armies." Baltimore:Joseph Cushing; 1814:156-164.

14f. Manson PN, Jesudass R, Marzella L, Bulkley GB, Im MJ, Narayan KK. "Evidence for an early free radical-mediated reperfusion injury in frostbite." Free Radical Biol & Med 1991;10:7-11.

15f. Mehta RC, Wilson MA. "Frostbite injury: prediction of tissue viability with triple-phase bone scanning." Radiology 1989;170:511-514.

16f. Murphy JV, Banwell PE, Roberts AHN, McGrouther DA. "Frostbite: pathogenesis and treatment." J Trauma 2000;48:171.

17f. Salimi Z, Wolverson MK, Herbold DR, Vas W, Salimi A. "Treatment of frostbite with IV streptokinase: an experimental study in rabbits." Am J Roentgen 1987;149:773-776.

18f. Skolnick AA. "Early data suggest clot-dissolving drug may help save frostbitten limbs from amputation." JAMA 1992;267:2008-2010.

19f. Weatherby-White RCA, Sjostrom B, Paton BC. "Experimental studies in cold injury II: the pathogenesis of frostbite. J Surg Res 1964;4:17-22.

20f. Zdeblick TA, Field GA, Shaffer JW. "Treatment of experimental frostbite with urokinase." J Hand Surg 1988;13:948-953.

21f. Zimmerman BJ, Granger DN. "Mechanisms of reperfusion injury." Am J Med Scien 1994;307:284-292.

22f. Zook N, Hussmann J, Brown R, Russell R, Kucan J, Roth A, Suchy H. "Microcirculatory studies of frostbite injury." Ann Plast Surg 1998;40:246-253.

NOTES

CHAPTER 9

OSTEORADIONECROSIS IN THE MAXILLOFACIAL REGION

J.P.R. van Merkesteyn

INTRODUCTION

Osteoradionecrosis of the facial bones, particularly of the mandible, is still one of the major complications of radiotherapy in the treatment of malignant tumors in the head and neck [28,30,34,43,44,45,53]. Treatment remains difficult, leading to resection of the mandible (Figure 1) in a considerable percentage of the patients [14,47].

The reported incidence of osteoradionecrosis of the jaws in recent literature varies from 2.6%-10.4% [59]. In a review of the literature Clayman [7] found a mean of 5.4%. Although the techniques of radiotherapy have changed, the incidence of osteoradionecrosis has not decreased in the last decades [59].

The majority of the cases of osteoradionecrosis occur within two years after radiation [9,38,54,59] but it may occur as late as 20 years post-radiation [8]. In recent large series on osteoradionecrosis of the jaws [9,54], 95% was found in the mandible and 5% in the maxilla. This difference has been known for a long time and is explained by the difference in bone structure and vascularisation between mandible and maxilla.

In a series of 536 cases of osteoradionecrosis of the mandible Marx and Johnson [38] found 39% to be spontaneous (Figure 2) and 61% to be surgery-related. Of the trauma-related osteoradionecrosis 51% was related to extraction of teeth, 38% due to post-radiation extractions, 11% due to pre-radiation extractions and 2% due to extractions during radiation. The other trauma-related causes were surgery in 9% and prosthetic appliances in only 1%. These figures correspond more or less with the more recent study of Thorn et al. [54] who found spontaneous osteoradionecrosis in 29% of the cases and trauma-related osteoradionecrosis in 72%, of which 55% was related to removal of teeth, 14% to surgery and 3% to injury from prosthetic devices.

The exact pathogenesis of osteoradionecrosis is still under debate. Due to the late effects of radiation, soft tissue and bone changes such as obliterative endarteritis and fibrosis occur [3,11,22,38]. These changes may, in a small percentage of the patients, lead to bone and/or soft-tissue necrosis. Although several predisposing and initiating factors are known [9,38] it is still difficult to predict whether a patient is really at risk for development of osteoradionecrosis or not.

The histopathologic sequence of events after exposure of normal tissue to radiation can be divided into four phases [5]:

Phase I: Characterized by the development of acute damage to cells and tissues. Initial damage to small blood vessels and connective tissue.

Phase II: Characterized by processes of recovery from acute damage. There may be some persisting evidence of cell necrosis or tissue hypoplasia and evidence of beginning of chronic or permanent tissue damage. Replacement fibrosis may already be evident. Atypical repair processes representing the beginning of an increase in arteriocapillary fibrosis.

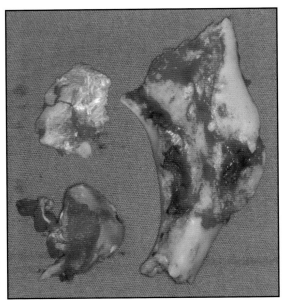

Figure 1.

Resected coronoid, fibrotic periosteum and mandibular angle, showing necrotic bone and resorption defects due to advanced osteoradionecrosis in a 64-year-old patient, three years after radiotherapy with a total dose of 70 Gy.

Phase III: An intermediate phase with little or no change in parenchymal cellularity. Degenerative changes in fine vascularity and interstitial fibrosis may progress slowly.

Phase IV: Delayed or late parenchymal degeneration, either in the form of gradual premature involution of tissues, with hypoplasia, atrophy, and replacement fibrosis, as in premature aging; or in the form of a more rapid breakdown or necrosis of tissues. At the histologic level, most of these types of delayed effects in parenchymal tissues seem to be sequentially secondary to progessively increasing degrees of degeneration of the fine vasculature and increasing density or quantity of fibrous connective tissue. In general, the larger the dose the earlier and more rapidly these delayed parenchymal effects develop.

Although the pathogenesis was not completely understood, osteoradionecrosis of the mandible was, for a long time, considered an osteomyelitis in irradiated bone as a result of a triad of radiation, trauma and infection [48].

In 1983 Marx [35] showed by means of microbial analysis of the so-called "infected bone" of osteoradionecrosis, that microorganisms play only a contaminant role in the pathophysiology of osteoradionecrosis. Furthermore it was found that 35% of the cases could not be correlated with an episode of trauma, thus showing that trauma is only one mechanism of

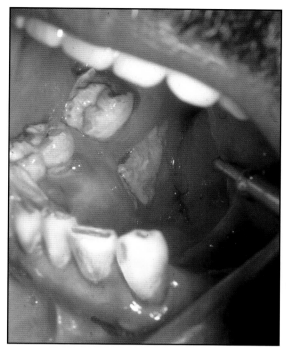

Figure 2.

Spontaneous osteoradionecrosis at the lingual surface of the right mandible in a 44-year-old patient, one year after radiotherapy of a carcinoma of the oropharynx with a total dose of 70 Gy.

tissue breakdown leading to osteoradionecrosis. According to Marx, osteoradionecrosis is not a primary infection of irradiated bone but a metabolic and tissue homeostatic deficiency created by radiation-induced cellular injury and characterized by the sequence: radiation, formation of hypoxic, hypovascular and hypocellular tissue, followed by tissue breakdown (cellular death and collagen lysis exceed synthesis and cellular replication) and resulting in a chronic, non-healing wound (the "three H" principle) [35].

More recently Bras et al. [4] reported on a study in which resection and sequestrectomy specimen of patients with osteoradionecrosis of the mandible were compared to irradiated non-osteoradionecrotic mandibles and non-irradiated mandibles. The authors conclude that osteoradionecrosis of the mandible is an ischemic necrosis caused by radiation-induced obliteration of the inferior alveolar artery, whereas revascularization from the facial artery is disturbed by radiation-induced vascular disease and periosteal damage. The most vulnerable part of the mandible is the buccal cortex of the premolar, molar and retromolar regions [4].

In other reports in recent literature osteoradionecrosis is also considered an ischemic necrosis of bone [14,54].

Due to these changes in concept on the pathogenesis of osteoradionecrosis, the treatment of osteoradionecrosis has changed considerably in recent years and is focussed on revascularisation of irradiated tissues [11,15,36,38,39,41].

DEFINITION OF OSTEORADIONECROSIS

One of the major problems in the diagnosis and treatment of osteoradionecrosis is that a proper definition or description is lacking. Wong [59] found 11 different clinical definitions in the recent literature. The most important differences concern the time the lesion is present, the extent of the disease, and the progression of the disease. It seems likely that these factors will lead to different biological behaviour and treatment response.

Concerning the time the lesion is present, reports using no limitation, three months or six months can be found in the literature. Since several authors report healing of denuded bone lesions after conservative therapy or spontaneously [3,13,59], the use of a minimum time seems to be relevant.

The extent of the disease is rarely clear. Except for the definition of Marx [35] in 1983 (case selection on an area greater than one centimeter of exposed bone), none of the authors used a minimum size of a lesion in the clinical definition. This may lead to comparison of lesions of denuded bone of several millimeters to lesions measuring one to several centimeters. The same goes for radiological criteria: except for the staging protocol in treatment of osteoradionecrosis of Marx [36] and his clear definition of advanced disease (Fig.3), often none are reported and lesions with hardly any pathology on the radiographs may end up in the same series as lesions with diffuse osteolysis of several centimeters of mandibular bone.

Epstein [13] proposed a classification to provide a guide for treatment selection and to allow classification for research purposes. He recognised chronic persistent (nonprogressive) and active progressive osteoradionecrosis [13,14] and reported that chronic nonprogressive osteoradionecrosis can remain stable without extensive intervention [14].

Unfortunately, this proposal and others [59] for a classification of osteoradionecrosis do not seem to have succeeded. This means that a general definition of osteoradionecrosis as "any exposed bone in a field of irradiation (>50 Gy), which is resistant to conservative treatment and has failed to heal for at least three months," still seems to be the best. When combined with radiological findings (not visible, limited to the alveolar process, throughout the height of the mandibular body) a good indication is given. Advanced disease may best be defined as reported by Marx [36]: patients who initially present with a pathologic fracture, osteolysis of the inferior border of the mandible on the orthopantomogram, or an orocutaneous fistula (Figure 3).

TREATMENT OF OSTEORADIONECROSIS

Treatment options for osteoradionecrosis of the mandible in the recent literature are still variable. The range varies from conservative non-surgical/non-hyperbaric oxygen treatment [59], free omental transfers [29], cancellous bone grafting [23] to surgery with or without adjunctive HBO [10,33]. However, the highest rates of resolution are found in series of a combined surgical and HBO approach (Marx 100% resolution [39], Wood 100% resolution [60], Vudiniabola 100% resolution [57], Curi 78% resolution [10], van Merkesteyn 69% resolution [47]).

Hyperbaric Oxygen

The rationale for the use of hyperbaric oxygen in radiation tissue damage is to revascularize irradiated tissues and to improve the fibroblastic cellular density, thus limiting the amount of non-viable tissue to be surgically removed, enhancing wound healing and preparing the tissues for reconstruction when indicated [27,36,38,39].

Revascularization in irradiated tissues by HBO has been demonstrated in an irradiated rabbit model by Marx et al. [41]. Six months after radiation of the mandible to an equivalent of 60 Gy, 14 rabbits were treated

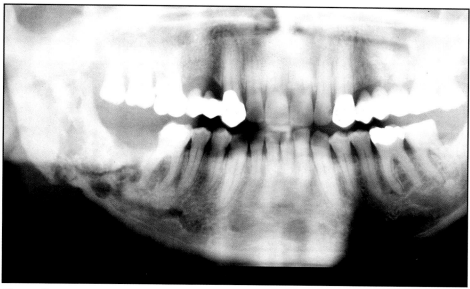

Figure 3.

Advanced osteoradionecrosis: osteolytic changes throughout the height of the mandibular body and pathological fracture in the mandibular angle in a 59-year-old patient six years after radiotherapy because of a squamous cell carcinoma of the oropharynx with a total dose of 72 Gy.

with hyperbaric oxygen, 2.4 ATA, 90 minutes daily, for 20 sessions, 14 rabbits received 20 sessions of normobaric oxygen and 7 rabbits served as controls. Microangiographic and histologic studies of the jaw and surrounding tissues, showed no differences in vascularization of the tissues between the normobaric oxygen and the control groups. The microangiograms of the hyperbaric oxygen group showed a sevenfold increase in vascular density compared to the other groups.

The vascular density was studied histologically at three levels: subcutaneous tissue, periosteum and mandibular cancellous marrow space. The vascular density at the subcutaneous level showed a four- to fivefold increase in the hyperbaric oxygen group compared to the normobaric oxygen and control groups. At the periosteal level a fourfold increase was found and in the marrow space a twofold increase in vascular density was found.

These results show that hyperbaric oxygen increases the vascular density throughout the tissues with the highest reponse in the subcutaneous tissue level.

Several clinical studies preceeded and confirmed the above-mentioned concept of revascularisation of irradiated tissues [35,36,37,39]. In one of those studies, the transcutaneous oxygen pressure ($TcPO_2$) in 34 patients from skin overlying osteoradionecrotic bone, was compared to the $TcPO_2$ from the left second intercostal space (a control site away from the radiation field) [37]. The $TcPO_2$ recordings over the osteoradionecrosis sites averaged only 30% of those of the control sites, indicating the difference in vascularization of the tissues. After eight sessions of HBO treatment, the TcPO$_2$ of the irradiated tissues started to rise rapidly to approximately 80% of the control values in the second left intercostal space after a total of 20 sessions. No further rise of the TcPO$_2$ was found during completion of the treatment to a total of 30 sessions. This effect was maintained for at least three years [37]. According to the authors this represented hyperbaric oxygen-induced angiogenesis in irradiated tissue.

Osteoradionecrosis of the Mandible

Marx developed a clinical staging protocol for the treatment of osteoradionecrosis of the mandible that has been reported in several publications [27,36,39]. This so-called "Miami protocol" or "30/10 protocol" selects patients who are able to respond to HBO treatment only or to less agressive surgery with a minimum of HBO treatment, and prepares patients who need aggressive surgery for hard tissue reconstruction.

In Stage I of the protocol all patients receive 30 sessions of HBO. Antibiotics can be discontinued but may be used if there is evidence of soft tissue infection. Local wound care is continued. After 30 sessions the exposed bone is examined for response, which is shown by softening of the bone and formation of granulation tissue. If the response is good, another 10 sessions are given. When the exposed bone does not show a good response, the patient is advanced to Stage II.

In Stage II, after at least 30 sessions of HBO, the patient undergoes a transoral resection of the exposed and non-viable bone (Figure 4). Care must be taken to reflect the periosteum as little as possible to prevent further devascularization of the bone. The wound is closed in layers over a base of bleeding bone. After surgery the patient receives another 10 sessions of HBO.

Stage III patients are those who have failed to respond to the treatment in Stage II and patients who initially present with a pathologic fracture, osteolysis of the inferior border on the orthopantomogram, or an orocutaneous fistula. It is believed that in these cases too much non-viable bone is present to respond to anything less than partial jaw resection. In Stage III the patient already has received 30 sessions of HBO and subsequently undergoes a transoral continuity resection of the mandible. The margins of the resection are determined by the presence of bleeding bone. The remaining segments of the mandible are stabilized with external pin fixation or maxillomandibular fixation. The soft tissues are closed primarily. After surgery the patient receives another 10 sessions of HBO.

Three months after resection the mandible may be reconstructed (Figure 5) with an allogeneic crib (rib, mandible, iliac crest) and autogenous cancellous bone grafts [42].

Marx reported in 1988 on 331 cases of osteoradionecrosis of the mandible treated by this protocol. The osteoradionecrosis was resolved in stage I in 13% of the patients. In Stage II 18% of the cases was resolved and 69% of the cases was resolved in Stage III, meaning a continuity resection of the mandible [40].

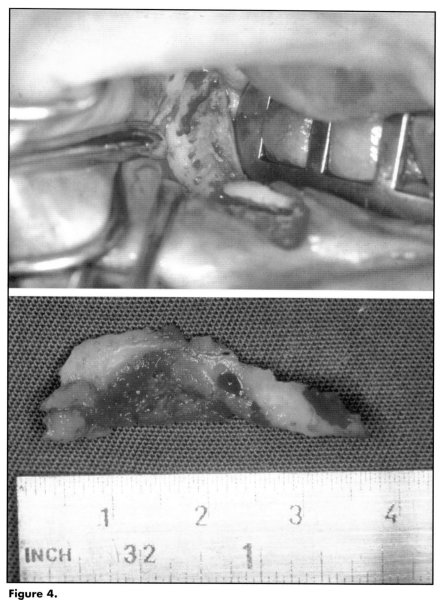

Figure 4.

Trans-oral resection of necrotic bone in osteoradionecrosis of the mandible limited to the alveolar process.

Marx also showed that reconstruction of the mandible after radiotherapy with particulate bone and cancellous marrow grafts showed good results when used in combination with HBO therapy [36]. However, some patients do not want to undergo additional reconstructive surgery, thus limiting the possibilities of an extensive surgical protocol as described above. Fortunately in selected patients a functional result may be achieved even without reconstruction (Figure 6).

The rate of resolution of osteoradionecrosis in a series of 29 patients with osteoradionecrosis of the mandible reported by van Merkesteyn et al. was 69% [47]. These patients were treated with the 30/10 protocol but indications for resection and reconstruction were used less aggressively, thus saving continuity of the mandible in some of the cases with advanced osteoradionecrosis [46]. Series reported by Epstein et al. [13] in which HBO was used in selected cases only and not in combination with surgery, reported less favourable results: 15% resolution and 42% stabilisation of osteoradionecrosis.

More recently Wood [60] and Vudiniabola [57] also reported on a series of patients treated with a protocol similar to that of Marx, starting treatment with HBO followed by surgery when necessary. Both series showed resolution of osteoradionecrosis in all cases. Surgery was needed in 80% and 64% of the cases respectively.

Unfortunately there are, even in recent literature, no prospective randomized trials to support the results of the abovementioned retrospective studies.

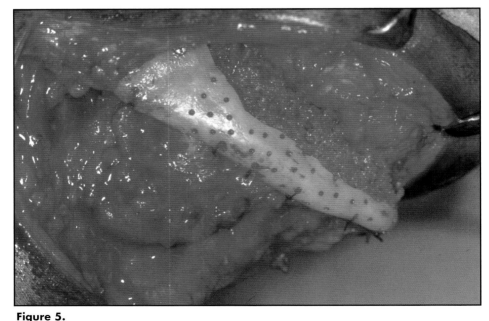

Figure 5.

Reconstruction of the mandible with a freeze-dried allogeneic human mandible filled with an autogenous particulate bone and cancellous marrow graft. Fixation is performed with miniscrews.

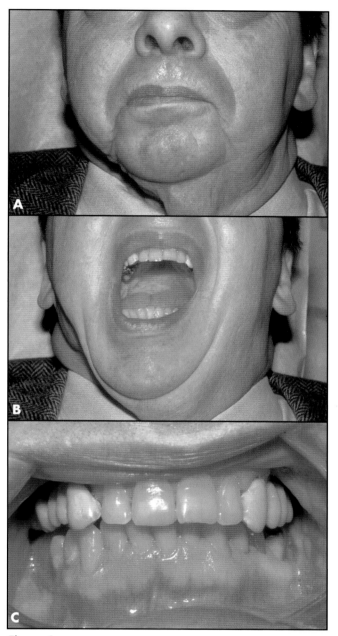

Figure 6.

Resection of the right mandibular angle because of osteo-radionecrosis (see also Figure 4), in a 59-year-old patient who declined reconstruction. After six weeks of intermax-illary fixation and traction with elastic bands a satisfacto-ry result is achieved with limited asymmetry (A), sufficient opening of the mouth with limited deviation (B), and acceptable occlusion (C).

Osteoradionecrosis in Other Sites

Although most of the reports on osteoradionecrosis in the literature concern lesions of the jaws, other sites of clinical significance are the skull, chest wall and pelvis [21,22,32,45,57].

No large series or controlled studies are available but clinical reports suggest that HBO is a useful adjunct in the treatment as has been shown in osteoradionecrosis of the jaws.

PREVENTION OF OSTEORADIONECROSIS

Dental Extractions

Development of osteoradionecrosis of the mandible is closely related to dental extractions [3,13,36,53,56]. Therefore, prevention of dental extractions is of the utmost importance.

When dental extractions have to be performed in irradiated patients (Figure 7), recent studies suggest that hyperbaric oxygen should be considered an adequate prophylactic measure. A study of Vudiniabola et al. [56] showed that prophylactic HBO treatment reduced the risk of osteoradionecrosis following surgery to irradiated jaws. However, since this study was not randomized, no firm conclusions can be drawn. Chavez and Adkinson [6] reported on a very low incidence of osteoradionecrosis after dental extractions of 1.5% in 40 consecutive patients treated with the HBO 20/10 protocol. This seems very low in comparison to the average reported incidence of 5.4% [7]. Unfortunately the radiation dose in this series of patients varied from 35 to 85 Gy, thus including patients with less than 50 Gy, and together with the fact that no separation was made between extractions in maxilla and mandible, no firm conclusions can be drawn from this study either.

Marx et al. [37] reported in 1985 on a randomized prospective clinical trial, comparing HBO to penicillin in the prophylaxis of osteoradionecrosis after tooth extraction in irradiated patients. Seventy-four patients having received irradiation to doses of 60 to 68 Gy were randomized in two groups. One group of 37 patients, in whom a total of 135 teeth had to be removed, received 1 million units of penicillin G intravenously just before surgery and 500 mg of phenoxymethyl penicillin four times daily for ten days after surgery. The other group of 37 patients, in which a total of 156 teeth had to be removed, received no antibiotics but 20 sessions of hyperbaric oxygen before tooth removal and ten sessions after tooth removal. For this study, osteoradionecrosis was defined as the presence of exposed bone after six months. In the penicillin group eleven patients (29.9%) developed osteoradionecrosis, whereas in the HBO group only two patients (5.4%) developed osteoradionecrosis.

In conclusion it seems that enough evidence is available to suggest that HBO should be considered as a prophylactic measure when post-irradiation dental extractions are necessary.

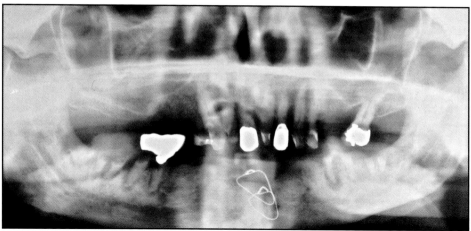

Figure 7.

A 74-year-old patient received 60 Gy of radiotherapy 10 years earlier, in which multiple extractions are indicated in a mandible showing numerous apical pathologic changes and diffuse changes in bone density.

DENTAL IMPLANTS IN IRRADIATED BONE

The use of osseointegrated dental implants in the rehabilitation of patients with cancer in the maxillofacial region has been a great step forward. Where osseointegration is highly successful in normal tissues or patients with acquired surgical defects in the craniofacial region, the results of implants in irradiated bone seem to be less successful. Several reports in the literature show an increased rate of implant loss when implants are placed in previously irradiated craniofacial bones [19,24,52]. However, other authors show no increase of implant loss in irradiated bone [1,2,12,16,26,51,58]. Unfortunately, in some of these reports no clear data of the radiotherapy were given [1,51]. In the report of Franzen et al. [16] only six of the 20 implants were placed in bone that received more than 50 Gy. In the report of Andersson et al. [2], 10 of the 15 patients received 50 Gy or less. This shows that the local radiation dose may vary considerably throughout the mandible and that it is important to check this local radiation dose before the placement of dental implants (Figure 8).

The use of a perioperative HBO protocol to reduce implant loss in irradiated bone has been reported in several series [17,19,20,23,31,49,50]. In a review of the literature by Larsen [31] an increase of the success rate of maxillofacial implants in all anatomical regions was found when adjunctive HBO was used. Granstrom [20] showed in a case-controlled study that HBO reduced the failure rate of implants inserted in irradiated bone. Experimental studies [18,25] also suggest a better osseointegration of implants in irradiated bone after HBO therapy.

In conclusion both experimental [18,25] and clinical [19,20,49,50,55] studies suggest that implant loss in irradiated bone will be reduced when HBO is used as adjunctive treatment, but further studies are needed to evaluate the exact value of HBO.

So far no series of patients have been published on osteoradionecrosis after placement of dental implants. However, considering the radiation-induced changes in bone and soft tissues, individual cases are likely to occur (Figure 9) and the use of perioperative HBO to prevent osteoradionecrosis is recommended by several authors [31,42].

SUMMARY

Treatment of osteoradionecrosis is still a major problem. Comparison of the different treatment modalities in the literature is difficult because of the many different manifestations of the disease (active, slowly progressive, superficial, advanced, with pathologic fracture etc.).

The use of HBO in the treatment of osteoradionecrosis has been well documented and it seems to be a useful adjunct. Although no prospective randomised trials have been reported, the amount of large series with favourable results, the experimental studies and the prophylactic studies seem to justify the use of HBO in the treatment of osteoradionecrosis. In the prevention of osteoradionecrosis in relation to dental extractions, a

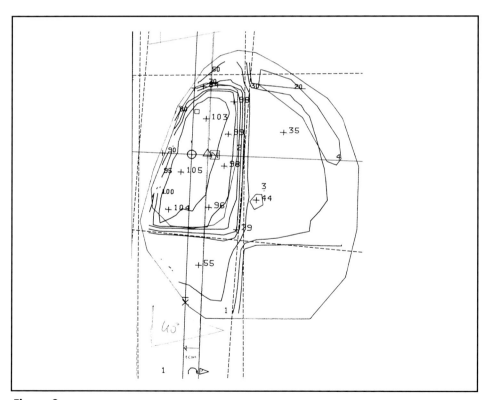

Figure 8.

Isodose curves in a patient who received radiotherapy of 60 Gy on the left (resected) mandible because of a squamous cell carcinoma. The isodose curves (100%=60 Gy) show that the remaining mandible received a dose less than 30% (20 Gy). Therefore the placement of dental implants in the right mandible seems to be possible without risk of osteoradionecrosis.

prospective randomised trial has clearly shown the benefits of HBO in comparison to antibiotic prophylaxis. The use of HBO as an adjunct to implantology in irradiated jaws is less well defined.

Several studies suggest a reduced failure rate of the implants but only experimental and one case-controlled study are available to support this.

SUGGESTED PROCEDURES

Hyperbaric Oxygen

In radionecrosis a series of treatment sessions at 2.4 ATA oxygen in a monoplace chamber or 2.4-2.6 ATA in a multiplace chamber, breathing by tight-fitting oronasal mask, head-tent or endotracheal tube, 90 minutes, once a day, five to seven days a week is recommended.

Osteoradionecrosis

Recommended hyperbaric oxygen treatment consists of:
- 30 sessions HBO followed by evaluation of tissue response.
- When wound healing occurs, 10 or more additional sessions are given. If the lesion does not respond to treatment, surgical debridement is indicated, followed by 10 additional sessions of HBO.

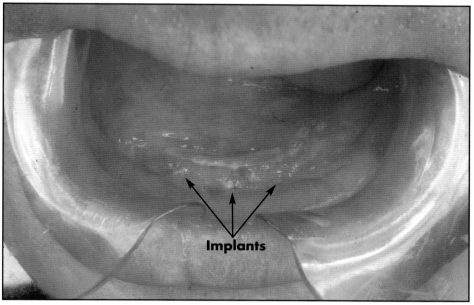

Figure 9.

Necrotic lingual cortex in a patient who received 20/10 HBO sessions to prevent radionecrosis after placement of implants in the mandible. The patient received radiotherapy (60 Gy) two years earlier because of a squamous cell carcinoma of the floor of the mouth. No implants were lost and the denuded bone was treated successfully by sequestrectomy under local anaesthesia.

- In severe cases of osteoradionecrosis of the mandible, resection of the affected part of the mandible is performed after the inital 30 sessions, followed by 10 sessions of HBO. Three months after resection, reconstruction may be performed without additional HBO treatment.

Prevention of (Osteo)Radionecrosis

Recommended treatment for prevention of osteoradionecrosis after surgery (dental extractions, reconstructive surgery, implantology) in irradiated tissues (without previous HBO treatment) consists of:

- 20 sessions of HBO followed by 10 post-operative sessions.

REFERENCES

1. Albrektsson T. A multicenter report on osseointegrated oral implants. J Prosthet Dent 1988;60:75-84.

2. Andersson G, Andreasson L, Bjelkengren G. Oral implant rehabilitation in irradiated patients without adjunctive hyperbaric oxygen. Int J Oral Maxillofac Impl 1998: 13:647-654.

3. Beumer J, Harrison R, Sanders B, Kurrasch M. Osteoradionecrosis: Predisposing factors and outcomes of therapy. Head & Neck Surg. 1984;6:819-27.

4. Bras J, Jonge HKT de, Merkesteyn JPR van. Osteoradionecrosis of the mandible: Pathogenesis. Am J Otolaryngol 1990;11:244-50.

5. Casarett GW. Radiation histopathology Vol. I, II. CRC Press 1980 Boca Raton, Florida, pp. 39-49.

6. Chavez JA, Adkinson CD. Adjunctive hyperbaric oxygen in irradiated patients requiring dental extractions: outcomes and complications. J Oral Maxillofac Surg 2001;59:518-22.

7. Clayman L. Management of dental extractions in irradiated jaws: A protocol without hyperbaric oxygen therapy. J Oral Maxillofac Surg 1997;55:275-281.

8. Constantino PD, Friedman CD, Steinberg MJ. Irradiated bone and its management. Otolaryngol Clin North AM 1995;28:1021-38.

9. Curi MM, Dibb LL. Osteoradionecrosis of the jaws: a retrospective study of the back ground factors and treatment in 104 cases. J Oral maxillofac Surg 1997;55:540-4.

10. Curi MM, Dib LL, Kowalski LP. Management of refractory osteoradionecrosis of the jaws with surgery and adjunctive hyperbaric oxygen therapy. Int. J. Oral Maxillofac. Surg 2000;29:430-434.

11. Davis JC. Soft tissue radiation necrosis: The role of hyperbaric oxygen. HBO Rev 1981;2:153-67.

12. Eckert SE, Desjardins RP, Keller EE, Tolman DE. Endosseous implants in an irradiated tissue bed. J Prosthet Dent 1996;76:45-49.

13. Epstein JB, Wong FLW, Stevenson-Moore P. Osteoradionecrosis: Clinical experience and a proposal for classification. J Oral Maxillofac Surg 1987;45:104-10.

14. Epstein J, Meij E van der, Mckenzie M, Wong F, Lepawsky M, Stevenson-Moore P. Postradiation osteonecrosis of the mandible; a long term follow-up study. Oral Surg 1997;83:657-62.

15. Fattore L, Strauss RA. Hyperbaric oxygen in the treatment of osteoradionecrosis: A review of its use and efficacy. Oral Surg Oral Med Oral Pathol 1987;63:280-86.

16. Franzén L, Rosenquist JB, Rosenquist KI, Gustafsson I. Oral implant rehabilitation of patients with oral malignancies treated with radiotherapy and surgery without adjunctive hyperbaric oxygen. Int J Oral Maxillofac Impl 1995:10:183-187.

17. Granström G, Jacobsson M, Tjellström A. Titanium implants in irradiated tissue: Benefits from hyperbaric oxygen. Int J Oral Maxillofac Implants 1992;7:15-25.

18. Granström G, Hansson A, Johnsson K, Jacobsson M, Albrektsson T, Tureson I. Hyperbaric oxygenation can increase bone to titanium implant interface strength after irradiation. 1992; Proc 18th Annual Meeting EUBS:151-155.

19. Granström G, Tjellström A, Branemark PI, Fornander J. Bone-anchored reconstruction of the irradiated head and neck cancer patient. Otolaryngol Head Neck Surg 1993;108:334-343.

20. Granström G, Tjellström A, Brånemark P-I. Osseointegrated implants in irradiated bone: A case-controlled study using adjunctive hyperbaric oxygen therapy. J Oral Maxillofac Surg 1999:57:493-499.

21. Hart GB, Strauss MB. Hyperbaric oxygen in the management of radiation injury. In: Schmutz J. (ed) Proceedings 1st Swiss symposium on hyperbaric medicine. Stiftung Hyperbare Medizin, Basel, 1986, pp.31-51.

22. Heimbach RD. Radiation effects on tissue. In: Davis JC, Hunt TK Eds. Problem wounds. The role of oxygen. Elsevier, Amsterdam, 1988;53-63.

23. Jisander S, Grenthe B, Salemark L. Treatment of mandibular osteoradionecrosis by can celloous bone grafting. J Oral Maxillofac Surg 1999;57:936-42.

24. Jacobsson M, Tjellström A, Thomsen P, Albrektsson T, Turessson I. Integration of titanium implants in irradiated bone. Histologic and clinical study. Ann. Otol. Rhinol. Laryngol. 1988;97:337-340.

25. Johnsson K, Hansson A, Granström G, Jacobsson M, Turesson I. The effects of hyperbaric oxygenation on bone-titanium implant interface strength with and without preceeding irradiation. Int J Oral Maxillofac Implants 1993;8:415-419.

26. Keller EE, Placement of dental implants in the irradiated mandible: a protocol without adjunctive hyperbaric oxygen. J Oral Maxillofac Surg 1997;55:972-80.

27. Kindwall EP. Hyperbaric oxygen's effect on radiation necrosis. In: Clin Plast Surg 1993;20:473-83.

28. Kluth EV, Jain PR, Stuchell RN, Frich JC. A study of factors contributing to the development of osteoradionecrosis of the jaws. J Prosth Dent 1988;59:194-201.

29. Kobayashi W, Kobayashi M, Hirota W, Kimura H. Free omental transfer for osteoradionecrosis of the mandible. Int J Oral Maxillofac Surg 2000;29:201-6.

30. Koka VN, Deo R, Lusinchi A, Roland J, Schwaab G. Osteoradionecrosis of the mandible: Study of 104 cases treated by hemimandibulectomy. J Laryngol Otol 1990;104:305-7.

31. Larsen PE. Placement of dental implants in the irradiated mandible: A protocol involving adjunctive hyperbaric oxygen. J Oral Maxillofac Surg 1997:55:967-971.

32. London S, Park SS, Gampper TJ, Hoard MA. Hyperbaric oxygen for the management of radionecrosis of bone and cartilage. Laryngoscope 1998;108:1291-6.

33. Maier A, Gaggl A, Klemen H, Santler G, Anegg U, Fell B, Karcher H, Smolle-Juttner FM, Friehs GB. Review of severe osteoradionecrosis treated by surgery alone or surgery with post-operative hyperbaric oxygenation. Brit J Oral Maxillofac Surg 2000;38:173-6.

34. Marciani RD, Ownby HE. Osteoradionecrosis of the jaws. J Oral Maxillofac Surg 1986;44:218-23.

35. Marx RE. Osteoradionecrosis: A new concept of its pathophysiology. J Oral Maxillofac Surg 1983;41:283-8.

36. Marx RE. Osteoradionecrosis of the jaws: Review and update. HBO Review 1984; 5:78-126.

37. Marx RE, Johnson RP, Kline SN. Prevention of osteoradionecrosis: A randomized prospective clinical trial of hyperbaric oxygen versus penicillin. JADA 1985;111:49-54.

38. Marx RE, Johnson RP. Studies in the radiobiology of osteoradionecrosis and their clinical significance. Oral Surg Oral Med Oral Pathol 1987;64:379-90.

39. Marx RE, Johnson RP. Problem wounds in oral and maxillofacial surgery. In: Davis JC, Hunt TK. Eds. Problem wounds: The role of oxygen. Amsterdam, Elsevier Publishing, 1988;65-123.

40. Marx RE. Oral cancer and jaw tumors. Proc. first International congress on oral cancer and jaw tumors, Singapore, November 1987. Prof. Postgraduate Serv. 1988. pp. 164-6.

41. Marx RE, Ehlers WJ, Tayapongsak P, Pierce LW. Relationship of oxygen dose to angiogenesis induction in irradiated tissue. Am J Surg 1990;160:519-24.

42. Marx RE. Radiation injury to tissue. In: Kindwall EP (ed.). Hyperbaric medicine practice. Best Publishing Company, Flagstaff AZ, 1994, pp.448-503.

43. Maxymiw WG, Wood RE, Liu FF. Postradiation dental extractions without hyperbaric oxygen. Oral Surg Oral Med Oral Pathol 1991;72:270-4.

44. Merkesteyn JPR van, Bakker DJ, Dellemijn HL. The use of hyperbaric oxygen in the treatment of osteomyelitis and osteoradionecrosis of the jaw. In: Bakker DJ, Schmutz J. Eds. Proc 2nd European Conf Hyperbaric Med, Foundation Hyperbaric Medicine, Basel 1990:151-4.

45. Merkesteyn JPR, Bakker DJ. Treatment of radiation damage in the head and neck in 66 patients: the value of hyperbaric oxygen. In: Schmutz J, Wendling J. Eds. Proc. Joint meeting on diving and hyperbaric medicine. Basel, Foundation for Hyperbaric Medicine, 1992:156-9.

46. Merkesteyn JPR, Balm AJM, Bakker DJ, Borgmeijer-Hoelen AMMJ. Hyperbaric oxygen treatment of osteoradionecrosis of the mandible with repeated pathological fracture. Report of a case. Oral Surg 1994;77:461-4.

47. Merkesteyn JPR, Bakker DJ, Borgmeijer-Hoelen AMMJ. Hyperbaric oxygen treatment of osteoradionecrosis of the mandible: Experience in 29 patients. Oral Surg 1995; 80:12-6.

48. Meyer I. Osteoradionecrosis of the jaws. The Year Book Publishers Inc. Chicago, 1958, 17-27.

49. Niimi A, Fujimoto T, Nosaka Y, Ueda M. A Japanese multicenter study of osseointegrated implants placed in irradiated tissues: A preliminary report. Int J Oral Maxillofac Implants 1997:12:259-264.

50. Niimi A, Ueda M, Keller EE, Worthington P. Experience with osseointegrated implants placed in irradiated tissues in Japan and the United States. Int J Oral Maxillofac Implants 1998:13:407-411.

51. Palmisano D, Guerra L, Finger I. Radiated bone and dental implants (abstract). J Dental Res 1991;70 (special issue).

52. Parel S, Tjellström A. The United States and Swedish experience with osseointegration and facial prosthesis. Int J Oral Maxillofac Implants 1991;6:75-79.

53. Sanger JR, Matloub HS, Yousif NJ, Larson DL. Management of osteoradionecrosis of the mandible. In: Clin Plast Surg 1993;20:517-30.

54. Thorn JJ, Hansen HS, Specht L, Bastholt L. Osteoradionecrosis of the jaws: clinical characteristics and relation to the field of irradiation. J Oral Maxillofac Surg 2000;58:1088-93.

55. Ueda M, Kaneda T, Takahashi H. Effect of hyperbaric oxygen therapy on osseointegration of titanium implants in irradiated bone: A preliminary report. Int J Oral Maxillofac Implants 1993;8:41-44.

56. Vudiniabola S, Pirone C, Williamson J, Goss AN. Hyperbaric oxygen in the prevention of osteoradionecrosis of the jaws. Aus Dent J 1999;44:243-247.

57. Vudiniabola S, Pirone C, Williamson J, Goss AN. Hyperbaric oxygen in the therapeutic management of osteoradionecrosis of the facial bones. Int J Oral Maxillofac Surg 2000;29:435-8.

58. Wagner W, Esser E, Ostkamp K. Osseointegration of dental implants in patients with and without radiotherapy. Act Oncol 1998:37:693-696.

59. Wong JK, Wood RE, McLean M. Conservative management of osteoradionecrosis. Oral Surg 1997;84:16-21.

60. Wood GA, Liggins SJ. Does hyperbaric oxygen have a role in the management of osteoradionecrosis? Brit J Oral Maxillofac Surg 1996;34:424-7.

NOTES

CHAPTER **10**

SELECTED AEROBIC AND ANAEROBIC SOFT TISSUE INFECTIONS

CLASSIFICATION, BACTERIOLOGY, DIAGNOSIS, AND
THE USE AND ROLE OF SURGERY AND ADJUNCTIVE
HYPERBARIC OXYGEN IN THE TREATMENT

D.J. Bakker

INTRODUCTION

Necrotising soft tissue infections caused by aerobic, anaerobic and mixed bacterial floras are an increasing problem in surgical and medical practice. They occur with increasing frequency and seriousness, especially in immune-compromised patients.

The suppression of the immune system may be caused by underlying systemic diseases, mainly: diabetes mellitus, malignancies, vascular insufficiency, and alcoholism; by the use of immunosuppressive drugs as in transplant recipients; in drug addicts; and in neutropenic patients. These infections occur after trauma (sharp and blunt), around foreign bodies in surgical wounds, or even "spontaneously" as is seen sometimes in scrotal and penile necrotising fasciitis (Fourniers gangrene). A large number of these infections have even been reported after a volcanic cataclysm (103) and also in children (15, 38, 65, 112, 141, 142).

Necrotising fasciitis is also seen postoperatively, i.e., after caesarean delivery in young women without risk factors (no diabetes or peripheral vascular disease) (54), after such "sterile" operations such as suction lipectomy (59, 132), and in Crohn's disease (99). As in gas gangrene every operation can be followed by necrotising fasciitis and a high index of suspicion is necessary for the diagnosis, especially after so-called "sterile" operations.

The clinical picture can vary considerably from patient to patient. Treatment is difficult, often irrational and very often "one step behind the facts," because early recognition is difficult and aetiology, bacteriology, and the clinical course are sometimes not well understood or expected to evolve in a different and more favourable way.

Considerable morbidity occurs and mortality can be very high, from 20% up to 70 or 80%. The highest mortality is found in the group of older debilitated diabetic patients with synergistic necrotising cellulitis (127).

HISTORY

For a proper understanding of these infections, a short historical review is necessary. In 1883, Jean Alfred Fournier, a French venereologist, described five cases of "gangrene foudroyante de la verge," later called Fourniers gangrene. Five healthy young men (ages 24-30 years) developed penile and/or scrotal gangrene, "spontaneously or after a superficial erosion, and despite large incisions and eschar excision, mortality was 60%" (51).

Even before that time descriptions of the same clinical entity can be found in the works of Hippocrates from the 5th century BC. He described "erysipelas, which was at its worst when it reached the private parts, the pubes and the genitals. Flesh, sinews and bones fell away in large quantities" (62).

After Hippocrates the first description of a possible case of necrotising fasciitis came from Baurienne in 1764 (16) in an adult, and thereafter a case in a young baby boy reported by Hebler in 1848 (57).

Also the work by the Confederate Army Surgeon Joseph Jones must be mentioned who described a variant of this disease in 1869 and 1870 during the Civil War in the United States, which he called "hospital gangrene" (67, 108).

Extensive reviews of the literature on necrotising soft tissue infections including Fourniers gangrene have been published by McCrea (89), Jones (68), and Stevens (117), as well as by Loudon (84), Sutherland (129), Chapnick and Abter (28), Weiss and Lavardière (138), Smith et al. (116), Eke (46), Capelli-Schellpfeffer and Gerber (27), and also by Wienecke and Lobenhoffer (140). Capelli-Schellpfeffer (27) investigated the role of hyperbaric oxygen in the treatment of these infections in urology.

Meleney, 1924, found the cause of this gangrene to be "a pure invasion of haemolytic streptococci" (92). Fourniers gangrene could thus be considered as a special form of haemolytic streptococcus gangrene. In the same article Meleney described this haemolytic streptococcus gangrene or "Meleney's ulcer," also caused by haemolytic streptococci (92). This publication was based on Meleney's experience in the Imperial Hospital in Peking (Beijing).

Cullen, also in 1924, gave a description of the so-called "postoperative progressive bacterial synergistic gangrene," in a patient after an appendectomy (34).

At first a confusing variety of microorganisms was found. But in studying the spreading periphery of the lesion, both clinically and experimentally (in guinea pigs), the interaction of a microaerophilic non-haemolytic streptococcus and a haemolytic staphylococcus aureus was found to be synergistic (21).

The confusion in the nomenclature started here, because Meleney described Cullen's ulcer and since then Meleney's and Cullen's ulcer were often regarded in the literature as the same disease. Sometimes this was even considered to be a variant of Fourniers gangrene.

This confusion is clearly shown by Kingston and Seal, who stated that "this animal model of Brewer and Meleney (anaerobic streptococcus and staphylococcus aureus) was unrelated to the disease Meleney's postoperative synergistic gangrene, which it was developed to explain" (72).

From this historical review it must be clear that they refer to "Cullen's postoperative progressive bacterial synergistic gangrene" and call that "Meleney's gangrene."

Brewer and Meleney described very clearly for the first time the very important mechanism of bacterial synergy for these infections. By bacterial synergy we mean that mixtures of organisms (two or more) can cause more severe infections than each of the organisms alone. This must be different-iated from the term "mixed infections," often with different aerobes and anaerobes, meaning that the net pathogenic effect is no greater than the sum of the damage caused by infection with each of the organisms alone (21).

This bacterial synergism was reason for Meleney to propose the first classification for these necrotising soft tissue infections with special reference to this phenomenon (93, 94). Meleney distinguished acute (for example, haemolytic streptococcal gangrene) and chronic infectious skin gangrene, an example of the latter are postoperative progressive bacterial synergistic gangrene. Kingston and Seal based the conclusions in their article on the division of these infections into three different categories, based on the rates of progression (from slow to rapid) (72).

Since 1926 a great variety of synergistic microorganisms both in humans and in animals have been found (for a review see Bakker, 1984, pages 74-90) (9). The bacteriology of these diseases has apparently changed considerably through the years. Meleney mentioned "associated organisms next to streptococci, concomitants, not adding to the development of the dis-ease, in a minority of cases"(92). Wilson found streptococci in 58% of his patients, (141) Crosthwait in 57%, (33) Ledingham and Tehrani in 8.5% (79), and in our series we initially found streptococci in 13.3% of our patients (9).

When necrosis of the deep fascia was recognised as essential in haemolytic streptococcal gangrene or Meleney's ulcer in 1948 by Wilson, the disease was renamed "necrotising fasciitis" in 1952 (141). Giuliano et al. (53) thought that two bacteriologic types of necrotising fasciitis could be recog-nized and Lamerton (78) even suggested three bacteriologic groups whose clinical pictures, however, largely overlap. Also, many microorganisms were suggested as causing postoperative progressive bacterial synergistic gangrene throughout the years. (9)

The problem is that we seldom see patients at the onset of the disease. Time elapsed since the onset and initial treatment, for example antibiotics given and possible surgical interventions are of course very important to explain later findings, especially later bacteriological culture results. Remarkably this is never mentioned in the literature whether about necrotising fasciitis or about progressive bacterial gangrene. Stone and Gorbach give a very detailed description of the microbiological findings without mentioning what we stated above (128). Smith et al. wonder why normal urethral, rectal, and cutaneous flora of otherwise low to moderate virulence are able to cause severe infections of this type (116). Well, maybe they do not. Is it possible that Meleney was right after all when he mentioned "concomitants, not adding to the development of the disease" (92)? Not every microorganism that is cultured is automatically causative to the disease.

Another thing seldomly mentioned is the location from where the cultures are taken. It can make a big difference if one takes a swab from the center of the wound or culture tissue biopsies at the spreading periphery of the disease. Brewer and Meleney mentioned that already in their first experiments on bacterial synergy (21). Recently a case of Fourniers gangrene was described where only Candida as the primary organism was cultured from the urine and later from perianal debrided tissue (66).

In the spring of 1994, a cluster of seven cases of invasive group A streptococcal (GAS) infections, including four cases of necrotising fasciitis occurred in Gloucestershire (England). When the British media reported this outbreak, the stories resembled Edgar Allan Poe's horror stories at its best. Expressions like "flesh-eating bacteria or virus," "galloping gangrene," and "killer bugs" were used to describe the process, and the impression was given that a whole new disease was discovered here. From the historical review given above it may be clear that this was not the case. A description of this outbreak can be found by Efstratiou et al. (45) and Monnickendam et al. (96).

Kujath and Eckmann (77) state that streptococci cause only a minority of necrotising fasciitis cases (three to four times less than cases caused by a polymicrobial flora). Podbielski et al. (106) found 10-18% group A streptococci and 51% "other" streptococci in their cultures of necrotising fasciitis. In 75-85% peptostreptococci were isolated (peptostreptococci cause a gas-forming infection). Group A streptococci and staphylococci were cultured when only a monoculture was found. All other microorganisms that were found were parts of a polymicrobial flora. In both articles nothing is mentioned about the time of culture in relation to the time of onset of the disease and if the patients were previously treated already. This makes it very difficult to show what the real causative microorganisms are.

A historical review of streptococcal infections with special emphasis on necrotising fasciitis and the use of hyperbaric oxygen is given by Bakker (12). Our conclusion is that interpretation and misinterpretation of historical facts and microbiological culture results have caused confusion and have added to the present difficulty in understanding the bacteriology, etiology, and clinical findings in these soft tissue infections.

CLASSIFICATION

An exact classification of necrotising soft tissue infections is difficult because the distinctions between many of the clinical entities are blurred and a great variety of names have historically been given to the same clinical entity.

Classification of these infections is usually made on the basis of:
a. The assumed causative microorganism(s) (50, 53, 55, 78, 92, 107)
b. The kind of tissue involved (2, 3, 50, 79, 81, 82, 141)
c. The kind of required therapy (50)
d. The rate of progression (72)
e. The initial clinical findings (49)

Each of these classifications has its advantages and its disadvantages because they are based on only one part of the problem. It is difficult to determine the causative microorganism(s) out of the wide variety of aerobes and anaerobes that can be cultured in these infections, and it can be equally difficult to diagnose the tissue primarily involved in the advanced stages of these infections when we usually see the patients.

The best therapy is almost always a combination of surgery, antibiotics, and adjunctive hyperbaric oxygen.

In our experience the rate of progression of these infections can change considerably from patient to patient and seems to be more dependent on the associated diseases of the patient and/or other systemic or local factors that affect the immune status, metabolism, and local vascularisation than on other factors (9, 86).

Following Ledingham and Tehrani (79) we proposed the Amsterdam classification of soft tissue infections (Table 1), based on the fact if the infections are superficial (as in progressive bacterial gangrene) or involving deeper tissues (as in necrotising fasciitis and myositis and myonecrosis). (Fig. 1 & 2)

TABLE 1. AEROBIC/ANAEROBIC SOFT TISSUE INFECTIONS & HYPERBARIC OXYGEN AS ADJUNCT

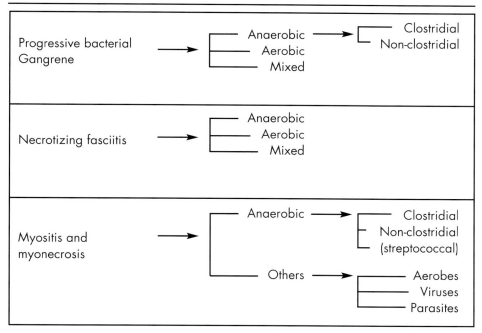

Amsterdam classification of soft tissue infections. In order to systematize the classification (following Ledingham and Tehrani (58)), we divided these infections into three groups, based on the anatomic location at the onset of the infection:
   1. progressing bacterial gangrene,
   2. necrotizing fasciitis, and
   3. myositis and myonecrosis.

ETIOLOGY

In these infections anaerobic microorganisms are often found in combination with aerobic Gram-negative organisms. In the traumatically, surgically, or medically compromised patient, local tissue hypoxia and a decreased oxidation-reduction potential (Eh) is usually present, thus promoting the growth of anaerobic microorganisms. The vast majority of these necrotising soft tissue infections have an endogenous anaerobic component.

Hypoxic conditions also allow the proliferation of facultative aerobic organisms since polymorphonuclear leukocytes function poorly under decreased oxygen tensions. The growth of aerobic microorganisms further lowers the Eh; more fastidious anaerobes become established and the disease process can rapidly accelerate. Clinically the most important signs of these infections are tissue necrosis, a putrid discharge, gas production, and the tendency of the process to burrow through fascial planes and in many cases the absence of the classical signs of tissue inflammation (86).

The variable quantity of gas in the tissues can be used in the differential diagnosis of these infections (10, 100, 101). Carbon dioxide and water are the end products of aerobic metabolism; carbon dioxide rapidly dissolves and rarely accumulates in tissues. The major tissue gases found in mixed aerobic and anaerobic soft tissue infections are probably H_2 and CH_4, less water-soluble end products of incomplete oxidation of energy sources. Nitrogen and hydrogen sulfide can also be found (101). Presence of these gases indicates a rapid bacterial multiplication at a low Eh (80, 101).

The etiology, in summary, in necrotising soft tissue infections is multifactorial and includes local and systemic factors as well as aerobic and anaerobic microorganisms. Even fungi have been found (66, 103).

1. **Local tissue trauma and bacterial invasion** follow operations such as abdominal surgery for intraperitoneal infections, drainage of ischiorectal and perianal abscesses, and minor and major traumatic lesions (blunt and sharp), and are also seen after intramuscular injections and intravenous infusions. Initially, streptococci play an important role in necrotising fasciitis, but very soon the bacteriologic pattern changes by colonization of the infected area and the use of antibiotics.

   Much of the recent work by Stevens describes the re-discovered importance of streptococci, especially the invasive group A streptococci (GAS) in these diseases (121, 122). Also Morantes mentions the return of an old nemesis in connection with streptococcal infections, when these infections are sometimes "rediscovered" (97). Bisno and Stevens (18) and Stevens (123) reviewed the streptococcal infections of skin and soft tissues.

   Bacterial synergism is an important mechanism in the onset of progressive bacterial gangrene but here again, no specific bacterial combination could be found underlying the disease and the bacteriologic pattern is changing very quickly as well.

2. **Local ischemia** frequently occurs in patients with diabetes mellitus, arteriosclerosis, and after amputations which are necessary for diabetic and arteriosclerotic vascular insufficiency. Moreover, a relative avascularity of the fascial planes in necrotising fasciitis can be noticed. We showed that secondary gangrene of subcutaneous tissues and skin could be caused by thrombosis of the subcutaneous blood vessels (5). (Fig. 16)

3. **Reduced host defense**. In almost all patients, serious underlying systemic diseases are present, mainly diabetes mellitus. This is reported in many series in the literature, also in necrotising fasciitis in other locations than perianal, such as cervical (30, 53, 78, 79, 110, 139, 139).

   Necrotising fasciitis occurs uncommonly in the head and neck region. Chen Lin et. described an analysis of 47 cases in 12 years (83). However, immunologic defects specific for necrotising soft tissue infections or specifically predisposing for these infections could not be found (11). (Fig. 12 & 13)

The importance of these different etiologic factors can vary from patient to patient and the factors are not necessarily present in every patient in the abovementioned order.

DIAGNOSIS

The diagnosis of these infections must primarily be made on the macroscopic appearance of the diseased area, which will be described below. The general condition of the patient, the clinical course of the disease, and the bacteriologic findings, unless in a very early stage, are not decisive in this respect. One has to realize that the classical local signs of tissue inflammation (rubor, calor, dolor, and tumor) are often absent. There are, however, general signs including evidence of fever, elevated white blood cell count, and a severe systemic reaction.

Wall et al. (136) tried to develop a simple model to help distinguish necrotising fasciitis from non-necrotising soft tissue infections. They found that a white blood cell count (WBC) at admission above 15,4 x 109/l or a serum sodium Na lower than 135 mmol/l were useful parameters to distinguish between both infections. However, since 70% of their patients were I.V. drug users, an evaluation in other settings to prove the value of their model remains necessary (90). A high index of suspicion and careful clinical examination is always necessary.

Locally, bulla, severe pain, rapid spread, and eventually gas formation can be noticed. Gas-forming infections can be caused by both aerobic and anaerobic soft tissue infections. A very useful algorithm or decision-tree on gas-producing infections has been published by Nichols (101). The initial diagnosis must be followed by immediate antibiotic and, if necessary, surgical, therapy, with adjunctive hyperbaric oxygen in selected cases (see "Therapy"). A Gram stain is taken initially but provides less information than is necessary or hoped for, because the real causative microorganisms can only be found by culturing tissue biopsies from the spreading periphery of the lesion or from the deeper tissues that are reached only when surgical debridement is performed.

An interesting publication by Ault et al. mentions a rapid streptococcal diagnostic kit, with which the authors were able to identify group A ß-haemolytic Streptococcus pyogenes as the presumptive causative microorganism in cases of necrotising fasciitis (5).

If the anatomic site of involvement is not clear, computed tomography (CT) scanning can provide this information (10) as well as sonography (97). One must, however, not lose too much time in diagnosis before surgical therapy is started.

The same goes for magnetic resonance imaging. Some find this useful for an early diagnosis (41); others found the images by MRI non-specific and conclude that the preoperative diagnosis must be based on the clinical picture and the evolution of the clinical status (4).

In most patients, direct inspection or inspection of the fascia after an incision to the level of the deep fascia under local anesthesia is sufficient for determining the diagnosis; exploration and debridement under general anesthesia can follow immediately.

For a differential diagnosis on clinical signs see Table 2. In rapid spreading "closed" infections, needle aspiration and Gram stain can provide more reliable information on the microbiological cause of the infection. It is a well-known fact that haemolytic bacteria (for example streptococci) play an important role in these disease processes and do not grow in open wounds (122, 141).

CLINICAL PICTURE AND BACTERIOLOGY

Progressive Bacterial Gangrene

Progressive bacterial gangrene, originally described as postoperative progressive bacterial synergistic gangrene or Cullen's ulcer (34) and as chronic infectious skin gangrene (93,94), is generally a slow advancing infectious process involving the epidermis, the dermis, the subcutaneous tissue including lymphatic channels (14, 17) and hair follicles, but never the deep fascia (the fascial plane that envelops the muscle compartment).

Progressive bacterial gangrene includes:
- Anaerobic crepitant or clostridial cellulitis, (91) (Fig. 4 & 5)
- Ecthyma gangrenosum or gangrenous impetigo,
- Pyoderma gangrenosum, (26) (Fig. 10 & 11)
- Erysipelas,
- Gangrenous or necrotising erysipelas, (105) (Fig. 3)
- Symbiotic gangrene (103), and
- Phagedena geometrica (18).

Progressive bacterial gangrene is directly related to skin infection. Around the site of an injury or infection, cellulitis occurs with redness, edema, and a slight swelling followed by a centrifugal necrosis of skin and subcutaneous tissues. This frequently capricious extension of necrosis is preceded by patchy, purplish discoloration of the skin. It is highly characteristic that the deep fascia, which envelops the muscle compartment, is never involved. Around the afflicted area, a 1-2 cm wide erythematous, raised border zone is present.

TABLE 2. CLINICAL SIGNS OF NECROTISING SOFT TISSUE INFECTIONS

	Progressive Progressive Bacterial Synergistic Gangrene	Bacterial Gangrene Anaerobic Crepitant or Clostridial Cellulitis	Necrotizing Steptococcal and Mixed (Fournier)	Fasciitis Synergistic Necrotizing Cellulitis	Myositis/Myonecrosis Non-Clostridial Strepticoccal
Incubation	1-3 Weeks	1 Week	1-4 Days	1-2 Days	1-3 Days
Onset	Gradual	Gradual/Acute	Acute	Acute	Acute
Sytem Toxicity	$\pm$	$\pm$	++	+++	++
Pain	Severe	Moderate	Moderate to Severe (Initially)	Severe	Severe
Exudate	Slightly Serious	Slightly Serious	Profuse Serosanguinous	Dishwater Pus Profuse	None or Slight
Odor Or Exudate	Foul	Foul	Foul	Foul	None
Gas	May Be Present	Abundant	Usually Not Present	May Be Present	Not Present
Muscle	No Change	No Change	Viable	Viable	Marked Change
Skin	Ulcer and Gangrene	Gangrene	Cellulitis + Secondary Gangrene	Cellulitis + Secondary Gangrene	Minimal Change
Mortality	5 - 15%	5%	15-25%	75%	2535%
Treatment: • Surgery • Antibiotics • Adjunctiive Hyperbaric Oxygen (HBO)	Necrotomy and Skingrafting Yes (Not Always) Yes (Compromised) Host and Systemic Toxicity	Incision and Drainage Yes Yes (Compromised Host and System Toxicity)	Yes Yes (Compromised Host)	Yes Yes Yes (Compromised Host)	Muscle Removal Yes Yes (Compromised Host)

Clinical signs in differential diagnosis of necrotizing soft tissue infections (Mod. from Lefrock, Molavi 1982, Mader 1988, Bakker 1998).

The speed of the extension may vary from weeks or even months to a few hours. Fresh granulation tissue with re-epithelialization may occur in the center while the centrifugal spread of necrosis still proceeds. The area is always very painful.

Bacteriological the cause can be anaerobic, as in crepitant clostridial cellulitis, aerobic, or mixed. Bacterial synergism plays an important role, but no specific combination can be held responsible for this disease. In order to find the causative microorganisms one has to culture from the spreading periphery, preferably tissue biopsies, and not from the necrosis or the granulating center, where a great variety of concomitant microorganisms can be found that do not cause nor add to the infection.

The usual primary pathogens are group A streptococci (GAS) and *Staphylococcus aureus* (alone or in synergism). We found streptococci in 92% in needle aspirates or tissue biopsies in progressive bacterial gangrene followed by multiple other aerobic and anaerobic microorganisms such as bacteroides species, Clostridium species and Enterobacteriaceae, Coliforms, Proteus, and Pseudomonas (in ecthyma gangrenosum).

Bacteroidaceae as *Bacteroides fragilis* are rarely seen as a single pathogen but always as part of a mixed polymicrobial flora. The role of Bacteroidaceae is not a direct one in causing soft tissue infections, but it influences the immunology of the host in diminishing the interferon production and the phagocytic capacity of macrophages and polymorphonuclear neutrophil granulocytes. Clinically *Bacteroides fragilis* is often seen in combination with *Escherichia coli* (95).

Crepitant Anaerobic Cellulitis (Fig. 4 & 5)

Crepitant anaerobic cellulitis involves clostridial and nonclostridial cellulitis and has often been misdiagnosed as gas gangrene. In general it is a more benign disease than gas gangrene. Clostridia can be found in pure culture and there can be marked tissue necrosis but no involvement of the deep fascia or muscles is seen until it is in a very advanced stage. There can be abundant soft tissue gas.

In case of extensive soft tissue damage or marked vascular insufficiency of an extremity, clostridial cellulitis can change into a true clostridial myositis with myonecrosis. Multiple aerobic and anaerobic organisms have been cultured including Enterobacteria-ceae, Clostridium species, Bacteroides species and Peptostreptococcus species. In our experience, in over 90% of cases of progressive bacterial gangrene there are serious underlying systemic diseases, most frequently diabetes mellitus. Malignancies and arteriosclerosis were also found, but less frequently.

Necrotising Fasciitis

Necrotising fasciitis (141), originally called haemolytic streptococcal gangrene, Meleney's ulcer, or acute dermal gangrene (92,93) is a progressive, generally rapid spreading, inflammatory process located in the deep fascia with secondary necrosis of subcutaneous tissues and skin. (Fig. 2)

The speed of skin involvement is directly related and proportional to the thickness of the subcutaneous tissue layer. The infection tends to spread very rapidly along the deep fascial plane.

Necrotising fasciitis includes:
- Hospital gangrene (67),
- Suppurative fasciitis (88),
- Fourniers gangrene or disease (51),
- Synergistic necrotising cellulitis (127), and
- Haemolytic streptococcal gangrene or Meleney's ulcer (92).

Necrotising fasciitis may start in a surgical wound, postoperatively, after a trivial injury like an insect bite, an abrasion, or contusion and may even show up spontaneously, in children (15, 38, 79, 92, 93, 142). Usually there is a sudden onset of pain and swelling at the site of or at a certain distance from the injury with a nonspecific redness, swelling, and edema. Initially the area may be very painful but later becomes numb and anesthetic.

During the next hours and/or days the redness rapidly spreads, the margins fade out into the normal skin but are not raised or very sharply outlined as seen in erysipelas. These signs and symptoms are already secondary to the most pathognomonic feature, the fascial and subcutaneous necrosis. This necrosis manifests itself as an extensive undermining of the skin and subcutis. If there is an opening in the skin, probes or gloved fingers can be passed under the skin and subcutis. In case of intact skin, the only way for diagnosis is incision into the deep fascia. This can be done at the bedside under local anesthesia.

Once the incision is made, the yellowish-green necrotic fascia becomes visible and after removal of this fascia, healthy, red, normal, bleeding muscle tissue is seen. If the fascia is left untouched, secondary involvement of the muscles with myositis and myonecrosis can be seen in a later phase. This must be prevented, if possible, by early incision and excision of all necrotic fascia ("fillet procedure"). (Fig. 17)

Without treatment a dusky discoloration of the skin appears as a small purple patch with irregular and initially ill-defined margins. This may occur at a certain distance from the injury or the operative wound. Identical patches may develop in the neighborhood which ultimately fuse and form a large plaque of gangrenous skin while the diffuse redness continues to spread. As a rule the patient is seriously ill: septic with a high fever (124). It is highly characteristic that the spread of the fascial necrosis is more extended than the visible changes of the skin. The apparently normal skin and subcutaneous tissue are loosened from the underlying necrotic fascia over a great distance from the original wound. Skin necrosis occurs secondary to thrombosis of subcutaneous blood vessels and the whole area may become anesthetic by necrosis of nerve fibers. In our series, the site of necrotising fasciitis showed an equal distribution between trunk and extremities. The head and neck were less frequently involved (139).

Fourniers gangrene or Fourniers disease (51), in its original form as scrotal gangrene, is a form of necrotising fasciitis. Careful observation shows that the process starts with necrosis of the scrotal fascia, tenderness, local edema, and redness of the scrotal skin. Very soon thereafter the skin becomes necrotic and the diagnostic "black spot" can be seen. When the infectious process extends from the penal-scrotal region to the abdomen or upper legs, the characteristic picture of necrotising fasciitis is seen. The scrotal subcutaneous layer is so thin that the majority of the patients are seen when the skin is already necrotic. In women "Fourniers gangrene" is recognized less easily as necrotising fasciitis, because of the thicker subcutaneous layer. In the literature however Fourniers gangrene in women is more and more recognized (43). Stephenson et al. describes 29 female patients with necrotising fasciitis of the vulva. Twenty patients or 69% were diabetic and the mortality in the diabetic patients was 78,6% (126). (Fig. 18)

Synergistic Necrotising Cellulitis (Fig. 25)

Synergistic necrotising cellulitis has been described as a different clinical entity (127). Because of the wide involvement of deeper tissues (necrosis of fascia and in a later stage, but very rapidly thereafter, involvement of subcutaneous tissue and muscles as well) together with severe systemic toxicity, we consider this to be a form of necrotising fasciitis. Mader considers this disease to be a nonclostridial myonecrosis (86). In our opinion the disease is the same, necrotising fasciitis, but the clinical course of the disease differs from patient to patient, dependent on general condition, the immune status, age, associated systemic diseases, and the time elapsed from the beginning of the disease to the moment when the patient is first examined. These infections are frequently located in the perianal region after improperly treated perianal and ischiorectal abscesses. About 75-80% of the mainly elderly patients have diabetes mellitus. Diabetes mellitus, besides age, malnutrition, hypertension, and intravenous drug abuse have been recognized as considerable risk factors for mortality in necrotising fasciitis (52). The simple fact that the patients were mainly elderly and that a high percentage of systemic sepsis was present in the series of Stone and Martin (127) may explain the unusually high mortality of 75%, compared with the mean mortality of 38.5% in a review of 15 reports including 272 patients (3) and 3-45% in the large review of 1726 patients by Eke (46).

There is confusion and uncertainty about the exact bacteriologic cause of necrotising fasciitis. Meleney (92) described the disease as haemolytic streptococcal gangrene and considered the cause to be "a pure invasion of haemolytic streptococci. This bacteriologic pattern seems to have changed as described before (9, 33, 79, 141). Wilson was the first to consider the name "haemolytic streptococcal gangrene" inappropriate because in his patients haemolytic staphylococci were frequently cultured (141).

Mader has stated that better culture techniques have demonstrated that Streptococcus pyogenes only occasionally causes these infections. This, however, cannot alter the fact that Meleney indeed found only streptococci, strongly suggesting at least an important role for this organism. Mader explains this by saying that although most infections are mixed aerobic and anaerobic, a type of necrotising fasciitis caused solely by Streptococcus pyogenes has been reported (86).

Careful bacteriologic techniques have shown anaerobes and aerobes: Peptostreptococcus species, Bacteroides species, Fusobacterium species together with Streptococcus pyogenes, *Staphylococcus aureus*, *Klebsiella pneumoniae*, *Pseudomonas aeruginosa*, Enterobacteriaceae, and even fungi (14, 30, 47, 53, 66, 78, 79, 80, 143).

Also Clostridia have been described in 90% of cases where Fourniers disease was accompanied by myositis. Again from the description it is not clear if gas gangrene was involved. The same authors describe a large variety of microorganisms which, apparently, they all consider causal (134). Even a very rare case of necrotising fasciitis after blunt trauma caused by a penicillin-resistant *Streptococcus pneumoniae* is reported (13).

It is, however, still very difficult to distinguish the real causative microorganisms from the concomitants. Giuliano described two bacteriologic types of necrotising fasciitis (53) and Lamerton even suggested three different groups (78). We could not confirm their findings in our patients (11). A very important observation that is not mentioned in any publication is the time the organisms are cultured in relation to the time of onset of the disease and the eventual previous treatment, surgery, antibiotics, or both. We mentioned this earlier. In our experience a pure and very early case of Fourniers gangrene, still without skin necrosis, showed streptococci in pure culture after needle aspiration. We found the same in other early cases of necrotising fasciitis.

The bacteriologic pattern changes during the clinical course of the disease and seems to be more dependent on the previous use of antibiotics, the extent and frequency of debridement, the use (or non-use) of diverting colostomies, the age and immune status of the patient, and associated systemic diseases. These pattern changes make it difficult to show that the cultured bacteria can, with certainty, be declared to be causative.

Brunet et al. (125) published a study on a total of 81 patients with perineal gangrene. They advocate very systematic microbiological investigations from specific locations and repeat that after every operative debridement. They start with an antibiotic regimen directed against anaerobes, Gram-positive cocci, and Gram-negative bacilli. This regimen is changed when later culture results so indicate. They stress the importance of a systematic exploration of the ischiorectal fossae.

We are convinced that for the onset of necrotising fasciitis, streptococci play a very important role and that the reported changes in the bacteriologic pattern are mainly caused by other factors mentioned above.

Stevens gave a review of invasive group A streptococcal infections both clinically (119, 123, 125) and historically (120) where he also describes the ongoing research in streptococcal virulence factors; important for eventual development of new vaccines.

Recent work on streptococcal virulence factors and their possible influence on the onset of soft tissue infections can be found in Unnikrishnan et al. (133) and Norrby-Teglund et al. (102). Dele Davies and Schwarz reviewed these infections in children (38). Stevens (124) also underlined the importance of a rapidly progressive Streptococcal Toxic Shock Syndrome that can accompany necrotising fasciitis (strep TSS). Mortality, even with adequate therapy, is 30-60% of patients in 72-96 hours. The bacteriology of synergistic necrotising cellulitis is largely the same as in other forms of necrotising fasciitis (86, 127).

Nonclostridial Myonecrosis

The most frequent and devastating anaerobic myositis and myonecrosis is clostridial myonecrosis or gas gangrene. We saw that some forms of synergistic necrotising cellulitis have been categorized as nonclostridial myonecrosis (80, 86, 127) and other forms as necrotising fasciitis. We consider muscle involvement to be a later stage of true necrotising fasciitis (11).

Other forms of nonclostridial myonecrosis caused by anaerobic streptococci (91) are found mainly in drug addicts in our patient series. Differential diagnosis between gas gangrene and streptococcal myositis can be very difficult. The muscles in streptococcal myositis have in general a more inflamed appearance than in gas gangrene. Muscle necrosis is seen later than in gas gangrene and the necrotic muscles are more greenish in color than the black muscle necrosis in gas gangrene. Also, gas production is less abundant and differently situated in streptococcal myositis. Severe systemic toxicity, however, can be the same in both diseases. (Fig. 24)

Myositis caused by aerobic microorganisms, viruses, or certain parasites is known and described but very rare and will not be discussed here (114).

THERAPY

Introduction

Treatment of aerobic, anaerobic, and mixed necrotising soft tissue infections is a combination of surgical debridement (timely, limited, or aggressive), appropriate antibiotics, good nutritional support, and optimal oxygenation of the infected tissues. In selected cases where ambient oxygen is insufficient, hyperbaric oxygen must be used.

Surgical treatment can vary in these infections from simple incision and drainage procedures to very aggressive "fillet" procedures and even amputations can become necessary.

Essential in the management is the administration of appropriate antibiotics.

The problem with this is twofold:

1. Late culture results, and
2. Treating the causative and not the concomitant microorganisms.

My policy is to initially choose those antibiotics that cover the suspected causative pathogens (aerobic and anaerobic). Usually we start in the early stages with penicillin-G (or clindamycin or both), metronidazole and gentamycin or tobramycin (9). Sometimes a third generation cephalosporin is indicated (86).

As early as 1952 Eagle already described the problem of treatment failure with penicillin in streptococcal infections in mice (42). Stevens repeated this phenomenon in 1988 in streptococcal myositis in a mouse model (118). Group A streptococci at the site of inoculation remained highly sensitive to penicillin only as long as the streptococci continued to grow at a rapid rate. The same was found to be true for erythromycin but not for clindamycin.

Zamboni and coworkers found penicillin therapy to be ineffective when started more than two hours after onset of a myositis in a mouse model. Although erythromycin resulted in higher survival rates, survival after clindamycin was still 70% even when treatment was started 16,5 hours after onset of the myositis (80% after 6 hours) (144). It is important to keep these data in mind when choosing a particular antibiotic treatment scheme. It seems that clindamycin is nowadays more appropriate than penicillin-G.

Hyperbaric oxygen is indicated when other measures (ambient oxygen) fail to oxygenate the infected tissues sufficiently. This must be monitored by transcutaneous or, even better, by direct intraphlegmonous and/or intramuscular pO_2-measurements (73, 113). The rationale for the use of adjunctive hyperbaric oxygen and the mechanisms have been outlined extensively by Mader and Thom (85, 86, 130).

The main goals are: (a) improvement of tissue pO_2, necessary for normal wound healing, (b) improvement of phagocytic function by stimulating the oxygen-dependent killing mechanisms, either direct or indirect, (c) the diminishing of edema and improvement of the circulation in the affected areas, (d) stimulation of fibroblast growth, and (e) increased collagen formation. This can be roughly summarized as stimulation of the host defense and repair mechanisms.

A useful algorithm or decision tree concerning the possible use of hyperbaric oxygen in soft tissue infections has been published by Bell (17).

Because of multiple variables, clinical studies using adjunctive hyperbaric oxygen are very difficult to evaluate. The wide variety in patients makes a randomized controlled trial virtually impossible. No patient is the same or presents him- or herself with the same symptoms. The variety in the bacteriological findings has been outlined sufficiently in this chapter. Almost all patients are compromised hosts. From some of the descriptions it is very difficult, if not impossible, to know which of the different clinical entities is involved. In this way it is very difficult to respond to the criticism of Tibbles and Edelsberg in their review stating that more prospective trials are necessary in order to prove the value of hyperbaric oxygen in necrotising fasciitis (131). Maybe that clinical evidence based on large numbers is sufficient to convince our adversaries. Even in gas gangrene, other gas-producing infections are mixed with the true clostridial myonecrosis. The rationale for adjunctive hyperbaric oxygen, however, is clear and based on animal studies, case reports, retrospective studies, and a few prospective studies (64, 110).

Korhonen (75, 76) showed in animal experiments, in healthy volunteers, and in patients with necrotising soft tissue infections that hyperbaric oxygen raised arterial oxygen tensions seven-fold and that oxygen tensions in the vicinity of the infected area were generally higher than in healthy tissues, thus establishing a hyperoxygenated zone around the infection. The CO_2 tensions rose only slightly during exposure to hyperbaric oxygen. Combining early and extensive surgery, broad-spectrum antibiotics, hyperbaric oxygen, and surgical intensive care gave the best results in the treatment of Fourniers disease with a mortality of 9%. In three publications the use of honey to improve the rate of wound healing is advocated in necrotising fasciitis (44, 46, 61).

Progressive Bacterial Gangrene

Prognosis in progressive bacterial gangrene is generally better than in necrotising fasciitis and is mainly determined by associated systemic diseases.

- **Surgery**: Surgery can be limited to necrotomies, limited excisions in the margin of the process, the necessity of which must be judged on a day-to-day basis. Normal wound care, including temporary artificial skin substitution (for example with a polyvinylalcohol foam) may be necessary (98). When a good granulating surface is obtained, split skin grafting can be performed. We have never been forced to more extensive excisions. If the gangrene is not responsive to the combined treatment scheme, amputation of an extremity may be necessary. Heinle et al. (58) claim superior results post-grafting, with a trend to lower mortality and morbidity, by the use of 5% Mafenide Acetate Solution. (Fig. 6 & 7)

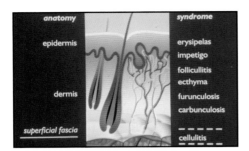

1. Anatomy of skin and soft tissues. Superficial layer. Deep layer is shown below (2). On the left side are the different anatomical layers and on the right side are the various infectious syndromes that we know in those respective layers.
(See page 253)

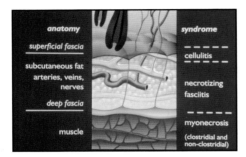

2. Anatomy of skin and soft tissues. Deep layer. Superficial layer shown above (1). On the left side are the different anatomical layers and on the right side are the various infectious syndromes that we know in those respective layers.
(See pages 253 & 258)

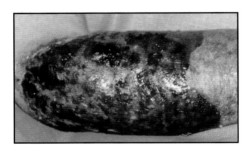

3. Gangrenous or necrotising erysipelas (a rare syndrome first described by Pfanner in 1918, lit. Nr. 105).
(See page 256)

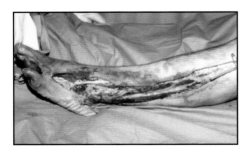

4. Patient with diabetes mellitus and a clostridial cellulitis of the left lower leg.
(See pages 256, 258 & 270)

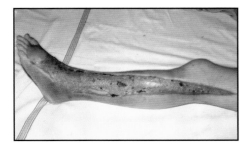

5. Treatment consisted of incision and drainage, hyperbaric oxygen and split skin grafting.
(See pages 256 & 258)

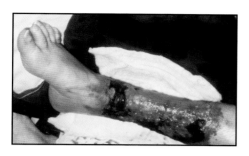

6. Progressive bacterial gangrene of the left lower leg in a patient with diabetes mellitus. She was treated for seven months without result in another hospital and sent to us to consider amputation. (See page 263)

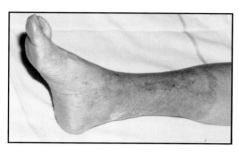

7. In our hospital we treated her (same patient as shown above, #6) with hyperbaric oxygen and penicillin-G (six times 1 million units per day for 14 days). Result after two months. (See page 263)

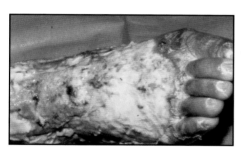

8. Immune compromised patient (steroids) and diabetes mellitus with progressive bacterial gangrene resistant to any form of therapy. (See page 269)

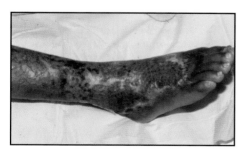

9. Penicillin G (two weeks 1 million U/day, and daily hyperbaric oxygen resulted after four weeks. (Same patient as above, #8, was sent to us for amputation). (See page 269)

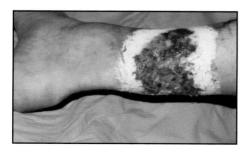

10. Pyoderma gangrenosum in a patient with ulcerative colitis. Treated with hyperbaric oxygen, while continuing steroids. The result after six weeks is shown in #11 on next page. (See page 256).

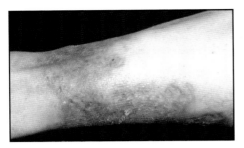

11. Treated with hyperbaric oxygen, while continuing steroids and the result after six weeks, same patient as shown in #10 on previous page. (See page 256)

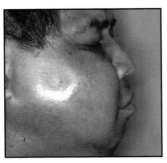

12. Immunocompromised patient, kidney transplant recipient on anti-rejection therapy. Patient shown below, #13. (See page 255)

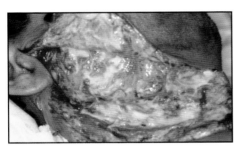

13. Example of a necrotising fasciitis in the face and neck. (See page 255)

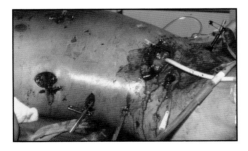

14. Necrotising fasciitis after an appendectomy. After referral, prompt excision, colostomy, antibiotics, and hyperbaric oxygen therapy. (See page 270)

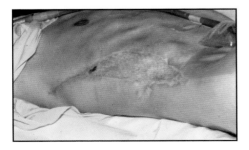

15. Same patient as #14, result after three months (14 sessions of hyperbaric oxygen). (See page 270)

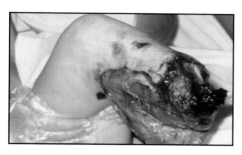

16. Example of a necrotising fasci-
    itis in an amputation stump
    after lower leg amputation.
    (See page 255)

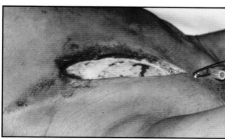

17. Diagnosis of necrotising fasciitis
    after an incision unto the deep
    fascia in the right lower
    abdomen. Note the necrotic
    deep fascia. (See page 259)

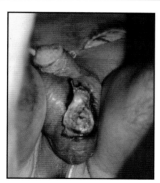

18. Fourniers gangrene and
    necrotising fasciitis of the
    lower abdomen. Fournier is
    synonymous with necrotising
    fasciitis. (See page 259)

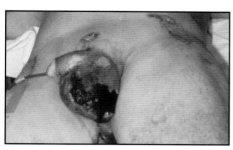

19. Necrotising fasciitis and
    Fourniers gangrene, unsuccess-
    fully treated for three days with
    inadequate incision-and-
    drainage procedures.
    (See pages 270 & 273)

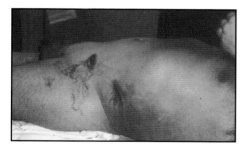

20. Same patient as seen in
    #19. (See pages 270 & 273)

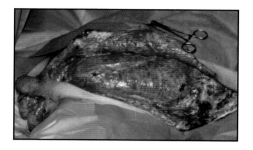

21. Wide incision and excision of all necrotic tissue. Note that the overlying skin is saved. This procedure was repeated four times in 48 hours. Hyperbaric oxygen treatment according to the "gas gangrene scheme." Same patient as #19 - 23. (See pages 270 & 273)

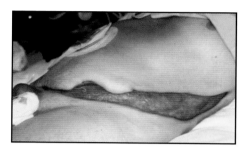

22. Same patient as #19 - 23, result after three weeks. Ready for grafting. (See pages 270 & 273)

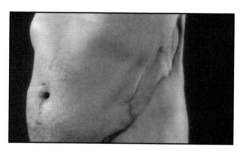

23. End result after three months. Same patient as shown above, #19 - 22. (See pages 270 & 273)

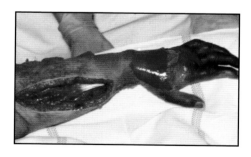

24. Streptococcal myositis of the right arm. Amputation proved to be necessary. (See pages 261 & 274)

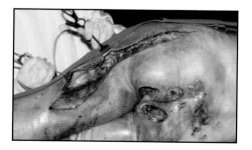

25. Example of a synergistic necrotising cellulitis (Stone and Martin 1992, lit.127). This is in fact an improperly treated necrotising fasciitis, four weeks after onset. (See pages 259 & 274)

- **Antibiotics**: Antibiotics should be directed to the causative and not to concomitant microorganisms. This can be very difficult because a wide variety can usually be cultured from these infections. In one of the author's patients, a 43-year-old male with a progressive bacterial synergistic gangrene of the abdominal wall postoperatively, a flora with *E. coli*, *Pseudomonas aeruginosa*, *Enterobacter cloacae*, Enterococci, Bacteroides species, and *Acinetobacter anitratum* was cultured. The clinical picture, however, professed that none of the microorganisms needed any treatment. With only local care, wound healing was uneventful. This underlines the significance of close cooperation between the clinical bacteriologist and surgeon. Since in 92% of the tissue biopsies taken from the margin of the process, streptococci were cultured followed by staphylococci, coliforms, proteus, pseudomonas, and clostridia, we usually start with penicillin-G, one million IU every three to four hrs I.V. and change this regimen only when indicated by the clinical course supported by bacteriologic evidence. Because of unresponsiveness of streptococci depending on the stage of the process, we use more and more clindamycin (118).
- **Hyperbaric oxygen**: Ledingham and Therani reported for the first time in literature that the adjunctive use of hyperbaric oxygen contributed to the arrest of the infection in four out of five of their patients (79). (Fig. 8 & 9)

    Experience with hyperbaric oxygen is reported more and more in the literature. The working mechanism makes it clear, why it is useful in treating necrotic soft tissue infections. All our patients reacted favorably when hyperbaric oxygen was added to the therapeutic regimen of surgery and antibiotics. We added hyperbaric oxygen when other treatment modalities failed. No proper prospective randomized trials are known which is a definitive disadvantage when advocating hyperbaric oxygen.

    From 1978-1987, 89 patients were treated with progressive bacterial gangrene. The mortality was 5.6%. All patients had serious associated diseases, diabetes mellitus being the most frequent (74 patients or 83.1%). Some patients had been treated for as long as four to six months with all known treatment modalities. Despite this, the gangrene extended progressively although slowly. At the time that amputation was considered to be unavoidable, the addition of hyperbaric oxygen stopped the progression and resulted in a clean, granulating wound, suitable for grafting after approximately three weeks of daily treatments (14-42 days in 84 patients).

    We recommend the adjunctive use of hyperbaric oxygen in progressive bacterial gangrene in cases where other treatment modalities fail, in cases with serious underlying systemic diseases and symptoms of general toxicity and in other immune-compromised patients.

Treatment Protocol for Progressive Bacterial Gangrene

- **Multiplace chamber**: 3 ATA 100% O_2, 90 minutes per treatment with appropriate air breaks, one to two treatments per day. If the response is favorable, this can be diminished to three to four

treatments per week. It is advisable to continue treatment for 10 days postgrafting.
- **Monoplace chamber**: In a monoplace chamber the same scheme can be used.

The question if the same results can be reached with lower oxygen pressures is difficult to answer since we do not have a clear definition of a dose of oxygen. In our experience these protocols are safe and side effects are absent or minimal. The most important thing is to establish in an oxygen challenge test that the pO_2 at the wound margin and/or in the wound itself is too low to expect normal wound healing; the next step is to show that this pO_2 can be raised by hyperbaric oxygen and not by 100% oxygen at one bar. Treatment schemes with 2,4 - 2,6 ATA O_2 report the same results.

Anaerobic clostridial cellulitis, sometimes misdiagnosed as gas gangrene, is a more benign disease than gas gangrene. Clostridia can be found in pure culture and there can be marked tissue necrosis. The deep fascia and the muscles however are not affected. With extensive tissue damage and/or in a seriously compromised host, a true clostridial myositis with myonecrosis can arise. (Fig. 4 & 5)
- **Surgical treatment** can be limited to incision and drainage followed by excision of the necrotic tissue.
- **Antibiotics**: Penicillin-G, 8-12 million IU per day I.V.
- **Hyperbaric oxygen**: Adjunctive hyperbaric oxygen is recommended in immune-compromised patients and in patients with systemic toxicity. In these patients the "gas gangrene" scheme is used:
  - **1st day**: 3 x 90 min. 3 ATA 100% O_2 in a multiplace or 2.5-2.8 ATA 100% O_2 in a monoplace chamber.
  - **2nd day**: 2 x.
  - **3rd day**: 2 x.
  - From the fourth day on, continue with one treatment per day until the wound starts granulating. Maximal treatment time is 10 days. We than found normal oxygen tissue tensions for wound healing when breathing normal air at sea level. This is the sign that hyperbaric treatment can be discontinued.

Necrotising Fasciitis
- **Surgery**: Primary and aggressive surgical debridement is the cornerstone in the management of this disease. Early and extensive incision of skin and subcutaneous tissue wide into healthy tissue, followed by excision of all necrotic fascia and nonviable skin and subcutaneous tissue is necessary. This has to be repeated as often as necessary. (Fig. 14 & 15) Within the first 24 hours repeated inspection of the whole infected area under general anesthesia is obligatory, with excision of further necrotised fascia, if present. These progressive necrotising surgical infections need a unified approach as soon as possible. It is of no use trying to determine the type of infection first by culturing the infected tissue because every delay in the start of treatment causes a significant higher mortality (32, 35, 37, 47, 52, 60, and 70, 135). (Fig. 19 - 23)

In most of our patients with a necrotising fasciitis of the peniscrotal and perianal area we performed a diverting colostomy. The extent of fascial necrosis can easily be determined by blunt finger dissection over the deep fascial plane through the incision and by direct inspection. Viable skin flaps need not be excised and can be saved. If no further fascial necrosis is seen, the process can be considered arrested. Usually, at least in our experience, from one to five debridements are necessary with a mean of three (in 40 patients between 1985-1990). A systematic exploration of the ischiorectal fossa in every case of a perianal soft tissue infection is very important (25).

- **Antibiotics**: Antibiotic treatment has an important place in the combined management of necrotising fasciitis, although second to surgery. Recommendations of drugs have changed with the development of new antibiotics and the risk of resistance. Colonization and selection of microorganisms by a former therapeutic or prophylactic regimen plays an important role (for example: antibiotic prophylaxis in large bowel surgery or treatment of a perianal abscess). If at the time of clinical diagnosis a polymicrobial flora is present, one has to be very careful not to treat a concomitant agent instead of the causative microorganisms.

  The present—confusing—bacteriologic findings in soft tissue infections are in part caused by the unnecessary, nondirected use of antibiotics. Streptococci have been identified as a major pathogen in these diseases. Kaul et al. gave a recent review on the incidence of necrotising fasciitis in Ontario, Canada (71) as did Smith et al. (116) and Corman et al. (32); the largest review, on 1726 cases, is published by Eke (46). Five cases in trauma patients were reported by Schwarz et al. (112).

  The drug of choice is penicillin-G, 8-10 million IU/24 hours I.V., with clindamycin more and more as the alternative. The other pathogens can be treated by metronidazole (anaerobes) and/or third generation cephalosporins (anaerobes, Entero-bacteriaceae) (49). *Bacteroides fragilis* can be treated with clindamycin or metronidazole (or covered by a third generation cephalosporin). A useful scheme for the initial choice of antibiotics is given by Mader (86).

- **Hyperbaric oxygen**: Clinical reports indicate an adjunctive role for hyperbaric oxygen in necrotising fasciitis. Although no large controlled randomized series have been published so far, hyperbaric oxygen provides a valuable adjunct in the overall treatment management (27, 37, 63, 104). An interesting discussion on the value of adjunctive hyperbaric oxygen can be found in the Deutsche Medizinische Wochenschrift by Bock et al. and Kujath et al. (19, 77). Kujath (77) underestimates the advantages and greatly exaggerates the disadvantages of hyperbaric oxygen in necrotising fasciitis. A useful discussion follows in a later issue of the same journal (40) (see "Discussion" in the reference list). The overall mortality figures in this disease range from 20-75%.

  a)   Only Ledingham reported poor results with hyperbaric oxygen (overall mortality 8/12 = 67%, in the hyperbaric oxygen group

8/9 = 89%). However, his initial surgical management is suspect and was probably not extensive enough. Adjunctive hyperbaric oxygen cannot be successful if surgery is inappropriate (79).

b) Riegels-Nielsen reported five patients with a mortality of 1/5 = 20%. All five patients had necrotising fasciitis of the external genitals and the lower abdominal wall and were treated with aggressive surgery, appropriate antibiotics, and adjunctive hyperbaric oxygen (109).

c) We treated 27 patients before 1985 with necrotising fasciitis, including 7 patients with Fourniers disease. Mortality was 5/27 = 18%. In another 40 patients (1985-1990) mortality was 5/40 = 12.5%. Patients were treated with a combination of surgery, antibiotics, and hyperbaric oxygen (9).

d) Eltorai et al. reported no mortalities in nine patients in which hyperbaric oxygen was added to the standard therapy (48).

e) Mader reported on a retrospective evaluation of 33 patients, of which 22 had involvement of the scrotum and perianal region. Of the 22, mortality in the hyperbaric oxygen group was 25% compared with a mortality of 67% in the non-hyperbaric oxygen group. All patients were seriously compromised hosts and 14 had diabetes mellitus (86).

f) Zamboni et al. treated six patients with one late death due to complications of pneumonia (143).

g) Riseman et al. reported on 29 patients with necrotising fasciitis treated between 1980 and 1988. Group I (n=12) received standard therapy and in group II (n=17) hyperbaric oxygen was added. Although group II patients were more seriously ill at admission, the mortality in this group was significantly lower (23%) than in group I patients (66%). Their conclusion was that the addition of hyperbaric oxygen to the surgical and antimicrobial treatment of necrotising fasciitis significantly reduced mortality and wound morbidity (number of necessary debridement). In their view, hyperbaric oxygen should be used routinely in the treatment of necrotising fasciitis. Following their results they conclude that withholding hyperbaric oxygen to patients when it is available will cause unnecessary deaths and is thus unethical (110).

h) Brown et al. reported on a retrospective review of the efficacy of hyperbaric oxygen. They looked only at truncal necrotising fasciitis and identified 54 patients (30 in the HBO group and 24 without HBO). There was a trend to better survival in the HBO treated group but without statistical significance (23).

i) Shupak et al. in a retrospective study of 37 patients over a rather long period, from 1984 - 1993 also did not find statistical difference between treatment with and without hyperbaric oxygen (115).

j) Hirn presented 11 patients treated with HBO in a clinical and experimental study and found a mortality of 1 patient (9%). He advocates HBO as an adjunct in the overall treatment of necrotising soft tissue infections (63).

k) Korhonen et al., in a retrospective study of 33 patients with Fourniers gangrene, found a mortality of 3 patients or 9%. They found that adjunctive hyperbaric oxygen reduced systemic toxicity, prevented extension of the necrotising infection and increased demarcation, thereby improving the overall outcome (74).

l) Hollabaugh et al. reported 7% mortality in a group of patients with Fourniers gangrene when treated with adjunctive hyperbaric oxygen (n=14). In the group without hyperbaric oxygen the mortality was 42% (n=12). This difference was statistically significant. A total of 38% of their patients had diabetes mellitus; 35% had alcoholabuses. Hyperbaric oxygen was given to patients solely on the basis of institution availability. Although the number of patients is still limited there is a good statistical paragraph concerning survival chances with and without hyperbaric oxygen (64).

m) Clark and Moon (29) underline the importance of adjunctive hyperbaric oxygen in the treatment of life-threatening soft-tissue infection.

n) Dahm et al. (36) found that the extent of the infection as measured by the BSA (Body Surface Area) involved was a highly statistical significant independent predictor of outcome and that Fourniers gangrene with an extension of 5% BSA or greater appeared to be an indication for adjunctive hyperbaric oxygen. Their results in 50 patients did not, however, reach statistical significance.

Compromised hosts with necrotising fasciitis have extreme morbidity and mortality. From these reports it is clear that adjunctive hyperbaric oxygen in these patients is a very valuable therapeutic tool.

Treatment Protocol for Necrotising Fasciitis

Proper, early, and aggressive surgical debridement remains the cornerstone of the treatment. These are surgical diseases that can only be treated with appropriate surgery first (6, 20, 35, and many others). (Fig. 19-22) Hyperbaric oxygen cannot compensate for bad surgery. However, the best results can only be obtained with a combination of surgery, antibiotics, and hyperbaric oxygen. The same conclusion was reached at a Consensus Conference in 2000 by the French Society of Dermatology, however without the use of hyperbaric oxygen which was still considered controversial (6, 20, 35). Mathieu (87), answering, stated that the controversy on the use of hyperbaric oxygen as a treatment for necrotising fasciitis is more caused by the difficulty to dispose of a hyperbaric equipment that is suited for the treatment of critical patients than by doubt on its real efficiency.

HBO treatment scheme (necrotising fasciitis): After the first surgical debridement, three treatment sessions are given in the first 24 hours.

- **In a multiplace chamber**: 3 ATA, 100% O_2 for 90 minutes per session. Appropriate air breaks are given as necessary.
- **In a monoplace chamber**: the same scheme can be used.
- After the first day continue treatment twice daily and if the improvement of the patient permits this, once daily until granulation is obtained (10-15 treatments in total).

Nonclostridial Myonecrosis (Fig. 25)

Synergistic necrotising cellulitis: The name "cellulitis" suggests progressive bacterial gangrene, but the disease is categorized by some as myonecrosis while, in fact, it is a necrotising fasciitis. This clearly demonstrates the difficulty of classification of this disease in its advanced stages when literally every kind of tissue is involved. The therapy is the same as described under necrotising fasciitis, but because more tissue is involved and the infection is especially fulminant, mortality reaches 75% without hyperbaric oxygen (127). This is not so much the result of the necrotising fasciitis itself, but of the extremely serious immune compromise of the patients, secondary to age, renal failure, arteriosclerosis, diabetes mellitus, malignancies, deficient nutrition, etc. These factors determine the danger and the rapid spread of this soft tissue infection. In light of the above and the grim prognosis of this disease, it is only logical to give adjunctive hyperbaric oxygen where possible.

Treatment Protocol for Non-Clostridial Myonecrosis

Again, hyperbaric oxygen has to be adjunctive to appropriate antibiotics (clindamycin or penicillin) and surgical incision and drainage, followed by excision of necrotic muscle. Prognosis worsens progressively when muscle tissue is involved. Aggressive surgery, appropriate antibiotics, and adjunctive hyperbaric oxygen following the "gas gangrene protocol."

- **1st day**: 3 x 90 min 3 ATA 100 % O_2 in a multiplace or a mono place chamber (appropriate air-breaks as mentioned before).
- **2nd day**: 2 times
- **3rd day**: 2 times.

Because the myositis started in most of our patients as a "closed" disease (after drug injection in addicts), there is an early need for decompressing fasciotomy and hyperbaric oxygen.

Anaerobic streptococcal myositis and myonecrosis: This infection is rare. (Fig. 24) The author has seen only seven patients since 1978. The mortality was 2/7 = 28.6%. The disease can be very fulminant, mimicking clostridial myonecrosis. Because we have demonstrated hypoxia through intramuscular pO_2 monitoring (73), we recommend the use of adjunctive hyperbaric oxygen. In cases of fulminant disease, systemic toxicity, and a compromised host, the gas gangrene protocol may be used. Stevens gives a recent review of invasive streptococcal disease including streptococcal myositis. The incidence, reading his report, is clearly much higher than in our experience (122, 125). Adams et al. (1) described 19 cases from the literature and added 2 of his own cases. In all cases the infection was caused by group A ß-haemolytic streptococci. Despite aggressive surgical and medical treatment, 18 out of 21 patients (85.7%) died. Demey et al. reported another two cases from Belgium (39). Zamboni et al. found in a mouse myositis model using streptococcus pyogenes that HBO alone did not decrease mortality or bacterial proliferation *in vivo* significantly, but the combined treatment of penicillin with HBO exerts at least additive effects in both decreasing bacterial counts *in vivo* and increasing survival in this model (144).

REFERENCES

1. Adams EM, Gudmundsson S, Yocum DE, Haselby RC et al. "Streptococcal myositis". Arch Int Med 1985: 145; 1020-1023.

2. Ahrenholz DH. "Necrotising soft tissue infections." Surg Clin North Am. 1988;68:199-2`14.

3. Ahrenholz DH. "Surgical spectrum. Clinical skin and soft tissue infection. Physicians World Communications (Monograph). West Point, Pa.: Merck, Sharpe and Dohme, 1988;16-24.

4. Arslan A, Jerome CP, Borthne A. Necrotising fasciitis: unreliable MRI findings in the pre operative diagnosis. Eur J Radiol 2000: 36(3); 139-143.

5. Ault MJ, Geiderman J, Sokolov R. "Rapid identification of Group A Streptococcus as the cause of Necrotising Fasciitis". Ann Emerg Med 1996: 28(2); 227-230.

6. Baier VP, Imdahl A. Nekrotisierende Fasciitis. Hier hilft nur radikales Debridement. MMW-Fortschr Med 2001: 143(15); 332-333.

7. Bakker DJ. "De hyperbare zuurstofbehandeling van acuut huidgangreen (necrotiserende fasciitis en progressief bacterieel gangreen)." Ned Tijdschr Geneeskd. 1980;124: 2164-2170.

8. Bakker DJ. "The treatment of acute dermal gangrene with hyperbaric oxygen." Proc VIIth Int Congr Hyperbaric Medicine. Moscow, Publishing Office "Nauka": 1983;238-240. (Russian)

9. Bakker DJ. "The use of hyperbaric oxygen in the treatment of certain infectious diseases especially gas gangrene and acute dermal gangrene." Drukkerij Veenman BV. Wageningen. University of Amsterdam, 1984;74-90.

10. Bakker DJ. Ibid, 42-44.

11. Bakker DJ, Kox C. "Classification and therapy of necrotising soft tissue infections: The role of surgery, antibiotics and hyperbaric oxygen." Current Problems in General Surgery. 1988;5(4):489-500.

12. Bakker DJ. "Streptococcal infections and hyperbaric oxygen". In M Gennser (ed) "Diving and hyperbaric medicine". Proc XXIV Ann Meeting of the EUBS. Stockholm Aug 12-15. 1998. FOA report: FOA-B-98-00342-721-SE; p 140-145. Print Elanders-Gotab, Stockholm, Sweden.

13. Ballon-Landa GR, Gherardi G, Beall B et al. Necrotising fasciitis due to penicillin-resistant Streptococcus pneumoniae: Case report and review of the literature. J Infect 2001: (42); 272-290.

14. Bartlett JG. "Necrotising soft tissue infections." Nichols RL, Hyslop NE, Bartlett JG (Eds.) Decision Making in Surgical Sepsis. Decker, Philadelphia, 1991;62-63.

15. Barton LL, Jeck DT. "Necrotising Fasciitis in Children. Report of two cases and a review of the literature". Arch Pediatr Adolesc Med 1996: 150; 105-108.

16. Beaurienne M. "Observation sur une plaie du scrotum." J de Med Chir Pharm: 1764 (20) ; 251-256.

17. Bell WH. "Use of hyperbaric oxygen in anaerobic soft-tissue infection." Nichols RL, Hyslop NE, Bartlett JG (Eds.) Decision Making in Surgical Sepsis. Decker, Philadelphia, 1991;78-81.

18. Bisno AL, Stevens DL. "Streptococcal infections of skin and soft tissues". New Eng J Med 1996: 334(4); 240-245.

19. Bock KH, Lampl L, Frey G. "Diagnose und Therapie der nekrotisierende Fasziitis. Hyperbare Oxygenation als ergänzende Therapieform". Deutsche Med Wochenschr 1996: 121(4); 116-117.

20. Brandt MM, Corpron CA, Wahl WL. Necrotising soft tissue infections: A surgical disease. Am Surg 2000: 66(10); 967-970.

21. Brewer GE, Meleney FL. "Progressive gangrenous infection of the skin and subcutaneous tissues, following operation for acute perforative appendicitis." Ann Surg. 1926;84: 438-450.

22. Brocq L. "Nouvelle contribution à l'étude du phagedenisme geometrique." Ann Dermatol Syph (Paris). 1916/1917;6:1-39.

23. Brown DR, Davis NL, Lepawsky M, Cunningham J, Kortbeek J. "A multicenter review of the treatment of major truncal necrotising infections with and without hyperbaric oxygen therapy". Am J Surg 1994: 167; 485-489.

24. Brun-Buisson C. Stratégie de prise en charge des fasciites nécrosantes. Conference de consensus. Texte des experts : quatrième question. Ann Dermatol Venereol 2001 : 128 ; 394-403.

25. Brunet C, Consentino B, Barthelemy A et al. Gangrènes périnéales: nouvelle approche bactériologique. Résultats du traitement médicochirurgical (81 cas). Ann Chir 2000 : 125 ; 420-427.

26. Brunsting LA, Goeckerman WH and O'Leary PA. "Pyoderma gangrenosum (Ecthyma). Clinical and experimental observations in five cases." Arch Dermatol Syph (Paris). 1930;22:655-680.

27. Capelli-Schellpfeffer M, Gerber GS. The use of hyperbaric oxygen in urology. J Urol 1999: 162; 647-654.

28. Chapnick EK, Abter EI. "Necrotising soft-tissue infections". Inf Dis Clin N Am 1996: 10(4); 835-855.

29. Clark LA, Moon RE. "Hyperbaric Oxygen in the Treatment of Life-Threatening Soft-Tissue Infections". Resp Care Clin N Am 1999: 5 (2); 203-219.

30. Clayton MD, Fowler JE Jr., Sharifi R, Pearl RK. "Causes, presentation and survival of fifty-seven patients with necrotising fasciitis of the male genitalia." Surg Gynecol Obstet. 1990;170:49-55.

31. Conférence de consensus de la Société Française de Dermatologie. Erysipèle et fasciite nécrosante : prise en charge. Texte court. Ann Med Int 2000 : 151(4); 465-470.

32. Corman JM, Moody JA,Aronson WJ. "Fourniers gangrene in a modern surgical setting: improved survival with aggressive management". BJU Int 1999: 84; 85-88.

33. Crosthwait RW Jr, Crosthwait RW and Jordan GL. "Necrotising fasciitis." J Trauma. 1964;4:149-157.

34. Cullen TS. "A progressively enlarging ulcer of abdominal wall involving the skin and fat, following drainage of an abdominal abscess apparently of appendiceal origin." Surg Gynecol Obstet. 1924;38:579-582.

35. Cunningham JD, Silver L, Rudikoff D. Necrotising fasciitis: A plea for early diagnosis and treatment. Mount Sinai J Med 2001: 68 (4&5); 253-261.

36. Dahm P, Roland FH, Vaslef SN et al. Outcome analysis in patients withprimary Necrotising Fasciitis of the male genitalia. Urol 2000: 56(1); 31-35.

37. Dellinger EP. "Severe necrotising soft tissue infections. Multiple disease entities requiring a common approach". JAMA 1981: 246(15); 1717-1721.

38. Dele Davies H, Schwartz B. Invasive Group A Streptococcal Infections in Children. In: Advances in Pediatric Infectious Diseases 1999: vol 14, Ch 6 ; 129-145. Mosby, Inc.

39. Demey HE, Goovaerts GC, Pattyn SR, Bossaert LL. "Streptococcal myositis. A report of two cases". Acta Clin Belgica 1991: 46 (2); 82-88.

40. Diskussion: Schmidt H, Welslau W, Hencke J, Siekmann U, Scharfe U, Tirpitz D, Kujath P, Eckmann C. "Die nekrotisierende Fasziitis und schwere Weichteilinfektionen durch Gruppe-A-Streptokokken". Dt Artztebl 1998: 95 (39); A-2395-2401.

41. Drake DB, Woods JA, Bill TJ et al. Magnetic Resonance Imaging in the early diagnosis of group A ß Streptococcal Necrotising Fasciitis: A case report. J Em Med 1998: 16(3); 4403-407.

42. Eagle H. "Experimental approach to the problem of treatment failure with penicillin. I.Group A streptococcal infection in mice". Amer J Med 1952; 13; 389-399.

43. Ecker KW, Derouet H, Omlor G, Mast GJ. "Die Fournier'sche Gangrän". Chirurg 1993: 64; 558-62.

44. Efem SEE. "Recent advances in the management of Fourniers gangrene: Preliminary observations". Surg 1993: 113; 200-204.

45. Efstratiou A, George RC, Tanna A et al. "Characterisation of Group A streptococci from necrotising fasciitis cases in Gloucestershire, United Kingdom". Adv Exp Med Biol 1997: 418: 91-93.

46. Eke N. "Fourniers Gangrene: A review of 1726 cases". Br J Surg 2000: 87; 718-728.

47. Elliott D, Kufera JA, Myers RAM. The microbiology of necrotising soft tissue infections. Am J Surg 2000: 179(5); 361-366.

48. Eltorai IM, Hart GB, Strauss MB, Montroy R, Juler GL. "The role of hyperbaric oxygen in the management of Fourniers gangrene." Int Surg. 1986;71:53.

49. Fildes J, Bannon MP, Barrett J. "Soft tissue infections after trauma." Surg Clin North Am. 1991;71:371-384.

50. Finegold SM, Bartlett JC, Chow AW, et al. "Management of anaerobic infections." Ann Intern Med. 1975;83:375-389.

51. Fournier A. "Gangrène foudroyante de la verge." Semaine Medicale. 1883;3:345-347;1884;4:69-70.

52. Francis KR, Lamaute HR, Davis JM et al. Implications of risk factors in necrotising fasciitis. Am Surg. 1993; 59 (5): 304-308.

53. Giuliano A, Lewis F Jr, Hadley K, Blaisdell FW. "Bacteriology of necrotising fasciitis." Am J Surg. 1977;134:52-57.

54. Goepfert AR, Guinn DA, Andrews WW, Hauth JC. "Necrotising fasciitis after Cesarean delivery". Obst Gynec 1997: 89(3); 409-412.

55. Gorbach SL, Bartlett JG, Nichols RL. Manual of Surgical Infections, Ch 9, Skin and Soft Tissue Infections. Brown, Boston, 1984.

56. Green RJ, Dafoe DC, Raffin TA. "Necrotising fasciitis". Chest 1996: 110 (1); 219-229.

57. Hebler. "Brand des Hodensackes und vollständiger Wiederersatz." Med Zeitung 1848: 41; 188.

58. Heinle EC, Dougherty WR, Garner WL, Reilly DA. The use of 5% Mafenide Acetate Solution in the postgraft treatment of necrotising fasciitis. J Burn Care Rehab 2001: 22; 35-40.

59. Heitmann C, Czermak C, Germann G. Rapidly fatal necrotising fasciitis after aesthetic liposuction. Aesth Plast Surg 2000: 24; 344-347.

60. Heitmann C, Pelzer M, Bickert B et al. Chirurgisches Konzept und Ergebnisse bei nekro tisierender Fasciitis. Chirurg 2001: 72; 168-173.

61. Hejase MJ, Simonin JE, Bihrle R, Coogan CL. "Genital Fourniers gangrene: Experience with 38 patients". Urology 1996: 47(5); 734-739.

62. Hippocrates. Hippocratic writings. Ed GER Lloyd. Epidemics Book I: Publ Penguin Classics. Middlesex England, 108-109, transl 1983. Idem: Book III: 121-122.

63. Hirn M. "Hyperbaric oxygen in the treatment of gas gangrene and perineal necrotising fasciitis. A clinical and experimental study". Academic Dissertation. Eur J Surg (Acta Chir) 1993: suppl 570.

64. Hollabaugh RS, Dmochowski RR, Hickerson WL, Cox CE. "Fourniers gangrene: Therapeutic impact of hyperbaric oxygen". Plast Reconstr Surg 1998: 101 (1); 94-100.

65. Hsieh T, Samson LM, Jabbour M, Osmond MH. Necrotising fasciitis in children in eastern Ontario: a case-control study. CMAJ 2000: 163(4); 393-396.

66. Johnin K, Nakatoh M, Kadowaki T et al. Fourniers gangrene caused by candida species as the primary organism. Urol 2000: 56(1); 153.

67. Jones J. "Investigations upon the nature, causes and treatment of hospital gangrene as it prevailed in the Confederate armies 1861-1865, New York." U.S. Sanitary Commission. Surgical Memoirs of the War of Rebellion. 1871.

68. Jones RB, Hirschmann JV, Brown GS, Tremann JA. "Fourniers syndrome: necrotising soft tissue infection of the male genitalia." J Urol 1979: 122; 279-282.

69. Käch K, Kossman T, Trentz O. "Nekrotisierende Weichteilinfekte". Unfallchirurg 1993: 96; 181-191.

70. Kaiser RE, Cerra FB. "Progressive necrotising surgical infections-A unified approach". J Trauma 1981: 21(5); 349-353.

71. Kaul R, McGeer A, Low DE et al. "Population-based surveillance for group A streptococcal necrotising fasciitis: Clinical features, prognostic indicators and microbiologic analysis of seventy-seven cases". Am J Med 1997: 103; 18-24.

72. Kingston D, Seal DV. "Current hypotheses on synergistic microbial gangrene." Br J Surg. 1990;77:260-264.

73. Kley AJ vd, Bakker DJ, Lubbers MJ, Henny CP. Skeletal muscle pO_2 in anaerobic soft tissue infections during hyperbaric oxygen therapy. Adv Exp Med Biol 1992: 317; 125-129.

74. Korhonen K, Hirn M, Niinikoski J. Hyperbaric oxygen in the treatment of Fourniers gangrene. Eur J Surg. 1998; 164 (4): 251-255.

75. Korhonen K. Hyperbaric oxygen therapy in acute necrotising infections. Ann Chir Gyn 2000: suppl 214; 7-36.

76. Korhonen K, Kuttila K, Niinikoski J. Tissue gas tensions in patients with necrotising fasciitis and healthy controls during treatment with hyperbaric oxygen: A clinical study. Eur J Surg 2000: 166; 530-534.

77. Kujath PE, Eckmann C. "Die nekrotisierende Fasziitis und schwere Weichteilinfektionendurch Gruppe-A-Streptokokken. Diagnose, Therapie und Prognose". Dt Artztebl 1998:95 (8); A-408-413.

78. Lamerton AJ. "Fourniers gangrene: non-clostridial gas gangrene of the perineum and diabetes mellitus." J R Soc Med. 1986;79:212-215.

79. Ledingham IM, Tehrani MA. "Diagnosis, clinical course and treatment of acute dermal gangrene." Br J Surg. 1975;62:364-372.

80. Lefrock JL, Molavi A. "Necrotising skin and subcutaneous infections." J Antimicrob Chemother 9 (Suppl A). 1982;183-192.

81. Lewis RT. "Necrotising soft tissue infections." Meakins JL (Ed.) Surgical Infection in Critical Care Medicine, Ed 20. London, Churchill Livingstone: 1985;153-171.

82. Lewis RT. "Soft tissue infection." Wilmore DW, Brennan MF, Harken AH, et al (Eds). Care of the Surgical Patient, Ed 21. New York, Scientific American: 1989;1-15.

83. Lin C, Yeh FL, Lin JT et al. Necrotising fasciitis of the head and neck : An analysis of 47 cases. Pals Reconstr Surg 2001: 107(7): 1684-1693.

84. Loudon I. "Necrotising fasciitis, hospital gangrene, and phagedena". Lancet 1994: 344; 1416-1419.

85. Mader JT, Adams KR, Sutton TE. "Infectious diseases: Pathophysiology and mechanisms of hyperbaric oxygen." J Hyp Med. 1987;2:133-140.

86. Mader J. "Mixed anaerobic and aerobic soft tissue infections." Davis JC, Hunt TK, (Eds.) Problem Wounds: The Role of Oxygen. New York: Elsevier, 1988;153-172.

87. Mathieu D. Place de l'oxygénotherapie hyperbare dans le traitement des fasciites nécrosantes. Conference de consensus de la Société Française de Dermatologie. Ann Dermatol Venereol 2001 : 128 ; 411-418.

88. McCafferty EL, Lyons C. "Suppurative fasciitis as the essential feature of haemolytic streptococcus gangrene." Surgery. 1948;24:438-442.

89. McCrea LE. "Fulminating gangrene of the penis." Clinics 1945: 4 (3); 796-829.

90. McGreer AJ. Commentary on Wall et al. A 2 factor model helped to rule out early stage necrotising fasciitis. Evidence Based Med 2001: 6; 96.

91. McLennan JD. "The histotoxic clostridial infections of man." Bact Rev. 1962;26:177-276.

92. Meleney FL. "Haemolytic streptococcus gangrene." Arch Surg. 1924;9:317-364.

93. Meleney FL. "A differential diagnosis between certain types of infectious gangrene of the skin, with particular reference to haemolytic streptococcus gangrene and bacterial synergistic gangrene. Surg Gynecol Obstet. 1933;56:847.

94. Meleney FL. "Bacterial synergism in disease process, with confirmation of the synergistic bacterial etiology of a certain type of progressive gangrene of the abdominal wall." Ann Surg. 1933;94:961-981.

95. Modai J. "Empiric therapy of severe infections in adults." Am J Med. 88 1990;(Suppl 4A):12S-17S.

96. Monnickendam MA, McEvoy MB, Blake WA et al. "Necrotising fasciitis associated with invasive group A streptococcal infections in England and Wales". Adv Exp Med Biol 1997: 418; 87-89.

97. Morantes MC, Lipsky BA. "Flesh-eating bacteria: Return of an old nemesis". Int J Dermat 1995: 34(7); 461-463.

98. Mutschler W, Bakker DJ. "Temporärer Hautersatz (temporary skin replacement)." Z für Allg.med. 1088;64(24):714-720.

99. Neuber M, Rieger H, Brüwer M et al. Fulminante Fasciitis necroticans bei Morbus Crohn-assoziiertem Verlauf. Chirurg 2000: 71; 1277-1280.

100. Nichols RL, Smith JW. "Gas in the wound: What does it mean?" Surg Clin North Am. 1975;55:1289-1296.

101. Nichols RL. "Gas-producing infections." Nichols RL, Hyslop NE, Bartlett JG, (Eds.) Decision Making in Surgical Sepsis. Decker, Philadelphia, 1991;60-61.

102. Norrby-Teglund A, Thulin P, Gan BS et al. Evidence for superantigen involvement in severe group A streptococcal tissue infections. J Infect Dis 2001: 184; 853-860.

103. Patino JF, Castro D, Valencia A, Morales P. "Necrotising soft tissue lesions after a volcanic cataclysm." World J Surg. 1991;15:240-247.

104. Paty R, Smith AD. "Gangrene and Fourniers Gangrene. Urol Clin N Am 1992 :19(1); 149-162.

105. Pfanner W. "Zur Kenntnis und Behandlung des nekrotisierenden Erysipels. Kriegschirurgische Mitteilungen aus dem VÜlkerkrieg 1914/1918, nr 81." Dtsch Z Chir. 1918;144:108-119.

106. Podbielski A, Rozdzinski E, Wiedeck H, Lütticken R. "Gruppe-A-Streptokokken und die nekrotisierende Fasziitis". Dt Artztebl 1998: 95 (8); A-414-420.

107. Pruitt BA. "Burns and soft tissues." Polk HC Jr (Ed.) Infection in the Surgical Patient. Clinical Surgery International 4. London, Churchill Livingstone: 1982;113-131.

108. Quirk WF, Sternbach G. " Joseph Jones: Infection with flesh eating bacteria". J Em Med 1996: 14 (6); 747-753.

109. Riegels-Nielsen P, Hesselfeldt-Nielsen J, Bang-Jensen E, Jacobsen E. "Fourniers gangrene: Five patients treated with hyperbaric oxygen." J Urol. 1984;132:918-920.

110. Riseman JA, Zamboni WA, Curtis A, Graham DR, Konrad HR, Ross DS. "Hyperbaric oxygen therapy for necrotising fasciitis reduces mortality and the need for debridements." Surg. 1990;108:847-850.

111. Rodloff AC, Montag TH, GÜrtz G, Harnoss B-M, Ehlers S. "Mikrobiologische Aspekte von Anaerobierinfektionen." Hau T (Ed.) Anaerobierinfektionen in der Chirurgie. Upjohn Heppenheim (Germany), 1991.

112. Schwarz N, Redl H, Grasslober H, Krebitz B. "Necrotising soft tissue infection- An increasing problem in orthopedic trauma". Eur J Trauma 2000: 2; 62-68.

113. Sheffield PJ. "Tissue oxygen measurements." Davis JC, Hunt TK, (Eds.) Problem Wounds: The Role of Oxygen. New York: Elsevier. 1988;37-44.

114. Sherris JC. "Skin and wound infection." Sherris JC (Ed.) Medical Microbiology. New York, Elsevier. 1984;555-561.

115. Shupak A, Shoshani O, Goldenberg I, Barzilai A, Moskuna R, Bursztein S. "Necrotising fasciitis: An indication for hyperbaric oxygen therapy"? Surgery 1995: 118 (5); 873-878.

116. Smith GL, Bunker CB, Dinneen MD. "Fourniers gangrene". Brit J Urol 1998: 81; 347- 355.

117. Stevens BJ, Lathrop JC, Rice WT, Gruenberg JC. "Fourniers gangrene: Historic (1764-1978) versus contemporary (1979-1988) differences in etiology and clinical importance. Am Surg 1993: 59 (5); 149-154.

118. Stevens DL, Gibbons AE, Bergstrom R, Winn V. "The Eagle effect revisited: Efficacy of clindamycin, erythromycin and penicillin in the treatment of streptococcal myositis. J Inf Dis 1988: 158 (1); 23-28.

119. Stevens DL. "Invasive Group A Streptococcus infections". Clin Inf Dis 1992; 14: 2-13.

120. Stevens DL. "Invasive group A streptococcal infections: the past, the present and future". Pediatr Inf Dis J 1994; 13: 561-566.

121. Stevens DL. "Streptococcal Toxic Shock Syndrome: Spectrum of disease, pathogenesis and new concepts in treatment". Em Inf Dis 1995; 1(3); 69-78.

122. Stevens DL. Review: "Invasive Group A Streptococcal Disease". Infec Agents and Dis 1996: 5; 157-166.

123. Stevens DL. "The Flesh-Eating Bacterium: What's next?" J Infect Dis 1999; 179(Suppl 2): S366-374.

124. Stevens DL. "Streptococcal Toxic Shock Syndrome associated with necrotising fasciitis". Ann Rev Med 2000: 51; 271-288.

125. Stevens DL. "Invasive streptococcal infections". J Infect Chemother 2001:7; 69-80.

126. Stephenson H, Dotters DJ, Katz V, Droegemueller W. "Necrotising fasciitis of the vulva". Am J Obstet Gynecol 1992: 166 (5); 1324-1327.

127. Stone HH, Martin JG,Jr. "Synergistic necrotising cellulitis." Ann Surg. 1992;175: 702-711.

128. Stone DR, Gorbach SL. "Necrotising fasciitis. The changing spectrum". Inf Dis Dermat. Dermat Clin 1997: 15(2); 213-220.

129. Sutherland ME, Meyer AA. "Necrotising soft-tissue infections". Surg Clin N Am 1994; 74(3); 591-607.

130. Thom SR. "Hyperbaric oxygen therapy in septicemia." J Hyp Med. 1987;2(3):141-146.

131. Tibbles PM, Edelsberg JS. Hyperbaric oxygen therapy. N Eng J Med 1996 : 334(25) ; 1642-1648.

132. Umeda T, Ohara H, Hayashi O et al. Toxic shock syndrome after suction lipectomy. Plast Reconstr Surg 2000: 106(1); 204-207. Discussion by R.A.Mladick 208-209.

133. Unnikrishnan M, Cohen J, Sriskandan S. Complementation of a speA negative Streptococcus pyogenes with speA: effects on virulence and production of streptococcal pyrogenic exotoxin A. Microb Pathogen 2001: 31; 109-114.

134. Vick R, Carson CC. Fourniers Disease. Urol Clin N Am 1999: 26(4); 841-851.

135. Voros D, Pissiotis C, Georgantas D et al. "Role of early and extensive surgey in the treatment of severe necrotising soft tissue infections". Br J Surg 1993: 80; 1190-1191.

136. Wall DB, Klein SR, Black S, Virgilio de C. A simple model to help distinguish necrotising fasciitis from nonnecrotising soft tissue infection. J Am Coll Surg 2000: 191(3); 227-231.

137. Webb R, Berg E. "Symbiotic gangrene due to Pseudomonas pyocyanea and E. coli." Austr NZ J Surg. 1966;36:159-160.

138. Weiss KA, Lavardière M. Group A streptococcus invasive infections: A review". Can J Surg 1997: 40(1); 18-25.

139. Whitesides L, Cotto-Cumba C, Myers RAM. Cervical necrotising fasciitis of odontogenic origing: A case report and review of 12 cases. J Or Max Surg 2000: 58(2); 144-151.

140. Wienecke H, Lobenhoffer P. Nekrotisierende Weichteilinfektionen. Chirurg 2001: 72; 320-337.

141. Wilson B. "Necrotising fasciitis." Am Surgeon. 1952;18:426-431.

142. Wilson DH, Haltalin KC. "Acute necrotising fasciitis in childhood." Am J Dis Child. 1973;125:591-595.

143. Zamboni WA, Riseman JA, Kucan JO. "Management of Fourniers gangrene and the role of hyperbaric oxygen." J Hyp Med. 1990;5(3):177-186.

144. Zamboni WA, Mazolewski PJ, Erdmann D et al. "Evaluation of Penicillin and Hyperbaric Oxygen in the treatment of streptococcal myositis". Ann Plast Surg 1997: 39(2); 131-136.

NOTES

CHAPTER 11

CLOSTRIDIAL MYONECROSIS

D.J. Bakker

INTRODUCTION

Gas gangrene is an acute, rapidly progressive, nonpyogenic, gas-forming, and necrotizing infection of muscles, subcutaneous tissues, and skin. The infection is caused by anaerobic, spore-forming bacteria of the genus Clostridium, primarily *Clostridium welchii* or *C. perfringens.* Untreated, the disease characteristically has a rapidly fatal outcome.

Traditionally, gas gangrene is associated with war [3, 60]. However, a low incidence of gas gangrene (0.016% = 22 cases) was found during the Vietnam conflict, and at least 27 cases of clostridial infection were reported in a 10-year period in a metropolitan community in Miami, Florida. [14] Early and adequate debridement and delayed wound closure in frontline surgery explain the recent low incidence of gas gangrene in war surgery [19]. Although Hippocrates described gas gangrene [45], we owe the most impressive description in early history to Fabricius Hildanus [42]. Also, Pare's well-known description of the wounded at the Siege de Rouen is suspect for gas gangrene [64]. Excellent reviews on the history of gas gangrene can be found in the literature [8, 50, 64, 58].

The first report on organisms that can live and reproduce in the absence of free oxygen comes from Pasteur [78]. In 1871 Bottini demonstrated the bacterial nature of gas gangrene, but he could not isolate the causal microorganism. In 1892 Welch and Nuttall isolated *Bacillus aerogenes capsulates (Clostridium perfringens* or *C. welchii,* the microorganism most frequently involved in gas gangrene [106]). Novyi isolated the *Bacillus oedematiens* or *Clostridium novyi* [74].

Treatment of gas gangrene with hyperbaric oxygen was introduced in 1960 by Boerema and Brummelkamp from Amsterdam [12].

ETIOLOGY AND PATHOPHYSIOLOGY

Clostridial spores instead of the vegetative form of the bacterium are responsible for contamination. The source of bacterial spores is either exo- or endogenous. Nearly all exogenous infections occur in patients with compound and complicated fractures with extensive soft tissue injuries after street accidents. Only a minority are seen after a "sterile" operation, intravenous infusion, intramuscular injection, criminal abortion, etc. [15].

Clostridial myositis as an endogenous infection is caused by contamination from a clostridial focus in the body, i.e., infection of the abdominal wall after gallbladder or colon surgery and also after urinary tract operations in patients with clostridial contamination of bile or urine. Great amounts of clostridia were found to be present in faeces (10^6–10^9/g faeces). In 44% of normal individuals clostridia were found to be present on the perineal skin. In the female genital tract clostridia were present in 5% of cases. In a review of 3,027 investigated wounds, contamination with *Clostridium perfringens* ranged from 3.8 to 39%, whereas in 187, 936 serious open wounds with extensive soft tissue damage gas gangrene developed in 1.76% of cases.

More advanced surgical techniques, such as external fixation techniques in trauma surgery, improved transport facilities, better initial wound care, and intensive medical care, have reduced this percentage to less than 0.5% [8, 34, 35, 38].

For the onset of gas gangrene two conditions are necessary: (a) the presence of clostridial spores, and (b) an area of lowered oxidation-reduction potential caused by circulatory failure in a local area or by extensive soft tissue damage and necrotic muscle tissue, an area with a low pO_2 where clostridial spores can flourish into the vegetative form.

The clostridial bacteria surround themselves with toxins. Local host defense mechanisms are abolished when the toxin concentration is sufficiently high, and then begins the ever-increasing tissue destruction and further clostridial growth. The progressive nature of gas gangrene depends on the continuous production of alpha-toxin by clostridia. Unless toxin production and bacterial multiplication are stopped, the patient will die.

The local condition of the wound is far more important than the presence of clostridia and can be considered as the clinically deciding factor for the onset of gas gangrene.

Gas gangrene has been recorded after:
- Soft tissue trauma
- Foreign bodies, hemorrhage, or necrotic tissue in the wound
- High-velocity missile wounds
- Compound fractures
- Deep contamination of wounds
- Prolonged delay in surgery
- Traumatic or surgical interruption of blood supply
- Criminal and spontaneous abortion
- Too-tight plaster casts or dressings
- Postoperative (after any kind of operation)
- After intramuscular, intravenous, and/or intra-arterial injections of any substance
- Other (and often minor) causes in otherwise healthy people and/or in the immune-compromised host like superficial traumatic abrasions, and other small wounds and also after liver transplantation [33, 37]

An extensive review of the literature on all initiating causes of gas gangrene is given by Heimbach [39].

BACTERIOLOGY

Gas gangrene is caused by anaerobic, spore-forming Gram-positive encapsulated bacilli of the genus clostridium. They are motile or nonmotile depending on the species. Since Pasteur described *Clostridium butyricum*, more than 150 species of Clostridium have been recognized, but only 6 are regularly associated with human disease: *C. perfringens*, *C. septicum*, *C. bifermentans*, *C. sporogenes*, *C. fallax*, and *C. novyi*.

C. perfringens is the most important and most frequently cultured species in gas gangrene in 80-90% of wounds [8,39]. It is particularly ubiquitous in nature because, except in the North African deserts, it is found naturally all over the world in soil and dust, and can be isolated in healthy persons from stomach, gallbladder, small and large intestine, vagina, and skin. *C. perfringens* is not a strict anaerobe; it grows freely in oxygen tensions up to 30 mm Hg and has restricted growth in tensions up to 70 mm Hg [8, 59]. It does not form spores in tissues. Laboratory identification of *C. perfringens* is performed by either the Nagler reaction or the Lecito-vitellin (LV) reaction [107]. More than 20 different exotoxins produced by clostridia have been identified; 9 of these exotoxins are responsible for local and systemic changes in gas gangrene and are produced by *C. perfringens:* alpha-toxin or phospholipase C, theta-toxin or perfringolysin, kappa toxin, mu-toxin, nu-toxin, fibrinolysin, neuraminidase, "circulating factor" and bursting factor. Alpha-toxin, the most important, is an oxygen-stable lecithinase-C or phospholipase-C, that is hemolytic, tissue-necrotizing, and lethal. Alpha-toxin hydrolyzes the intact lecithin molecule to produce phosphoryl choline and a water-insoluble diglyceride. Alpha-toxin is chemically related to lecithinase-A, which is present in a variety of snake venoms and poison of bees and scorpions, lecithinase-B and D [39].

The other toxins are probably ancillary to alpha-toxin and give rise to hemolysis, causing anemia, jaundice, and renal failure by hemoglobinuria, tissue necrosis, and serious systemic effects such as cardiotoxicity and brain dysfunction. Other exotoxins are synergistic and enhance a rapid spread of infection by destroying, liquifying, and dissecting healthy tissue.

Stevens and Bryant investigated the role of theta-toxin in the pathogenesis of clostridial gas gangrene. They found evidence for the suggestion that theta toxin in high concentrations is a potent cytolysin and promotes direct vascular injury at the site of infection. At lower concentrations theta-toxin activates PMNs and endothelial cells, and in so doing promotes vascular injury distally by activating adherence mechanisms by PMN-dependent adherence molecules such as the integrin CD 11/CD 18 [94].

The rapid tissue necrosis associated with *C. perfringens* infection may be related to progressive vascular compromise orchestrated by dysregulated host cell responses induced by theta-toxin [94]. Both alpha- and theta-toxin are necessary for vascular leukostasis to occur [24]. Alpha-toxin can be fixed to susceptible skin cells in 20-30 min and is detoxified within two hours of its elaboration, and causes active immunity with production of a specific antitoxin [60,109]. The progressive nature of gas gangrene depends on the continuous production of alpha-toxin.

In an earlier paper, Stevens et al. [93] already described the lethal effects and cardiovascular effects of purified alpha- and theta-toxins from *C. perfringens.*

Awad et al. [6] showed genetic evidence for the essential role of alpha-toxin in gas gangrene. Stevens [96] also showed that alpha- and theta-toxins differentially modulate the immune response and induce acute tissue necrosis in clostridial gas gangrene. This is further supported by the work of Ninomiya et al. [70] and Alapa-Giron et al. [1], who showed that alpha-toxin plays a key role in the systemic intoxication of clostridial myonecrosis, probably by affecting the functions of platelets and phagocytes. Also Awad et al. [7] showed the synergistic effects of both alpha-toxin and theta-toxin (perfringolysin).

The fulminant nature of shock in these patients is caused by alpha-toxin (direct effect on myocardial contractility) and the combined effect of alpha- and theta-toxin on the induction of the production of potent endogenous mediators of shock [97].

Bryant et al. [16,17] showed that tissue destruction in gas gangrene is related to profound attenuation of blood flow initiated by activation of platelet responses by alpha-toxin. This is responsible for rapid tissue destruction. Therefore, without hyperbaric oxygen, radical amputation as soon as possible was advocated. Alpha-toxin stimulated platelet/neutrophil aggregation in a gpIIbIIIa-dependent fashion (a platelet fibrinogen receptor). Bryant therefore suggests as a therapeutic strategy to target gpIIaIIIb to prevent vascular occlusion and maintain tissue viability so that radical surgery may not be necessary. Hyperbaric oxygen is another way to prevent radical surgery in the treatment of gas gangrene, not mentioned at all by Bryant.

A very informative review on a cellular and molecular model of the pathogenesis of clostridial myonecrosis including the abovementioned data is given by Stevens [98].

A further subdivision can be made in clostridia that are toxogenic, i.e., *C. perfringens, C. septicum, C. novyi,* and clostridia that are believed to be only proteolytic, i.e., *C. histolyticum, C. bifermentans, C. sporogenes,* and *C. fallax,* which augment an infection by their proteolytic capabilities, but do not cause the classical gas gangrene syndrome. *C. tertium, C. sphenoides,* and *C. sordelli* can be considered as contaminants. It is not known if and what these microorganisms add to the disease process. The essential role of alpha-toxin in the pathogenesis of gas gangrene was confirmed by Williamson and Titball who developed a genetically engineered vaccine against alpha-toxin. This vaccine proved to be of value in animal experiments [108].

CLINICAL PRESENTATION OF GAS GANGRENE

Altemeier [3] described four forms of necrotizing clostridial disease:

1. Clostridial myonecrosis with toxicity (true gas gangrene)
2. Localized clostridial myonecrosis
3. Clostridial cellulitis with toxicity
4. Clostridial cellulitis without toxicity (#3 and 4 are discussed under Progressive Bacterial Gangrene in the chapter on Necrotizing Soft Tissue Infections)

The incubation time of gas gangrene varies from one hour [62] to 41 days [5]. Kiranov studied gas gangrene in Bulgaria between 1964 and 1977. In 87% of cases in wartime, gas gangrene started four days or less after injury. Time between injury and onset of gas gangrene in peacetime was longer [4,26,52,105].

Patients who are at risk for infection in general (i.e., patients with predisposing factors such as ischemia, diabetes mellitus, lowered resistance, foreign bodies etc.; patients with underlying systemic diseases; elderly people; debilitated patients with gastrointestinal, biliary, or genitourinary tract infections; drug addicts; etc. are also more vulnerable to gas gangrene. Even a case of intracardiac gas gangrene can be found in the literature [18]. From time to time cases of intracerebral gas gangrene are reported as well [10]. A high index of suspicion and the knowledge that however rare and trivial the occasion, gas gangrene may occur, are imperative.

Although not mentioned very frequently in the literature, gas gangrene can occur in young children also. We had no patients under the age of five but twenty patients between five and fifteen years of age. A review is given by Roloff [82,83].

The local picture of gas gangrene is not like that of other pyogenic infections, which usually begin with a red erythematous discoloration of skin. In gas gangrene the erythematous discoloration is subtle. Then, later, a rapidly progressive phlegmone appears. One of the first signs is extreme pain in the wound area, which is in sharp contrast to the minor local signs. Upon examination, at first one cannot imagine that the patient suffers such severe pain. The wound area appears quiet. This disproportional pain was noticed already by Fabricius Hildanus [42]. In a very short time the extremity, when we take this as an example, swells enormously, and the initially pale skin becomes tight and shiny. A watery thin, red-brownish wound exudate may appear. The gas produced by the bacteria (from carbohydrates) is so delicately dispersed in the muscle tissues that it cannot be felt. At this stage the gas can only be seen on X-ray as feather-like air figures between the muscle fibers. This was observed by Savill as early as 1916 [85]. (Fig. 8-13)

The next phase is the highly progressive and centripetal bronze- or copper-like discoloration, also known as bronze erysipelas, which is darkest in colour near the wound area while the wound margins and protruding muscle tissues are brown-black, showing myonecrosis. Tension in the tissues may be great enough to restrict arterial circulation and lymph drainage. (Fig. 3-7) From that moment on there is an even more aggressive progression of the phlegmone. The progression of skin discoloration with tissue necrosis and hemolysis, together with the deeper localized myonecrosis that lies a bit behind, can be astounding. In one patient we measured a 25-cm progression in 45 min. Progression is most aggressive in arteriosclerotic, diabetic, or traumatic vascular insufficiency. In this phase of the disease the border of gas forming in the tissues is often ahead of discoloration and necrosis. The gas is palpable, with a crackling sensation, like walking in dry snow, in the tense tissues proximal to the discoloration. Soon thereafter, the skin may become dark brown and blue-black bullae filled with clostridia-containing serosan-guinolent fluid may appear. The extremity spreads a typical sickly sweet odor, also called "mousy." Without treatment the patient dies quickly in septic shock.

Signs and symptoms depict an overwhelming process. After the initial stage of extreme pain in the wound area, the body temperature rises within 12 hours to about 41°C. This is still the early edematous stage without discoloration of tissues. Blood pressure falls, pulse rate quickens, and septic shock develops. The erythrocyte sedimentation rate (ESR) is low and the leukocyte count is increased to $20\text{-}30/10^9/l$.

Moreover, there is a kind of psychiatric-neurological complex of symptoms characterized as toxic psychosis or symptomatic psychosis. The patient becomes dull and confused, which may progress into coma or delirium. Nora and cooperators [73] demonstrated a direct effect of alpha-toxin (phospholipase C) on phospholipids of the tissues of the central nervous system. They concluded that symptomatic or toxic psychosis is caused by the direct influence of circulating alpha-toxin on the central nervous system. This view is supported by our experience that the condition of patients improves rapidly when they are treated with hyperbaric oxygen. Edematous swelling of brain tissue and degenerative cell destruction have been described. Jaundice, partly caused by hemolysis by alpha-toxin and partly by hepatic insufficiency, can be found in 25-50% of patients [80]. Clostridia are also found in blood cultures. The overall picture of a hemorrhagic state after alpha-toxin injection is caused by diminution of platelets, alteration of clotting activity, liberation of heparinoid substances, damaged capillary and epithelial cells throughout the body, and by the influence of the toxin on the liver and alteration of plasma proteins.

Impairment of kidney function is frequently seen in gas gangrene and varies from a slight to moderate increase of blood urea, oliguria, or complete anuria, necessitating (hemo)- dialysis. One of the most important factors in the onset of impaired kidney function is the hemolytic-uremic syndrome (HUS) [80]. Septic shock degrades kidney function still further. Almost every patient with gas gangrene is anemic because of hemolysis by circulating alpha-toxin. Close monitoring and, if necessary, immediate correction of the electrolyte and fluid balance are mandatory. Many other complications due to the primary disease can be expected and must be adequately treated as early as possible. Complications such as adult respiratory distress syndrome (ARDS) after severe trauma, fat embolism syndrome in long bone fractures, deep vein thrombosis in patients who are immobilized for a long time, myocardial irritability by circulating clostridial endotoxins, and disseminated intravascular coagulopathy (DIC) are often seen in these serious infections.

DIFFERENTIAL DIAGNOSIS

McLennan [60] divided histotoxic infections of humans into those that are traumatic and those that are non-traumatic. In this classification a distinction was made between anaerobic cellulitis (See chapter on Selected Aerobic and Anaerobic Soft Tissue Infections) and anaerobic clostridial myonecrosis. He defined anaerobic cellulitis as a clostridial infection that involves only necrotic tissue killed by ischemia and by direct trauma and does not invade healthy tissue. Anaerobic clostridial myonecrosis (true gas gangrene) was described as an acute invasion of healthy living tissue not damaged by previous trauma or ischemia. He proposed the classifications in Table 1.

TABLE 1. TRAUMATIC AND NONTRAUMATIC WOUND INFECTIONS

Traumatic wound infections	Nontraumatic wound infections
Simple contamination Anaerobic cellulitis Anaerobic myonecrosis Clostridial Nonclostridial	Idiopathic Infected vascular gangrene

"The infected vascular gangrene has frequently, if inexcusably, been confused with gas gangrene and in view of its benignity, chronicity, and ease of treatment, must be carefully excluded" [60]. (Fig. 15)

It should, however, be born in mind that vascular gangrene infected with clostridial organisms may, under certain circumstances, i.e., as a complication of an operation upon an extremity, give rise to acute clostridial cellulitis or myonecrosis in the previous healthy part of that extremity [77]. (Fig. 14)

Hitchcock et al. [47] differentiated clostridial infections into (a) spreading diffuse myositis, (b) localized myositis, and (c) cellulitis. Although this division may be of value, there is still the possibility that an apparently localized myositis can progress into a spreading diffuse myositis. Altemeier's classification of clostridial infections is similar to that of Hitchcock, but he added tetanus, which is no longer an indication for hyperbaric oxygen [3,31]. Brightmore [13] described a number of nonclostridial gas-forming infections in the perianal region, besides Fournier's gangrene. A third classification was proposed by Darke et al. [21], who differentiated gas gangrene and related infections as (a) clostridial gas forming, (b) clostridial non-gas forming, (c) clostridial uterine, and (d) nonclostridial, with a distinction between streptococci and *Eschericia coli*.

AMSTERDAM CLASSIFICATION OF SOFT TISSUE INFECTIONS (TABLE 2)

Since clostridial myositis with myonecrosis is generally called gas gangrene, we may assume that the formation and presence of gas in the tissues are valuable diagnostic tools in establishing the diagnosis. All bacterial and nonbacterial disorders with tissue emphysema should therefore be included in the differential diagnosis.

Nonbacterial Causes

All traumatic and chemical nonbacterial causes of soft tissue gas should be investigated when soft tissue crepitance is present without local or systemic signs of infection. Mechanical and traumatic sources of gas include excessive undermining of tissue planes during operation, which results in air entrapment. Air can also leak into tissues from defects in the oesophagus, respiratory tract, and gastrointestinal tract. Excessive manipulation during surgery may cause gas in the operative site; however, this gas

TABLE 2. AEROBIC/ANAEROBIC SOFT TISSUE INFECTIONS & HYPERBARIC OXYGEN AS ADJUNCT

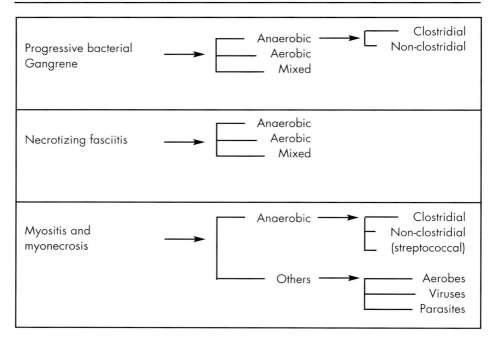

Amsterdam classification of soft tissue infections. In order to systematize the classification (following Ledingham and Tehrani (58)), we divided these infections into three groups, based on the anatomic location at the onset of the infection:
  1. progressive bacterial gangrene,
  2. necrotizing fasciitis, and
  3. myositis and myonecrosis.

decreases rapidly. Air leakage after perforation of the oesophagus is usually closely related to endoscopy and/or dilatation, or to spontaneous perforation.

Air leakage from the respiratory tract is usually caused by trauma or by chest tube insertion. We have seen three patients with soft tissue gas after wound irrigation with hydrogen peroxide who had been referred on suspicion of gas gangrene.

Bacterial Causes

There are several other severe nonclostridial crepitant infections, both aerobic *(E. coli, Klebsiella, Enterobacter,* and *Pseudomonas)* anaerobic *(Peptostreptococcus, Bacteroides),* and mixed [2,11,21,27,37,68,101]. In almost all cases of gas-forming infectious processes, soft tissue gas can be ascertained by clinical investigation alone. Upon examining the infected area, a crackling is felt. Sometimes an X-ray of the infected area is necessary to confirm the diagnosis. We obtain X-ray pictures as a standard procedure, because we consider the specific feather-like distribution of gas in the muscle tissue to be a significant diagnostic tool. (Fig. 8-13)

DIAGNOSIS

The diagnosis is based on clinical and bacteriological findings. Myositis and myonecrosis are important clinical signs, as is gas on X-ray. Only in the case of infection with *Clostridium novyi (C. oedematiens)* is gas in the muscles absent [35]. Because the novyi alpha-toxin affects specifically and more seriously vascular permeability [62] , edema is more prominent. In gas gangrene caused by *C. novyi*, discoloration of the skin may be more purple than the copper- or bronze-like colour present in other clostridial infections. (Fig. 1) Blood and/or wound cultures must be positive for at least one of the pathogenic clostridia. Most of the time myositis and myonecrosis are so overwhelming that, if present, other microorganisms hardly play a role in the early stage of the disease. After the gas gangrene is cured, these micro-organisms may become more significant [15]. A Gram stain shows many, Gram positive, short, clubshaped rods, sometimes with terminal spores, without leukocytes. Samples for culture and specimens for histology should preferably be taken at a distance proximal to the center of infection or wound area, and not from apparently dead or healthy muscles. Samples for bacteriology should be taken from deep muscle tissue because superficial smears are of little value. For diagnosis in a gas-forming infection, needle aspiration can be done from the involved area together with careful clinical inspection of the extent of infection. Needle aspiration has to be performed under sterile conditions from deep-lying muscle tissue and should be stored immediately in a special transport vial for anaerobes. Gaschromatography can show alpha-toxin in the blood of patients with gas gangrene. This method has not yet been routinely used [56].

Roggentin et al. [81] developed an immunoassay for rapid and specific detection of *Clostridium perfringens*, *C. septicum*, and *C. sordelli* by determining their sialidase activity (neuraminidase) in serum and tissue homogenates. Sialidases produced by these three clostridia were bound to polyclonal antibodies raised against the respective enzymes and immobilized onto microtiter plates. Applied to nine samples from patients there was a high correlation between the results of the immunoassay and the bacteriological analysis of the infection.

Scheven [86] described identification of *C. perfringens* in clinical materials from patients with a mixed infection by means of a modified reversed CAMP-test.

PROPHYLAXIS OF GAS GANGRENE

Prevention of gas gangrene can be achieved by measures directed against the source of infection and by proper wound management and wound care. General hygienic measures for both patient and doctor, combined with prophylactic treatment of the patient, to reduce contamination with clostridia to an ultimate minimum, are essential. The best prophylaxis against gas gangrene in wartime was a "good soap bath and clean clothing the night before an attack" [41]. In this regard, showering drastically reduces the number of microorganisms [27].

Prophylactic treatment consists of proper wound care and antibiotics; gas gangrene antitoxin is obsolete. In exceptional cases hyperbaric oxygen can be used as a prophylactic.

GENERAL WOUND CARE AND MANAGEMENT

Etiologic factors in the onset of gas gangrene are generally the same as those in non-clostridial surgical infections. They are (a) the presence of microorganisms, (b) dead space, and (c) necrotic tissue including collections of bile, serum, and lymph. In particular, wounds involving deep muscle areas with extensive laceration and devitalization with impairment of the main blood supply are highly vulnerable; so are injuries of the buttocks, thighs, legs, and finally, to a lesser extent perhaps, the shoulders.

The condition of the wound is far more important for the onset of gas gangrene than is the presence of clostridial spores. Circulatory insufficiency in the wound area causes a lowered oxidation-reduction potential, thus creating favorable conditions for clostridial spores to develop into the vegetative form. A basic element for the prevention of infections is proper surgical management, together with antibiotics (preferably a combination of antibiotics directed to both anaerobes and aerobes).

As prophylaxis against gas gangrene, penicillin-G in high dosages can be recommended (10-20 million units/day). If used, antibiotics should be continued for at least five days because, although the risk of gas gangrene decreases, it still remains present during the whole period of wound healing.

The following guidelines in wound management should be considered:

- Adequate, particularly early and meticulous debridement of wounds, especially in high-risk patients
- Meticulous hemostasis
- Deep wounds left open and adequately drained
- Tight dressings and tight casts avoided
- Frequent and early use of colostomies in patients with deep-penetrating wounds of buttocks and/or upper legs, decubitus ulcers, and perianal and ischiorectal abscesses
- Delayed closure in traumatic wounds and after lower-leg amputation, especially in patients at risk, perhaps even when the blood supply to the level of amputation has been considered to be sufficient at operation

A general rule as to the initial treatment of open fractures is difficult to make. The best policy seems to be to refrain from immediate internal fixation in patients at risk, unless a completely stable general and local situation can be reached. In these circumstances it is better to use a form of external fixation, because stabilization of fractures is necessary in the prevention of infections.

Delayed osteosynthesis has been advocated as a safe and tissue-saving way of treatment. This involves a few days' delay, during which time the soft tissues can recover from local shock and can be properly judged for viability, whether or not treated with hyperbaric oxygen during this period. If early osteosynthesis is preferred or high-risk conditions are present, delayed wound closure is advisable. Every surgeon has to realize that the possibility of gas gangrene always exists, despite all of the therapeutic and prophylactic measures outlined here.

ANTIBIOTIC PROPHYLAXIS

Penicillin in high quantities is the best prophylactic agent, although clostridial myositis has developed in patients treated with it. Chloramphenicol and erythromycin are also being used. In theory vancomycin and metronidazole are effective, although the results of their clinical application are not known. Tetracycline and clindamycin are not recommended because of the relatively common resistance of clostridia, although there are studies mentioning a 100% sensitivity of clostridia to clindamycin. When risk factors indicate, penicillin prophylaxis should be given as early as possible.

The question remains, what should be considered a severe wound prone to develop gas gangrene? The answer is difficult because of the characteristic unpredictability of gas gangrene. We often encounter totally unexpected gas gangrene, i.e., after operations that could be considered completely "sterile" (stripping of varicose veins). Penicillin also has its risks. Very high doses (over 20 million units/day) may cause hemolytic anemia and very serious coagulation disorders [100,103].

As a rule short-term high dosage of antibiotics is recommended in wounds prone to infection. Although penicillin is the drug of choice, complications, as well as the risk of allergic reactions, make it not advisable to treat all serious wounds with this antibiotic. The attending surgeon must individualize each case to weigh the risk of gas gangrene against the risk of penicillin complications. Ertmann et al. [25] recommended the use of the broad-spectrum antibiotic mezlocillin both prophylactically and therapeutically. In their patient series many mixed infections were found.

HYPERBARIC OXYGEN

Although prophylaxis with hyperbaric oxygen is not recommended in every patient at risk for gas gangrene, this modality may be considered in patients with serious anaerobic contamination and in cases where the circulation is either disturbed or at risk. In particular, hyperbaric oxygen should be considered after reimplantation of extremities, reconstructive vascular surgery for open fractures with vascular damage (i.e., high-velocity bullet wounds), amputation for arteriosclerotic and/or diabetic gangrene, in heavy contaminated wounds with soil and mud etc. Also serious immune-compromised patients can be candidates for prophylactic hyperbaric oxygen.

PATIENTS AT RISK

Factors putting patients at risk for the onset of gas gangrene are: ischemia, traumatic vascular damage, and arteriosclerotic and/or diabetic arterial insufficiency; lowered resistance by drugs (addicts); starvation; systemic underlying disease such as diabetes mellitus, lupus erythematodes, rheumatic fever, inflammatory bowel disease (Crohn's disease, ulcerative colitis), malignancies, immunodeficiencies (either idiopathic or caused by corticosteroids, as in transplantation patients with liver and/or kidney function failure); foreign bodies (plates and screws after osteosynthesis, bone cement, sutures etc.). Special attention should be given to patients who underwent:

- Osteosynthesis after an open, compound fracture with contamination of the wound area
- Lower-leg (or even upper-leg) amputation for diabetic and/or arteriosclerotic arterial insufficiency
- High-risk surgery especially in elderly patients
- Large bowel surgery
- Surgery for acute cholecystitis and/or cholangitis
- Repeated injections with epinephrine or epinephrine-containing compounds (contraindicated in areas with already-compromised circulation)
- Operations for small and large bowel ileus
- Drug addicts with infections (including streptococcal myositis or myonecrosis) that can be accompanied by compartment syndromes, postabortion infections, and perineal and ischiorectal abscesses

TREATMENT OF GAS GANGRENE

General Supportive Measures

In almost all cases we are faced with seriously ill patients in need of intensive care treatment. In addition to the specific treatment directed to the causative microorganisms, general supportive measures are to be taken. Generally, these concern the maintenance of tissue perfusion and oxygenation (!), monitoring of fluid and electrolyte balance as well as blood pH, control of central venous pressure or pulmonary wedge pressure, etc. The end of a central venous line should not enter the right atrium. Patients with gas gangrene easily develop myocardial irritability and uncontrollable arrhythmia can be induced by a catheter within the right atrium [39]. Particularly in gas gangrene, clinical estimation of fluid loss by wounds, mucous membranes, etc. is important. Patients are invariably in need of blood transfusion, due to hemolysis caused by clostridial α-toxin. Whole blood or an adequate composition of blood components should be given. Specific deficits should be corrected by specific blood components.

Other supportive measures are directed to the cardiac and pulmonary status of the patient, adequate immobilization of the infected and injured part (including fractures), relief of pain, management of renal failure, and treatment of thrombophlebitis (which is a frequent and prominent manifestation of anaerobic infection). The use of anticoagulants should be weighed against the risk of septic hemorrhage.

Patients with gas gangrene run an increased risk of developing tetanus, because tissues with *C. perfringens* are equally suitable for *C. tetani*. Tetanus prophylaxis is necessary according to the guidelines of the Committee on Infections of the American College of Surgeons (and other specific guidelines in other countries).

Gas gangrene antitoxin, abandoned as a prophylactic modality, is controversial as far as the curative application is concerned. There is no consensus as to the results and very serious side effects are encountered in more than 10% of cases [79]. A total of 57% adverse effects and a fatal outcome were reported in a series of 81 patients [57].

We discontinued gas gangrene antitoxin treatment in 1964. Also, the U.S. Army no longer uses gas gangrene antitoxin [8].

Before hyperbaric oxygen therapy became available, the treatment of gas gangrene was almost entirely surgical. The main objective was to excise or amputate as soon as and as generously as possible in order to remove all diseased tissue; even disarticulations were considered. Limb-saving operations were discarded in favor of life-saving procedures directed at radical extirpation of the site of infection. Removal of all compromised tissue was thought to prevent clostridial growth and thus arrest onset and spread of gas gangrene. Although the mortality decreased, it still remained between 20 and 50%. (Fig. 2) Even when the disease was discovered early, the mortality remained well over 10%. Moreover, patients who survived were often disabled and subjected to long-lasting physical and psychological rehabilitation programs. Initially after discovery of the causative anaerobic microorganisms, application of hydrogen peroxide and zinc peroxide creams was tried. These efforts changed the pO_2 at the surface and in superficial layers, but not in deeper tissue layers and certainly not in the center of the infection. Slightly better results were reached with other modalities of local application of oxygen such as: (a) allowing oxygen to penetrate the wounded tissues by inserting tubes, or (b) injecting oxygen into the wound and into the tissues at the borderline of a progressing infection. (Fig. 2) But still there were parts of the body (i.e., intra-abdominal and intracranial) that were not suitable for injection therapy. During World War I, German surgeons warned against this injection therapy, which was sometimes complicated by fatal gas embolism [58,90]. Local oxygen therapy was disappointing and could not be recommended [32]. In a survey of 607 patients with gas gangrene treated with all kinds and combinations of treatment modalities, the mean mortality was 49.7% (range 19-55%). The patients were treated by incision, drainage, debridement, amputation, disarticulation, serum therapy, rib resections, charcoal therapy and irrigations with hydrogen peroxide and/or Dakin's solution. In serious cases, 50% mortality is still reported without hyperbaric oxygen therapy [110]. Roloff [82] reported a mean mortality between 1966 and 1988 of 68.2% (even 92% in postoperative gas gangrene and 40% in the post-traumatic group). During World War I the mortality of gas gangrene in the American Expeditionary Force in France was 48.5% (674 of 1389 patients with gas gangrene) [64]. The present treatment for gas gangrene includes surgery, antibiotics, general resuscitative and ancillary measures, and hyperbaric oxygen.

Surgery

Surgery has an important place in gas gangrene, but it has undergone changes in timing and extent since hyperbaric oxygen became available. In clostridial cellulitis it is generally sufficient to perform large incisions and, if necessary (because of tissue necrosis), excisions only as deep as the deep fascia.

In clostridial myositis and myonecrosis the main objective is the removal of dead tissue and blood because erythrocytes, containing catalase, counteract the influence of hyperbaric oxygen. However, the problem in gas gangrene is not dead nor healthy tissue, but the quickly advancing phlegmone in between the two. This phlegmone of infected but potentially viable tissue is best treated primarily by hyperbaric oxygen instead of surgery. Initial surgery can be limited to wound opening in traumatic and postoperative patients and sometimes decompressing fasciotomy; no ablative surgery is necessary, in our experience. (Fig. 19 & 20) Minimal debridement and fasciotomies can be performed, if this is necessary and to save time, in a multiplace hyperbaric chamber while pressurizing and at pressure.

In most cases removal of necrotic tissue can be delayed until after the second or third hyperbaric oxygen session, or even until hyperbaric treatment is completed, depending on the general condition of the patient. (Fig. 16 & 17)

Cristoferi et al. [20] recommend the use of spore elements and of a special frequency soft-tissue laser in helping wound healing, besides other already mentioned measures, especially in gas gangrene patients.

After gas gangrene is successfully treated, of course normal principles of wound healing including the necessary support by surgical measures apply (secondary wound closure, split skin and full thickness grafts, and other kinds of plastic and reconstructive measures). These can be found in every surgical textbook and will not be discussed in detail here.

Antibiotics

General consensus has been reached as to treatment of the life-threatening clostridial myonecrosis with high doses of antibiotics. Penicillin is preferred in combination with one or two other antibiotics directed against mixed superinfections [25,29,34,35,38,60,79].

Erttmann and colleagues [25] recommend the use of broad spectrum antibiotics from the start and even for peri-operative antibiotic prophylaxis. In their experience the quantity of mixed infections was such that penicillin-G alone was not sufficient. This is certainly true when you get patients in advanced stages of the disease. In the beginning the "clostridium factor" is so overwhelmingly present that to start with penicillin is justified. However, nothing speaks against the start with broad spectrum antibiotics including high doses of penicillin.

Chloramphenicol is suggested as a reasonable alternative for patients with severe penicillin allergy, because of the sensitivity of most anaerobes to this drug [63]. The potentially lethal hematologic complications of chloramphenicol prompted many clinicians to use erythromycin, lincomycin, and clindamycin for anaerobic infections in general [9].

For the treatment of myonecrosis and clostridial cellulitis with toxicity, the best choice after penicillin-G is probably clindamycin, vancomycin, and metronidazole [28]. Clostridia other than *C. perfringens* are less sensitive to clindamycin and vancomycin. In our patients *C. perfringens* was responsible for gas gangrene in 95.8% of cases. In order to minimize the potassium load in patients already at risk for hyperkalemia, sodium penicillin is proposed for use instead of potassium penicillin according to the following schedules: 6-20 million units penicillin/day and clindamycin intravenously (in adults, 600 mg/6 h; in children, 5 mg/kg body weight/6 hrs) as well as gentamycin (or tobramycin) (in adults, 1.5 mg/kg bodyweight/8 hrs; in children, 2.5 mg/kg body weight/8 hrs, depending on renal function). We consider antibiotics as an adjuvant in the treatment of gas gangrene with hyperbaric oxygen.

Hyperbaric Oxygen

The action of hyperbaric oxygen on clostridia and other anaerobes is based on the formation of oxygen free radicals in the absence of free-radical degrading enzymes such as superoxide dismutases, catalases, and peroxidases. The first clinical results in gas gangrene were remarkable, but were difficult to reproduce in the animal model [43,44,46,67]. This can be explained in part by the fact that pressures used in some of the experiments were too low, because the resistance of small laboratory animals against a high pO_2 is different from that of human beings. Hyperbaric oxygen is, however, bacteriostatic and bactericidal for *Clostridum welchii* [43,44]. Local application of oxygen is of no use in the treatment of gas gangrene. Nora et al. [72] showed that hyperbaric oxygen at 3 atmospheres absolute pressure (ATA) had no effect on cell-free preformed alpha-toxin. Van Unnik [102] showed that a pO_2 of 250 mm Hg in the tissues is necessary to stop alpha-toxin production completely, although this does not kill all *Clostridium welchii*.

A tissue pO_2 over 250 mm Hg can be reached with 100% oxygen breathing at 3 ATA [53,87,89]. Already circulating toxin is fixed to the living cells within 30 min of its elaboration [44]. Free-circulating toxins or tissue-bound toxins are not affected by high O_2 levels but they are rapidly detoxified by normal host factors [49,60,61,72,73].

The conclusion can be that when the patient is at 3 ATA and breathing 100% oxygen, virtually all dangerous alpha-toxin has disappeared after 30 min. Because the progressive nature of gas gangrene depends on the continuous production of alpha-toxin, hyperbaric oxygen is the quickest way initially to break that vicious circle.

Animal experiments (in mice, rabbits, guinea pigs, and dogs) and clinical data show that a combination of hyperbaric oxygen, local debridement, and antibiotics led to less mortality and morbidity than any of these treatment modalities alone [22,35,35,47,51,54,55,66,84,91,92].

A little more cautious are Tibbles and Edelsberg [99] in a review article stating that "the available clinical and experimental evidence suggests that multiple early treatment sessions with hyperbaric oxygen at the advised pressures are beneficial." Mitton and Hailey [65], weighing the evidence, conclude that there is strong rationale for the use of hyperbaric oxygen. The evidence suggests significant reductions in both mortality and morbidity when treatment includes hyperbaric oxygen treatment.

Mortality in the series of Hirn [46] was 28%. He concluded that mortality and morbidity could be reduced if the disease is recognized early and appropriate therapy applied promptly. He recommends adequate operative debridement, antibiotics, hyperbaric oxygen, and surgical intensive care.

Heimbach [40] reports a literature review of cases since 1961. He found 117 articles with a total of 1200 patients. There are more, because our 500 cases are not mentioned in his review. The mean mortality was 25%; the disease-specific mortality was 15%. When the treatment started within the first 24 hours the disease-specific mortality decreased to 5%.

In experimental monomicrobial gas gangrene the combination therapy of surgery and HBO started 45 min after the inoculation of bacteria reduced the mortality to 13% compared with 38% with surgery alone.

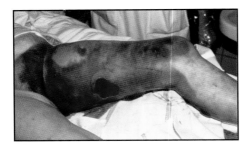

1. Clinincal picture of a gas gangrene caused by *clostridium novyi*. There is more vascular damage and edema. (See page 291)

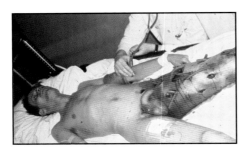

2. Classic gas gangrene after a closed femur fracture. In the picture, from the early days in 1961, you can see how the referring surgeon tried initially to treat this patient, by multiple incisions and insertion of tubes to get oxygen into the tissues. (See page 295)

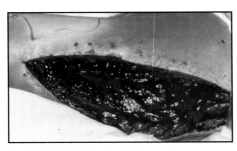

3. Gas gangrene after a hip operation. Note the inflamed and dead muscle tissue protruding from the incision wound. (See page 287)

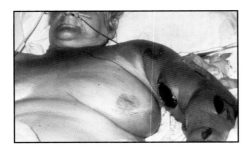

4. Gas gangrene after a bee sting in the hand. Note the copper-like discoloration of the skin and the dead muscle tissue protruding from multiple incision wounds made in the referring hospital. Patient was admitted in deep septic shock and died before the first hyperbaric session. (See page 287)

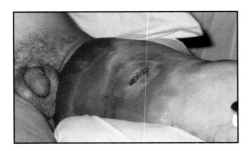

5. Gas gangrene after a complicated femur fracture, conservatively treated with a Kirscner wire traction. (See page 287)

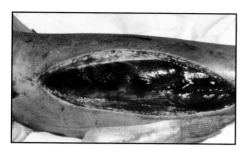

6. So-called spontaneous gas gangrene. Incision of the lower leg skin and subcutaneous tissue and fascia. Note the dead muscle tissue. (See page 287)

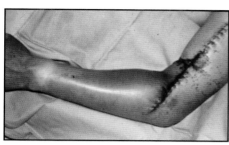

7. Gas gangrene of the lower arm after operative treatment of an upper arm fracture with radial nerve damage. (See page 287)

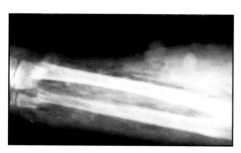

8. X-ray picture of a gas gangrene of the lower arm after a Colles fracture of the wrist. Note the feather-like air figures in the muscles which are very characteristisc of gas gangrene. (See pages 287 & 290)

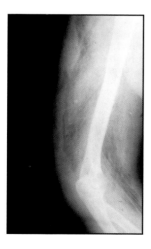

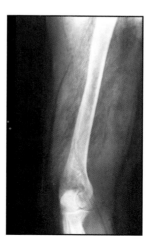

9. X-ray picture of gas in the tissures in gas gangrene of lower and upper arm. Feather-like air figures same as in photo #8. (See pages 287 & 290)

10. Idem upper arm. (See pages 287 & 290)

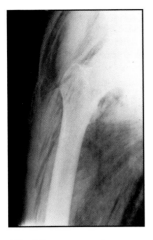 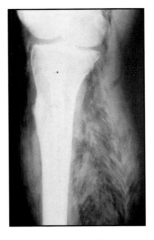 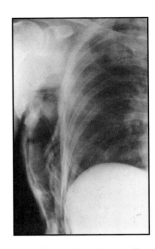

11. Idem upper leg.
   (See pages 287
   & 290)

12. Idem lower leg.
   (See pages 287 & 290)

13. Idem thoracic wall
   and axilla. (See pages
   287 & 290)

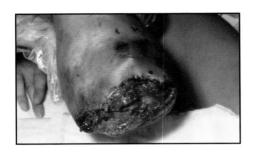

14. True gas gangrene in a trau-
   matic amputation stump in a
   young patient. (See page 289)

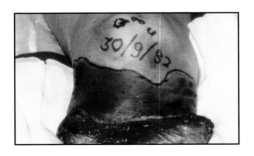

15. Infected vascular gangrene in
   a old patient after a lower leg
   amputation. (See pages 289
   & 305)

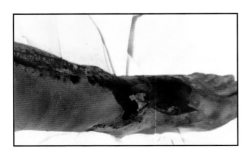

16. This is an example of the
   demarcating effect of hyper-
   baric oxygen treatment. It is a
   picture of an ankle fracture in a
   43-year-old lady treated with
   osteosythesis and followed by
   gas gangrene. Treatment only
   hyperbaric oxygen.
   (See pages 296 & 302)

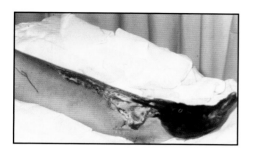

17. This photo is of the same patient above (photo #16), taken only 26 hours later. Also the tissue saving effect; only a Symes-type amputation was necessary. (See pages 296 & 302)

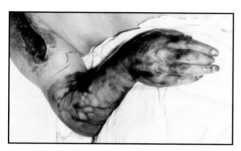

18. Demarcating effect of hyperbaric oxygen. Life-saving but an upper arm amputation was necessary. (See page 302)

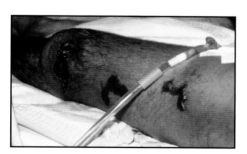

19. Gas gangrene of the upper leg after a contusion of the skin. Hyperbaric oxygen and limited excision of tissue. (See page 296)

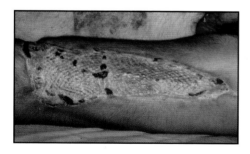

20. Same patient as above (photo #19). End result after split skin grafting. (See page 296)

The combination therapy appeared to be especially effective in wound healing and in prevention of morbidity compared with surgical debridement alone. The effectiveness of the combination therapy was strongly time-dependent. In the multi-microbial gas gangrene model the addition of hyperbaric oxygen to surgery tended to reduce mortality, but the difference between the groups was not statistically significant. However, the combined therapy with surgery and hyperbaric oxygen was highly effective in reducing morbidity and improving wound healing compared with survival debridement alone [46]. The timing and extent of surgical treatment remains controversial and is very difficult to determine on the basis of retrospective analysis alone.

Erttmann et al. [26] concluded from a retrospective analysis of 136 patients treated between 1970 and 1990 that operative treatment, i.e., debridement and fasciotomies, should be done before hyperbaric oxygen therapy. Delayed surgery gave worse results in their patients. In our experience, it is very important that hyperbaric oxygen therapy starts as early as possible, because the best treatment results are achieved in the earliest possible stage of the infection [26,34,35]. Results worsen progressively when hyperbaric oxygen treatment is delayed or not given at all [23,36]. Early and aggressive surgery and late hyperbaric oxygen treatment led to a significantly higher mortality and morbidity [69,76,88]. The performance of time-consuming procedures before hyperbaric oxygen treatment is contraindicated, because it further endangers the life of the patient. In our experience, it was nearly always possible to delay more definitive surgery until one to four hyperbaric oxygen treatment sessions were completed. Of course, if you have a large multiplace hyperbaric chamber at your disposal, you can operate these patients under pressure during hyperbaric oxygen treatment. The two largest and oldest centers with experience in this field are the University Medical Centers in Amsterdam and Graz [91].

The advantages of early hyperbaric oxygen treatment are that:
- It is *life-saving*, because less heroic surgery needs to be performed in very ill patients and the cessation of alpha-toxin production is rapid.
- It is *limb-and tissue-saving*. No major amputations or excisions are done in advance and, when demarcation becomes clear, far less tissue appears to be lost than initially thought.
- It *clarifies the demarcation* so that there is a clear distinction between dead and still-living tissue within 24-30 hours [8]. (Fig. 16-18)

Advocated pressures vary from 2.5 ATA in a monoplace chamber to 3.0 ATA in a large multiplace chamber during 90 min of 100% O_2 breathing per treatment session. Frequency of treatment varies from three to four times during the first 24 hours up to a total of seven treatments in three days (3-2-2), to continuation of two treatments daily after 48 hrs until the infection is completely controlled. We have never used more than seven treatments in three days. During this time infection was controlled or the patient died. As soon as the patient is breathing 100% O_2 at the required pressure, the tissue pO_2 around and even inside the infected area rises to values over 250 mm Hg, so that the production of alpha-toxin stops completely [87]. Within 30 min the circulating toxin is fixed to the living cells [60] and the growth of clostridia is limited. After a short interval the hemolytic, tissue-necrotizing, and lethal activity of the clostridia is stopped.

Between hyperbaric oxygen sessions when the patient is at sea-level pressure, alpha-toxin production starts again, but before a dangerous level is reached, the next session stops production once more. The intermittent periods without alpha-toxin production and the rapid destruction of circulating alpha-toxin enable the body to utilize its own host-defense mechanisms. The temporary arrest of alpha-toxin production may lead to a change in the environment of the clostridia, which consequently no longer meets the requirements for optimum function of the clostridia. The transiently increased pH, the arrest of the activity of proteolytic enzymes in the tissue, and the consequent arrest of the release of amino acids in the lesion may result in a condition of the surrounding tissues that is not ideal for the functioning and multiplication of anaerobic microorganisms. In the infected area the circulation is improved by diminished edema and compression of gas bubbles. It goes without saying that already necrotic tissue is lost, but the quantity of tissue that is lost is, in our experience, always far less than initially expected before hyperbaric oxygen treatment.

Amsterdam Therapeutic Regimen

A patient suspected of having gas gangrene must be transferred to a hyperbaric unit as soon as possible.

Doctors in the referring hospital are asked to do two things:

1. Give the patient 2 million units of sodium-penicillin I.V.
2. Remove the sutures and open the wound in postoperative and post-traumatic patients.

After admission to the hyperbaric unit:

*   Wound inspection to evaluate the clinical picture, discoloration of skin, muscle necrosis, swelling of the infected area, discharge and smell from the wound, in order to ascertain the clinical diagnosis gas gangrene.
*   Removal of sutures and opening of the wound, when not done so already, and determine whether complete opening has been performed. In cases of gas gangrene after injections or minor injuries, wounds are not surgically handled initially.
*   Bacteriology, including a direct smear for Gram staining, aerobic and anaerobic blood and wound cultures, and tissue specimens for culture and histology. A Gram stain with Gram-positive spore-bearing rods and without leukocytes supports the clinical diagnosis of gas gangrene and hyperbaric oxygen treatment is indicated. This treatment is started before the results of the cultures are known, because cultures take time and alpha-toxin production has to be stopped as soon as possible.

3. Demarcation of the boundaries of discoloration and crepitance
4. Blood sampling for laboratory investigations, including hemoglobin, hematocrit, leukocytes, electrolytes, kidney and liver function tests, arterial blood gases, coagulation parameters, etc.

5. Infusion therapy and shock treatment as soon as the patient arrives in the hospital
6. X-rays for signs of clostridial myositis
7. Antibiotics: 8-10 million sodium penicillin units I.V. per day. This can be extended later if a broader coverage is required. In the first hours of a gas gangrene infection, mixed infections are not that important
8. Adequate patient sedation, if necessary before starting hyperbaric treatment. Interaction of sedatives and their use under hyperbaric conditions have been outlined by Walsh [104]
9. Myringotomy is performed in patients who are not capable of "clearing the ears"; to equalize the pressure differences on both sides of the eardrum during treatment (in small children, in very old and in very sick patients). Myringotomy is easily and quickly performed under local anaesthesia and is virtually without complications. The opening in the eardrum remains competent during the three days of treatment. If further treatments have to be given tympanostomy tubes can be inserted
10. Hyperbaric oxygen treatment. Advocated pressures vary from 2.5 ATA in a monoplace chamber to 3.0 ATA in large multiplace chambers during 90 min of 100% oxygen breathing per treatment session. Frequency of treatment sessions varies from three to four times during the first 24 hrs twice daily during the next 48 hrs; a total of seven treatments. After this period the infection is controlled or the patient has died (within 24 hrs after admission in our series). As a control of the treatment we use transcutaneous and intramuscular pO_2 measurements before, during, and after treatments
11. Between treatments the patient is admitted to the ICU if necessary and wound dressing changes are performed as indicated above

The actual decision on termination of treatment depends on the patient's response to HBO. If the patient remains toxic the treatment profile needs to be extended. Utilization review is indicated after 10 treatments.

Results

Between October 1960 and January 1994, 618 patients suspected of gas gangrene were admitted to our department. In 462 cases (74.8%) the diagnosis of gas gangrene could be confirmed both clinically and bacteriologically. Bacteriological confirmation of blood and/or wound cultures for at least one pathogenic *Clostridium* species invariably followed the first 24 hrs of hyperbaric oxygen therapy. A positive clinical picture and a Gram-stained smear with Gram-positive spore-bearing rods and without leukocytes were arguments to start treatment immediately. The lack of initial bacteriological confirmation of the diagnosis gas gangrene should not delay treatment in cases of clinical gas gangrene. However, only those patients with the clinical picture of gas gangrene and positive wound/tissue and/or blood culture are included in the series of 462 patients.

In the years after 1994 the number of patients decreased to approximately 5-7 patients annually in our center. The results with the treatment modality mentioned above remained the same as described.

Gender and Age Distribution

The group of 462 patients with proved gas gangrene consisted of 347 men (75.1%) and 115 women (24.9%) with a mean age of 44.6 years (range 5-94 years).

Classification of Patients with Gas Gangrene

Our patients were classified into three groups according to the cause of gas gangrene: group 1 (n = 281; (60.8%)), accidents; group 2 (n = 145; (31.4%)), operations; group 3 (n = 36; (7.8%)), other causes.

The majority in group 1 acquired gas gangrene after a traffic accident (n = 203); in second place were industrial or agricultural accidents (n = 40). Only in seven cases were sports accidents involved. Finally, in 31 cases gas gangrene was caused by another kind of accident.

In group 2, 145 patients acquired gas gangrene postoperatively, either after acute or elective surgery. Every operation can be complicated by gas gangrene. A sudden rise in temperature within the first 24 hrs after the operation, together with the onset of disproportional wound pain, may be a sign of gas gangrene, even after the most elective and "sterile" operation (Table 3). Most patients (n = 71) developed gas gangrene after amputation for arteriosclerotic and/or diabetic gangrene. As a result of seriously impaired circulation, these patients already suffer from tissue ischemia or necrosis, which are important factors in the aetiology of gas gangrene.

A clear distinction should be made between the so-called infected vascular gangrene (non-traumatic, histotoxic infection) and true gas gangrene. Infected vascular gangrene is generally a much more chronic, (Fig. 15) relatively benign infection without symptoms of general toxicity. The patient is not very ill, has no high fever, and the soft tissue infection without myonecrosis is located in the amputation stump. Clostridia can be present in this usually mixed aerobic-anaerobic infection. The slight degree of myositis or myonecrosis usually has an appearance that is different from that of true clostridial myonecrosis and runs a different course as well. Only clostridial myonecrosis in a seriously ill patient with a fulminant progressive disease involves gas gangrene and needs hyperbaric oxygen treatment. In view of the possible endogenic source of clostridial spores, there is a slight prevalence of gas gangrene after surgery of the colon (n = 11), gallbladder (n = 10), perineum (n = 6), and for ileus (n = 6).

The third group (n = 36) is probably the most difficult, but also the most interesting, category; it has a variety of causes (Table 6) of which intramuscular injections take the greatest part (n = 11). It is clear that clostridial growth may be expected in areas of ischemia caused by an injected substance with a vasoconstrictive effect, i.e., epinephrine. In one case of I.V. infusion, gas gangrene developed 1.5 hrs after venipuncture. Two exceptional cases of gas gangrene occurred after an insect sting while the patients were gardening.

TABLE 3. TYPE OF OPERATION PRECEDING GAS GANGRENE (N = 145) AND MORTALITY (N = 26) DUE TO GAS GANGRENE

Type of operation	N	Mortality
Amputation for arteriosclerotic and/or diabetic gangrene	71	11
Colonic surgery and trauma	11	4
Cholecystectomy	10	3
Sympathectomy	6	–
Perineal abscess and wound	6	–
Ileus	6	3
Appendectomy	6	2
Vascular surgery (no trauma)	5	1
Osteosynthesis (not acute)	3	1
Amputation after trauma	3	–
Gastric surgery	2	–
Radical mastectomy	2	–
Arthrotomy knee joint	2	–
Herniotomy	2	–
Varicetomy	1	–
Prostatectomy	1	–
Mitral commissurotomy	1	–
Caesarian section	1	–
Pyelotomy	1	–
Pacemaker implantation	1	–
Embolectomy	1	1
Liver/kidney biopsy	1	–
Arthrotomy ankle joint	1	–
Nonclostridial intracranial abscess drainage	1	–

TABLE 4. MORTALITY OF GAS GANGRENE FOR GROUPS 1-3 FROM OCTOBER 1960 THROUGH JANUARY 1994

Group	No. of patients	Mortality		
		Overall	Manifest gas gangrene	After full treatment
1	281	31 (11.0%)	18 (6.3%)	13 (4.6%)
2	145	44 (30.3%)	26 (18.0%)	18 (12.4%)
3	36	20 (55.6%)	10 (27.8%)	10 (27.8%)
Total	462	95 (20.6%)	54 (11.7%)	41 (8.9%)

TABLE 5. DISTRIBUTION AND TYPE(S) OF CLOSTRIDIA FOUND IN WOUND CULTURES (N = 462)

Type	No. of patients
C. *perfringens*	403
C. *septicum*	9
C. *bifermentans*	3
C. *sporogenes*	3
C. *fallax*	2
C. *novyi*	1
C. *perfringens* + C. *sporogenes*	12
C. *perfringens* + C. *sordelli*	10
C. *perfringens* + C. *sphenoides*	4
C. *perfringens* + C. *bifermentans*	5
C. *perfringens* + C. *tertium*	2
C. *perfringens* + C. *novyi*	2
C. *perfringens* + C. *fallax*	1
C. *perfringens* + C. *septicum*	2
C. *septicum* + C. *sphenoides*	1
C. *perfringens* + C. *sporogenes* + C. *sphenoides*	1
C. *perfringens* + C. *septicum* + C. *sporogenes*	1

Bacteriology

Clostridium perfringens was the major representative, either in pure culture (403 of 462, 87.2%) or in combination with other pathogenic clostridia (41 of 462, 9.7%) (Table 5). In 91.1% of cases only one *Clostridium* species was cultured. Positive blood cultures were found in 115 cases (24.9%).

Mortality

In order to gain clear insight into the results of hyperbaric oxygen therapy and the survival of patients, it is important to make a distinction between two categories in considering mortality. The first category deals with patients who actually died from gas gangrene during the active phase of the disease and have positive cultures, and the second category involves those who die from other causes after gas gangrene is considered cured. Even in this latter group with cured gas gangrene, it is possible to find positive cultures that can possibly be explained by the difference between the full bacterial life of clostridia with toxin production and the somehow restricted life of clostridia that are still living, but not capable of toxin production any more after hyperbaric oxygen treatment.

An interesting observation was reported by O'Brien and Melville [75] about the possible ability of *Clostridium perfringens* to escape the phagosome of macrophages under aerobic conditions. Thus it can be possible that persistence inside macrophages of *C. perfringens* is an important factor in the early stages of a gas gangrene infection.

In our series 400 patients survived during the active phase of the disease (mortality 54 of 462; 11.7%) and 367 ultimately survived. A total of 41 patients died from causes other than gas gangrene (pulmonary embolism, cardiac infarction, metastases of a colon carcinoma, etc.) four days or more after therapy. Mortality for the three groups of patients is shown in Table 4. In group 1 gas gangrene was mainly located in the extremities and was diagnosed at a relatively early stage. In group 2 the infection was generally located on the trunk or proximally on an extremity. In group 3 the high mortality (10 of 36, 27.8 %) was caused by late diagnosis. These patients were admitted in an advanced stage of infection—septic shock—and consequently could not stand the first 24 hrs of therapy.

Table 7 shows mortality in relation to the number of hyperbaric sessions. If patients survived until the fourth hyperbaric session (which started 24 hrs after the first treatment), there was no more mortality from gas gangrene. All 48 patients died within 24 hrs after the start of hyperbaric oxygen therapy before the fourth session. It is hardly possible to show more clearly than in Table 7 how important time is in the treatment of gas gangrene.

AMPUTATIONS

Between October 1960 and January 1994 the total number of patients with gas gangrene of the extremities was 365. A total of 88 patients had already undergone amputations elsewhere for arteriosclerotic and/or diabetic vascular insufficiency [104], gas gangrene [21], or trauma [12]. Amputations for gas gangrene (13 of 355, 3.7%) were mostly performed between 1960 and 1965. During that period surgeons were not acquainted with the fact that

TABLE 6. KIND OF INCIDENT PRECEDING GAS GANGRENE IN GROUP 3 PATIENTS *(N = 36)* **AND MORTALITY** *(N = 10)* **DUE TO GAS GANGRENE** *(N = 10)*

Causitive Incident	N	Mortality
Intramuscular injection	11	4
Criminal abortion	3	–
Knee-joint puncture	3	–
Intravenious infusion	4	–
Bladder catheterization	1	–
Ulcus cruris	2	–
Insect sting	2	1
Cowhorn attack	1	–
Mudbath	1	–
Acute pancreatitis	1	1
Fournier	1	–
No port of entry	6	4

TABLE 7. MORTALITY FROM MANIFEST GAS GANGRENE (54 OF 462) DURING HYPERBARIC OXYGEN THERAPY. (OCTOBER 1960 THROUGH JANUARY 1994)

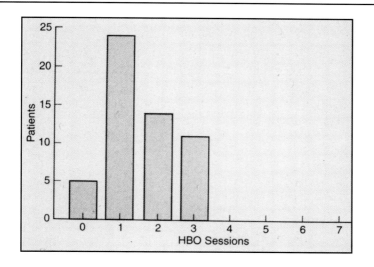

primary surgery was not necessary if hyperbaric oxygen facilities were available. Between 1975 and 1985 only two amputations for gas gangrene were performed before sending the patient to us. After completion of hyperbaric oxygen therapy, 70 amputations were necessary (70 of 355, 19.7%), reamputation or stump correction was carried out 17 times in primary amputated patients (17 of 67, 25.4%), and in 22 cases the extremity was already considered to be lost because of frank necrosis at the time of admission. In the other 26 cases (26 of 355, 7.3%) amputation had to be carried out despite hyperbaric oxygen therapy. This clearly demonstrates a lower amputation rate than that after primary surgery, reported to be 50-55% [88]. Based on these results, we postulate that primary ablative surgery to treat gas gangrene of the extremities is contraindicated.

REFERENCES

1. Alapa-Giron A, Flores-Diaz M, Guillouard I et al. Identification of residues critical for toxicity in Clostridium perfringens phospholipase C, the key toxin in gas gangrene. Eur J Biochem 2000: 267(16); 5191-5197.

2. Altemeier WA, Culbertson WR (1948) Acute non-clostridial crepitant cellulitis. Surg Gynec Obstet 87: 206-212

3. Altemeier WA (1966) Diagnosis, classification and general management of gas producing infections, particularly those produced by *Clostridium perfringens*. Proc Third International Conference on Hyperbaric Medicine, Brown IW jr, Cox BG (eds) Natl Acad Sci Natl Res Counc Pub11404, Washington DC; 481

4. Altemeier WA, Fullen WD (1971) Prevention and treatment of gas gangrene. JAMA 217:806-813

5. Arapov DA (1956) Die anaerobe Infektion. In: Grosse Med Enzyklopaedie: 1130, Moskou Medgis

6. Awad MM, Bryant AE, Stevens DL, Rood JI. Virulence studies on chromosomal alpha-toxin and theta-toxin mutants constructed by allelic exchange, provide genetic evidence for the essential role of alpha-toxin in *Clostridium perfringens*-mediated gas gangrene. Mol Bol 1995: 15(2); 191-202.

7. Awad MM, Ellemor DM, Boyd RL et al. Synergistic effects of alpha-toxin and per fringolysin O in *Clostridium perfringens*-mediated gas gangrene. Infect Immun 2001: 69(12); 7904-7910

8. Bakker DJ (1984) The use of hyperbaric oxygen in the treatment of certain infectious diseases especially gas gangrene and acute dermal gangrene. Thesis, University of Amsterdam, Veenman Wageningen

9. Bartlett JG, Sutter VL, Finegold SM (1972) Treatment of anaerobic infections with lincomycin and clindamycin. N Engl J Med 287:1006-1010

10. Bele S, Fiedler A, Woertgen C et al. Fatal intracerebral gas gangrene in a 10-month-old child. Zentralbl Chir 2000: 125(8); 688-690

11. Bessman AN, Wagner W (1975) Non-clostridial gas gangrene; report of 48 cases and review of the literature. JAMA 233: 958

12. Boerema I, Brummelkamp WH (1960) Behandeling van anaerobe infecties met inademing van zuurstof onder een druk van 3 atmosferen. Ned Tijdschr Geneesk 104; 2548-2550

13. Brightmore J (1972) Perianal gas producing infection of non-clostridial origin. Br J Surg 59:109-116

14. Brown PM, Kinman PB (1974) Gas gangrene in a metropolitan community. J Bone Joint Surg 56A:1445-1451

15. Brummelkamp WH, Bakker DJ (1978) Gas gangrene. In: Cost WS, Mandema E (eds): Spoedeisende Gevallen in de Interne Kliniek. Elsevier Amsterdam Brussel, pp 73-88

16. Bryant AE, Chen RYZ, Nagata Y et al. Clostridial gas gangrene. I. Cellular and molecular mechanisms of microvascular dysfunction induced by exotoxins of *Clostridium perfringens*. J Inf Dis 2000: 182; 799-807

17. Bryant AE, Chen RYZ, Nagata Y et al. Clostridial gas gangrene II. Phospholipase C-induced activation of platelet gpIIaIIIb mediates vascular occlusion and myonecrosis in *Clostridium perfringens* gas gangrene. J Inf Dis 2000: 182; 808-815

18. Chowdhury PS, Timmis SBH, Marcovitz PA. *Clostridium perfringens* within intracardiac thrombus. A case of intracardiac gas gangrene. Circulation 1999: 100; 2119.

19. Coenen H (1919) Der Gasbrand. Ergeb Chir Orthop 11: 235

20. Cristoferi G, Fabris G, Ronconi AM et al. La gangrène gazeuse. Considerations cliniques, pronostic et perspectives thérapeutiques selon notre expérience. J Chir (Paris) 1991 : 128 (5) ; 243-246

21. Darke SG, King AM, Slack WK (1977) Gas gangrene and related infections: Classification, clinical features and aetiology, management and mortality. A report of 38 cases. Br J Surg 64:104-112

22. Demello FJ, Haglin JJ, Hitchcock CR. Comparative study of experimental *Clostridium perfringens* infection in dogs treated with antibiotics, surgery and hyperbaric oxygen. Surg 1973 : 73; 936-941.

23. Eckmann C, Kujath P, Shekarriz H, Staubach K-H. Clostridiale myonekrose als Folge intramuskulärer Injektionen – Beschreibung dreier fatales Verläufe. Langenb Arch Chir 1997: Suppl II (Kongressbericht 1997); 553-554

24. Ellemor DM, Baird RN, Awad MM et al. Use of genetically manipulated strains of *Clostridium perfringens* reveals that both alpha-toxin and theta-toxin are required for vascular leukostasis to occur in experimental gas gangrene. Inf Immun 1999: 67(9); 4902-4907

25. Erttmann M, Hobrecht R, Havemann D (1992) Ist Penicillin-G das Mittel der Wahl beim Gasödem? Zentral BI Chir; 117:509-514

26. Erttmann M, Havemann D (1992) Behandlung des Gasödems. Unfallchirurg 95:471-476

27. Finegold SM (1975) Anaerobic bacteria in human disease. New York: Academic Press, pp 21-27

28. Finegold SM, Bartlett JG,Chow AW et al. (1975) Management of anaerobic infections. UCLA conference. Ann Intern Med 83:375

29. Florey HW, Cairns H (1943) Investigation in war wounds: penicillin. A Preliminary Report of the War Office and the Medical Research Council on Investigation Concerning the Use of Penicillin in War Wounds. War Office publ Bethesda: US Dept *AMD7/90D*

30. Godsick WH, Hermann HL, Jonas G et al. (1954) Uterine gas gangrene: review with recent advances in therapy and report of three cases. Obstet GynecoI 3:408-415

31. Gottlieb SF (1977) Oxygen under pressure and micro-organisms. In: Davis JC, Hunt TK (eds): Hyperbaric oxygen therapy. Bethesda: Undersea Medical Society, p 79-99

32. Graf A (1939) Umspritzungen mit H_2O_2 bei Gasbrand? Munch Med Wochenschr 86:28

33. Hall TR, Poon A, Yaghscian H et al. (1991) Gas gangrene: an unusual cause of graft failure in an orthoptic pediatric liver transplant. Paediatr RadioI 22:579-581

34. Hart GB, Lamb RC, Strauss MB (1983) Gas gangrene: I. A collective review. J Trauma 23:991-995

35. Hart GB, Lamb RC, Strauss MB (1983) Gas gangrene II: a 15-Year experience with hyperbaric oxygen. J Trauma 23:995-1000 .

36. Hearty W, Schelling G, Haller M et al. Generalisierte Gasbrandinfektion mit Rhabdomyolyse nach Cholezystektomie. Anaesthesist 1997: 46; 207-210

37. Hedström SA (1975) Differential diagnosis and treatment of gas producing infections. Acta Chir Scand 141: 582-589

38. Heimbach RD (1980) Gas gangrene: review and update. HBO Rev 1:41-61

39. Heimbach RD (1994) Gas gangrene. In: Kindwall (ed): Hyperbaric Medicine Practice. 2nd Ed. Best Publ.Comp. Flagstaff (Az), 1999, Ch.21, pp 549-573

40. Heimbach R. Gas Gangrene. In: Kindwall EP, Whelan HT eds. Hyperbaric Medicine Practice, 2nd ed Best Publishing Company Flagstaff Az. 1999: chapt. 21; 549-573

41. Henry MG (1946) Emergency surgical measures aboard an APA during an amphibious invasion. US Nav Med Bul146:1057

42. Hildanus WF (1914) (reprinted 1968) Ausgewählte observationes. In: Schaefer RJ (ed): Klassiker der Medizin, Vol. 11. Leipzig: Barth

43. Hill GB, Osterhout S (1966) In vitro and in vivo experimental effects of hyperbaric oxygen on Clostridium perfringens. In: Brown IW, Cox BG (eds): Proc Third International Conference on Hyperbaric Medicine, pub11404, Washington DC: National Academy of Science, National Research Council, p 538

44. Hill GB, Osterhout S (1971) Experimental effects of hyperbaric oxygen on selected clostridial species.I.In vitro studies. J Infect Dis 115: 17-15

45. Hippocrates (1983) Hippocratic writings.In: Lloyd GER (ed): Epidemics book I. Middlesex: Penguin Classics, pp 108-109

46. Hirn M (1993) Hyperbaric oxygen in the treatment of gas gangrene and perineal necrotizing fasciitis. A clinical and experimental study. Eur J Surg (Suppl) 570: 9-36

47. Hitchcock CR, Haglin JJ, Arnar O (1967) Treatment of clostridial infections with hyperbaric oxygen. Surgery 61:759-769

48. Jantsch H, Barton P, Függer R et al. (1991) Sonographic demonstration of septicaemia with gasforming organisms after liver transplantation. Clin Radiol 43: 397- 399

49. Kaye D. Effect of hyperbaric oxygen on clostridia in vitro and in vivo. Proc Soc Exp Biol Med 1967: 124; 360-366.

50. Kellett CE (1939) The early history of gas gangrene. Ann Med Hist, pp 452-459

51. Kelley HG, Pace WG. Treatment of anaerobic infections in mice with hyperpressure oxygen. Surg Forum 1963: 14; 46-47.

52. Kiranow IG (1980) Inkubationsperiode der anaeroben Gasbrand-infektion. Unfallheil-kunde 83:76-79

53. Kivisaari J, Niinikoski J. Use of silastic tube and capillary sampling technique in the measurement of tissue pO_2 and pCO_2. Am J Surg 1973: 125; 623-627.

54. Klopper PJ. Hyperbaric oxygen treatment after ligation of the hepatic artery in rabbits. In: Boerema I, Brummelkamp WH, Meijne NG, eds. Clinical application of hyperbaric oxygen. Proceedings of the First International Congress on Hyperbaric Medicine. Amsterdam: Elsevier, 1964: 31-35.

55. Korhonen K, Klossner J, Hirn M, Niinikoski J. Management of clostridial gasgangrene and the role of hyperbaric oxygen. Ann Chir Gynecol 1999: 88; 139-142.

56. Krull W (1981) Gaschromatographischer Toxinnachweis im Blut. Presented at the "Arbeitstagung. Die Behandlung der Gasbrandinfektion-Resignation oder neue Ansätze". Kiel, May 9-10

57. Langley FH, Winkelstein LB (1945) Gas gangrene, a study of 96 cases treated in an evacuation hospital. J Am Med Assoc 128: 783- 792

58. Linton DS. The obscure object of knowledge: German military medicine confronts gas gangrene during World War I. Bull Hist Med 2000: 74; 291-316

59. McLeod JW. Variations in the periods of exposure to air and oxygen necessary to kill anaerobic bacteria. Acta Pathol Microbiol Scand 1930: 3(suppl); 255.

60. McLennan JD (1961) The histotoxic clostridial infections of man. Bacteriol Rev 16: 177-276

61. McLennan JD, McFarlane RG (1945) Toxin and antitoxin studies of gas gangrene in man. Lancet ii:301-305

62. Martin PGC (1941) A case illustrating the early onset of gas gangrene. J R Nav Med Serv 28:388

63. Martin WJ. Gardner M, Washington JA (1972) In vitro antimicrobial susceptibility of anaerobic bacteria isolated from clinical specimens. Antimicrob Agents Chemother 1:148-158

64. Millar WM (1932) Gas gangrene in civil life. Surg Gynecol Obstet 54:232-238

65. Mitton C, Hailey D. Health technology assessment and policy decisions on hyperbaric oxygen treatment. Int J Tech Ass Health Care 1999: 15(4); 661-670

66. Morgan MS. The place of hyperbaric oxygen in the treatment of gas gangrene. Br J Hosp Med 1995: 53(9); 424-426

67. Muhvich KH, Anderson LH, Mehm WJ. Evaluation of antimicrobials combined with hyperbaric oxygen in a mouse model of clostridial myonecrosis. J Trauma 1994: 36(1); 7-10.

68. Nichols RL, Smith JW (1975) Gas in the wound: What does it mean? Surg Clin North Am 55:1289-1296

69. Nier H, Kremer K. Der Gasbrand: Weiterhin ein diagnostisches und therapeutisches Problem. Zentralbl Chir 1984: 109; 402-417.

70. Ninomiya M, Matsushita O, Minami J et al. Role of alpha-toxin in *Clostridium perfringens* infection determined bu using recombinants of *C.Perfringens* and *Bacillus subtilis*. Inf Immun 1994: 62 (11); 5032-5039.

71. Noble WC (1961) The size distribution of airborne particles carrying *Cl. welchii*. J Pathol 81:513

72. Nora PF, Mousavipour M, Laufman H (1966) Mechanism of action of high pressure oxygen in Clostridium perfringens exotoxin toxicity. In: Brown IW Jr, Cox BG (eds): Hyperbaric Medicine Publ 1404 Washington, DC: National Academy of Science. National Research Council, p 565

73. Nora PF, Mousavipour M, Mittlepunkt A et al. (1966) Brain as target organ in *Clostridium perfringens* toxicity. Arch Surg 92: 243- 246

74. Novyi FG (1894) Ein neuer anaerober Bacillus des malignen Oedems. Z Hyg Infekt 17: 209-232

75. O'Brien DK, Melville SB. The anaerobic pathogen *Clostridium perfringens* can escape the phagosome of macrophages under aerobic conditions. Cell Microbiol 2000: 2(6); 505-519

76. Pailler JL, Labeau F. La gangrène gazeuse : Une affection militaire ? Acta Chir Belg 1986 : 86 ; 63.

77. Palomba P, Schacht U (1974) Das Gasödem bei durchblutungsgestörten Extremitäten (Hyperbare Sauerstofftherapie). Aktuel Chir 9: 67-70

78. Pasteur L (1861) Animal infusoria living in the absence of free oxygen and the fermentations they bring about. Animacules infusoires vivant sans gaz oxygène libre et determinant des fermentations. CR Acad Sci 52:344-347.

79. Rifkind D (1963) The diagnosis and treatment of gas gangrene. Surg Clin North Am 43:511-517

80. Roding B, Groeneveld PHA, Boerema I (1972) Ten years of experience in the treatment of gas gangrene with hyperbaric oxygen. Surg Gynecol Obstet 134:579-585

81. Roggentin T, Kleineidam RG, Majewski DM et al. (1993) An immuno assay for the rapid and specific detection of three sialidase-producing clostridia causing gas gangrene. J Immunol Methods 157: 125-133

82. Roloff D (1991) Voraussetzungen für die Verlegung Gasbrandkranker in eine spezialisierte Einrichtung. Anaesthesiol Reanimat 16: 49-58

83. Roloff D. Gasbrandinfektionen im Kindesalter – Eine übersicht. Pädiatr Grenzgeb 1991: 30 (3); 193-203

84. Rudge FW. The role of hyperbaric oxygenation in the treatment of clostridial myonecrosis. Mil Med 1993: 58 (2); 80-83

85. Savill (1916) X-ray appearances in gas gangrene.Arch Radiol Electroth 21: 201

86. Scheven M. Nachweis von Clostridium perfringens aus mischinfiziertem Patientenmaterial mittels modifizierten reversen CAMP-test. Z gesammte Hyg 1991: 37(2); 90-91.

87. Schoemaker G (1964) Oxygen tension measurements under hyperbaric conditions. In: Boerema I, Brummelkamp WH, Meijne NG (eds). Clinical application of hyperbaric oxygen. New York: Elsevier, pp 330-335

88. Schott H (1979) Die Gasbrand Infektion (Prinzipien der Behandlung,Ergebnisse). Hefte zur Unfall 138:179-186

89. Sheffield PJ (1988) Tissue oxygen measurements. In: Davis JC, Hunt TK (eds). Problem wounds: the role of oxygen. New York: Elsevier, pp 37-44

90. Simmonds M (1915) Gasembolie bei Sauerstoffinjektion. Münch Med Wochenschr 19:662.

91. Smolle-Jüttner FM, Pinter H, Neuhold K-H et al. Hyperbare Chirurgie und Sauerstofftherapie der clostridialen Myonekrose. Wien Klin Woch 1995: 107(23); 739-741

92. Stephens MB. Gas Gangrene. Potential for hyperbaric oxygen therapy. Postgrad Med 1996: 99(4); 217-224

93. Stevens DL, Troyer BE, Merrick DT et al. Lethal effects and cardiovascular effects of purified alpha- and theta-toxins from *Clostridium perfringens*. J Inf Dis 1988: 157; 272-279.

94. Stevens DL, Bryant AE, Adams K, Mader JT. Evaluation of therapy with hyperbaric oxygen for experimental infection with *Clostridium perfringen*. Clin Infect Dis 1993 ;17:231-237

95. Stevens DL, Bryant AE. Role of α-toxin, a Sulfhydryl-activated Cytolysin, in the pathogenesis of clostridial gas gangrene. Clin Inf Dis 1993: 16(suppl 4); S195-199.

96. Stevens DL, Tweten RK, Awad MM et al. Clostridial gas gangrene: Evidence that alpha- and theta-toxins differentially modulate the immune response and induce acute tissue necrosis. J Inf Dis 1997: 176; 189-195.

97. Stevens DL, Bryant AE. Pathogenesis of *Clostridium perfringens* Infection: Mechanisms and mediators of shock. Clin Inf Dis 1997: 25(suppl 2); S160-164

98. Stevens DL. The pathogenesis of clostridial myonecrosis. Int J Med Microbiol 2000: 290; 497-502

99. Tibbles PM, Edelsberg JS. Hyperbaric-oxygen therapy. Review article. N Eng J Med 1996: 334(25); 1642-1648

100. Unsworth lP (1976) High-dose penicillin and gas gangrene. Lancet ii : 417

101. Van Beek A, Zook E, Yaw P et al. (1974) Non-clostridial gasforming infections. Arch Surg 108:552

102. Van Unnik AJM (1965) Inhibition of toxin production in *Clostridium perfringens* in vitro by hyperbaric oxygen. Antonie van Leeuwenhoek 31: 181-186.

103. Vreeken J (1984) Verlenging van de bloedingstijd door gebruik van antibiotica. Ned Tijdschr Geneesk 128:1480-1481

104. Walsh JF (1980) Interaction of drugs in the hyperbaric environment. Bethesda: Undersea Medical Society

105. Weinstein WM, Onderdonk AD, Bartlett JG et al. (1975) Antimicrobial therapy of experimental intra-abdominal sepsis. J Infect Dis 132: 282-286

106. Welch WH, Nuttall GH (1892) A gas producing bacillus capable of rapid development in the blood vessels after death. Bull Johns Hop Hosp 3: 81-91

107. Whitby L, Hynes M (1961) The clostridia of gas gangrene. In: Medical bacteriology, 7th ed. London: Churchill Ltd, pp 300- 307

108. Williamson ED, Titball RW. A genetically engineered vaccine against alpha-toxin of *Clostridium perfringens* protects mice against experimental gas gangrene. Vaccine 1993: 11(12); 1253-1258

109. Willis AT (1969) Clostridia of wound infection. London: Butterworth

110. Zierott G, May E, Harms H (1973) Changes in the evaluation and therapy of gas edema through the administration of hyperbaric oxygenation. A clinical comparative study of 31 cases of gas edema. Bruns Beitr Klin Chir 220:292-296

NOTES

CHAPTER 12

HYPERBARIC OXYGEN THERAPY IN THE MANAGEMENT OF NON-HEALING WOUNDS

D. Mathieu

INTRODUCTION

A chronic (non-healing) wound or the so-called "problem wound" is defined as any wound which fails to heal within a reasonable period by the use of conventional medical or surgical methods (1).

As defined, this is a common clinical situation, which induces multiple medical visits, prolonged hospitalization, and fastidious nursing care. Its economic and social cost is largely unknown but is surely enormous.

In this chapter, we will consider mainly non-healing wounds, located in the lower limb, even if most of the concepts exposed may be applied to any non-healing wound. Healing problems due to burn, cold, radiation, or toxin injury are discussed in others chapters.

PATHOPHYSIOLOGICAL BASES OF HEALING PROCESS IMPAIRMENT

Healing is a highly integrated biological process resulting from several separated but related steps (Table 1). In order for a wound to heal, haemostatic and inflammatory mechanisms must be intact, mesenchymal cells must migrate to and proliferate in the wounded area, angiogenesis and epithelialization must occur, and collagen must be synthesized, cross linked, and aligned properly to provide strength to the healed area. In open wounds, contraction must take place as well. All these processes must occur in proper sequence and time for optimal wound healing (2, 3).

The non-healing wound is a result of an impairment of one or more of these processes. Multiple factors may lead to impaired healing. They can be classified as intrinsic, or local, factors which are characteristics of the wound itself and extrinsic, or constitutional which are characteristics of the patient (Table 2) (1). Many of these factors are related and most of the extrinsic factors act through intrinsic changes.

TABLE 1. NORMAL WOUND HEALING PROCESS

A normal wound healing response (type non-closed skin incision) can be divided in different phases:

Day 0	Haemostasis	• vascular contraction • platelet aggregation and degranulation • fibrin formation (thrombus)
Day 0 – 3	Inflammatory phase	• vascular exudation • neutrophil infiltration • monocyte conversion to macrophage • matrix enrichment in proteoglycans
Day 3 – 6	Proliferative phase	• angiogenesis • fibroblast infiltration and proliferation • collagen formation
Day 3 – 15	Remodelling phase	• vascular maturation • fibroblast conversion to fibrocyte • collagen degradation and formation

TABLE 2. FACTORS THAT IMPAIR HEALING

Intrinsic Factors	Extrinsic Factors
Infection	Hereditary healing disorders
Foreign bodies	Nutritional deficiencies
Ischemia	Distant malignancies
Cigarette smoking	Old age
Venous insufficiency	Diabetes
Radiation	Jaundice
Mechanical trauma	Alcoholism
Local toxins	Uraemia
Cancer	Glucocorticoid steroids
	Chemotherapeutic agents
	Other medications

The most commonly involved factors for impaired healing are ischemia and infection.

Infection increases the inflammatory process, inducing wound hypoxia through high oxygen consumption and local blood flow impairment due to tissue edema. The inflammatory phase is prolonged, delaying the whole healing process. Collagen deposition, epithelialization, and contraction do not occur or occur in a very limited fashion (4, 5).

Ischemia is another common factor in non-healing wound, resulting in tissue hypoxia, a pivotal characteristic of healing limitation or arrest. Oxygen is required for aerobic metabolism and energy production. Although anaerobic metabolism is possible in a hypoxic wound environment, the quantity of energy that can be generated by this mechanism is inadequate for normal healing (6).

The rate of fibroblast proliferation is likewise influenced by the oxygen concentration (7). Oxygen is also required for hydroxylation of lysine and proline during collagen synthesis (8). Without adequate hydroxylation, collagen thermal stability is significantly impaired, leading to diminished wound strength. The overall rate of collagen synthesis has also been demonstrated to be inhibited *in vitro* by hypoxia (9). The only aspect of healing facilitated by hypoxia is the induction of angiogenesis (10), but correct maturation of the new capillary network requires a normal oxygen tissue pressure.

Hypoxia impairs healing in several wound models. Niinikoski first demonstrated that collagen accumulated in cellulose sponges in rats at a rate correlated with inspired oxygen tension (7), and Hunt and Pai obtained similar results using a wound cylinder model (11). Stephens and Hunt showed that the tensile strength of incision wounds varied with inspired oxygen tension (12).

In addition to its direct effect on wound healing biology, hypoxia also impairs the body's defense mechanisms against bacterial invasion. Oxygen is required by neutrophils for the creation of oxygen free radicals that kill bacteria (13). The susceptibility of wounds to infection was found to directly correlate with oxygen concentration in two experimental models (4, 14).

RATIONALE FOR HYPERBARIC OXYGEN THERAPY IN NON-HEALING WOUND MANAGEMENT

Evidence that HBO May Correct Tissue Hypoxia

If wound hypoxia is the cause of healing failure, then to provide oxygen is an aetiological treatment. Hyperbaric oxygen increases tissue oxygen pressures by increasing arterial oxygen pressure (PaO_2). Using the Krogh's mathematical model (15), oxygen partial pressure in any point of a tissue may be predicted in relation to the distance of this point to the capillary and to the oxygen pressure over the whole length of the capillary. Factors that influence capillary oxygen pressure are tissue oxygen consumption, capillary blood flow, intercapillary distance, and arterial oxygen pressure. If the Krogh's model is applied to the hyperbaric condition, when arterial oxygen pressure is increased from 100 torr (with the patient breathing air at atmospheric pressure) to 2000 torr (with the patient breathing pure oxygen at 3 atm abs), there is a corresponding fourfold increase in the oxygen diffusion distance at the capillary arterial end and a twofold increase at the venous end.

These theoretical predictions were confirmed experimentally by Hunt (16), Hunt and Pai (11), Kivisaari and Niinikoski (17), and Niinikoski and Hunt (18) who demonstrated by direct tissue oxygen measurements using a tonometric technique via silastic tube implantation that tissue oxygen pressure is increased from 50 torr to over 400 torr during an HBO therapy session at 2 atm abs.

Using the Krogh's model, it is possible to predict the ability of HBO to increase tissue oxygen pressure in different kinds of hypoxia: increase in intercapillary distance such as in edema, vascular destruction as in infection, or radionecrosis. However, in all these situations HBO is only able to increase tissue oxygen pressure provided that local circulation has not completely disappeared. This point is important to consider because it is from that remaining local blood flow that the oxygen reaches the target area.

Evidence that HBO May Favor the Healing Process

The rationale for using HBO in non-healing wounds has been regularly reviewed (19-22) and may be summarized as follows:

- HBO corrects wound hypoxia by increasing blood content in dissolved oxygen, by reallocating blood flow to hypoxic areas due to the hyperoxic vasoconstriction in normal tissue (23), by favorizing microcirculatory blood flow in increasing red blood cell deformability (24).
- HBO enhances cell metabolism (25), preserves intracellular adenosine triphosphate content (26), decreases oxidative cell aggression (27).
- HBO stimulates fibroblast proliferation (28, 29) and extracellular matrix synthesis (30), increases collagen formation and deposition (7, 28), promotes more rapid growth of capillaries and formation of functional microcirculatory network (31, 32).
- HBO reduces edema formation (33) and increases wound tensile strength (32).
- HBO reduces wound infection by its direct effect on anaerobic bacteria and its indirect effect in enhancing the microbicidal ability of polymorphonuclears (5).

However, two points are important to consider:

The effect of oxygen pressure on healing processes varies according to the phase. Hypoxia is a potent stimulus for the initial events: secretion of angiogenetic factors, migration of fibroblasts, induction of procollagen synthesis. Alternatively, a normal oxygen pressure is needed to obtain formation of a normal capillary network (32), proliferation and maturation of fibroblasts (7, 34), formation of a mechanically resistant collagen (7, 32). In that respect, alternance of hypoxic and hyperoxic periods as realized during an HBO treatment given in repeated HBO sessions may be of a particular interest for optimizing healing processes.

HBO only acts as a corrective measure on some factors involved in the healing impairment. It exerts its positive effects only in ischemic wounds and had no effect on the healing of a normal wound (35). It cannot be looked at as the unique therapeutic measures but has to be integrated in the whole management of the patient.

Evidence that HBO May Be Clinically Effective in the Treatment of Non-healing Wounds

HBO has been used in multiple types of wounds and ulcers (36). In many of those, HBO efficacy has been reported only in anecdotal reports and following the Evidence Based Medicine methodology, the level of evidence on which is based the recommendation to use HBO is often too low. Efforts to raise this level are urgently needed.

Central to the indication of HBO is tissue hypoxia as the main or as an important factor in the delayed healing.

Ulcer Due to Arterial Insufficiency

Peripheral vascular disease (PVD) is a common cause of non-healing ulcers. The most common cause of PVD is arteriosclerosis obliterans. Most often, it becomes manifest between the age of 50 to 70 years. Smoking, diabetes, hyperlipemia, and familial history are the main risk factors. It produces segmented narrowing or obstruction of the lumen in the arteries supplying the lower limb, which leads to tissue hypoxia. Ulcers are the key mark of the 4th stage in the Fontaine's classification and are an imperative finding to consider revascularization procedure.

Thrombo-angiitis obliterans is a less frequent cause of PVD, which predominates between the ages of 20 to 40 years. It causes arterial obstruction by segmental inflammatory and proliferative lesions of the medium and small vessels of the lower limb. The aetiology is unknown, but there is a strong association with cigarette smoking.

Some studies have been published reporting favorable results but good randomized controlled studies are still lacking (37-39).

In our own experience, provided that HBO can increase $TCPO_2$ above 50 torr, all patients healed with an average number of 46 HBO sessions (40). In that respect, HBO may be considered for a non-healing ulcer:

- When no possibility of revascularization is possible.
- In association with a revascularization procedure (either surgical or endovascular) in case of infected ulcer.

Diabetic Foot Ulceration

Diabetic foot ulceration (DFU) is a major complication, which affects 4 to 10 percent of the diabetic population (41, 42). As such, foot problems represent one of the most common reasons for hospital admission among diabetic patients. Despite numerous prevention and treatment protocols in the last two decades, the rate of lower extremity amputation is 15 times greater in diabetic patients than compared with non-diabetic patients (43). More over, 50 percent of the diabetic amputees may require an amputation of the contralateral limb during the first four years after an amputation of the first limb (44).

Beside the human cost, economic cost is also very high. Hospitalization for amputation in a diabetic patient has been estimated to a mean direct cost of 18,000 Euros and a mean duration of 42 days (45).

Pathophysiology of Diabetic Foot Ulceration

Sensory neuropathy, ischemia, and infection are the principal pathogenic factors in DFU (46).

Peripheral neuropathy has a central role and is present in more than 80 percent of diabetic patients with foot lesions (47). In most cases, ulceration is a consequence of the loss of protective sensation allowing small injuries to often go unnoticed (48, 49). However, the most common mechanism appears to be unperceived, excessive, and repetitive pressure on plantar bony prominences, like metatarsal heads (50). That explains why non-weight bearing measures are mandatory in the overall treatment of DFU.

Ischemia is the other major factor contributing to DFU. Peripheral vascular disease has a high incidence in diabetic patients and has been shown to be a pathogenic factor in 60 p. cent of diabetic patients with non-healing ulcers and 46 p. cent of those undergoing major amputation (51). Ischemia weakens local defenses against infection because of reduced blood flow and tissue supply in oxygen, essential nutrients and growth factors. Transcutaneous oxygen measurement ($TCPO_2$), but not a reduced ankle-arm blood pressure index, has been shown to be an independent predictor of lesion and a level of 30 mmHg in ambient air is critical in predicting DFU healing (52). Evaluation of revascularisation possibility is therefore mandatory in the overall treatment of DFU.

Infection is a frequent complication favored by neuropathy and ischemia. Its severity may range from a mild, localized infection to a limb-threatening necrotizing process with fasciitis (46). Beside these devastating infections leading often to amputation, bone and joint involvement has been shown to be a factor of delayed healing and subsequent amputation even when ischemia has been relieved by a revascularisation procedure (53).

Clinical Studies

Many factors cause an impaired oxygenation in the diabetic foot (54-56). Measurements of tissue oxygen tensions ($TCPO_2$) in non-healing diabetic wounds showed values far below those where wound healing could be expected. Even breathing 100% O_2 did not raise the $TCPO_2$ enough. Hyperbaric oxygen therapy has been shown to be able to increase tissue O_2 tension in certain diabetic patients with chronic wounds (57, 58). A direct response and a response over time were demonstrated. This HBO-induced increase in $TCPO_2$ has been shown to be predictive for healing success even in the presence of a low $TCPO_2$ in ambient air and a lack of increase in normobaric oxygen (59).

The first study on HBO in DFU treatment was done by Hart et al in 1979 (60) and was followed by several other anecdotal or retrospective studies. Prospective trials were reported by Doctor (61) and Zamboni (62) but the largest prospective, randomized study so far was published by Faglia et al. (63). A total of 70 patients with Wagner grades 2, 3, and 4 were treated; 35 with HBO and 33 without HBO. Variables in patients did not differ significantly in any item of clinical characteristics. The presence of neuropathy and vasculopathy did not differ significantly in both groups. As to the results, in the HBO group there were three major amputations (1 AKA and 2 BKA) which is 8.6%, and in the non-HBO group 11 (4 AKA and 7 BKA) which is 33.3%. The reduction of the amputation relative risk (RR = 0.25) was statistically significant. The significance was highest in the group of patients with a Wagner classification of 4 (2/22 HBO, 11/20 non-HBO).

Considering these evidences, the Jury of the ECHM Consensus Conference on hyperbaric oxygen in the treatment of foot lesion in diabetic patients, held in London, the 4th and 5th of December, 1998, stated (64):

There is some evidence from a number of trials, each of which suffers from methodological problems, to support the use of HBO in ischaemic limb-threatening problems in diabetic patients. This is Level 2 evidence.

A result of the meeting is the recognition of urgent need for a collaborative international trial for the application of HBO in diabetic foot lesions. Patients with diabetic foot problems warrant treatment by foot care teams with careful evaluation of metabolic, neuropathic and vascular factors. Potential candidates for HBO may include those with Wagner grade 3 to 5 lesions treated unsuccessfully by standard methods when amputation seems a possibility.

Pre-treatment evaluation should include an assessment of the probability of its success which might include: TCPO2 & O2 challenge at pressure, assessment of peripheral circulation by invasive /non-invasive methods.

Such a randomized controlled study is currently running in the frame of the European Research Program COST Action B14 (information may be found on the web site: www.oxynet.org).

Venous Stasis Ulcer

Up to 1% of the general population will suffer from a chronic venous ulcer at some point of their lives. Venous stasis ulcer is one of the manifestations of chronic venous insufficiency, which is defined as hypertension involving either the superficial or both the superficial and deep venous system. Edema is frequently associated. Due to the prolonged evolution, this process leads to chronic inflammation and tissue sclerosis. Transcutaneous oxygen measurements and laser Doppler flowmetry have shown decrease in microcirculatory perfusion and tissue hypoxia.

Conventional treatment is generally effective when correctly applied. It includes physical therapy with leg elevation and compression, ulcer dressing, and surgery when indicated.

The role of HBO seems to be very limited. Some authors have reported favorable results (39, 65-67) but it is generally agreed that these ulcers heal without any special HBO treatment. However, a double-blind, randomized study has demonstrated a decrease in the size of chronic leg ulcers that had no healing tendency despite correct treatment (68).

Decubitus Ulcer

The cause of decubitus ulcers is pressure on the skin, which interferes with the circulation at the point of contact. Prolonged rest or immobilization in one position, as with hemiplegics and paraplegics, may lead to this within a few hours. Poor skin hygiene, malnutrition, and debility are contributing factors. These ulcers are usually located over bony prominences such as the sacrum and the heel. The ulcer results from breakdown of the ischemic skin and subsequent bacterial invasion and inflammatory reaction. Persistence of the latter leads to microvascular thrombosis, which further aggravates ischemia.

Conventional treatment includes pressure limiting measures, infection control, and management of secondary contributing factors such as spasticity, skin maceration, and malnutrition.

Th role of HBO is very limited. Eltorai (69) reported a study of 28 patients with a 65 percent success rate. But HBO cannot obviate the nonprescription or the ill application of pressure relief measures.

However, HBO may be used as an adjunct to surgery either for the preparation of patients with infected pressure ulcer or following a skin graft or flap.

Chronic Leg Ulcer in Sickle-cell Anemia

Sickle-cell anemia is consecutive to the presence of high concentrations of hemoglobin-S (70). Clinical manifestations occur mainly in homozygous (SS) patients, and heterozygous patients with another associated abnormal hemoglobin (hemoglobin-C disease, beta-thalassemia). Deoxygenation of this abnormal hemoglobin, acidosis, dehydratation, and temperature variations induce the sickling of erythrocytes. Sickling is responsible of chronic hemolytic anemia, and of three kinds of acute events: thrombosis, infections, and paroxysmal anemia. Oxygen transport is also impaired, because hemoglobin-S has a lower affinity for oxygen than hemoglobin A. P50 of hemoglobin-S is high and the mild hypoxemia found in sickle-cell anemia is related to a low oxygen saturation and a low oxygen arterial content (71).

Sickle-cell anemia is responsible for chronic alteration of various organs: brain, lungs, liver, kidneys, eyes, and skin. Legs ulcers are known to be very difficult to treat using conventional therapies (71). HBO has been proposed in order to increase oxygen tissue delivery (72).

Medhaoui (73) reported a study in 15 patients, all homozygous SS, presenting 23 ulcers. The average session number was 11 ± 9. Healing was obtained in all patients but recurrence occurred in eight patients.

MANAGEMENT OF A PATIENT WITH A NON-HEALING WOUND

An accurate diagnosis of all the factors impairing healing is a prerequisite for the success of the treatment in a non-healing wound. This means that a patient referred to a hyperbaric center for a non-healing wound has to under go an extensive evaluation, if not made previously.

Management of Factors Impairing the Healing Process

Once the contributory factors have been identified, treatment can be instituted. Benefit may be derived from improved management of contributing factors, even though the primary disease cannot be cured. For example, diabetes will benefit from careful dietary management and infection may respond to optimal treatment. Once local conditions have been optimized, some wounds will heal by secondary intention. This emphasizes the need to correctly select patients for HBO after an extensive evaluation and an opti-mization of the treatment. HBO alone may be a futile treatment if not inte-grated in the whole management of the patient.

Local Wound Management

Optimal local wound management depends on the nature of the wound (Table 3) (74). Surgical debridement is indicated for wounds contain-ing non-viable tissue, or foreign material. For infected wounds, the goal of treatment is to decrease the bacterial count of the wound tissue without any disequilibrium in the bacterial flora, or selection of multiresistant strains. It has been shown that systemic antibiotics are not effective to lower bacterial counts and must not be prescribed except in the case of surrounding cellulitis or bone/joint infection.

Topical agents with antibacterial activity have been utilized for a long time but evidence of efficacy are not many and some agents have been shown to cause cell toxicity. Dressing must be chosen in order to provide an optimal healing milieu. This is based principally on the manipulation of hydration and oxygen tension within the wound. Because of their high water content and their liquefying properties, hydrogels are preferred for wounds where there exist large desiccated areas or scabs not easily removed by mechanical detersion. Hydrocolloids are indicated when large areas covered by fibrinous exudates persist. Film or gauze is used on clean and well-granulating wounds.

Patient Management

Nutritional status is a key factor for healing. A deficiency in protein intake will impair collagen synthesis and alter cellular functions. Inadequate intake of carbohydrate or fat slows all normal metabolic function and diverts proteins from cell synthesis to cell energy supply. Selective deficiencies in vitamins or minerals may also impair various aspects of healing. Correction of nutritional deficiencies must be obtained as improvement in nutritional status has been demonstrated to reverse malnutrition-induced healing defects.

Cessation of smoking or alcoholic intemperance must also be empha-sized even if it is usually not often obtained. Discontinuation of drugs impairing the healing process such as glucocorticoid steroids or chemo-therapy agents must also be considered if allowed by the patient's condition.

TABLE 3. WOUND CARE STRATEGY

- Deal with underlying pathology (including infection)
- Cleanse and debride wound
- Determine wound type, depth, and degree of exudation
- Absorb exudation by appropriate dressing
- Occlude the wound as soon as possible
- Appose the wound edges as soon as possible (in healing by primary intention)

Metabolic control of diabetes is an important goal to achieve. Diabetic patients are particularly at risk for wound healing complications and infection that may induce uncontrolled hyperglycemia. On the other hand, uncontrolled diabetes has been demonstrated to impair wound healing. Thus, reinforcement of dietetic measures and switching to insulin are often required.

Constant effort is required to eliminate or reduce pressure on wound areas. In many cases, undue pressure on insensible areas induces wounds that do not heal as long as the pressure is not relieved (diabetic patient with neuropathic foot lesion, pressure ulcers). Non-weight-bearing measures are mandatory in the management of these patients.

Venous insufficiency has to be taken into account. Persistent venous hypertension and its consequences are often the cause of non-healing ulcers. Proper evaluation is required in order to evaluate surgical possibilities. Edema control has been shown helpful in obtaining healing in this setting.

Arterial insufficiency is a major factor inducing healing impairment and has to be looked at in any patient with a non-healing wound. Patient history, physical and Doppler examinations have to be analyzed in respect to potential surgical indication. Rest pain, disabling claudications, and non-healing wounds are indications to consider surgery in these patients. An arteriogram is required and will provide necessary information regarding the surgical or endoluminal revascularization possibilities. If possible, revascularization must always be realized prior or associated with HBO.

Selection of Patients for HBO Therapy

The use of HBO in non-healing wounds is based on the assumption that wound tissues are hypoxic and this hypoxia is the major factor impairing healing. The validity of this assumption has been largely demonstrated and commonly accepted indications of HBO include diabetic foot lesion, arterial ulcer, skin graft and flap, and radionecrosis.

However, in all these situations, conventional therapy as exposed above may have a certain rate of success and the need for HBO becomes less evident. Therefore, objective criteria to select patients for HBO are needed.

Rationale for Using Transcutaneous Oxygen Pressure Measurements for Selecting HBO-prescribed Cases

Tissue hypoxia is the common denominator for numerous HBO indications. Tissue hypoxia has to be corrected during the HBO session to get consequent beneficial effects for healing or defense against infection. Therefore, selecting a patient for HBO needs to demonstrate the tissue hypoxia and its correction using HBO.

Although the advantages of measuring oxygen pressure during hyperbaric sessions are generally accepted, the invasive (arterial puncture, implanting of electrodes) and complex (radioactive oxygen, magnetic resonance imaging) nature of such measurements has this far dissuaded physicians from carrying out direct measurements of tissue oxygen pressure. Transcutaneous oxygen measurement is a non-invasive method and represents an opportunity whose application to HBO therapy is rich in possibilities (75).

Transcutaneous Oxygen Pressure Measurements

History

At the beginning of the 1950s, Baumberger and Goodfriend (76) showed that when a subject immersed his finger in a buffer solution heated to 45°C, the partial oxygen pressure of this solution became, within 60 min, the same as the subject's arterial pressure. Some years later, Clark (77, 78) developed a polarographic electrode capable of measuring partial oxygen pressure in the blood both *in vitro* and *in vivo*. Huch (79, 80) adapted Clark's electrode to measure $TCPO_2$ with the aim of evaluating arterial oxygen pressure in a non-invasive way. Monitoring PaO_2 by measuring $TCPO_2$ is presently a widespread practice in neonatology (81, 83), but has not been extended to adult medicine given the numerous factors that exist in the $PaO_2/TCPO_2$ relationship.

In intensive care units it was quickly realized that a drop in $TCPO_2$ could be related either to a drop in PaO_2 or to a drop in blood flow rate (84). This eliminated $TCPO_2$ as a non-invasive method for monitoring PaO_2. However, Shoemaker and Vidyssagar (85) drew attention to the interest of $TCPO_2$ as an indicator of overall blood flow. Measurement of $TCPO_2$ or $TCPO_2/PaO_2$ gradient has been used in evaluating the peripheral circulatory state either in shock (86-88) or during localized ischemia such as in arterial trauma (89), peripheral vascular disease (90-93), musculocutaneous flap and graft (94, 95), and more recently, in hyperbaric medicine (96-99).

Technique

Transcutaneous oxygen pressure measurement uses a Clark's polarographic electrode modified to incorporate a heating element and a thermistor. The principle of the measurement is based on an electrochemical reduction at the cathode.

The current generated by oxygen reduction is proportional to the number of oxygen molecules entering in the chamber between anode and cathode. The heating element maintains a constant temperature between 42°C and 44°C under thermistor monitoring (Figure 1). A phosphate-buffered potassium chloride solution ensures contact between the surface of the electrode and the oxygen-pervious membrane. The electrode is fixed to the skin via an adhesive ring filled with a contact solution (Figure 2). When the electrode is heated, heat is transferred to the surface of the underlying skin. This has three effects: a vasodilatation of arterioles and capillaries located immediately beneath the electrode, an increase in the size of cutaneous pores, and a better oxygen permeability of the stratum corneum, all these effects decreasing the obstacle to oxygen transcutaneous diffusion.

Transcutaneous oxygen pressure measurement has several advantages: It is a non-invasive method that gives good patient compliance; it is easy to use; and it can be repeated at several points without bacterial contamination. However, the method has several limitations. Skin properties influence $TCPO_2$ measurements because of differences in skin oxygen permeability (localization, thickness) or in oxygen consumption (sudation). Heating is critical because there is a constant relationship between the

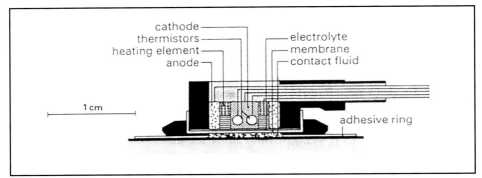

Figure 1. Diagram of a TCPO$_2$ Electrode

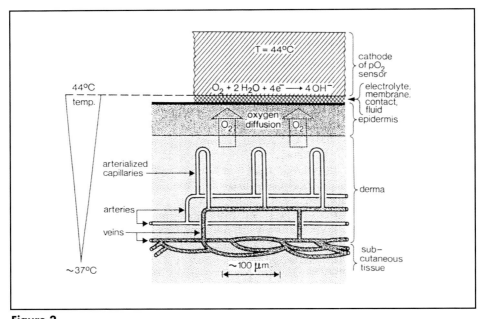

Figure 2.

Cross section of skin showing the oxygen diffusion path from dermal capillaries to measurement chamber of TCPO$_2$ electrode.

electrode temperature and the recorded TCPO$_2$. Heating also modifies skin properties in particular in inducing a vasodilatation and in increasing oxygen permeability. Temperature profiles created in tissue by heating may be different from one site or from one subject to another, leading to false difference between TCPO$_2$. Mechanical pressure onto the electrode also alters TCPO$_2$ producing a drop in recorded value. Anaesthetic gases may affect TCPO$_2$. Finally, electrode response time influences the time that needs to be waited before reading. All theses factors have to be taken into account before interpreting a TCPO$_2$ value; in particular, these parameters have to be reported: heating temperature, site of measurement, TCPO$_2$ value at a reference site (usually subclavicular area), and time allowed before reading.

Measurement in Hyperbaric Environment

Before taking any measurement, the electrode must undergo strict calibration. Ordinary calibration in the ambient environment assuming that atmospheric PO_2 is 150 torr, as is usually advised by manufacturers, is grossly insufficient in hyperbaric medicine. Although electrode response has been checked to be linear in a range between 0 and 2000 torr, inaccurate calibration may lead to major error when high oxygen pressure is used. The one-point calibration technique has to be rejected, because the electrode response line cannot be fixed. We use a two-point calibration technique: zero adjustment is done using pure nitrogen with the electrode in a calibration chamber. Electrical zero is not sufficient. The second calibration point is determined using a calibration gas with 22% oxygen. The calibration is checked by measuring the oxygen pressure in a third gas with a known percentage of oxygen.

In our practice this procedure takes approximately 30 min for simultaneous calibration of ten electrodes and is carried out after each new electrode preparation (approximately once a week). On the other days calibration is only checked by measuring the oxygen pressure of the standard gas. If there is any significant discrepancy, the whole calibration process is repeated.

With regard to $TCPO_2$ measurement, selected areas are carefully shaven, cleaned, and degreased. A double-sided fixation ring is placed on the chosen spot and the electrode attached after application of an electrolytic contact solution. Sensors are placed near the wound and at different levels of the limbs. The heating temperature is set to 43.5°C. A reference electrode is placed on the upper front part of the thorax. Simultaneous readings are made after equilibration (the length of time depending on the oxygen inhaled pressure, usually 10-15 min at 2.5 atm abs). Measurements are performed under three successive conditions: patient breathing normal air, normobaric pure oxygen by facial mask, and pure oxygen at 2.5 atm abs in the hyperbaric chamber.

The use of $TCPO_2$ measurements in hyperbaric oxygen raises some specific problems. One problem is the electrical safety when the device is brought in the chamber. This is best solved by leaving the electronic device outside the chamber, the probes being connected by special wires passed through the chamber wall. A second problem is that high $TCPO_2$ cannot be recorded, because the display window is limited to three digits or is misinterpreted by the software that sends an over range error message. To obviate this difficulty it is often advised to do a calibration at mid-scale (i.e., to set the 150 torr point at 75 torr recording). Unfortunately, this significantly increases the uncertainty in the high PO_2 range. Because the Clark's electrode has a linear response even at these high values, a specific electronic and/or software adaptation has to be made to allow measurements over 1000 torr. Unfortunately, few manufacturers have marketed this hyperbaric adaptation.

Interpreting Transcutaneous Oxygen Pressure Measurement

Many studies have been reported that allow interpretation of $TCPO_2$ measurement. In patients with both normal cardiac output and cutaneous circulation, $TCPO_2$ gives a reliable indication of PaO_2, but correlation reduces with age. The $TCPO_2/PaO_2$ ratio is equal to 1.0 in a newborn child and 0.79 in a young adult. This estimation of arterial oxygen pressure via $TCPO_2$ is commonly used in neonatology (81, 83).

In adults, on the other hand, numerous factors interfere in the $PaO_2/TCPO_2$ relationship. Local skin properties and blood flow are especially important (101). No direct comparison may be done between absolute values of $TCPO_2$ taken in two different sites on the same subject or between two different subjects. However, given that the subject has a normal PaO_2, and that measurements are done in the same site, $TCPO_2$ is a reliable index of local blood flow (102).

An unusually low $TCPO_2$ may be due to a cutaneous vasoconstriction (hypovolemia, vasoconstricting drugs, cold environment, etc.) or to insufficient heating of the electrode. On the other hand, a too-high heating temperature will induce a phlycten, which decreases the $TCPO_2$. An unusually high $TCPO_2$ would indicate that the electrode has become loose and displayed PO_2 is the ambient one, or that a gas bubble was formed when the electrode was being prepared or during decompression.

Protocol for Patient Selection

In our center we follow this protocol for patient selection in cases of problem wounds (Figure 3):

1. Transcutaneous oxygen pressures are first recorded in atmospheric air. The patient is lying on his back, comfortably installed, in a medium-warm environment (22-24°C). Measurements are done at least at three sites: subclavicular area for reference, close to the wound, and contralaterally in a mirror-like fashion. Electrode calibration is checked before each test in measuring oxygen concentration in a standard gas. Probe heating is set up to 43.5°C.

    a. $TCPO_2$ at the reference site has to be over 50 torr. If not, examination has to be done to rule out a technical problem (electrode calibration, skin preparation and electrode fixation, heating, mechanical pressure, etc.). Then patient condition has to be checked: previous lung or heart disease, skin vasoconstriction (cold, stress, drug, etc.), hypovolemia (particularly in acute conditions such as crush syndrome or limb ischemia). Arterial blood gas determination may be necessary. After careful examination, supplemental oxygen may be needed to get a sufficient level of $TCPO_2$ at the reference site.

    b. $TCPO_2$ at the wound site is recorded after a sufficient time to allow equilibrium (5-10 min in atmospheric air).

      i. $TCPO_2$ at the wound site is normal or slightly decreased ($TCPO_2$ > 20 torr). Tissue hypoxia is not the main cause of the lesion and HBO is not indicated, at least for oxygen supplementation; it may be indicated because of another effect (i.e., anaerobic infection).

      ii. $TCPO_2$ at the wound site is reduced (< 20 torr). Tissue hypoxia is present in normal conditions. Then the patient undergoes compression up to 2.5 atm abs.

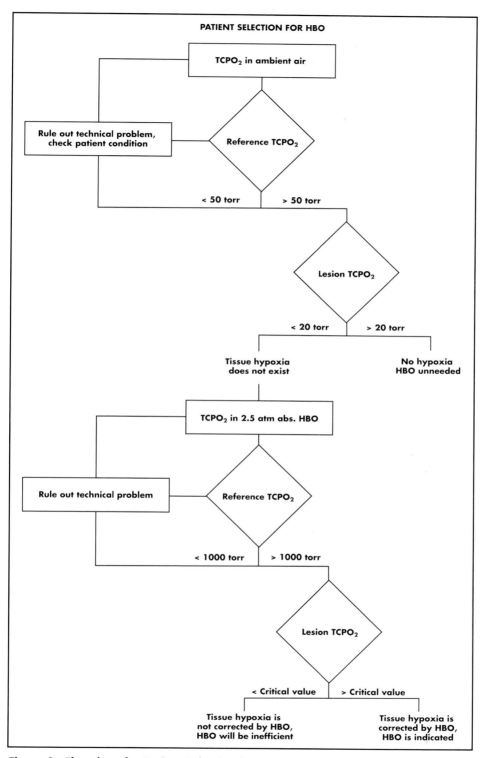

Figure 3. Flowchart for Patient Selection for HBO Using TCPO$_2$

2. Transcutaneous oxygen pressure is then recorded, patient breathing pure oxygen at 2.5 atm abs. Measurement is done in the same three sites. For the best, three different electrodes and devices have to be used to avoid any variation in the technical part of the measurement. After compression and oxygen breathing, the patient is allowed some time to be comfortably accustomed to the hyperbaric ambience.

   a. $TCPO_2$ at the reference site has to be over 1000 torr. Of course, on a theoretical basis, $TCPO_2$ should be over 1800 torr, but because of hyperoxic vasoconstriction, mean reference values are between 1000 and 1200 torr with a trend to be lower in elderly patients. If low $TCPO_2$ is obtained, mask congruity first has to be checked. Then a blister formation induced by electrode heating has to be ruled out.

   b. $TCPO_2$ at the wound site is recorded after equilibrium has been reached (10-15 min slightly longer than in atmospheric air).

   i. $TCPO_2$ at the wound site increases and overpasses a critical level depending on the indication. The HBO will induce a normalization of tissue oxygen pressure and then will exert its healing effects. This situation may be considered as a good indication for HBO.

   ii. $TCPO_2$ does not increase or insufficiently increases tissue oxygen pressure. Tissue hypoxia will not be corrected by HBO and there is no justification for use of HBO in this case.

Critical TCPO$_2$ Values for HBO Patient Selection

Based on our experience, we have tried to determine critical values of $TCPO_2$ for HBO patient selection in different clinical settings (Table 4). We report here these values together with the clinical background on which they have been based.

Refractory Arterial Skin Ulcer (40)

A total of 20 patients with arterial skin ulcer persistent after proper medical treatment were evaluated. $TCPO_2$ measured close to the ulcer did not differ according to outcome (healing or failure) in atmospheric air or normobaric oxygen.

TABLE 4. CRITICAL VALUES OF TCPO$_2$ IN HBO

Arterial trauma	20 mmHg
Musculocutaneous flap	50 mmHg
Arterial ulcer	50 mmHg
Diabetic foot lesion	100 mmHg

Note: Failure of HBO treatment is highly probable if $TCPO_2$ measured in HBO (2.5 atm abs. pure oxygen) near the lesion is lower than these critical values.

A $TCPO_2$ of less than 50 torr when breathing pure oxygen at 2.5 atm abs is constantly associated with failure, whereas $TCPO_2$ over l00 torr in HBO is consistent with success.

Diabetic Foot Lesion (102)

A total of 38 patients with diabetic foot lesions were evaluated. $TCPO_2$ measured close to the wound did not differ according to outcome (healing or failure) in atmospheric air or normobaric oxygen. $TCPO_2$ in HBO (2.5 atm abs) is significantly higher in patients who heal than in patients who do not. In contrast, with patients with arterial ulcer, $TCPO_2$ of less than 100 torr is specifically associated with failure. Such a difference in critical $TCPO_2$ level demonstrates that local ischemia is not the sole factor in the resistance to healing of diabetic foot lesions.

Musculocutaneous Skin Flap (103)

A total of 15 patients with pedicle musculocutaneous flap were evaluated by clinical examination and $TCPO_2$ measurements; 12 had clinical evidence of total flap ischemia and 3 of partial flap ischemia. In ambient air neither absolute value of $TCPO_2$ (2.6 ± 3.6 vs 11.7 ± 12.6 torr, n. s.) nor difference in the ratio between $TCPO_2$ of the flap and the subclavicular reference shows any significant difference according to the outcome (failure or success). Normobaric oxygen measurements are the same. Conversely, in HBO there is a significant difference in $TCPO_2$ between the two groups (12 ± 12 vs 378 ± 385 torr; $p < 0.02$).

A $TCPO_2$ higher than 50 torr in hyperbaric oxygen (2.5 atm abs) is the best cut-off value to discriminate success from failure.

Transcutaneous Oxygen Pressures in Monitoring of Evolution

After the first $TCPO_2$ evaluation for patient selection, repetition of $TCPO_2$ measurement may be useful to follow evolution. It allows early detection of any vascular complication occurring during treatment that might require medical or surgical intervention.

It also allows an estimation of the angiogenetic progression by comparing the $TCPO_2$ repeatedly measured at fixed intervals (75).

Transcutaneous Oxygen Pressure and HBO Treatment Quality

The goal in hyperbaric oxygen therapy is essentially to increase tissue oxygen pressure by increasing the pericapillary diffusion gradient. Numerous factors may influence the quality of oxygen supplied to the patient, particularly in cases of incorrect mask application, poor patient compliance, or preexisting pulmonary pathology (58). Measurement throughout the HBO session of transcutaneous oxygen pressure in a reference zone may detect insufficient oxygen pressure increase. Quality of oxygen administration has to be checked by the personnel (rate, relaxation threshold, mask tightness, etc.). If persistent, a new evaluation of pulmonary function has to be done (looking for arteriovenous shunting, alveolar capillary block, etc.).

CONCLUSION

A large body of pathophysiological evidence supports the potential beneficial role of HBO to increase a delayed healing process. Daily experience supports it's use in the clinical management of patients with non-healing wounds. However, following the Evidence Based Medicine methodology there are still not enough good positive randomized controlled studies to issue a strong recommendation.

The European Committee for Hyperbaric Medicine, in its 1st Consensus Conference (104), stated:

HBO might be adjunct to conventional management in patients with ischemic lesions (ulcers or gangrene) without surgically treatable arterial lesions or after vascular surgery:
- *In the diabetic patient, the use of HBO is recommended in the presence of a chronic critical ischemia as defined by the European Consensus Conference on Critical Ischemia, if transcutaneous oxygen pressure readings under hyperbaric conditions (2.5 ATA, 100% oxygen) are higher than 100 torr (Type 2 recommendation).*
- *In the arteriosclerotic patient the use of HBO is recommended in cases of a chronic critical ischemia, if transcutaneous oxygen pressure readings under hyperbaric conditions (2.5 ATA, 100% oxygen) are higher than 50 torr (Type 2 recommendation).*
- *HBO is recommended in compromised skin grafts and myo-cutaneous flaps (Type 2 recommendation).*
- *In every other case, the measurement of transcutaneous oxygen pressure is recommended as an index for the definition of the indication and of the evolution of treatment (Type 2 recommendation).*

Further studies are urgently needed in order to improve the level of evidence of such recommendations.

*Chronic Critical Ischemia: periodical pain, persistent at rest, needing regular analgesic treatment for more than two weeks, or ulceration or gangrene of foot or toes with ankle systolic pressure < 50 torr in the non-diabetic or toes systolic pressure < 30 torr in the diabetic (Second European Consensus on Critical Ischemia: Circulation 1991, 84, IV, 21-26).

46. Caputo GM, Cavanagh PR., Ulbrecht JS, Gibbons GW, Karchmer AW. Assessment and management of foot disease in patients with diabetes. N Engl J Med 1994 ; 331 : 854-860.

47. Pecoraro RE, Reiber GE, Burgess Em. Pathways to diabetic limb amputation : basis for prevention. Diabetes Care. 1990 ; 13 : 513-521.

48. Boulton AJ, Kubrusly DB, Bowker JH et al. Impaired vibratory perception and diabetic foot ulceration. Diabet Med. 1986 ; 3 : 335-337.

49. Sosenko JM, Kato M, Solo R, Bild DE. Comparison of quantitative sensory-threshold measures for their association with foot ulceration in diabetic patients. Diabetes Care 1990; 13 : 1057-1061.

50. Brand PW. Repetitive stress in the development of diabetic foot ulcers. In : Levin ME, O'Neal LW, eds. The diabetic foot. 4th ed. St Louis : C.V. Mosby, 1988 : 83-90.

51. Pomposelli FR Jr, Jepsen SJ, Gibbons GW et al. Efficacy of the dorsal pedal bypass for limb salvage in diabetic patients : short-term observations. J Vasc Surg 1990 ; 11: 745-752.

52. McNeely MJ, Boyko EJ, Ahroni JH, Stensel VL, Reiber GE, Smith DG et al. The independent contributors of diabetic neuropathy and vasculopathy in foot ulcerations. Diabetes Care, 1995 ; 18 : 216-219.

53. Carsten CG, Taylor SM, Langan EM, Crane MM. Factors associated with limb loss despite a patent infrainguinal bypass graft. Am Surg. 1998 ; 64 : 33-37.

54. Cianci P., Hunt TK. Adjunctive hyperbaric oxygen therapy in treatment of diabetic foot wounds. In : Levin ME., O'Neal LW., Bowker JH. (eds). The diabetic foot 5th ed. Mosby-year book, Saint-Louis. 1993 : 305-319.

55. Brakora MJ, Sheffield PJ. Hyperbaric oxygen therapy for diabetic wounds. Clin Pod Med Surg. 1995 ; 12 : 105-117.

56. Williams RL. Hyperbaric oxygen therapy and the diabetic foot. J Am Pod Med Ass. 1997 ; 87 : 279-292.

57. Sheffield PJ. Tissue oxygen measurements with respect to soft tissue wound healing with normobaric and hyperbaric oxygen. Hyperbaric Oxygen. 1985 ; 6 : 18-46.

58. Sheffield PJ. Tissue Oxygen measurements. In : Davis JC, Hunt TK (eds). Problem wound, the role of oxygen. Elsevier, Amsterdam. 1988 ; 17-51.

59. Wattel F, Mathieu D, Fossati P et al. Hyperbaric oxygen in the treatment of diabetic foot lesions. J Hyp Med. 1991 ; 6 : 263-268.

60. Hart GB, Strauss MD. Response of ischemic ulcerative conditions to OHB. In Smith G (ed). Proceedings of the Sixth International Congress on Hyperbaric Medicine. Aberdeen. Aberdeen University Press. 1979 : 312-314.

61. Doctor N, Pandya S, Supe A. Hyperbaric oxygen therapy in diabetic foot. J Postgrad Med 1992 ; 38 : 112-114.

62. Zamboni Wa, Wong HP, Stephenson LL et al. Evaluation of hyperbaric oxygen for diabetic wounds: a prospective study. Undersea and Hyperb Med. 1997 ; 24 : 175-179.

63. Faglia E, Favales F, Aldeghi A et al. Adjunctive systemic hyperbaric oxygen therapy in treatment of severe prevalently ischemic diabetic foot ulcers. A randomized study. Diab Care 1996 ; 19 : 1338-1343.

64. Fourth Consensus Conference of the European Committee on Hyperbaric Medicine. London. December 4-5, 1998. Hyperbaric oxygen in the management of foot lesions in diabetic patients. Diabetes Nutr Metab. 1999 ; 12 : 47-48.

65. Slack WK., Thomas DA., Dejode LRJ. Hyperbaric oxygen in treatment of trauma, ischemic disease of limbs and varicose ulcerations. In Brown IW., Cox B. (eds). Proceedings of the 3rd international congress on hyperbaric medicine. National Academy of Sciences – National Research Council, Washington D.C. 1966 : 621-624.

66. Bass BH. The treatment of varicose leg ulcers by hyperbaric oxygen. Postgrad Med J. 1970 ; 46 : 407-408.

67. Fischer BH. Treatment of ulcers on the legs with hyperbaric oxygen. J Dermatol Surg. 1975 ; 1 : 55-58.

68. Hammerlund C., Sundberg T. Hyperbaric oxygen reduced size of chronic leg ulcers: a randomized double-blind study. Plast Reconstr Surg. 1994 ; 93 : 829-833.

69. Eltorai I. Hyperbaric oxygen in the management of pressure sores in patients with injuries to the spinal cord. J Dermatol Surg Oncol. 1981 ; 7 : 737-740.

70. Steinberg MH. Pathophysiology of sickle cell disease. Baillieres Clin Haematol. 1998 ; 11 : 163-184.

71. Ballas SK. Sickle cell disease : clinical management. Baillieres Clin Haematol. 1998 ; 11 : 185-214.

72. Laszlo J., Obenour W. Jr., Saltzman HA. Effects of hyperbaric oxygenation on sickle syndromes. South Med J. 1969 ; 62 : 453-456.

73. Mehdaoui H., Elisabeth L. Sickle-cell anemia. In : Oriani G., Marroni A., Wattel F. Handbook on hyperbaric medicine. Springer, Berlin. 1996 : 830-833.

74. Wiseman DM., Rovee DT., Alvarez OM. Wound dressings : design and use. In : Cohen IK., Diegelman RF., Lindblad WS. (eds). Wound healing : biochemical and clinical aspects. Saunders, Philadelphia. 1992 : 562-580.

75. Mathieu D., Neviere R., Wattel F. Transcutaneous oxymetry in hyperbaric medicine. In : Oriani G., Marroni A., Wattel F. (eds). Handbook of hyperbaric medicine. Springer, Berlin. 1996 : 686-698.

76. Baumberger JP, Godfriend RB. Determination of arterial oxygen tension in man by equilibration trough intact skin. Fed Proc. 1951 ; 10 : 10-11.

77. Clark LC Jr, Wolf R, Granger D. Continuous recording of blood oxygen tensions by polarography. J Appl Physiol. 1953 ; 6 : 189-193.

78. Clark LC Jr. Monitor and control of blood and tissue oxygen tension. Trans Am Soc Artif Intern Org. 1956 ; 2 : 41-46.

79. Huch R, Lubbers DW, Huch A. Quantitative continuous measurement of partial oxygen pressure on the skin of adults and newborn babies. Pflugers Arch. 1972 ; 337 : 185-198.

80. Huch A, Huch R, Hollmann G, Hockerts T. Transcutaneous PO_2 of volunteers during hyperbaric oxygenation. Biotelemetry. 1977 ; 4 : 88-l00.

81. Eberhard P, Mindt W, Jahn F, Hammacher K. Oxygen monitoring of newborns by skin electrodes. Correlation between arterial and cutaneously determined PO_2. In : Bruley DF, Bicher HI (eds). Advances in experimental medicine and biology. Plenum Press, New York. 1973 ; 37B : 1097-1101.

82. Eberhard P, Mindt W, Jann F, Hammacher K. Continuous PO_2 monitoring in the neonate by skin electrodes. Med Biol Eng. 1975 ; 13 : 436-442.

83. Hohenauer L. Transcutaneous monitoring Of PO_2 ($TCPO_2$) in sick newborn babies : three years of clinical experience. In : Huch A, Huch R, Lucey JF (eds). Continuous transcutaneous blood gas monitoring. New York, Alan R. Liss. 1979 : pp 375-376.

84. Montgomery H, Horowitz O. Oxygen tension of tissues by polarographic method. J Clin Invest. 1953 ; 29 : 1120-1130.

85. Shoemaker WC, Vidyssagar D. Physiological and clinical significance of $PTCO_2$ measurements. Crit Care Med, 9 : 689-690.

86. Brantigan JW, Ziegler EC, Hynes KM, Dunn KL, Albo D. Tissue gases during hypovolemic shock. J Appl Physiol. 1974 ; 31 : 117-122.

87. Dennhardt R, Ricke MF, Huch A, Huch R. Transcutaneous PO_2 monitoring in anaesthesia. Eur J Intens Care Med. 1976 ; 2 : 29-33.

88. Podolsky S, Baraff LJ, Geeher E. Transcutaneous oximetry measurements during acute blood loss. Ann Emerg Med. 1982 ; 11 : 523-525.

89. Kram HB, Shoemaker WC. Diagnosis of major peripheral arterial trauma by transcutaneous oxygen monitoring. Am J Surg. 1984 ; 147 : 776-780.

90. Eickhoff JH, Engell HC. Transcutaneous oxygen tension measurement on the foot in normal subjects and in patients with peripheral arterial disease admitted for vascular surgery. Scand J Clin Lab Invest. 1981 ; 41 : 742-748.

91. Ratlift DA, Clyne CAC, Chant ADB, Webster JHH. Prediction of amputation wound healing : the role of transcutaneous PO_2 assessment. Br J Surg. 1984 ; 71 : 219-222.

92. White RA, Nolan L, Harley D, Shoemaker WC. Noninvasive evaluation of peripheral vascular disease using transcutaneous oxygen tension. Am J Surg. 1982 ; 144 : 68-75.

93. Wyss CA, Matsen FA III, Simmons CW, Burgess EM. Transcutaneous oxygen tension measurements on limbs of diabetic and nondiabetic patients with peripheral vascular disease. Surgery. 1984 ; 95 (3) : 339-345.

94. Achauer BM, Black KS, Litke DK. Transcutaneous PO_2 in flaps : a new method of survival prediction. Plast Reconstr Surg. 1980 ; 65 : 738-745.

95. Serafin D, Lesence CB, Mullen RY, Georgiade NG. Transcutaneous PO_2 monitoring for assessing viability and predicting survival of skin flaps : experimental and clinical correlations. J Microsurg. 1981 ; 2 : 165-178.

96. Sheffield PJ, Workman WT. Noninvasive tissue oxygen measurements in patients administered normobaric and hyperbaric oxygen by mask. Hyperb Oxygen. 1985; 6: 47-62.

97. Abbot NC, Swanson Beck J, Carnochan FM, Spence VA, James PB. Estimating skin respiration from transcutaneous PO_2/PCO_2 at 1 and 2 atm abs on normal and inflamed skin. J Hyperb Med. 1990 ; 5 : 91-102.

98. Wattel F., Mathieu D., Neviere R. Transcutaneous oxygen pressure measurements. A useful technique to appreciate the oxygen delivery to tissues. J Hyperbaric Med. 1991 ; 6 : 269-281.

99. Hart GB, Meyer GW, Strauss MB, Messina VJ. Transcutaneous partial pressure of oxygen measured in a monoplace hyperbaric chamber at 1.15 and 2 atm abs oxygen. J Hyperb Med. 1990 ; 5 : 223-229.

100. Dowd GSE, Linge K, Bentley G. Measurement of transcutaneous oxygen pressure in normal and ischaemic skin. J Bone Joint Surg. 1983 ; 65 : 79-83.

101. Evans NTS, Naylor PFD. The systemic oxygen supply to the surface of the human skin. Respir Physiol. 1967 ; 3 : 21-37.

102. Hauser CJ, Shoemaker WC. Use of a transcutaneous PO_2 regional perfusion index to quantify tissue perfusion in peripheral vascular disease. Ann Surg. 1983 ; 197 : 337-343.

103. Wattel F, Mathieu D, Fossati F, Neviere R, Coget JM. Hyperbaric oxygen in the treatment of diabetic foot. Undersea Biomed Res. 1990 ; 17 (Suppl) : 160-161.

104. Mathieu D, Neviere R, Pellerin P, Patenotre P, Wattel F. Pedicle skin flap. prediction of outcome by transcutaneous oxygen measurements in hyperbaric oxygen. Plast Reconstr Surg. 1993 ; 91 : 329-334.

105. European Committee for Hyperbaric Medicine. First Consensus Conference on Hyperbaric Medicine. University Press, Lille. 1994.

NOTES

CHAPTER 13

HYPERBARIC OXYGEN FOR CRUSH INJURIES AND COMPARTMENT SYNDROMES: SURGICAL CONSIDERATIONS

M.B. Strauss

INTRODUCTION

Crush injuries and skeletal muscle-compartment syndromes (SMCS) are two related conditions that arise as a consequence of trauma. Common features include ischemia and hypoxia at the injury site, a gradient of injury, and the potential for self perpetuation of the injury (Figure 1).[1] Management of the severe forms of these injuries almost always requires surgery. The mechanisms of hyperbaric oxygen (HBO) are logical interventions for the pathophysiology of these conditions and HBO should be used when the seriousness of the injuries results in high complication rates even with optimal surgical and medical interventions. Even so, HBO is not often used in their management. Reasons for this include the lack of clearly defined indications, the reluctance of traumatologists to use HBO, the logistics of providing HBO, costs, and the acceptance of, as standards of practice in severe injuries, outcomes with complication rates as high as 50% without using HBO.

Crush injuries and SMCS are approved indications for HBO according to Medicare and Undersea and Hyperbaric Medical Society guidelines.[2,3] It is considered an acute type 2 indication (recommended) by the European Consensus Conference on Hyperbaric Medicine.[4] Reimbursement by third party payers in the United States for HBO is rarely challenged when used as an adjunct for managing crush injuries and SMCS. Since appropriateness and reimbursement seem not to be questioned when using HBO for these conditions, a primary purpose of this chapter is to provide objective indications for its use.

An important consideration in making the indications for HBO objective is ascertaining the host status of the patient. Although Cierney and Mader utilize a 3-level host status evaluation (see chapter on Chronic Refractory Osteomyelitis), I propose a more comprehensive five criteria 10-point evaluation system be used in patients with crush injuries, SMCS, and

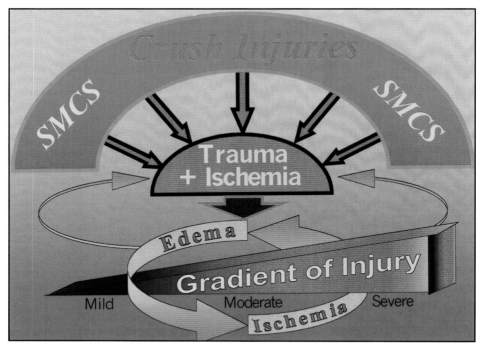

Figure 1.

Trauma plus hypoxia are the unifying features in crush injuries and skeletal muscle-compartment syndromes (SMSC). They lead to the self perpetuation (vicious circle) of edema and ischemia. Outcomes with appropriate interventions are a function of the seriousness of the injury which falls along a gradient.

problem wounds to help decide when to use HBO.[5,6] Each criteria is scored from 0-2 using objective, simple to grade findings (Table 1). If an observation is between two findings then half points are used. If the Host Score is 8-10, healing should occur as expected and HBO only be used in the severest of injuries. If the Host Score is 4-7, the patient is moderately compromised and HBO should be used in injuries of lesser severity. Finally, if the Host Score is 0-3, the patient is severely compromised and HBO should be used even in the mildest injuries if a decision is made to salvage the limb rather than doing a primary amputation. Thus, the lower the Host Score in crush injuries and SMCS, the greater the need for using HBO in the management. The matching of the Host Score with accepted grading criteria for crush injuries and SMCS provides objective indications to use HBO for these problems.

CRUSH INJURIES

Crush injuries occur when tissues are damaged due to transmission of energy from a moving object to body tissues that are stationary or moving at different rate or vice versa at the time of impact. The greater the energy exchange the more severe the tissue injury. If the energy exchange is too great, the tissues are immediately damaged beyond repair. In these situations management is directed at removal of nonviable tissue to the point of primary

TABLE 1. HOST STATUS

Criteria	Findings			Interpretation
	2 Points[1]	1 Point[1]	0 Points[1]	
Age	<40	40-60	>60	Healthy 8-10 Points
Ambulation[2]	Community	Household	None	
CV[3]/Renal[4]	Normal	Impaired	Decompensate	
Smoke/ Steroids[4]	None	Past	Current	Impaired 7-4 Points
Neuropathy/ Deformity[4]	None	Mild-to-Moderate	Severe	Marginal 3-0 Points

Notes: [1]Use 1/2 Points if observations are between two findings
[2]Subtract 1/2 point if walking aids required
[3]CV=cardiovascular
[4]Whichever gives the lower score

amputation and preserving the viability of the tissues at the margins of the injury. Invariably there is a gradient of tissue injury.[1] Edema, hypoxia, contamination, if the wound is open, and delayed host responses are factors which lead to death of the marginal tissues, delayed healing, infection, and nonunion of fractures. A widely accepted, yet easy to use open fracture-crush injury classification system (Gustilo) facilitates the comparison of treatment interventions with the severity of injury (Table 2a).[7] In the severest injuries, i.e., Gustilo Types III-B and C fractures, the complication rates approach 50% with current, "cutting-edge" surgical and orthopedic interventions.[8] Furthermore, if host healing responses are compromised, complication rates are even higher and/or these complication rates are observed even with lesser degrees of injury.

Effects of HBO which decrease morbidity in crush injuries include correction of tissue hypoxia and reduction of edema.[1] These effects help to provide a favorable environment for fibroblast function, neutrophil oxidative killing, and angiogenesis. Other beneficial effects of HBO for crush injuries include perturbation of the reperfusion injury and maintenance of red blood cell deformability.[9-11] The ability for blood cells to deform is essential for maintaining flow and preventing sludging in the microcirculation. Consequently, HBO is a logical intervention for those crush injuries where high complication rates can be anticipated. In a randomized, double-blind, placebo-controlled trial of open fractures with crush injuries, Bouachour showed statistically significant improvement in primary healing rates and a

TABLES 2A & 2B. GUSTILO CLASSIFICATION OF OPEN FRACTURES, CRUSH INJURIES AND OBJECTIVE INDICATIONS FOR USING HBO IN THESE SITUATIONS

Table 2a: Gustilo Classification of Open Fractures, Crush Injuries[7]

Grade	Findings	Complications (infections, non-healing, amputation)
I	Puncture type wound; Usually from inside to out	Almost nil
II	Laceration associated with the open fracture	10%
III	Crush component to the injury	Vary with the sub-type
-A	Sufficient soft tissue to cover the bone	~10%
-B	Exposed bone remains after debridement	~50%
-C	Concomitant major vascular injury to the extremity	>50%

Table 2b: Objective Indications for Using HBO in Open Fracture-Crush Injuries

Gustilo Grade	Host Status		
	Normal	Impaired	Marginal (Severely compromised)
I	-	-	Yes
II	-	Yes	Yes
III -A	-	Yes	Yes
-B	Yes	Yes	Yes/No[1]
-C	Yes	Yes/No[1]	Yes/No[1]

Notes: [1]Consider primary amputation

decreased number of returns to the operating room in the HBO treated arm.[12] In addition, when the host factor of age (which is one of the five criteria in my host score) over 40 years was considered, primary healing was significantly improved in the HBO group.

The Gustilo open fracture with crush injury classification matched with the Host Score provides objective indications for using HBO in crush injuries (Table 2b). Hyperbaric oxygen is recommended for all Gustilo Types III-B and III-C open fracture wtih crush injuries regardless of the host status because of the 50% complication rates that occur with fractures of this severity. However, a primary amputation must be considered in this group if the patient is a severely compromised host (Host Score 0-to-3). In the moderately compromised host (Host Score 4-to-7), HBO should be used for both Type-II fractures and Type III-A fractures. Finally, if the host is severely compromised adjunctive HBO should be considered for even the Type-I fracture.

Surgical and orthopedic interventions for crush injuries are based on the type of injury and should be independent of the decision whether or not to use HBO. That is, HBO should not be used as an excuse to delay surgery or not do surgery. However, when the decision to use HBO is made, it should be started as soon after the injury as possible. If there are delays in starting surgery, and HBO is available, it should be given while awaiting the availability of the operating room.

There is no single ideal protocol for using HBO in crush injuries. Treatment schedules are largely a function of clinical judgment and experience. The maintenance of tissue oxygenation is critical in the immediate post injury period. Consequently, I recommend HBO treatments three times a day at 2 to 2.4 atmospheres absolute (ATA) for two days. After 48 hours the treatments can be reduced to twice a day for two days and then daily for two days. By this time the host responses to injury are established, the metabolic state of the patient stabilized, and edema reduced. If at this time flaps or graft sites are threatened, then HBO is continued twice a day for a total of two weeks for its angiogenesis effect. Finally, if devitalized dead and/or infected bone is present in the wound, then HBO is continued for an additional two weeks for a total of 40 to 60 treatments. In this situation the mechanisms of HBO are directed toward bone remodeling and infection control (see Osteomyelitis chapter).

CASE REPORTS

Case 1. A 17-year-old male sustained a severe crush injury, open fracture (Gustilo Type III-B) to his right leg when he fell into a spinning drum used to extract water from wet towels at a car wash. Thirty or more comminuted fracture fragments were observed on plain X-rays (Figure 2a). A skin slough occurred and the foot was cool and hypesthetic. Leg amputation was recommended. The patient refused and was transferred for HBO treatments about 24 hours after injury. The wound tracted to bone; wound cultures were positive and appropriate antibiotics administered. Hyperbaric oxygen treatments began on a twice a day schedule. About the fifth post-injury day the fractures were aligned and stabilized with external fixation. The slough area was skin grafted. Hyperbaric oxygen continued for a total of 60 treatments. Antibiotics were stopped after three weeks due to leucopenia. The skin graft took fully. The fracture healed over a six-month period. Later a stress fracture developed but healed without complications. Subsequent X-rays showed remarkable remodeling of the severely comminuted fracture (Figure 2b).

Case 2. A 28-year-old male sustained a closed crush injury, fracture (Gustilo Grade-III-A/B) to his left leg. Infection developed after debridement and external fixation. A septic non-union persisted even after 19 debridements, bone grafting, and electrical stimulation (Figure 3a). Anytime the patient tried to use his limb the infection flared and he became septic. After 18 months of dealing with the problem he decided to have a leg amputation. However, his wife, a nurse at our hospital, persuaded him as a final attempt to save his leg to try HBO as an adjunct to additional orthopedic management. After two weeks of prepatory HBO treatments, the fracture site was debrided including removal of a large fibrocartilaginous interface and stabilized with external fixation. Ten days later the wound base was clean, and the bone covered with granulation tissue (Figure 3b). An open (Papineau) cancellous bone graft was used to bridge the bone deficit. Hyperbaric treatments

The following figures are anterior-posterior (AP) plain X-rays of a 17-year-old male with a comminuted Type III-B open fracture, crush injury:

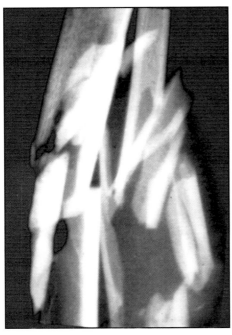 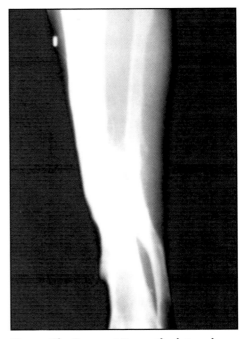

Figure 2a. Highly comminuted (30 or more fragments counted on the original films) Gustilo Type III-B open fracture crush injury. The amount of comminution and fracture displacement reflects high energy exchange to the tissues.

Figure 2b. X-rays 18 months later show remarkable healing and bone remodeling. The remodeling (as well as the delayed stress fracture) are attributed to the stimulating effects hyperbaric oxygen had on the osteoclast (the bone remodeling cell).

totaling 60 continued for approximately three weeks post-operatively. The open bone graft site epithelialized within two months. The bone-grafted fracture site healed in six months (Figure 3c).

Discussion of Case Reports 1 and 2: It is informative to compare the morbidity of Case 1 in which HBO was started immediately and in Case 2 in which it was delayed 18 months (Table 3). With the early use of HBO in Case 1, the patient with the exception of the delayed onset stress fracture essentially had a complication-free course, even though the injury was more severe than in Case 2. In Case 2, the infected non-union osteomyelitis protocol was used (see Osteomyelitis chapter) for salvage of a limb which had caused so much morbidity for the patient that he had decided to have it amputated. These comparative case reports support the recommendation for the early use of HBO in crush injuries and the obvious resulting cost-effectiveness that can be realized for fracture, crush injuries where the known complication rates are high.

SKELETAL MUSCLE-COMPARTMENT SYNDROMES

Skeletal muscle is enclosed by unyielding fascia, that is to say the fascia has very little elasticity. When edema develops within the intact fascial compartment, the pressure in the compartment increases. If the intracompartmental pressure secondary to the swelling exceeds the perfusion pressure of the microcirculation in the compartment (about 1/3 the systolic blood pressure), the microcirculation collapses and perfusion to the contents of the compartment is arrested. Ischemia results with loss of function of the compartment's nerve and muscle contents. The causes of increased compartment pressures include: (1) Post-traumatic edema, (2) Obstruction of venous outflow, (3) Increases in the contents of the compartment (i.e., after osteotomies and bone grafting), and (4) Decreased perfusion pressure (i.e., shock or inflow impairment). All of these causes can be associated with the acute effects of trauma. However, osteotomies and bone grafting may be done for reconstruction, delayed salvage, and/or deformity correction purposes. Blood flow impairment from prolonged limb compression in the "crush" syndrome from drug-induced or other types of comas is another cause of SMCS.

Management of the established SMCS is fasciotomy. This decompresses the muscle and immediately lowers the compartment pressure, thereby restoring perfusion to the contents of the compartment. If this is not done rapidly, irreversible damage occurs to the components of the compartment. Usually the injury and resultant hypoxic-anoxic injury to the compartment contents is diffuse and tends to worsen with time over the first 12 to 24 hours. This effect is due to self perpetuation (i.e., the injury worsens with time) of the ischemic edema pathophysiology cycle (Figure 1). Twenty-four hours or more may pass before the SMCS becomes established. Hence, fasciotomy, when indicated, should not be cancelled because the time from injury to the time of diagnosis exceeds the four to six hour period in which muscle tissue dies if it is totally deprived of oxygen. Conversely, irreversible damage may occur in only a few hours if injury is compounded by total ischemia of the compartment, such as with active bleeding into the compartment, occlusion of major blood vessels and/or moderate-to-severe compromise of the host exists.

The following figures are plain AP X-rays and an operating room photo of a 28-year-old male with a grade 3-A/B open fracture crush injury:

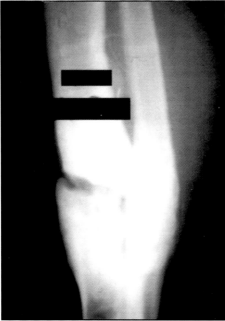

Figure 3a. Plain AP X-ray 18 months after a Gustilo Type IIII-A/B short oblique fracture of the tibia. A fibrocartilaginuous interface is present at the fracture site as well as a wire for electrical stimulation (unsuccessful) of the fracture. At this point the patient had had 19 surgical procedures for the injury.

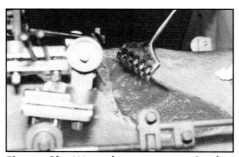

Figure 3b. Wound appearance in the operating room 10 days after debridement, external fixation, antibiotics, and hyperbaric oxygen. Healthy granulation tissue is present throughout the wound (including coverage of the bone ends). The surrounding skin is likewise healthy being free of cellulitis and induration. Open autologous cancellous bone grafting was done at this time.

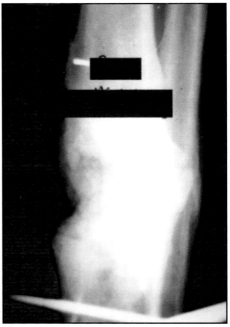

Figure 3c. Plain AP X-ray approximately six months later demonstrates consolidation of the bone graft and fracture healing. The external fixator was removed at this time.

Once function of the structures in the compartment is lost, full recovery occurs infrequently.[13,14]

Convincing laboratory studies show statistically significant reduction, in loss of muscle function, metabolites associated with muscle injury, edema and muscle necrosis with HBO (Figures 4a,b).[15-20] This makes HBO a logical intervention for the SMCS. Why then is HBO not used more with this condition? The answer is twofold: First, the prevalent attitude in the surgical communities is that the patient either has a compartment syndrome or does not have a compartment syndrome. If a compartment syndrome exists then fasciotomy is the treatment; if not, then the patient needs to be

TABLE 3. IMMEDIATE AND DELAYED USE OF HYPERBARIC OXYGEN FOR OPEN FRACTURES, CRUSH INJURIES OF THE LEG
(SEE CASE REPORTS)

Finding	Immediate	Delayed
Patient's Age	17	27
Etiology	Rotating drum water extractor	Motor Vehicle
Fracture Description	Highly comminuted entire shaft	Short oblique middle, distal thirds
Fracture Type (Gustilo)	III-B	III-A/B
Surgeries	2	22
Early Wound Infection	Yes	No
Cronic Refractory Osteomyelitis	No	Yes
Time to Union	9 months	24 months
Hospital Days	40	120

observed until surgery becomes necessary or the problem resolves. Second, there is lack of understanding when to use HBO during the self-perpetuation evolution of the SMCS. In order to resolve these questions and objectify when HBO is indicated in the compartment syndrome, it is helpful to divide the continuum of injury responses into three stages (Figure 5). First is the **Suspected** Stage. At this stage the SMCS is not present, but the severity of the injury or the circumstances (i.e., prolonged ischemia time) raise suspicions that a SMCS could develop. In this stage HBO is not recommended, but frequent neurocirculatory checks of the injured extremity are required to recognize the development of and progression into a SMCS. Of course, surgical interventions are done as required for the original injury.

If the edema-ischemia cycle perpetuates itself the **Suspected** Stage evolves into the **Impending** Stage of the SMCS. In this stage there are signs of a developing SMCS. Signs include pain with passive stretch, hypesthesia of toes (or finger tips if the problem is in the upper extremity), discomfort with passive stretch, and/or swelling in the compartment. If any of these exist, compartment pressure measurements are indicated. Unfortunately, controversy remains as to what pressure levels require a fasciotomy (Table 4).[14, 21-26] Again, clinical experience and the presence of frank neuropathy lead to the decision to decompress the compartment.

If the pressures are below the recommended levels for fasciotomy then HBO treatments should be initiated promptly (Table 5). Hyperbaric oxygen stops the progression of the SMCS by interrupting the self-perpetuating

The following figures show a comparison of the histological changes in compartment syndromes of dogs that were and were not treated with hyperbaric oxygen (HBO):

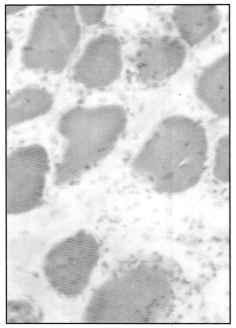 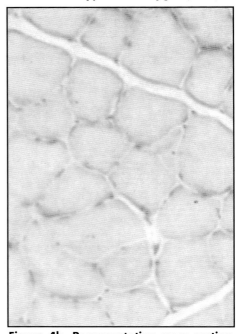

Figure 4a. Representative cross section of muscle from a compartment that was pressurized to 100 millimeters of mercury for eight hours but not treated with HBO. Note the variation in fiber size, perifascicular edema, hyalinization, leukocyte infiltration, and central migration of nuclei (original magnification, x 100).

Figure 4b. Representative cross section of muscle from a compartment that was pressurized to 100 millimeters of mercury for eight hours and then was treated with intermittent HBO. Normal structure of the skeletal muscle fibers, the nuclei, and connective-tissue planes is preserved, in contrast to the untreated control animal (original magnification, x 100).

edema-ischemia cycle. Reduction of muscle injury and edema with HBO were statistically significant in our canine model SMCS studies (Figures 4a,b).[18-20]

When making decisions whether or not to use HBO for the SMCS, the host status must be considered (Table 1). The more compromised the host, the lower the compartment pressure thresholds for using HBO (Table 5). When compartment pressure measurements are not available, then the decision to use HBO is based on clinical signs and symptoms alone (Table 5).

In the third stage of the SMCS the compartment syndrome is **Established**. Symptoms, signs, and/or pressure measurements confirm the diagnosis and dictate immediate fasciotomy be done. After surgery HBO should be used to reduce morbidity if one or more of the following is present (Table 5): (1) Ischemic muscle, (2) Demarcation of viable and non-viable muscle is unclear, (3) Threatening skin graft or flaps or grafts, (4) Residual neuropathy, (5) Massive swelling, and/or (6) Compromised host (Table 1).

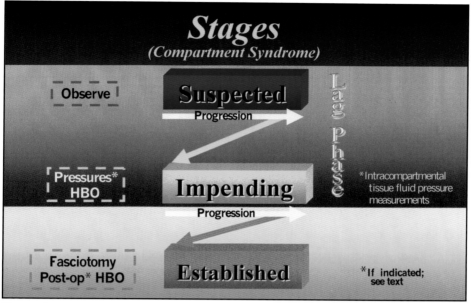

Figure 5.

Stages of the skeletal muscle-compartment syndrome (SMCS). The stages repre-sent identifiable "landmarks" for a problem like the SMCS that has a gradient of injury. Specific interventions (dotted squares) are indicated for each stage. The lag phase is the time from injury to the time the Established stage of the SMCS is reached. It, of course, varies with the etiology, the extent, and the management of the injury as well as the host status. Not all SMCS progress to the Established stage.

Fasciotomy restores perfusion to the contents of the compartment. Because between the diffuse injury at the microcirculation level, there is often a gradient between live, ischemic, and necrotic muscle. Naturally, the extent varies case-by-case. This makes randomized control trials particularly challenging and would perhaps subject the investigators to litigation if untoward outcomes occur with a particular arm of the protocol. Debridements of involved muscle in the SMCS should be conservative. With HBO there is often restoration of function of the injured, ischemic, undemar-cated (that is, living vs. dead) muscle after fasciotomy. In addition, HBO accelerates demarcation of live and dead muscle so at the time the patient is returned to the operating room for coverage and/or closure, the margins for debridements are more easily established.

As in crush injuries, HBO treatment schedules for SMCS are based on what is the suspected pathophysiology. During the **Impending** stage, one or two treatments with HBO at 2.0 to 2.4 ATA seem sufficient to stop the ischemia-edema cycle and arrest the progression of the SMCS. After fasciotomy (i.e., the **Established** stage), HBO should be used three times a day for edema reduction, support of threatened skin flaps, preservation of muscle viability, and restoration of function. By the third day, tapering of

TABLE 4. COMPARTMENT PRESSURE MEASUREMENT CRITERIA FOR FASCIOTOMY

Author (Year)[Reference]	Indication for Faciotomy (Intracompartmental tissue Fluid pressure in mmHg)
Whitesides (1975)[21]	Within 10-30 of diastolic blood pressure (DBP)[1]
Matsen (1976)[22]	40
Mubarak(1978)[23]	30
Matsen (1980)[14]	45
Heckman (1993)[24]	Within 10-20 of DBP[1]
Mateva (1994)[25]	Within 20 mm of DBP
McQueen (1996)[26]	Within 30 of DBP[2]

Note: 1. The more impaired the host the greater the difference should be between the DBP and the intracompartmental pressure for deciding to do a fasciotomy.
2. Post-traumatic in healthy hosts

HBO treatments is done until it is stopped after five to seven days. If deterioration occurs while reducing the number of daily HBO treatments, it is easily recognized and the frequency of HBO can be increased accordingly. This option is particularly useful when managing threatened flaps. For residual neuropathy one or two treatments daily should be given for ten to fourteen days. If the SMCS is in the Established stage, and the operating room is not available, HBO treatments at 2 ATA for 90 minutes should be given while awaiting surgery (see next case report).

CASE REPORTS

Case 3. A 17-year-old male was water skiing and used the tow rope to pull himself through the water by the calf of his leg. He spilled and was dragged through the water with tremendous force being applied to the calf area. The patient presented to the emergency department at our hospital shortly after the injury and was told that he had a contusion of the calf. Rest, ice, and elevation were prescribed. After 18 hours, increased swelling and pain developed in the leg. Numbness was noted in the bottom of his foot. He returned to the hospital. The deep posterior muscle compartment of the leg measured a pressure of 46 mmHg. Fasciotomy surgery was immediately scheduled. An operating room was not available due to lack of staffing. The decision was made to give the patient HBO while awaiting preparation of the operating room. Almost immediately upon reaching pressure the patient noted a marked improvement in his pain symptoms and clearing of the numbness symptoms from the bottom of his foot. A repeat measurement after

TABLE 5. CRITERIA FOR USING HBO FOR SKELETAL MUSCLE-COMPARTMENT SYNDROMES

I. **Impending Stage (See Figure 5)**
    (Use Clinical Signs and Symptoms and/or Pressure Measurements)

    A. **Signs and Symptoms**
        1. Pain in the muscle compartment
        2. Discomfort with passive stretch
        3. Swelling in and/or a "fullness" feeling of fascia over the compartment
        4. Hypesthesia of sensory areas distal to the compartment
        5. Encephalopathy, myelopathy, and/or neuropathy in the Suspected Stage
           with any of the above findings

    B. **Pressure Measurements**

Pressure (mmHg):	Host Status:
Increasing Serial Measurements	
>45	Regardless of host status
	Healthy
30-40	Impaired and/or hypotensive
<30	Marginal and/or shocky

II. **Established Stage, Post-Fasciotomy**
     (One or more of the following Residual Findings)

    A. Ischemic muscle
    B. Demarcation of viable and nonviable muscle is unclear
    C. Threatened skin flap or graft
    D. Residual neuropathy
    E. Massive swelling
    F. Compromised host (see Table 1)

the treatment showed that the pressure in the compartment had decreased to 40 mmHg. Since the patient was a healthy host, this pressure level, in the absence of symptoms, was low enough to avoid fasciotomy. Surgery was cancelled. The patient remained asymptomatic and was discharged the next day after the third HBO treatment.

    Comment. This patient was in the **Impending-Established** stages of the SMCS, that is, in the continuum between the two. It was serendipity that the operating room was not available immediately, since he met the criteria for a fasciotomy. The HBO treatment changed the patient's course by obviating the need for a fasciotomy. It must be emphasized that HBO should not be used as a substitute for fasciotomy when the indications for surgery exist. However, while awaiting availability of an operating room, HBO should be started. If symptoms resolve as in this case and compartment pressures decrease to safe levels, then surgery may be avoided.

Case 4. A wood sliver which lodged in the elbow region of an 8-year-old male became infected. Clostridia was cultured. However, myonecrosis was not present but because of massive swelling a compartment syndrome developed. The patient underwent fasciotomy. All tissues were viable. For the reason of post-fasciotomy massive swelling, HBO was started (Table 5) (Figure 6a). Over a ten-day period swelling decreased markedly (Figure 6b). Staged closures were done and obviated the need for skin grafting (Figure 6c). Full function returned to the upper extremity.

Comment. Hyperbaric oxygen was used in the post-fasciotomy period for the indication of massive swelling. The positive clostridial culture in the absence of myonecrosis was appropriately managed with surgery and antibiotics. Hyperbaric oxygen was used for the reason of residual, massive post-fasciotomy swelling. The rapid reduction in edema which was associated with post-operative HBO treatments made it possible to do a delayed primary closure of the extensive fasciotomy wound.

CONCLUSIONS

The use of HBO for crush injuries and SMCS has the potential to improve outcomes in conditions where high complication rates exist. It is a source of frustration to those of us in hyperbaric medicine that this modality is not used more often in these situations. The objective indications presented in this chapter provide guidelines for using HBO that are logical, based on accepted grading criteria and complement the other management efforts for the patient. The question is why in situations where complication rates are as high as 50% is HBO not used to lessen the morbidity. With Bouchaur's randomized controlled study and over 850 anecdotal case reports, the evidence for using HBO as an adjunct to surgical and orthopedic interventions for crush injuries is strong.[1,12,27] For the SMCS several hundred case-report experiences also attest to its usefulness.[28,30] To deny the use of HBO in crush injuries and SMCS because of lack of validated outcomes is as ridiculous as denying orthopedic surgical interventions for closed tibial fractures. A review of approximately 2,800 references on closed tibial fractures found only two that were randomized control trials.[31] To hold HBO to higher standards than other interventions is denying the patient the chances of improved outcomes in crush injuries and SMCS. As in the orthopedic management of these problems management guidelines for using HBO need to be tempered with consensus processes.[32]

Are there evidenced-based criteria to justify the use of HBO in crush injuries and SMCS? When the American Heart Association criteria are used, HBO meets the criteria for a Category 1 indication. With the ten-point evidenced-based evaluation system I devised, crush injuries receive seven points and compartment syndromes six points (Table 6). A score of five points or more qualifies the intervention as evidenced base.

Finally, are hyperbaric oxygen costs justifiable in crush injuries and SMCS? The additional expenses associated with HBO treatments need to be measured against the costs of dealing with the 50% complication rates of Gustilo Type III-B and C open fracture crush injuries. In 1977 Brighton reported that the cost to resolve the 100,000 crush type fractures that fail to

The following figures are clinical photos from an eight-year-old male after a skeletal-muscle compartment syndrome developed from a sliver contaminated with *Closridia perfringens* that lodged in his left elbow region:

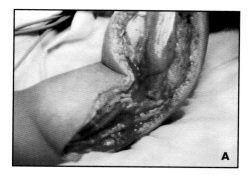

Figure 6a. Wound appearance after surgical decompression of the upper extremity. The swollen tissues are caused by massive edema. The histological appearance of edema in tissues can be appreciated from Figure 4a.

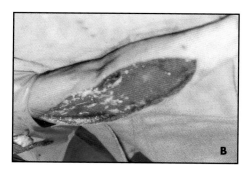

Figure 6b. Ten days after fasciotomy and twice a day hyperbaric oxygen treatments, the edema is resolved and the wound is ready for coverage, closure.

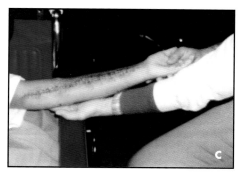

Figure 6c. Upper extremity appearance after delayed, staged primary closure (sutures still in place).

heal primarily in the United States each year was $140,000 for each case.[33] Today the costs would be many-fold higher. Amputation of the extremity is not inexpensive either. An amputation after a failed revascularization with prostheses and rehabilitation for 18 months may approach $50,000.[34] Even more devastating is the missed treatment of SMCS. In 1993 it was reported that the indemnity payment for the failure to diagnose a compartment syndrome was over $250,000.[35]

Certainly, the adjunctive use of HBO will not generate perfect outcomes in all of these situations. However, it does reduce morbidity by one-third or more in those crush injuries, open fractures where complication rates are 50% or higher. In a "head-to-head" comparison with Caudel's report, Matos showed overall complications were reduced by 49% and the percentage of amputations reduced by one-half with adjunctive use of HBO in Gustilo Type 3B and C open fracture, crush injuries.[8,36] For the SMCS we reported that the total costs (hospitalization, surgical, and HBO) were 75% less for treating the **Impending** stage as compared to the **Established** stage.[37] Consequently, objective, evidenced-based, and cost-effective indications exist for the use of HBO in crush injuries and SMCS. Hyperbaric oxygen has enormous potential for use in these conditions. The excuses for not using HBO for crush injuries and SMCS such as "50% complication rates in severe trauma are acceptable," "it is inconvenient to use," and "there is no evidence to show it is beneficial" are not valid today.

TABLE 6. EVIDENCE-BASED INDICATIONS (STRAUSS): CRUSH INJURIES AND SKELELTAL MUSCLE-COMPARTMENT SYNDROMES (SMCS)

Criteria (Score each from 0-2)[1]	Crush Injuries[2]	SMCS
1. Outcomes (Clinical and laboratory)	1	$1\frac{1}{2}$
2. Mechanisms (Appropriate for the pathysiology of the conditions)	2	1
3. Literature reviews/ meta-analyses	1	1
4. No other treatment available (Failures with previous interventions or outcomes poor with accepted interventions)	$1\frac{1}{2}$	$1\frac{1}{2}$
5. Randomized controlled trials and/or head to head studies	$1\frac{1}{2}$	0
Total[3]	**7**	**6**

Notes: 1. Scoring

  2=Overwhelming evidence

  1=Evidence is consistent with criterion

  0=No information, no benefit, or possible harm

  2. Use $\frac{1}{2}$ points when information is between two findings

  3. Five points or more qualiflies as an evidenced-base indication

REFERENCES

1. Strauss M. Crush injury compartment syndrome and other acute traumatic peripheral ischemias, in Hyperbaric Medicine Practice, 2nd Ed, Eds: Kindwall E, Whelan H. Best Publishing Company, Flagstaff, AZ, Chap 30, pp 753-771, 1999.

2. Medicare Bulletin 424. Hyperbaric Oxygen (HBO) Therapy. May 11, 1999.

3. Hyperbaric Oxygen Therapy: 1999 Committee Report, Ed. Hampson NB. Kensington, MD: Undersea and Hyperbaric Medical /Society, Inc., pp. 17-21.

4. Camporesi EM. Special meeting held during Annual Meeting in Cancun to discuss similarities and differences in indications for hyperbaric oxygen therapy approved by the UHMS Hyperbaric Oxygen Therapy Committee and the European Consensus Conference on Hyperbaric Medicine, Pressure, 1997;26(6):8-10, Nov-Dec.

5. Cierny G II, Mader JT, Penninck JJ. A clinical staging system for adult osteomyelitis. Contemp Orthop, 1985;10(5):17-37.

6. Strauss MB, Groner-Strauss WS. Wound scoring system streamlines decision-making. Biomechanics, 1999;VI(8):38-43.

7. Gustilo RB, Mendosa RM, Williams DN. Problems in the management of Type III (severe) open fractures. A new classification of Type III open fractures. J Trauma, 1984;24:742-746.

8. Caudle RJ, Stern PJ. Severe open fractures of the tibia. J Bone Joint Surg, 1987;69A(6):801-807.

9. Mathieu D, Coget J, Vinkier L, et al. Red blood cell deformability and hyperbaric oxygen therapy. HBO Review, 1985;6(4): 280 (Abstr).

10. Thom SR. Functional inhibition of leukocyte B2 integrins by hyperbaric oxygen in car bon monoxide-mediated brain injury in rats. Toxicol Appl Pharmacol, 1993;123: 248-256.

11. Zamboni WA, Roth AC, Russel RC, et al. The effect of acute hyperbaric oxygen therapy on axial pattern skin flap survival when administered during and after total ischemia. J. Reconstr Microsurg, 1989;5:343-3347.

12. Bouachour G, Cronier P, Gouello JP, et al. Hyperbaric oxygen therapy in the management of crush injuries: a randomized double-blind placebo-controlled clinical trial. J Trauma, 1996;41:333-339.

13. Bradley EL III. The anterior tibial compartment syndrome. Surg Gynecol Obstet, 1973;13:289-297.

14. Matsen FA III, Winquist RA, Krugmire RB Jr. Diagnosis and management of compartment syndrome. J Bone Joint Surg, 1980;62(A):286-291.

15. Bartlett RL, Stroman RT, Nickels M, et al. Rabbit model of the use of fasciotomy and hyperbaric oxygen in the treatment of compartment syndrome. Undersea and Hyperbaric Medicine, 1998;25(Suppl):29(#77).

16. Nylander G, Nordstr H, Franzen L, et al. Effects of hyperbaric oxygen in post-ischemic muscle. Scand J Plast Reconstr Surg, 1988;22:31-39.

17. Nylander G, Otamiri DH, Larsson J. Lipid products in postischemic skeletal muscle and after treatment with hyperbaric oxygen. Scand J Plast Reconstr Surg, 1989;23:97-103.

18. Skyhar MJ, Hargens AR, Strauss MB, et al. Hyperbaric oxygen reduces edema and necrosis of skeletal muscle in compartment syndromes associated with hemorrhagic hypotension. J Bone Joint Surg, 1986;68A:1218-1224.

19. Strauss MB, Hargens AR, Gershuni DH, et al. Reduction of skeletal muscle necrosis using intermittent hyperbaric oxygen in a model compartment syndrome. J Bone Joint Surg, 1983;60A:656-662.

20. Strauss MB, Hargens AR, Gershuni DH, et al. Delayed use of hyperbaric oxygen for treatment of a model compartment syndrome. J Orthop Res, 1986;4:108-111.

21. Whitesides TE Jr., Haney TC, Morimoto K, Harada H. Tissue pressure measurements as a determinant for the need of fasciotomy. Clin Orthop Rel Res, 1975;113:43-51.

22. Matsen FA, Mayo RA, Sheridan GW, Krugmire RB. Monitoring of intramuscular pressure. Surgery, 1976;79:702-709.

23. Mubarak SJ, Hargens AR. Acute compartment syndromes. Surg Clin North Am, 1983;63:539-565.

24. Heckman MM, Whitesides TE Jr, Grewe SR, et.al. Histologic determination of ischemic threshold of muscle in the canine compartment syndrome model. J Orthop Trauma, 1993;7:199-210.

25. Matava, MJ, Whitesides TE JR, Seiler JG III, Hutton WC. Determination of the compartment threshold pressure of muscle ischemia in the canine model. Orthopedic Transactions, 1993-1994;17(3):667-668.

26. McQueen, MM, Christie J, Court-Brown CM. Acute compartment syndrome in tibial diaphyseal fractures. J Bone Joint Surg, 1996; 78-B:95-98.

27. Malerba F, Oriani G, Farnetti A. HBO in orthopedic disorders. In: Oriani G, Marroni A, Wattel F. eds. Handbook on Hyperbaric Medicine. New York, NY: Springer-Verlag: 1996;416.

28. Fitzpatrick, DT, Murphy PT, Bryce M. Adjunctive treatment of compartment syndrome with hyperbaric oxygen. Military Medicine, 1998;163(8):577-579.

29. Oriani G. Acute indications of HBO therapy-final report, in: Oriani G, Marroni A, Wattel F. eds. Handbook on Hyperbaric Medicine, Springer, New York, 93-103, 1996.

30. Strauss MB, Hart GB. Hyperbaric oxygen and the skeletal-muscle compartment syndrome. Contemporary Orthopaedics, 1989;18:167-174.

31. Swiontkowski MF. Outcome assessment in lower extremity trauma: what have we learned? Orthopaedics Today, 2000;March, p.5.

32. Malcynski JT, Hoff WS, Reilly PM, et al. Practice management guidelines for trauma patients: where's the evidence? J Trauma, 2000;47:1170 (Abstr).

33. Brighton CT. "Quotation". Hospital Tribune, 1977;(9 May):4.

34. Mackey W, McCulloughs, Conlon TP, et.al. The costs of surgery for limb threatening ischemia. Surgery, 1986;99:26-35.

35. Templeman D, Schmidt RD, Varecka TF. The economic costs of missed compartment syndromes. Orthopedic Transactions, 1993-1994;17(4):989.

36. Matos LA, Hutson JJ, Bonet H, Lopez EA. HBO as an adjunct for limb salvage in crush injuries of the extremities. Undersea and Hyperbaric Med, 1999;20(Suppl):60-67 (#187).

37. Strauss MB. Editorial: Cost-effective issues in HBO therapy: complicated fractures. J Hyperbaric Med, 1988;3(4):199-205.

NOTES

CHAPTER 14

HYPERBARIC OXYGEN THERAPY AND LATE SEQUELAE OF RADIATION THERAPY: THE GENITOURINARY TRACT AND GASTROINTESTINAL TRACT

A.J. van der Kleij, J. Schmutz

INTRODUCTION

David Wals published the first paper related to side effects of radiation in 1897 entitled "Deep Tissue Traumatism from Roentgen Ray Exposure". Three theories were mentioned to the cause of radiation dermatitis. First, x-rays could cause the injury, or by something that constantly accompanies them. Secondly, ozone could be liberated in the surface-tissues. The third theory was from Gilchrist who conceived that the result of dermatitis could be due to actual particles of platinum carried by the cathode rays. Today it is generally accepted that the cell DNA-lesion, double-strand break, is the most important factor responsible for the radiation-induced cellular injury and/or cellular death. In clinical practice reactions occurring within the first three months after the initial radiation treatment are regarded as to be early radiation injuries and late radiation injuries occur three months following radiation. The clinical sequence of events after the DNA-lesion is related with histological findings (Rubin and Cassaret, 1968) and the most important functional deterioration is on microcirculatory level characterized by endarteritis and arteriole-capillary fibrosis (Figure 1). Hopewell (1975) demonstrated one consistent finding after irradiation of tissues: the appearance of irregularly spaced vascular constrictions, particularly in the walls of arterioles. The slowly progressive arteriolar fibrosis and interstitial fibrosis after irradiation contribute to the delayed parenchymal hypoplasia and cause the late effects of radiation (Figure 2). Further tissue atrophy can

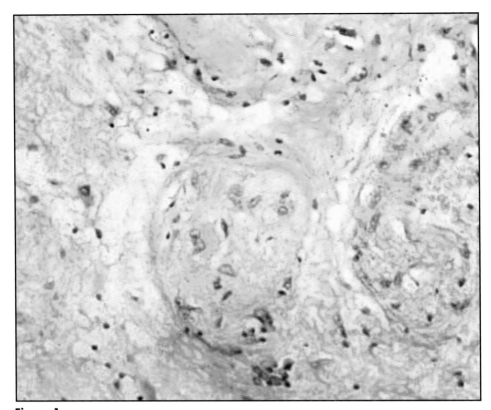

Figure 1.

High power; segmental sclerosis of vessels in the submucosa of the bowel.

be a result of direct cell hypoplasia or, secondarily, to a hyponutritional state in the tissue caused by the impaired microcirculation (Philip Rubin). Overall, these events finally result into late radiation injury, which is clinically characterized by tissue atrophy, contraction and fibrosis due malfunctions of fibroblasts. According Marx and Johnson (1987) microscopically it can be described as a "hypovascular-hypocellular-hypoxic" tissue complex. In the usual course of events late radiation injury is also characterized by a progressive course ending in tissue necrosis initiated by impaired cellular oxygen availability.

Consequently, the cornerstone to treat late radiation injury is restoration of impaired tissue oxygenation by an inducement of the (neo) angiogenesis. Angiogenesis can be described as a stimulus for the formation of collateral circulation, resulting in compensatory adaptation of tissue perfusion (Waltenberger et al., 1996). In the last decade angiogenesis research has remarkably increased especially in the field of experimental and clinical oncology (Gasparini, 1996).

Performing a survey in PubMed from 1966 until 2001 to the numbers of articles annually published on "angiogenesis" or "neovascularization" revealed from 1966 until 1971 a very low increase from 2 to 12 numbers,

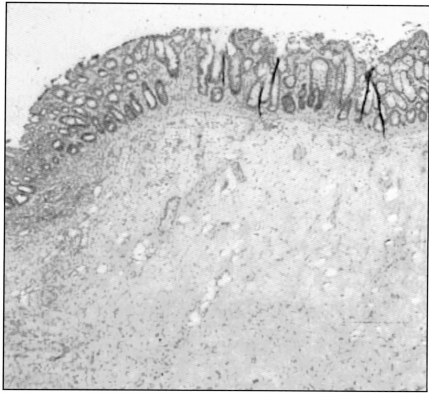

Figure 2.

Low power; radiation induced submucosal fibrosis. Note the hypocellular area submucosal.

whereas from 1991 until 2001 a steep increase from 1045 to 5258 is seen (Figure 3). A search for the same period on "hyperbaric oxygenation" revealed yearly a much less wider range of numbers between 576 and 246 with the top mainly at the end of the sixties (Figure 3). This actually reflects that in hyperbaric medicine during the last two decades no real revival of research has occurred. However most likely this will change in the future because controlled clinical trials are initiated within the frame of the European research network COST Action B14-Hyperbaric Oxygen.

The increase of the annually published articles on "angiogenesis" or "neovascularization" in the last decade is due to the discovery and molecular sequencing of endothelial growth factors, endogenous angiogenesis inhibitors, and other molecules of the extracellular matrix involved in the angiogenesis (Gasparini, 1996). In general angiogenesis is characterized by very complex multiple genetic and physiological control mechanisms. Physiological angiogenesis occurs mainly in embryonic development, the female menstrual cycle, and wound healing.

Hypoxia per se is able to stimulate vascular endothelial growth factor (VEGF-A)-induced angiogenesis. VEGF is a specific endothelial mitogen and chemoattractant inducing angiogenesis and it has been shown that the

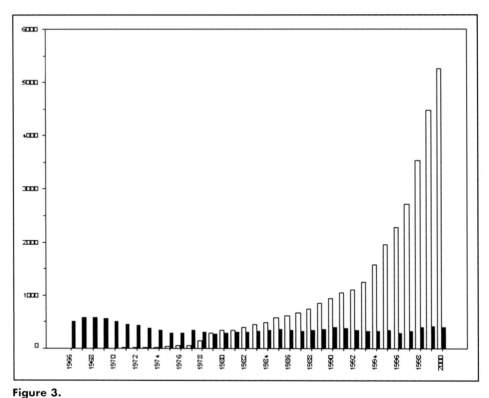

Figure 3.

Number of articles found on PubMed from 1966 until 2001. Open bars represent the number of articles related to angiogenesis or neovascularization. Solid bars represent the number of articles related to hyperbaric oxygenation.

endothelium plays an active role in hypoxia-induced angiogenesis. Hypoxia stimulates VEGF-dependent signaling not only by upregulation of VEGF ligand but also by functional upregulation of a specific signaling receptor (Waltenberger et al., 1996).

What about the opposite effect–increased tissue PO2 by hyperbaric oxygen therapy (hyperoxia) inducing a lessened angiogenesis? The effect of hyperoxia on VEGF levels was investigated in a wound model by Sheikh et al. (2000). In rats HBO therapy was administered for 90 minutes, twice daily with 100% oxygen at 2.1 atmospheres absolute in a randomized study with an HBO therapy and a control group. This treatment was continued for 7 days following wounding and VEGF, PO2, and lactate levels in wound fluid were measured on days 2, 5, and 10. The VEGF levels significantly increased with HBO by approximately 40% 5 days following wounding and decreased to control levels 3 days after exposures were stopped whereas wound lactate levels remained unchanged with HBO treatment. The authors concluded that increased VEGF production seems to explain in part the angiogenic action of HBO and hypoxia may be a less important stimulus for neovascularization of wounds than previously thought and finally VEGF production in wounds may be mediated by oxidants.

Treatment of late radiation injuries with hyperbaric oxygen (HBO) was introduced in 1973 by Greenwood and Gilchrist. Several years later the efficacy of HBO to induce angiogenesis was demonstrated in experimental (Knighton DR et al., 1981) and clinical studies (Marx and Johnson, 1988). Research has also shown that an increase in the transmucosal oxygen tension in irradiated tissue during HBO treatment is based on angiogenesis (Thorn et al., 1997).

In the following sections organ-related injuries will be discussed in more detail.

LATE RADIATION INJURIES OF THE GU TRACT AFTER PELVIC IRRADIATION

Late radiation injuries of the bladder are influenced by numerous factors such as the use of multiple fields, total dose, combined modality therapy, dose-response relationship, etc. The incidence of late bladder reactions associated with pelvic irradiation is difficult to assess because standardized criteria for grading "bladder" toxicities are not available (Marks LB et al., 1995). Depending on the site of injury, locally or the whole bladder, clinical symptoms can be haematuria, dysuria, frequency, incontinence, stream reduction, and pain in the suprapubic, pelvic, or perineal region. In other words a patient suffering from late radiation injury of the bladder will have not only one symptom but a variety of symptoms. Radiation-induced hemorrhagic cystitis is well known to the clinician because patients seek fast medical help since haematuria is associated with a recurrent tumor.

Treatment for minor symptoms can often be solved with medication. Radiation and chemotherapy account for the majority of severe hemorrhagic cystitis and can be defined as "insidious diffuse vesical bleeding" (de Vries et al., 1990). According Dean and Lytton (1978) approximately 20% of the patients treated with pelvic irradiation have bladder complications. Crew et al. (2001) report from a literature survey an incidence of less than 5%, which increased with time since irradiation. The histological bladder changes induced by pelvic irradiation are submucosal cell infiltrates, fibrosis, and luminal occlusion (Suresh et al., 1993).

The surgical approach to solve the clinical problem of intractable radiation-induced bladder injury is a urinary diversion, an ileocystoplasty, a colocystoplasty, a gastrocystoplasty or a cystectomy. However, performing a urinary diversion the complication rate may reach 60% and for cystectomy the rate may be as high as 20% (Neulander et al., 2000).

The optimal treatment for moderate to severe late radiation injury has not been elucidated and remains a discouraging problem for the clinician, who is not aware of the beneficial effect of HBO therapy for late radiation injuries. Several methods have been evolved to treat hemorrhagic radiation cystitis such as simple bladder irrigation, cystodiathermy, intravesical instillation of formalin (Ferrie et al., 1985), hydrodistention, bilateral hypogastric artery ligation (Goldstein et al., 1968), internal iliac embolization (Ferrer et al., 1998), urinary diversion and cystectomy (Neulander et al., 2000). All these treatments are associated with a high morbidity rate and have a great negative impact on health and quality of life.

HBO TREATMENT FOR HEMORRHAGIC RADIATION CYSTITIS

In 1986 Schoenrock and Cianci reported the first patient with radiation cystitis successfully treated with HBO therapy. Three years later Rijkmans et al. described in a retrospective study of ten patients the beneficial effect of HBO therapy. In this series all patients had massive refractory macro-haematuria with positive cystoscopy and histology findings. A mean of 20 HBO sessions at 3.0 ATA was given and two patients received 40 HBO sessions. Haematuria stopped in six patients and was less in four patients. Control-cystoscopy showed in all patients a reduction of the hemorrhagic radiation cystitis and it helped the demarcation and biopsy of tumor relapse.

In total 17 relevant reports were found in the literature related to HBO treatment for urinary disorders after pelvic irradiation. In total 236 patients were treated in three case reports, one prospective study, and thirteen retrospective studies (Table 1). The cure rate ranged between 27% and 92%. The only prospective study (Bevers et al., 1995) describes the experience with 40 patients. Since that time HBO therapy is an established method at the AMC for the urologists and oncologists to treat radiation-induced bladder injuries. From 1996 to 2000 an additional number of 63 patients have been treated of which fifteen are female and forty-eight male with a mean age of 70.7 years (ranging between 32.7 and 92 years). These patients were included in "The Lancet study" (n=40) in which the effect of HBO treatment for radiation cystitis was expressed in good, moderate, and no effect. The overall result of these 103 (40 + 63) patients revealed 60% of the patients with a good result, 28% with a moderate effect, and 12% with no effect (Table 2).

Until HBO therapy was introduced, treatments were aggressive and dangerous and very debilitating whereas adverse effects of HBO therapy are minimal. There is now enough evidence in the literature that HBO therapy can have a definitive place in the treatment of bladder injury after pelvic irradiation. Further studies are needed to determine the most appropriate treatment window and in the future protocols to treat radiation cystitis with HBO ought to be enrolled in cooperation with oncologists and urologists.

RADIATION-INDUCED INJURIES OF THE LARGE BOWEL AFTER PELVIC IRRADIATION

Late radiation injury of the rectum is most frequently seen after pelvic irradiation because the rectum is fixed in the pelvis. There are many other symptoms related to pelvic irradiation (i.e., ischemic bone complications) which are underestimated sequelae (Erickson et al., 2000) and are often very debilitating for the patient. Besides radiation-related factors the incidence of radiation injuries is also influenced by other factors (e.g., a combination with chemotherapy or diabetes mellitus). Herold et al. (1999) analyzed nine-hundred forty-four prostate cancer patients who were treated with three-dimensional conformal external-beam radiotherapy. Radiation morbidity was quantified using Radiation Therapy Oncology Group (RTOG) and modified Late Effects Normal Tissue Task Force (LENT) scales. Patients with a preexisting history of either Type I or Type II diabetes mellitus were

TABLE 1. REPORTS OF HBO TREATMENT FOR URINARY DISORDERS AFTER PELVIC IRRADIATION.

Study design	N	Symptoms	Nr.HBO sessions	Outcome	Author and source (in alphabetical order)
Case report	2	Severe hemorrhagic cystitis	?	Complete cure	Akiyama A. et al. Nippon Hinyokika Gakkai Zasshi 1994 Aug;85(8):1269-72
Prospective	40	Severe haematuria	20	37 (92%) cured	Bevers RF et al. Lancet 1995 Sep 23;346(8978):803-5
Retrospective	11	Intractable haematuria	40	3 (27%) complete cured, 3 persistent symptoms	Del Pizzo JJ et al., J Urol 1998 Sep;160(3 Pt 1):731-3
		Suprapubic pain		5 initially responded	
Retrospective	20	Hemorrhagic radiation cystitis	44	16 patients (80%) cured, 2 patients (10%) markedly decreased, 1 no-responder	Lee HC. Et al., Undersea Hyperb Med 1994 Sep;21(3):321-7
Retrospective	11	EORTC grading scale, 0 Grade 1, 3 Grade 2. 6 Grade 3, and 2 Grade 4.	26	Grade 2, one went to =0, one went to 1, one had inadequate treatment Grade 3, one went to 0, three went to 1, two went to 2, Grade 4, one went to 3, one stayed at 4 and had cystectomy	Mayer et al., Rad. and Oncol. 2001; 61: 151-6.
Retrospective	17	Hemorrhagic cystitis	14	11 (64%) cured, 2 residual microscopic hematuria 2 had improvement, but died of complications relating to cancer shortly after completion of treatment, 2 recurrence of gross hematuria	Mathews R. et al., J Urol 1999 Feb;161(2):435-7
Retrospective	20	Macrohematuria	25	11 healed, 5 recurrence, 3 died, 1 lost	McGinn-Merritt W et al. Late effect radiation injuries: a retrospective review. Undersea Hyperb Med. 2000; 27 (Supp.): 10.
Case report	1	Hemorrhagic cystitis, colitis	30	Haematuria cured, no more tarry stool	Miura M. et al., Int Urol Nephrol 1996;28(5):643-7
Retrospective	10	Hemorrhagic cystitis	20	7 (70%) cured, and improved urinary frequency	Miyazato T. et al., Nippon Hinyokika Gakkai Zasshi 1998 May;89(5):552-6
Retrospective	6	Hemorrhagic cystitis	45	5 (83%) cured	Nakada T. et al. Eur Urol 992;22(4):294-7
Retrospective	14	Confirmed hemorrhagic cystitis	28	8 (57%) cured, 2 (14%) had marked improvement 4 (29%) poor outcome of which 3 recurrent malignancy	Norkool DM., et al. J Urol 1993 Aug;150(2 Pt 1):332-4.
Retrospective	3	Urge-incontinence	40 or less	All improvement of urge-incontinence	Peusch-Dreyer D. Et al., Strahlenther Onkol 1998 Nov;174 Suppl 3:99-100
Retrospective	10	Severe macroscopic haematuria	20	5 (60%) cured, 4 (40%) decreased but had residual bladder malignancies	Rijkmans BG. Et al., Eur Urol 1989;16(5):354-6
Case report	1	Severe radition cystitis	?	Cured	Schoenrock GJ and Cianci P. Urology 1986 Mar;27(3):271-2
Retrospective	70	Hemorrhagic cystitis	25 (2-70)	Cured 40%, improvement 29%, no improvement 15%, drop out 10%, deaths 6%	Simao AG et al., Proc European Underwater and Baromedical Society. 2000, Ed. R. Cali-Corleo. Pp. 55-57.
Retrospective	3	Radition cystitis	?	Cured	Suzuki K. Et al., Int Urol Nephrol 1998;30(3):267-71
Retrospective	13	Hemorrhagic radiation cystitis	60	12 (92%) cured	Weiss JP. Et al., J Urol 1994 Jun;151(6):1514-7

coded as diabetics. One hundred twenty-one patients had diabetes (13% of total). Diabetics experienced significantly more late grade 2 GI toxicity (28% vs. 17%) and late grade 2 GU toxicity (14% vs. 6%).

The incidence of severe late bowel damage after radiation therapy for primary pelvic malignancies is around 5% (Emami et al., 1991, Cunningham et al., 1980) whereas the incidence of mild to moderate late bowel damage lies between 20%-25% (Gallagher et al., 1986). Treatment-induced bowel injury in rectal carcinoma of patients receiving perioperative external beam radiotherapy (EBRT) was assessed by Miller et al. (1999). The authors reviewed 304 records of patients undergoing radiotherapy for rectal carcinoma with or without chemotherapy (CT). Chronic proctitis was documented in 38 (12%) patients, including three patients with small bowel injury. The probability of developing treatment-induced bowel injury at five years following treatment was 19%. Variables associated with an increased risk of bowel injury were transanal excision, escalating radiation dose, and increasing age. Twenty of the affected patients required operative treatment, and two deaths occurred due to treatment-induced enteritis. Incidence of late intestinal side effects were assessed 3-4 years after pelvic radiotherapy for carcinoma of the endometrium and cervix (Bye et al., 2000). Compared with pre-treatment conditions, an increase in cases with pain in the lower back, hips, and thighs was observed. In addition pain and diarrhoea were associated with deterioration in HRQOL.

Late rectal complications are expressed in symptoms referring to the rectal reservoir-function (incontinence) and/or rectal bleeding. Chronic proctitis is clinically characterized by rectal irritation or urgency (tenesmus), presence of mucous or blood in the stool, and, in some patients, frequent loose bowel actions. However, Denham et al. (1999) questioned themselves "Is there more than one late radiation proctitis syndrome?" The authors investigated 244 patients, who were treated in the past for prostate cancer with radical irradiation, by examination and by questionnaire relating to late radiation-induced symptoms and their effects on normal daily life. The presence of symptoms of acute proctitis was the only factor to predict any of three late symptoms: urgency, frequency, and diarrhea. Urgency was a common late symptom which often had an important impact on normal daily life. Five subgroups of patients with varying combined different late rectal symptoms could be identified, including one group with minimal symptoms. The subgroups (one bleeding and rectal discharge and one fecal urgency and bleeding) were the two most important factors to impact on normal daily life.

TREATMENT OF RADIATION-INDUCED INJURIES OF THE LARGE BOWEL

The surgical treatment of radiation-induced injuries of the large bowel (e.g. proctitis) is in principle based on fecal stream diversion because it is thought that it decreases bowel irritation, resulting in decreased rectal bleeding. However, the underlying pathologies, submucosal injury, fibrosis, ischemia, and subsequent ulceration are not improved. Jao et al. (1986) reviewed 720 patients in which procto-scopically radiation-induced proctitis was diagnosed at the Mayo Clinic between 1950 and 1983. Sixty-two patients with severe colorectal symptoms were treated surgically. Sixty-two patients underwent a total of 143 operations with eight operative deaths (13%), and forty patients (65%) had sixty-one complications. The morbidity rate was lower after colostomy alone (44% in 27 patients) than after more aggressive operations (80% in 35 patients). Transverse loop colostomy and descending colostomy were safer than sigmoid colostomy. Dissection of adhesions, opening of tissue planes, and careless manipulation of intestine resulted in necrosis and perforation of the intestine, bladder, or vaginal wall and were the main causes of fecal and other internal fistulas according the authors. Severe late small bowel damage may become evident as small bowel obstruction, adhesions, or fistulas all requiring surgery. The incidence of mild to moderate late bowel damage such as chronic diarrhea due to mal-absorption of the small intestine is probably underestimated because most literature reports quote only severe late complications that require surgery.

It is clearly identifiable that non-surgical interventions prevail above surgical interventions because of the high mortality and morbidity rate. Denton et al. (2002) performed an extensive electronic survey (Cochrane Review) to the effects of various non-surgical treatment options for the management of late chronic radiation proctitis. They included studies (preferentially randomized controlled trials) of interventions for the non-surgical management of late radiation proctitis in patients who had undergone pelvic radiotherapy as part of their cancer treatment. This literature review revealed the following non-surgical treatments for the treatment of radiation proctitis: amino salicylic acid derivatives as anti-inflammatory agents (Baum et al., 1989); corticosteroids-steroids, orally or as enemas, for their anti-inflammatory properties (Kochhar et al., 1999). Sucralfate preparations, oral and rectal administration, a method which claims to prevent intractable post-radiation proctitis (Henriksson et al., 1992; Sasai et al., 1998); short chain fatty acid preparations (Pinto et al., 1999); formalin local application of formalin or irrigation with formalin (Roche et al.,1996); thermal coagulation, Argon laser as well as endoscopic coagulation (Swaroop et al., 1998). The reviewers could include only six controlled trials and none of the trials compared anti-inflammatory with placebo. Rectal sucralfate showed greater clinical improvement for proctitis than anti-inflammatories agents and the addition of metronidazole to the anti-inflammatory regime appeared to improve the response rate. Rectal hydrocortisone was more effective than rectal betamethasone for clinical improvement and short chain fatty acid enemas did not appear to be effective compared to placebo.

No randomized controlled trials (Table 3) were found related to hyperbaric oxygen therapy for late radiation-induced injuries of the large bowel. Using their search strategy eight references were identified of which seven were retrospective series and only one was a prospective observational case series (Williams et al., 1992). They registered two reports (Feldmeier et al., 1996; Gouello et al., 1999) with baseline assessments of the degree of chronic radiation proctitis with a score or a grade of the histological or symptomatic features. Quality of life data was not recorded in any of the reports. The authors concluded that HBO may be of value for large bowel chronic radiation changes refractory to other treatments; however, the degree of benefit and the cumulative effect or duration of response could not

TABLE 2.   RESULTS OF HBO FOR RADIATION CYSTITIS. THE LANCET STUDY + PERIOD 1996-2000 (N = 103).

Type of Cancer	Good	Moderate	No Effect	Total
Bladder	18	10	7	35
Prostate	29	11	3	43
Uterus	6	1	1	8
Cervix	8	5	1	14
Ovary	1	-	-	1
Urethra	-	1	-	1
Rectal	-	1	-	1
Total	62 (60%)	29 (28%)	12 (12%)	n=103

be quantified because of the methodology and quality of the data. Treatment-related morbidity was acceptable and the effect on quality of live could not be assessed in their survey (Denton et al., 2002). It is evident from the literature that there is no definitive intervention for radiation proctitis. In the era of evidence based medicine HBO may play a role in the future only when sufficient evidence is derived from randomized studies with clearly diagnostic criteria.

RADIATION-INDUCED FISTULAE/STRICTURES AND HBO

The prospective observational case series (Williams et al., 1992) evaluated the effect of HBO on radiation-induced soft tissue necrosis in patients who previously received treatment for gynecologic malignancy. Fourteen patients with radiation necrosis of the vagina alone or in association with recto-vaginal fistula were treated (15 HBO sessions). Only one treatment failed. This good outcome shows that HBO can also be applied in comp-romised post-operative healing. Hyperbaric oxygen given to five patients at risk of radiation-related complications before abdominal and pelvic surgery (Pomeroy et al., 1998) were prospectively treated with hyperbaric oxygen before a planned abdominal operation. In their experience HBO can even be used as preventive treatment to reduce the morbidity rate in these complicat-ed patients.

Due to late radiation injury chronic fibrotic strictures (Green et al., 1984) of the recto-sigmoid junction and rectum may cause large bowel obstructions which often require surgical resection with primary anastomosis

TABLE 3. REPORTS OF HBO TREATMENT FOR RADIATION INJURY OF THE RECTUM/SIGMOID

Study Design	N	Symptoms	Nr. HBO Sessions	Outcome	Authors
Prospective	7	EORTC graduation, 0 Grade 0, 0 Grade 1, 4 Grade 2, 6 Grade 3, 0 Grade 4	26 (2-60)	Grade 2, two went to =0, one went to 1, one had inadequate treatment. Grade 3, one went to 0, four went to 1, one went to 2	Mayer et al., 2000
Retrospective	38	Rectal bleeding		Improvement of rectal bleeding in 61% of cases	Aanderud et al., 2000
Case Study	2	Refractory severe pain, tenesmus, bleeding, foul-smelling purulent discharge unhealed in 1 patient and post operative non healing foul smelling discharge in the other one	60	Patient healed	**Bem et al., 2000**
Retrospective	4	3 patients with moderate to severe bleeding, typical rectoscopy findings, one had severe proctalgia	3 pat. 30 sessions, 1 pat. 60 sessions	Significant improvement in bleeding and rectoscopy findings for all patients, one bleeding relapse after 3 months, proctalgia patient no change	**Kitta et al., 2000**
Retrospective	36	All refractory, 9 chronic wounds, 19 rectorrhagia, 9 profuse diarrheas, 24 patients had abdominal surgery, blood transfusion before HBO2	67 (12-198)	9 cures, 12 improvements, 11 failures, 1 patient died from radiation injury, two from cancer, one from liver cirrhosis	Gouëllo et al., 1999
Retrospective	14	Symptoms were refractory in 11 patients, 11 had rectorrhagia, 5 diarrhea, 5 tenesmus or colic.	40 (20-72)	9 patients were healed, 3 patients improved and relapsed by end of follow up (months), 2 did not respond at all	**Warren et al., 1997**
Retrospective	18	All refractory, 17 rectorrhagia, 4 pain, 4 incontinence, 8 diarrhea	24 (12-40)	7 rectorrhagia, 2 pain, 3 incontinence, 4 diarrhea improved or healed	**Woo, 1997**
Case Study	1	Severe rectorrhagia	30	Cessation of rectorrhagia and reversal of histological findings	**Nakada, 1993**

Note: Authors in **bold** are included in the Denton et al., Cochrane review.

or colostomy but not without considerable mortality and morbidity. Dilatation with bougie or balloon or self-expanding metal stent (Piccinni and Nacchiero, 2001) has been attempted with differing rates of success and the risk of hemorrhage or perforation. The question remains: "Can HBO be applied for intestinal obstruction?" There are a few case reports in the literature where HBO was applied for intestinal obstruction. Yasuharu and Kanematsu (1998) describe their experience with a two-year-old girl with a enormous intra-abdominal tumor. During laparotomy it appeared that the tumor was impossible to remove because of invasion of large vessel. In the postoperative period she developed after a received chemotherapy regimen on day 42 an intestinal obstruction which despite standard treatment remained unchanged. Surgery was ruled out for several reasons. An alternative treatment was HBO which was given twice a day on days 45 and 48. After the initial treatment symptoms disappeared and after recovery surgery was possible on day 49. In adults the authors have a policy when postoperative paralysis or adhesive obstructions of the intestine are not improved after three dives surgery is considered. In our institution we also have experience with several cases in which chronic bowel obstruction was treated with HBO. One case will be presented here. A 31-year-old female diabetic patient had undergone a Wertheim-Okabayashi procedure for cervix malignancy at the age of 29 years. One year later she developed a bowel obstruction which required surgical resection with primary anastomosis. March 2000 she had complaints of a distended abdomen and frequently stools. A plain abdominal radiograph revealed a massive distended large bowel (Figure 4) caused by a stenotic region in the recto-sigmoid (Figure 5). She received 50 HBO treatments after which she fully recovered (Figure 6).

A new approach could be the use of HBO to prevent late radiation injuries. Feldmeier et al. (1995) demonstrated in an experimental study in rats who received HBO 7 weeks after irradiation of 30 Gy abdominopelvic in 10 fractions the beneficial effect of HBO. The HBO group had fewer gross signs of enteropathy, less narrowing, and less rigidity in their harvested bowel segments compared to the control group. However, in practice the treatment window is unknown because the clinician is unable to determine the optimal moment in time to initiate HBO treatment.

INFLAMMATORY BOWEL DISEASE AND HBO

Crohn's Disease

There are several reports describing the beneficial effect of HBO therapy as adjunctive treatment in severe perineal Crohn's disease (Brady et al., 1989, Nelson et al., 1990, Lavy et al., 1994, Colombel et al., 1995). The first patient was described by Brady et al. in 1989 who failed to heal after multiple surgical interventions. Of all 22 patients described in the literature, 16 (73%) had a complete response to HBOT, two (9%) a partial response, and four (18%) no response (Noyer and Brandt, 1999). To assess the effect of HBO treatment on colonic damage Rachmilewitz et al. (1998) studied in two models of experimental colitis, and examined whether this effect was mediated by modulation of NO synthesis.

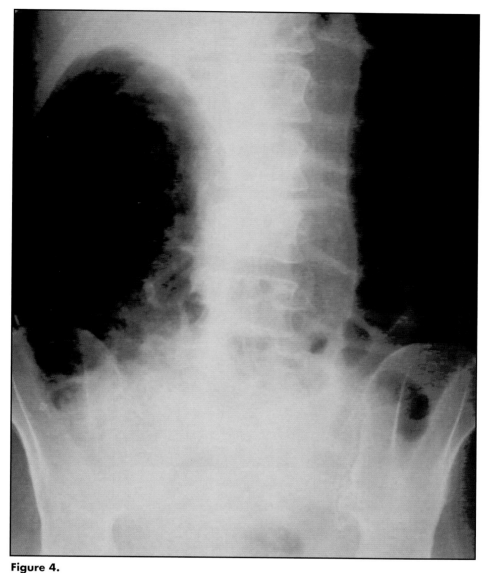

Figure 4.

Plain abdominal radiograph before HBO treatment.

Colitis was induced by either flushing the colon with 2 ml 5% acetic acid or intracolonic administration of 30 mg trinitrobenzenesulphonic acid (TNB) dissolved in 0.25 ml 50% ethanol. Rats were exposed to HBO (100% oxygen at 2.4 atmosphere absolute) for one hour twice on the day of colitis induction and once daily thereafter. Control rats were treated only with acetic acid or TNB. Rats were killed 24 hours after acetic acid administration or one and seven days after TNB treatment. It was found that HBO effectively decreases colitis induced by acetic acid and TNB. In addition the decreased

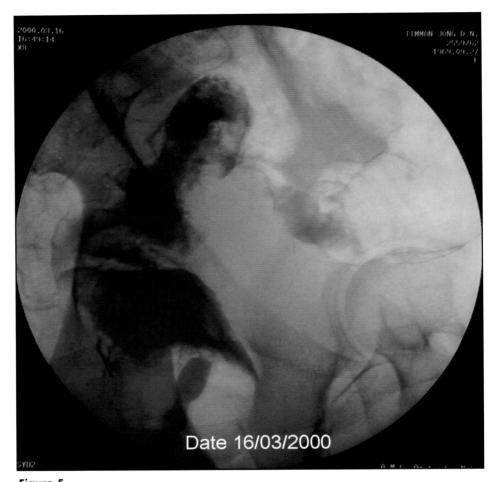

Figure 5.

Colonic double contrast radiograph. Note the stenotic region over several centimeters.

NO synthase activity induced by HBO suggests that reduction in NO generation may be among the mechanisms responsible for the anti-inflammatory effect of HBO. It may be concluded that HBO may be a useful adjunct in the therapy of only large non-healing Crohn's perineal lesions in patients refractory to conventional therapies.

ULCERATIVE COLITIS

In a case report Kuroki et al. (1998) describe their experience to treat a toxic megacolon non-surgically with HBO. HBO treatment resulted within 48 hours in a marked improvement and colectomy was not necessary. There are only a few reports in the literature in Bulgarian and Russian language available. Buchman et al. (2001) describe the first successful use of hyperbaric oxygen therapy in the treatment of ulcerative colitis. Therapy consisted of

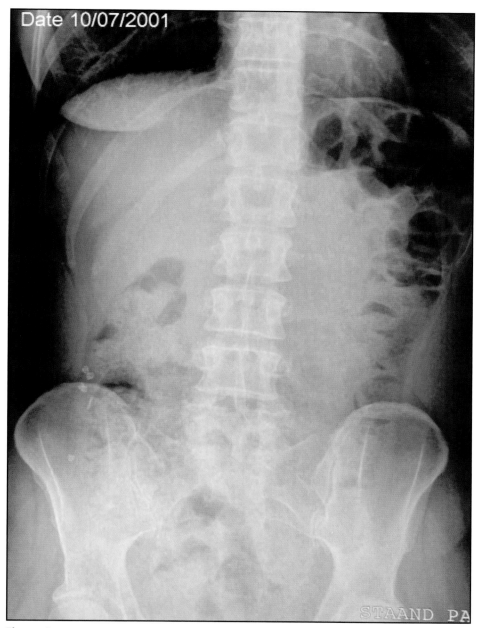

Figure 6.

Plain abdominal radiograph 14 months after the initiation of the HBO treatment.

30 courses of 100% oxygen at a pressure of 2.0 atm absolute. Clinical remission was achieved on the basis of the Truelove–Witts and disease activity index scores whereas corticosteroids were successfully tapered off once remission was achieved. It is understandable that these scanty reports are evidence that there is no place for HBO in the treatment for ulcerative colitis.

PNEUMATOSIS CYSTOIDES INTESTINALIS

Masterson et al. in 1979 were the first authors, followed by others (Grieve et al., Madsen et al., Paw and Reed, and Shimada et al.), who reported the use of HBO in the treatment of pneumatosis cystoides intestinalis (PCI). PCI is a benign air-filled cystic formation lying in submucosal or sub-serous digestive tissue and has been reported all along the digestive tract. PCI is a sign, not a disease. Fifteen percent of all cases of PCI are idiopathic. In the other cases, digestive tract or respiratory tract diseases are usually the underlying cause. Exceptionally systemic disease may be associated with PCI, particularly systemic sclerosis (Grasland et al., 1998). The most important task for the surgeon is differentiation between the benign non-complicated cases and the life-threatening forms such as bowel necrosis, perforation, and infections. Mathus-Vliegen et al. (........) describe the treatment for PCI in six patients with all cysts confined to the left colon. Two required surgical intervention (one bowel perforation and one resection of the sigmoid colon because of volvulus), two were treated with HBO for two weeks, one was treated with a fiber-enriched diet, and one did not receive any treatment but symptoms persisted for four years. Patients treated with HBO for PCI resulted in rapid relief of symptoms and early healing of pneumatosis but recurrence occurred after eight months and two months, respectively. PCI confined to the small intestine and treated with HBO was described by Paw and Reed (1996). This patient was treated in a monoplace chamber and each course consisted of a 60-min period at 100% oxygen at two atm abs, five courses a week for two weeks reduced to two courses a week for an other two weeks and finally one weekly basis for a further four weeks. Finally he fully recovered. There is a role for HBO in the treatment of PCI; however, the clinical judgment remains the cornerstone when and how to treat a patient with HBO.

REFERENCES

1. Aanderud L, Thorsen E, Brattebo G, Forland M, Kristensen G. Hyperbaric oxygen treatment for radiation reactions. Tidsskr Nor Laegeforen. 2000 Mar 30;120(9):1020-2.

2. Akiyama A, Ohkubo Y, Takashima R, Furugen N, Tochimoto M, Tsuchiya A. [Article in Japanese] [Hyperbaric oxygen therapy in the successful treatment of two cases of radiation-induced hemorrhagic cystitis]. Nippon Hinyokika Gakkai Zasshi 1994 Aug;85(8):1269-72.

3. Baerts et al. Br. J. Urology, 81(6): 929-30. 1998 Hyperbaric oxygen treatment for radiation ulcer of the bladder.

4. Baum CA, Biddle WL, Miner PB. Failure of 5-aminosalicylic acid enemas to improve chronic radiation proctitis. Digestive Diseases & Sciences 1989;34(5):758-69.

5. Bem, J, Bem S, Amarjit S. Use of hyperbaric oxygen chamber in the management of radiation related complications of the anorectal region. Report of two cases and review of the literature. Dis Colon Rectum. 2000 ;43: 1435-38.

6. Bevers RFM, Bakker DJ, Kurth KH. Hyperbaric oxygen treatment for haemorrhagic radiation cystitis. Lancet 1995 Sep 23;346(8978):803-5.

7. Brady CE, Cooley BJ, Davis JC. Healing of severe perineal and cutaneous Crohn's disease with hyperbaric oxygen. Gastroenterology 1989 Sep;97(3):756-60.

8. Buchman AL, Fife C, Torres C, Smith L, Aristizibal J. Hyperbaric Oxygen Therapy for Severe Ulcerative Colitis. J of Clinical Gastroenterology 2001;33:337-339.

9. Bye A, Trope´ C., Loge JH., Marianne Hjermstad M., Kaasa S. Health-Related Quality of Life and Occurrence of Intestinal Side Effects After Pelvic Radiotherapy. Acta Oncologica 2000; Vol. 39, No. 2, pp. 173–180.

10. Charneau J, Bouachour G, Person B, Burtin P, Ronceray J, Boyer J. Severe haemorrhagic radiation proctitis advancing to gradual cessation with hyperbaric oxygen. Digestive Diseases & Sciences 1991;36(3):373-5.

11. Colombel JF, Mathieu D, Bouault JM, Lesage X, Zavadil P, Quandalle P, Cortot A. Hyperbaric oxygenation in severe perianal Crohn's disease. Dis Colon Rectum 1995;38:609–14.

12. Crew, JP, Jephcott CR, Reynard, JM. Radiation-induced haemorrhagic cystitis. Eur Urol. 2001 Aug; 40(2):111-23.

13. Cunningham IGE: The management of radiation proctitis. Aust N Z J Surg 50:172-178, 1980.

14. Cunningham IGE: The management of radiation proctitis. Aust N Z J Surg 50:172-178, 1980.

15. Dean, RJ., Lynton B. Urologic complications of pelvic irradiation. J. Urol., 1978; 119:64.

16. Del Pizzo 11, Chew BH, Jacobs SC, Sklar GN. Treatment of radiation induced hemorrhagic cystitis with hyperbaric oxygen: long-term followup. J Urol1998 Sep;160 (3 Pt 1):731-3.

17. Denham JW, O'Brien PC., Dunstan RH., Johansen J., See A., Hamilton CS, Bydder S.,Wright S. Is there more than one late radiation proctitis syndrome? Radiother. Oncology 1999; 51: 43-53.

18. Denton A, Forbes A, Andreyev J, Maher EJ. Non surgical interventions for late radiation proctitis in patients who have received radical radiotherapy to the pelvis (Cochrane Review). In: The Cochrane Library, Issue 2, 2002. Oxford: Update Software.

19. Emami B, Lyman J, Brown A et al: Tolerance of normal tissue to therapeutic irradiation. Int J Radiat Oncol Biol Phys 1991; 21: 109-122.

20. Erickson BA, Murray KJ, Erickson SJ, Carrera GF. Radiation-induced pelvic bone complications: An underestimated sequelae of pelvic irradiation. Int J Radiat Oncol Biol Phys 2000; 48: 3, Supplement; 31.

21. Feldmeier JJ, Heimbach RD, Davolt DA, Court WS, Stegmann BJ, Sheffield PJ. Hyperbaric oxygen an adjunctive treatment for delayed radiation injuries of the abdomen and pelvis. Undersea and Hyperbaric Medicine 1996;23(4):205-13.

22. Feldmeier JJ, Jelen I, Davolt DA, Valente PT, Meltz ML, Alecu R. Hyperbaric oxygen as a prophylaxis for radiation-induced delayed enteropathy. Radiother Oncol 1995 May;35(2):138-44.

23. Ferrer Puchol MD, Borrel Palanca A, Gil Romero J, Pallardo Calatayud Y, Cervera de Val V, Laso Pablos MS, Nogues Pelayo E. Severe hematuria caused by radiation cystitis. Selective percutaneous embolization as an alternative therapy. Actas Urol Esp 1998 Jun;22(6):519-23.

24. Ferrie BG, Rundle IS, Kirk D, Paterson PI, Scott R. Intravesical formalin in intractable haematuria. J Urol (Paris) 1985;91(1):33-5.

25. Gallagher MJ, Brereton HD, Rostock RA et al: A prospective study of treatment techniques to minimize the volume of small bowel with reduction of acute and late effects associated with pelvic irradiation. Int J Radiat Oncol Biol Phys 1986 12: 1565-1573.

26. Gasparini G. Angiogenesis research up to 1996. A commentary on the state of art and suggestions for the future. Eur J of Cancer 1996; Vol 32A, No. 14, pp. 2379-2385.

27. Goldstein AG, D'Escrivan IC, Allen SD. Haemorrhagic radiation cystitis. 1968 r J Urol Aug;40(4):475-8.

28. Gouello JP, Bouachour G, Person B, Ronceray J, Cellier P, Alquier PH. Intérêt de l'oxygénothérapie hyperbare dans la pathologie digestive post-radique. 36 observations. Presse Med. 1999. 28(20):1053-7.

29. Grasland A, Pouchot J, Leport J, Barge J, Vinceneux P. Pneumatosis cystoides intestinalis. Presse Medicale 1998 27 (35): 1804-1812 Nov 14.

30. Green N, Goldberg H, Goldman H, Lombardo L, Skaist L. Severe rectal injury following radiation for prostatic cancer. J Urol 1984 131:701-704

31. Greenwood TW, Gilchrist AG. Hyperbaric oxygen and woundhealing in post irradiation head and neck surgery. Br J Surg 1973; 60:394-397.

32. Grieve DA, Unsworth IP. Pneumatosis cystoides intestinalis: an experience with hyperbaric oxygen treatment. Aust N Z J Surg 1991 Jun;61(6):423-6.

33. Henriksson R, Franzen L, Littbrand B. Prevention and therapy of radiation induced bowel discomfort. Scandinavian Journal of Gastroenterology 1992;Supplement 1992:7-11.

34. Herold DM, Hanlon AL, Hanks GE. Diabetes mellitus: a predictor for late radiation morbidity. Int J Radiat Oncol Biol Phys 1999; 43: 475-9.

35. Hopewell, JW. Early and late changes in the functional vascularity of the hamster pouch after local irradiation. Radiation Res. 1975; 63:157-164.

36. Jao SW, Beart RW Jr, Gunderson LL. Surgical treatment of radiation injuries of the colon and rectum. Am J Surg 1986 Feb;151(2):272-7.

37. Kindwall EP. Hyperbaric oxygen treatment of radiation cystitis. Clin Plast Surg 1993 Iul;20(3):589-92.

38. Kitta T, Shinohara N, Shirato H, Otsuka H, Koyanagi T. The treatment of chronic radiation proctitis with hyperbaric oxygen therapy in patients with prostate cancer. BJU International 2000;85:372-4.

39. Knighton, DR., Silver, IA., Hunt, TK. Regulation of wound-healing angiogenesis-effect of oxygen gradients and inspired oxygen concentration. Surgery. 1981 Aug;90(2):262-70.

40. Kochhar R, Sriram PV, Sharma SC, Gole RC, Patel F. Natural history of late radiation proctosigmoiditis treated with topical sucralfate suspension. Digestive Diseases & Sciences 1999;44(5):973-8.

41. Kuroki K, Masuda A, Uehara H, Kuroki A. A new treatment for toxic megacolon. The Lancet 1998 352: 782.

42. Lavy A, Weisz G, Adir Y, Ramon Y, Melamed Y, Eidelman S Hyperbaric oxygen for peri-anal Crohn's disease. J Clin Gastroenterol 1994;19:202-5.

43. Lee HC, Liu CS, Chiao C, Lin SN. Hyperbaric oxygen therapy in hemorrhagic radiation cystitis: a report of 20 cases. Undersea Hyperb Med 1994 Sep;21 (3):321-7.24.

44. Madsen S, Arnell P, Santesson B, Henning R. A case report. Hyperbaric oxygen cured a gastrointestinal disease. Lakartidningen 1995 May 3;92(18):1901-2.

45. Marks LB, Carrol P, Dugan TC, Anscher MS. The response of the urinary bladder, urethra and ureter to radiation and chemotherapy. Int J Radiation Oncology Biol Phys. 1995, vol 31;5: 1257-1280.

46. Marx RE, Johnson RP. Studies in the radiobiology of osteoradionecrosis and the clinical significance. Oral Surg Med Pathol 1987; 64:379-390.

47. Masterson JS, Fratkin LB, Osler TR, Trapp WG. Treatment of pneumatosis cystoides intestinalis with hyperbaric oxygen. Ann Surg 1978 Mar;187(3):245-7.

48. Mathews R, Rajan N, Iosefson L, Camporesi E, Makhuli z. Hyperbaric oxygen therapy for radiation induced hemorrhagic cystitis. J Urol 1999 Feb;161(2):435-7.

49. Mathus-Vliegen EMH, Bakker DJ, Tytgat GNJ, Pneumatosis cystoides intestinal: Clinical presentation, diagnosis and treatment in 6 patients. Undersea Hyperb Med.

50. Mayer R, Klemen H, Quehenberger F, Sankin O, Mayer E, Hackl A, Smolle-Juettner F-M. Hyperbaric oxygen – an effective tool to treat radiation morbidity in prostate cancer. Rad. and Oncol. 2001; 61: 151-6.

51. McGinn-Merritt W et al. Late effect radiation injuries: a retrospective review. Undersea Hyperb Med. 2000; 27 (Supp.): 10.

52. Miller AR, Martenson JA, Nelson H, Schleck CD, Ilstrup DM, Gunderson LL Donohue JH. The incidence and consequences of treatment-related bowel injury. Int. J. Radiation Oncology Biol. Phys., 1999; 43: 4, 817–825.

53. Miura M, Sasagawa I, Kubota Y, Iijima Y, Sawamura T, Nakada T. Effective hyperbaric oxygenation with prostaglandin El for radiation cystitis and colitis after pelvic radiotherapy. Int Urol Nephrol 1996;28(5):643-7.

54. Nakada T, Kubota Y, Sasgawa T et al. Therapeutic experiences of hyperbaric oxygen therapy in radiation colitis. Diseases of the Colon & Rectum 1993; 36:962-5.

55. Nakada T, Yamaguchi T, Sasagawa I, Kubota Y, Suzuki H, Izumiya K. Successful hyperbaric oxygenation for radiation cystitis due to excessive irradiation to uterus cancer. Eur Urol 1992; 22(4):294-7.

56. Nelson EW Jr, Bright DE, Villar LF. Closure of refractory perineal Crohn's lesion. Integration of hyperbaric oxygen into case management. Dig Dis Sci 1990 Dec;35(12):1561-5.

57. Neulander EZ, Rivera I, Eisenbrown N, Wajsman Z. Simple cystectomy in patients requiring urinary diversion. J Urol 2000 Oct; 164(4) : 1169-72.

58. Norkool DM, Hampson NB, Gibbons RP, Weissman RM. Hyperbaric oxygen therapy for radiation-induced hemorrhagic cystitis. J Urol 1993 Aug;150(2 Pt 1):332-4.

59. Noyer CM, Brandt LJ, Hyperbaric Oxygen Therapy for Perineal Crohn's Disease. The Amer J Gastroenterology 1999 94; 2: 318-321.

60. Ohno Y, Kanematsu T. Hyperbaric oxygen therapy for intestinal obstruction in children: An exceptional experience in a compromised child. J of Pediatric Surgery 1998 33; 10: 1543-1545.

61. Paw HG, Reed PN. Pneumatosis cystoides intestinalis confined to the small intestine treated with hyperbaric oxygen. Undersea Hyperb Med 1996 Jun;23(2):115-7.

62. Peusch-Dreyer D, Dreyer KH, Muller CD, Carl U. Management of postoperative radiation injury of the urinary bladder by hyperbaric oxygen (HBO). Strahlenther Onkol1998 Nov;174 SuppI3:99-100.

63. Philip Rubin. In: Clinical Oncology. A Multidisciplinary Approach for Physicians and Students. 7th Edition.1993. W.B. Saunders. ISBN 0-7216-3761-2.

64. Piccinni G, Nacchiero M. Management of narrower anastomotic colonic strictures. Case report and proposal technique. Surg Endosc. 2001 Oct;15(10):1227.

65. Pinto A, Fidalgo P, Cravo M et al. Short chain fatty acids are effective in short term treatment of chronic radiation proctitis. Diseases of the Colon & Rectum 1999;42:788-796.

66. Pomeroy BD, Keim LW, Taylor RJ. Preoperative hyperbaric oxygen therapy for radiation induced injuries. J Urol., 1998: Vol 159, 1630-1632.

67. Rachmilewitz D, Karmeli F, Okon E, Rubenstein I, Better OS. Hyperbaric oxygen: a novel modality to ameliorate experimental colitis. Gut 1998;43:512–518.

68. Rijkmans BG, Bakker Dl, Dabhoiwala NF, Kurth KH. Successful treatment of radiation cystitis with hyperbaric oxygen. Eur Urol 1989;16(5):354-6.

69. Roche B, Chautems R, Marti MC. Application of formaldehyde for treatment of haemorrhagic radiation-induced proctitis. World Journal of Surgery 1996;20(8):1092-4.

70. Rubin P, Casarett GW. Clinical radiation pathology. W.B. Saunders Company Philadelphia, London, Toronto 1968; Vol. I: 38-61.

71. Sasai T, Hiraishi H, Suzuki Y, Masuyama H, Ishida M, Terano A. Treatment of chronic post-radiation proctitis with oral administration of sucralfate. American Journal of Gastroenterology 1998;93(9):1593-5.

72. Schoenrock GI, Cianci P. Treatment of radiation cystitis with hyperbaric oxygen. Urology 1986 Mar;27(3):271-2.

73. Schultheis TE, Lee RW, Hunt MA, Hanlon AL, Peter RS, Hanks GE. Late GI and GU complications in the treatment of prostate cancer. Int J Radiation Oncology Biol Phys 1997 Jan 1;37(1):3-11.

74. Sheikh AY, Gibson JJ, Mark D, Rollins MD, Hopf HW, Hussain Z, Hunt TK. Effect of hyperoxia on vascular endothelial growth factor levels in a wound model. Arch Surg. 2000;135:1293-1297.

75. Shimada M, Ina K, Takahashi H, Horiuchi Y, Imada A, Nishio Y, Ando T, Kusugami K. Pneumatosis cystoides intestinalis treated with hyperbaric oxygen therapy: usefulness of an endoscopic ultrasonic catheter probe for diagnosis. Intern Med 2001 Sep; 40(9): 896-900.

76. Simao AG, Roque AF, Sousa A, Sampaio J, Torres P, Solva J. Radiation induced hemorrhagic cystitis and HBO. Proc European Underwater and Baromedical Society. 2000, Ed. R. Cali-Corleo. Pp. 55-57.

77. Suresh UR, Smith VI, Lupton EW, Haboubi NY. Radiation disease of the urinary tract: histological features of 18 cases. J Clin Pathol.1993 Mar;46(3):228-31.

78. Suzuki K, Kurokawa K, Suzuki T, Okazaki H, Otake N, Imai K, Yamanaka H. Successful treatment of radiation cystitis with hyperbaric oxygen therapy: resolution of bleeding event and changes of histopathological findings of the bladder mucosa. Int Urol NephroI1998;30(3):267-71.

79. Swaroop VS, Gostout CJ. Endoscopic treatment of chronic radiation proctopathy. Journal of Clinical Gastroenterology 1998;27:36-40.

80. Thorn JJ, Kallehave F, Westergaard P, Hansen EH, Gottrup F. The effect of hyperbaric oxygen on irradiated oral tissues: transmucosal oxygen tension measurements. Journal of Oral & Maxillofacial Surgery 1997; 55(10) 1103-1107.

81. Vries de CR, Freiha FS. Hemorrhagic cystitis : a review. J of Urology. 1990; vol 143; 1-9.

82. Wals D. Deep tissue traumatism from roentgen ray exposure. BMJ 1897; pp. 272.

83. Waltenberger J, Mayr U, Frank H, Hombach V. Suramin is a potent inhibitor of vascular endothelial growth factor. A contribution to the molecular basis of its antiangiogenic action. J Mol Cell Cardiol 1996 Jul;28(7):1523-9.

84. Warren DC, Feehan P, Slade JB, Cianci PE. Chronic radiation proctitis treated with hyperbaric oxygen. Undersea & Hyperbaric Medicine 1997;24(3):181-4.

85. Weiss IP, Boland FP, Mori H, Gallagher M, Brereton H, Preate DL, Neville EC. Treatment of radiation-induced cystitis with hyperbaric oxygen. J Urol1985 Aug; 134(2):352-4.

86. Weiss IP, Mattei DM, Neville EC, Hanno PM. Primary treatment of radiation-induced hemorrhagic cystitis with hyperbaric oxygen: 10-year experience. J Urol1994. Jun;151(6):1514-7.

87. Weiss IP, Neville EC. Hyperbaric oxygen: primary treatment of radiation-induced hemorrhagic cystitis. J Urol1989 Jul;142(1):43-5.

88. Williams JA, Clarke D, Denis EJ, Smith S. The treatment of pelvic soft tissue radiation necrosis with hyperbaric oxygen. American Journal of Obstetrics and Gynaecology 1992;167(2):412-6.

89. Woo TC, Joseph D, Oxer H. Hyperbaric oxygen treatment for radiation proctitis. International Journal of Radiation Oncology, Biology, Physics 1997;38(3):619-22.

NOTES

CHAPTER 15

HYPERBARIC OXYGEN AS AN ADJUNCT TO SURGICAL MANAGEMENT OF THE PROBLEM WOUND

M.B. Strauss

INTRODUCTION

There is little dispute that surgery is an important adjunct in managing the problem wound. Controversy arises when to use hyperbaric oxygen (HBO) even though it is the most frequent use of this therapy in the United States. The questions of what defines a problem wound and when to use HBO for problem wounds have heretofore not been clearly defined. The diagnosis "Problem Wound" is not an approved condition by Medicare even though "enhancement of healing in selected Problem Wounds" is listed as an approved condition by the Undersea and Hyperbaric Medical Society guidelines.[1,2] Consequently, reimbursement for HBO treatment for the majority of the wound care population, that is to say the Medicare group, is not given if the Problem Wound diagnosis is used. This poses several dilemmas. First, the definition of a problem wound is subject to interpretation. Second, how does one determine the indications for HBO when a myriad of interventions are available to deal with problem wounds? Third, how does HBO aid in the management of problem wounds? Finally, what surgical techniques can be used to optimize outcomes of problem wounds? This chapter addresses these dilemmas, and precisely defines the role of HBO as an adjunct to surgical management of the problem wound.

WOUNDS APPROVED FOR HYPERBARIC OXYGEN

Although the diagnosis of problem wounds itself is not an indication for HBO, there are several conditions that are associated with and/or are the cause of problem wounds which are "approved" indications for HBO according to Medicare and Undersea and Hyperbaric Medical Society guidelines (Table 1).[1,2] Acute conditions include wounds associated with acute arterial and/or traumatic ischemia, gas gangrene, necrotizing infections of soft

TABLE 1. NOMENCLATURE USED TO DEFINE PROBLEM WOUNDS FOR WHICH HYPERBARIC OXYGEN IS APPROVED

I. Acute Conditions

    a. Gas gangrene *, +
    b. Wounds Associated with Acute Traumatic Peripheral Ischemia*
    c. Crush Injury Wounds *, +
    d. Necrotizing Soft Tissue Infections *, +
    e. Wounds Associated with Acute Arterial Insufficiency *
    f. Preservation of Compromised Skin Grafts/Flaps *, +
    g. Wounds Associated with Actinomycosis *
    h. Thermal Burns +

II. Subacute and Chronic Conditions

    a. Chronic Refractory Osteomyelitis *, +
    b. Wounds Remaining After Failed Flaps or Grafts *, +
    c. Wounds Secondary to Delayed Radiation Injury (Soft Tissue and Bone Radiation Necrosis) *, +
    d. Enhancement of Healing in Select Problem Wounds +

Key: * MEDICARE (Center for Medicare/Medicaid Services) Guidelines[1]
      + Undersea and Hyperbaric Medical Society Guidelines[2]

tissues, mixed synergistic infections, nonhealing wounds associated with crush injuries, compromised/failed flaps and/or threatened skin grafts, and burns. Many of these conditions are specifically addressed in other chapters in this book. Subacute and chronic conditions associated with problem wounds include chronic refractory osteomyelitis, arterial insufficiency ulcers after failed flaps and/or grafts, and radiation injury of soft tissue and bone. Terminology such as nonhealing wound, venous stasis ulcer, diabetic ulcer, vasculitic ulcer, malperforans ulcer, and pressure sore should be eschewed as a diagnosis for using HBO.

    The hyperbaric medicine consultant and/or surgeon must select the appropriate terminology for describing the wound in order for HBO treatments to be reimbursed. This list of approved problem wound conditions offers many choices for such. Even more important, if the initial management is not improving the wound and/or has failed, then HBO should be used. It is essential to remember that HBO is an adjunct to optimizing host responsiveness and the wound environment and not a substitute for other measures to manage the wound.[3] In the majority of problem wounds, especially in the compromised host, wound hypoxia is a major cause of failure to heal.[4,5] Hence, HBO becomes a logical intervention with its hyperoxygenation effect for the hypoxic problem wound. This specific terminology is being proposed to the Center for Medicare/Medicaid Services as a new, specific indication for HBO.

TABLE 2. WOUND SCORE (STRAUSS):
SCORE BASED ON 5 CRITERIA, EACH GRADED FROM 2 TO 0 POINTS

2-0 Appearance (Red Base=2, White or Yellow Base=1, Black Base=0)
2-0 Size (<Thumb print=2, Thumb to Fist=1, >Fist=0)
2-0 Depth (Skin-Subcutaneous=2, Muscle-Tendon=1, Bone-Joint=0)
2-0 Infection (Colonized=2, Cellulitis=1, Septic=0)**
2-0 Perfusion (Palpable Pulse=2, Doppler Detected Pulse=1,No Pulse=0)***

TOTAL POINTS
(10 Score is Best; 0 Score is worst)

Healthy Wound:	**8 - 10**	**Points**
Problem Wound:	**4 - 7**	**Points**
Futile Wounds:	**0 - 3**	**Points**

Notes: *   Use 1/2 points when findings are intermediate between two descriptions
**   Septic is defined as cellulitis with leucocytosis, fever, positive blood cultures, and/or uncontrolled blood sugars
*** Supplemental evaluation techniques when edema or wounds may obscure pulse detection

2 Points: Warm foot, normal capillary refill and/or normal room air juxta-wound $P_{tc}O_2$ studies

1 Point: Cool foot, sluggish capillary refill and/or hypoxic room air juxta-wound $P_{tc}O_2$ studies that increase to over 200 mmHg with HBO

0 Points: Cold foot, no capillary refill and/or juxta-wound $P_{tc}O_2$ studies that show no or little effect with HBO

Abbreviations: $P_{tc}O_2$=Transcutaneous Oxygen
HBO=Hyperbaric Oxygen

DEFINING THE PROBLEM WOUND

Since there is a continuum in the severity of the previously listed wounds, how does one target the group, especially the sub-acute and chronic wound types, as problems for which HBO is needed? Clinical descriptions such as nonhealing, necrotizing, uncontrolled sepsis, and progressive deterioration are often used to justify HBO. Appropriate assessment is necessary to determine the seriousness of the wound and what interventions including HBO are appropriate. Above, the problem wound was defined qualitatively. Grading systems for wounds have been devised to help establish the severity and provide guidelines for treatments. I recommend using a grading system that is based on five objective criteria that readily classify the severity of the wound, and can be used to quantitate improvement (Table 2). Each criterion is graded using objective findings on a scale of 2 (best) to 0 (worst). Because the clinical assessment of perfusion may be difficult to measure in the presence of foot wounds, brawny edema, induration, and scaring, we use transcutaneous oxygen measurements and Doppler detection of pulses to help in the grading of this criterion. A healthy wound generates a score of 8-to-10, a problem wound 4-to-7, and a futile wound 0-to-2.

The wound score provides a quantitative method to define a problem wound and a logical approach to management (Figure 1). It can be used equally well with acute, sub-acute, or chronic wounds and in wounds over any part of the body. A healthy wound will heal with minimal attention. One hundred percent good outcomes are expected. A futile wound will probably not heal without angioplasty and/or revascularization, high patient motivation, and very concerted wound healing team efforts. The problem wound is the wound type in which healing is expected to occur in 90 percent or more of the cases with appropriate treatment strategies.[6]

Once a wound with a healing problem or anticipated healing problem is recognized, appropriate interventions precisely timed in the healing continuum are essential to achieve the best possible outcomes.[7] Four treatment strategies are used to optimize outcomes of problem wounds: (1) Preparation of the wound base, (2) Protection of the wound, (3) Selection of appropriate dressings, and (4) Wound oxygenation (Figure 1). Hyperbaric oxygen is one of the interventions to improve the wound oxygenation treatment strategy. The first and fourth strategies will be fully described as they directly apply to the thesis of this chapter; for the other two strategies, information can be obtained from the references for this chapter.[7,8]

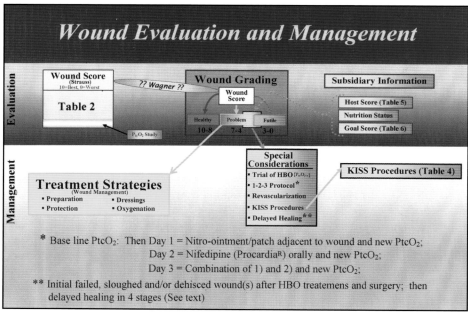

Figure 1. Algorithm for Evaluation and Management of Wounds

The Wound Score (Strauss) easily differentiates wounds into healthy, problem, or futile. The Wagner Score although well established does not provide this versatility. For problem wounds four treatment strategies are utilized to optimize results. When the wound score is in a transition zone between problem and futile, subsidiary information is needed to decide whether or not to attempt wound salvage. If the decision is made to attempt wound salvage, then the four treatment strategies plus the special considerations are utilized.

WOUND PREPARATION

The wound base must be prepared so that other strategies will be effective. It should be adequately debrided to facilitate optimal wound dressing techniques. Deformities, redundant tissue, avascular tissue, and bone extending beyond soft tissues should be removed so closure will be easy to do, minimally invasive, and durable. Management of the wound base is guided by the appearance criterion used for scoring a wound (see Table 1). If the wound base is red (a score of "2" on the appearance criterion of the wound score), normal saline or other physiological agents or coverings should be used to maintain a moist, healthy environment. If the wound base is white or yellow (a score of "1" on the appearance criterion), interventions are done to remove the exudate and/or superficially necrotic material. Enzymatic debriding agents are useful for this purpose. In-office or on-the-ward limited debridements with a scalpel are effective in removing necrotic debris over a vascular wound base. The debridements are "limited" inasmuch as the goal is to remove only obvious and easily accessible necrotic or mechanically inappropriate (i.e., in the way for dressing changes) material in a serial fashion. This is in contrast to an in-operating room debridement in which the goal is to establish surgical margins. Limited debridements conserve the most possible tissue and usually are well tolerated pain-wise due to the removal of only necrotic tissue. If a neuropathy is present as is frequently observed in diabetics, debridements to this extent can usually be done without the patient experiencing pain. With limited, repetitive debridements, blood loss is almost negligible. Hydrotherapy (whirlpool or pulsatile lavage) softens and hydrates the tissues so that limited debridements can be even more effective.

If the wound base is black (a score of "0" on the appearance criterion of the wound score), then debridement to viable vascularized tissues is required. If the wound site is septic with drainage, cellulitic margins, and absence of clear demarcation of viable from nonviable tissues, debridement in the operating room is usually required and closure needs to be delayed. If the black-based wound is mummified (i.e., a thin eschar) and the demarcation between healthy and necrotic tissues is sharp, this natural covering can be used as a biological dressing. After sufficient angiogenesis has occurred under the eschar coverage, closure of the wound can be done in the operating room with the expectation of good outcomes, or epithelialization of the wound can occur under the eschar margins. The angiogenesis effect from HBO requires a minimum of two weeks of treatments.

Mechanical problems such as deformities, contractures, and muscle imbalances must be corrected. Nonviable bone must be removed. Osteotomies, ostectomies, joint resections, joint manipulations, and tenotomies are surgical techniques used to achieve these goals. Frequently, these measures can be done in the nonoperating room setting with equipment as simple as scalpel, forceps, scissors, curettes, and/or bone ronguers by individuals familiar with their use. When anesthesia and an operating room are required, the debridement/wound preparation should be done by a surgeon with an interest in problem wounds.

Another important consideration regarding wound appearance is that of the nutritional status of the patient. Wounds in malnourished patients heal poorly, and if severely malnourished may not heal or even worsen while the wound is being treated. The status of the patient's nutrition is easily established by measuring albumin and prealbumin levels.[9] The clinical nutrition consultant can optimize the patient's diet especially if factors such as obesity, dysphagia, renal insufficiency, or combinations of these are present and complicate nutrition care. Nutrition is one problem that is almost always correctable (in contrast to wound perfusion) with oral supplements, nasogastric feeding, percutaneous endoscopic gastrostomy, and/or hyperalimentation.

WOUND OXYGENATION

Wounds require adequate perfusion to heal. Juxta-wound tissue oxygen tensions of 30-40 mm are required for wound healing and infection control.[10,11] Wound oxygenation strategies often complement each other.[6] An important consideration for achieving this strategy is edema reduction. Edema decreases oxygen availability by increasing the diffusion distance of oxygen from the capillary to the cell. If edema occurs in a confined space, circulation may be compromised due to collapse of the microcirculation from increased intracompartmental pressure. The foot has more closed spaces, potential compartments, and tendon sheaths than almost any other structure in the body. Edema reduction is achieved through elevation, elastic wraps, support hose, immobilization, pain control (so the leg is not kept in the dependent position for pain relief), pneumatic compression devices, and hydrotherapy. The requirement to dangle a leg continuously indicates severe occlusive vascular disease to the extremity. The dependent position increases blood flow due to the gravity effect, but the persistent dependent position of the legs causes edema, venous stasis, stasis dermatitis, and stasis ulcers. The foot wound is especially susceptible to edema formation due to its propensity to be in the dependent position for sitting, standing, and walking activities.

Optimization of cardiac and renal function are essential medical interventions for management of problem wounds. Improved perfusion augments oxygen, growth factors, and substrate delivery to the wound. Diuresis mobilizes extracellular fluid and reduces edema. The vascular surgeon may improve perfusion by revascularization and the radiologist by angioplasty. If outflow is poor and the arterial disease diffuse, benefits from these techniques alone may be inadequate to meet oxygenation and perfusion demands for wound healing.

Hyperbaric oxygen complements all the above methods of improving wound oxygenation and, in many situations, may be the only effective method for managing hypoxia in the problem wound. It increases plasma and tissue oxygen tensions 10-fold and oxygen diffusion distance through tissue fluids 3-fold.[12] With HBO, oxygen delivery is no more flow dependent (vs. red blood cell oxygen delivery) than the other substances physically dissolved in the plasma. Juxta-wound ($PtcO_2$) transcutaneous oxygen measurements supplement the wound score perfusion criterion and can indicate which wounds need and/or are benefited by HBO. They help to objectify the use of HBO. In our experiences, if $PtcO_2$'s increase to over 200 mmHg, healing occurs in more than 80% of the problem wounds managed with HBO regardless of the room air measurements.[5] Recently it was observed in *in vitro* studies that HBO enhances proliferation of fibroblasts from older adults to the same level of activity that is observed in the newborn.[13] This was attributed to enhancement of cellular proliferation and growth factor receptors by HBO treatments. In summary, HBO is one of the wound oxygenation treatment strategies for managing the problem wound (Figure 2). It is especially indicated in the hypoxic wound and/or the wound in the "special consideration" category. The fibroblast proliferation data helps to explain the benefits observed in healing of the problem wound in the host with impaired wound healing abilities.

Many pharmacological agents can improve flow and other rheological properties of blood. They include red blood cell deforming agents, blood vessel dilating agents (both local, i.e., nitroglycerin paste/patches, and systemic), and anticoagulants. We often use nitroglycerin patches adjacent to the wound if the PtcO2 studies with HBO do not exceed 200 mmHg. In most cases improved oxygen tensions are observed. Use of these agents requires judgment. Many have significant side effects and need to be monitored.

SURGICAL TECHNIQUES TO OPTIMIZE MANAGEMENT OF PROBLEM WOUNDS

When "pushing the envelope" to salvage problem wounds special surgical interventions are required. They need to be as gentle and non-invasive as possible. Invariably the patient has compromised wound healing abilities.

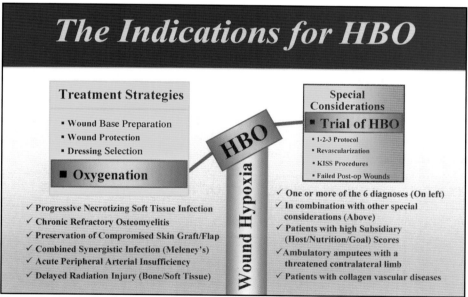

Figure 2. The Indications for Hyperbaric Oxygen (HBO)

Precise indications exist for using HBO as an adjunct to manage wounds. It is one of the wound oxygenation treatment strategies for problem wounds. Hyperbaric oxygen should be used if one or more of the six conditions under the oxygenation section of the treatment strategies are present. For the problem-futile transitional wound where a salvage attempt is indicated by subsidiary scoring (See Figure 1), HBO should be used as a special consideration if one or more of the six conditions under the special considerations strategies exist. The common denominator for using HBO is wound hypoxia.

These procedures have several objectives: (1) Make the wound clean and stable, (2) Manage deformities, muscle-tendon imbalances, and joint contractures, and (3) Minimize the insult to the wound environment and surrounding tissues as little as possible. Repetitive procedures, i.e., debridements, are preferable to establishing surgical margins which often require major amputations. The wound must establish its own line of demarcation. Healing of problem wounds, once optimal treatment strategies are started, evolve through three stages: (1) Resting (latency), (2) Granulation, and (3) Coverage (Table 3).[13] Appropriate timing of procedures is essential for each stage of healing.

Many of the surgical procedures used to manage problem wounds can be done in-office, on-the-ward, or in-clinic without the added time and expenses of using the operating room (Table 4).[14] Special surgeries which require the operating room can be selected to minimize tissue injury and the requirement of 20-fold or more increases in blood and oxygen that wound healing may require.[8] Most of these special procedures are done percutaneously or through wounds that are already open.

Customary amputations may not be appropriate when attempting to achieve closure, coverage of problem foot wounds. Unconventional procedures such as longitudinally oriented flaps for forefoot wounds, combinations of forefoot-midfoot amputations, dorsal flaps to cover forefoot-midfoot plantar amputation wounds, partial or complete medial and lateral ray resections, subtotal calcanectomies, split thickness skin grafts over granulated cancellous bone, and middle ray resections with foot narrowing are surgical options that can be effective in achieving wound healing, yet allow the patient to use the foot. For many of the patients with problem foot wounds the goal is to have a stable, healed foot platform for independent ambulation at the household or limited community level. Usually these unconventional procedures meet this goal. Pain is rarely a problem from these uncustomary procedures because of underlying sensory neuropathy.

Subsidiary information is required when making decisions to manage wounds that are in the transition zone between problem and futile wounds,

TABLE 3. STAGES IN THE HEALING OF THE PROBLEM WOUND

Stage	Findings	Goals	Approximate Duration	Comments
1. Latency	Non-healing, sepsis, and/or necrotic tissue	(1) Initiate an inflammatory response (2) Control sepsis (3) Prepare the wound bed for optimal dressing changes and later for coverage closure (4) Edema reduction	2 weeks	Use the four wound strategies described previously[7] plus organism-specific antibiotics. Hyperbaric oxygen (HBO) is used to augment wound oxygenation when indications exist (see Figure 2).
2. Granulation	Angiogenesis; resolution of cellulitis; normalization of nutrition	Healthy, granulating wound base	2 weeks	Obtain transcutaneous oxygen measurements; consider angioplasty and/or revascularization if indicated and feasible
3. Coverage, closure	Healthy vascular based wound	Durable coverage with flaps and/or grafts, or by secondary intention	2 weeks	Continue HBO if needed for threatened flaps or grafts

TABLE 4. "KISS" (KEEP IT SIMPLE...AND SPEEDY) PROCEDURES FOR MANAGING PROBLEM WOUNDS

In Office, in-clinic, or on-the-ward KISS Procedures:	Comment
1. Debridements (Calluses, crusts, eschars, ulcer margins, wound bases, etc.)	For size and depth documentation use these criteria from the wound score (Table 2). For complexity: Grade 1=scalpel, Grade 2=scalpel and forceps, Grade 3=these plus scissors, and Grade 4=the above plus ronguers
2. Percutaneous tenomities of toe tendons	Especially useful for clawed toe deformities
3. Joint manipulations	Usually in conjunction with tenotomies
4. Partial wound approximations ("Stay" sutures)	Effectively, instantly reduces size of a wound, yet still allows access for dressing changes
5. Toe nail trimming, debuking, and/or debridement of ingrown nail margins	Four grades[15]
6. Open amputations, osteotomies, and ostectomies	Usually the wound is open to the joint and/or bone protrudes beyond soft tissues

In-Operating room KISS procedures	Comment
1. Excision of ulcer; debridement of underlying bursa and bone	Effective technique for managing deformities which are very frequently the underlying cause of problem wounds
2. Drill and osteoclasis of depressed metatarsel head	For malperforans ulcer management with minimally invasive surgery[16]
3. Inner metatarsal resection and foot narrowing with temporary placement of a mini-external fixation	For necrotic middle rays in the dysvascular foot wound[17]
4. Percutaneous Achilles tendon lengthening	Effective for managing equinus contractures; use prophylactically for short forefoot and midfoot amputations
5. Percutaneous temporary pin stabilization of joints	Useful for correcting deformities, immobilization of joints, and optimally "resting" compromised flaps and grafts
6. Percutaneous intramedually ankle rodding	A technically demanding, but minimally invasive (2 1/2cm incision for rod insertion and 2 or 3 one cm incisions for interlocking screws) procedure

for example, scores in the 3-1/2 to 4-1/2 point range (Figure 1). This information should include the general health status of the patient (i.e., Host Score) and the patient's desires and expected cooperation (i.e., Goal Score). This information is quickly determined by using 0-to-10 point scores for each (Tables 5 and 6). If the subsidiary scores are 4 or greater then wound salvage is indicated and special considerations are done (Figure 1). In this group of patients we often observe initial dehiscence and sloughs (i.e., failed wounds) after HBO and surgery. However, over 90% of these wounds have healed secondarily progressing through four distinct stages: (1) Deterioration, (2) Latency, (3) Granulation tissue formation, and (4) Epithelialization.[18]

Failures resulting in lower extremity amputations have been observed in the following situations: (1) New vascular occlusive events, (2) Methicillin resistant *Staphylococcus aureus* infections in a subset of diabetics, (3) Patients with collagen vascular diseases especially if on steroids or antibiotics, (4) Patients with residual mechanical problems in the foot, and/or (5) Intractable pain. I have observed a subset of diabetics who are unable to eradicate Methicillin resistant *Staphylococcus aureus* infections from their foot wounds even with surgery, antibiotics, and HBO. The antibiotics and HBO suppress the infection. Once these are discontinued the infection flares necessitating amputations to at least one joint proximal to the involved tissue site. When the Methicillin resistant infection in this subset of diabetics occurs at midfoot or ankle level, a lower limb amputation is required to arrest the infection.

TABLE 5. HOST SCORE (STRAUSS): 5 CRITERIA EACH GRADED FROM 2 TO 0

Criteria	2 Points*	1 Point*	0 Points*	Assessment
Age	<40	40-60	>60	Normal Host Score = 8-10
Ambulation (Subtract 1/2 point if walking aids needed)	Community	Household	None	
Cardiovascular/ Renal Function**	Normal	Impaired	Decompensated	Impaired Host Score = 4-7
Smoking/Steroids	Never	Past	Current	
Neuropathy/Deformity	None	Mild to Moderate	Severe	Incompetent Host Score = 0-3

* Use 1/2 points if findings are between two descriptions
** Whichever item gives the lower score

TABLE 6. GOAL SCORE (STRAUSS): 5 CRITERIA EACH GRADED FROM 2 TO 0

Criteria	2 Points*	1 Point*	0 Points*	Assessment
Motivation (To keep limb)	Strong	Some	None	High Potential: 8-10 Points Likely to be successful in preventing new or recurrent wounds
Comprehension (Of problem)	Full	Some	None	
Compliance (Diet, skin care, glucose monitoring, activity)	Full	Some	None	Moderate Potential: 4-7 Points Close monitoring, frequent follow-ups required to prevent new or recurrent wounds
Family Support	Full	Some	None	
Independence (Activities of daily living, hygiene, etc.)	Full	Some	None	Poor or No Potential: 0-3 Points Likely to need early lower extremity amputation due to new or recurrent wounds after hospital discharge

*Use 1/2 points if findings are between two descriptions

DISCUSSION

After optimizing the four treatment strategies: 1) Wound base preparation, 2) Wound protection, 3) Wound dressing selections, and 4) In wound oxygenation, 90% or more of the wounds in the problem and problem-futile transition group will heal.[6] Surgeries are oftentimes required to achieve coverage, closure. Usually the surgical choices become obvious, but may require unconventional flaps and foot amputation levels. In the problem-futile transition group primary healing after surgery and HBO has been observed in about 50% of the cases, but in those that fail to heal primarily, nearly 90% heal by secondary intention progressing through four stages.[18] Hyperbaric oxygen, probably through its angiogenic effect, appears to "jump start" the secondary healing process.

This chapter also demonstrates where HBO fits into the comprehensive management of a problem wound (Figure 2). It is not a substitute for the other strategies, nor does it compete with them. However, as a wound oxygen improving strategy, it is one of the most effective. Likewise, with this approach the role for $PtcO_2$ studies becomes better defined and helps to provide objective criteria for the use of HBO.[5]

The effectiveness of HBO in diabetic foot wounds has been summarized previously.[19] Two additional randomized control trials for diabetic foot wounds have become available since the previously referenced summary was prepared.[20,21] With HBO the healing rates have increased from 48 to 85 percent and lower extremity amputation rates have been decreased from 46 to 18 percent (Table 7). It is important to appreciate from this analysis that the outcomes are remarkably similar whether they were randomized control, head-to-head, prospective, or retrospective studies. As an Evidenced Based Indication for problem diabetic foot wounds HBO qualifies as a level I condition according to the American Heart Association Guidelines.[32] With the 10 point Evidenced Base Indications system that I advocate using (see Table 2 in Osteomyelitis chapter), these conditions generate a score of 8-1/2 (Outcomes = 2, Mechanisms = 2, Literature = 1-1/2, No other interventions = 1-1/2, and randomized control trials, head-to-head studies = 1-1/2).[33] In summary, this chapter provides objective criteria for defining the problem wound, the appropriate indications for using HBO, special surgical considerations for optimizing wound healing, and two Evidenced Based Indication evaluation systems to justify the use of HBO.

TABLE 7. OUTCOMES OF DIABETIC FOOT WOUNDS MANAGED WITH (w) AND WITHOUT (w/o) HYPERBARIC OXYGEN

Author/Year (Reference)	Patients		Healed (%)		Amputations (%)		Comment
	w/HBO	w/o HBO	w/HBO	w/o HBO	w/HBO	w/o HBO	
Abida, 2001 (20)	19	14	13(68)	4(29)			Double-blind randomized control trial. At the 12-week end-point of the study, the median wound area decreased 96% in the HBO group vs. 41% in the control (p=0.43)
Lee, 2001 (21)	20	12	17(85)	6(50)			Randomized Control Trial: Those in HBO group had more severe wounds (Wagner Score NS, but Strauss Wound Score p=0.03). Healing: HBO=95.6 days; controls 138.1 days p=0.038
Stone, 1995 (22)	87	383	63(72)	203(53)	24(28)	179(47)	Retrospective study; HBO patients had more severe wounds. Wagner Scoring used
Faglia, 1996 (23)	35	33	-	-	3(86%)	11(33.3)	Randomized study; significant improvement in the $P_{tc}O_2$'s in the HBO Group
Wirjosemito, 1992 (24)	42	-	35(83)	-	5(12)	-	Five year follow-up; matched subject (head-to-head study) with Britton's (Reference 28) non-HBO treated patients
Wattel, 1991 (25)	59	-	52(88)	-	7(12)	-	HBO-healed group had significantly higher $P_{tc}O_2$'s than the failed group
Oriani, 1990 (26)	62	18	59(95)	12(67)	3(5)	6(33)	Controls refused HBO; retrospective study
Cianci, 1988 (27)	39	-	36(92)	-	3(8)	-	Retrospective study
Britton, 1987 (28)	-	64	-	29(45)	-	35(55)	Standard care but without HBO; see Wirjosemito study (Reference 24) above
Baroni, 1987 (29)	18	10	16(89)	2(11)	0(0)	4(40)	Prospective HBO series, matched retrospective controls; standard diabetic treatment for both groups
Davis, 1987 (30)	168	-	118(70)	-	50(30)	-	Retrospective study
Strauss, 1985 (31)	50	-	44(88)	-	3(6)	-	Retrospective study; 3 (6%) Remained unhealed, but remaining wound was small enough not to interfere with activities of daily living
TOTALS	599	533	453/535	256/534	98/560	235/507	
PERCENT			(85)	(48)	(18)	(46)	

REFERENCES

1. Medicare Bulletin 424. May 11, 1999, Hyperbaric Oxygen (HBO) therapy.

2. Hyperbaric Oxygen Therapy. 1999 Committee Report. Hampson NB, Chairman and Editor. Undersea and Hyperbaric Medical Society, Inc., Kensington, MD.

3. Strauss MB. Improving host factors. Hyperbaric oxygen secondary effects. Current Concepts in Wound Care 1987; 10(4):7-10.

4. Hunt TK, Pai MP. The effect of varying ambient oxygen tensions on wound metabolism and collagen synthesis. Surg Gynecol Obstet 1972; 135:561-567.

5. Strauss MB, Bryant BJ, Hart GB. Transcutaneous oxygen measurements under hyperbaric oxygen conditions as a predictor for healing of problem wounds. Foot & Ankle International, 2001 (In Press).

6. Borer KM, Borer RC Jr., Strauss MB. Prospective evaluation of a clinical wound score to identify lower extremity wounds for comprehensive wound management. Undersea Hyperb Med 2000; 27(Suppl):34.

7. Strauss MB, Pinzur MS. Treatment strategies for problem diabetic foot wounds. 68th Annual Meeting Proceedings, American Academy of Orthopedic Surgeons, 2001; 2:SE 64:675-676.

8. Strauss MB. Diabetic foot and leg wounds: Principles, management and prevention. Primary Care Reports 2001; 7(22):187-198.

9. Strauss MB, Syms MB, Borer KM, Strauss WG. Nutrition assessment in management of problem wounds. Undersea Hyperb Med 2000; 27(Suppl):35.

10. Hunt TK, Zederfeldt B, Goldstick TK. Oxygen and healing. Am J Surg 1969; 118:521-525.

11. Hohn DC. Oxygen and leucocyte microbial killing. In: Davis JC, Hunt TK, eds. Hyperbaric Oxygen Therapy. Bethesda, MD: Undersea Medical Society, Inc; 1997:101-110.

12. Strauss MB. Improving host responsiveness by hyperoxygenation. Current Concepts in Wound Care 1987; 10(3):11-16.

13. Reenstra WR, Buras JA, Svoboda KS. Hyperbaric oxygen increases human dermal fibroblast proliferation, growth factor receptor number and in vitro wound closure. Undersea Hyperb Med 1998; 25(Suppl):53, #164

14. Strauss MB, Hart JD. KISS (Keep It Simple and Speedy) procedures for problem foot wounds. Undersea Hyperb Med 2001; 28(Suppl):35-36.

15. Strauss MB, Hart JD, Winant DM. Preventive foot care. A user friendly system for patients and physicians. Postgrad Med J 1998; 103(5):223-245.

16. Strauss MB. Controlled osteoclasis for "dropped" metatarsal head problems. European Foot and Ankle Society, 3rd Congress, 2000. Stockholm, Sweden, Abstract p. 33.

17. Strauss MB, Bryant BJ. Forefoot narrowing with external fixation for problem cleft wounds. Foot & Ankle International 2001, 2002; 23 (5): 433-439

18. Strauss MB and JD Hart. Delayed healing of failed flaps in problem wounds after hyperbaric oxygen and surgery. Undersea and Hyperbaric Medicine 2001; 28(Suppl):65.

19. Strauss MB and Bryant BJ. The cutting edge: Hyperbaric oxygen. Orthopedics, 2002; 25 (3): 303-309.

20. Abidia A, Kuhan G, Laden G, et al. Role of hyperbaric oxygen therapy in ischaemic, diabetic, lower-extremity ulcers: a double-blind randomized control trial. Br J Surg 2001; 88(SRS Abstracts):744.

21. Thang LC, Ramiah R, Seng LC, Rajoo V. Adjunctive hyperbaric oxygen in diabetic foot ulcers. A preliminary report. Proceedings of the Malaysian Orthopaedic Association Meeting, April 2001.

22. Stone JA, Scott R, Brill LR, Levine BD. The role of hyperbaric oxygen in the treatment of diabetic foot wounds (abstract). Diabetes, 1995; 44(suppl):71A.

23. Faglia E, Favales F, Aldeghi A, et al. Adjunctive systemic hyperbaric oxygen therapy in treatment of severe prevalently ischemic diabetic foot ulcer. Diabetes Care, 1996; 19:1338-1343.

24. Wirjosemito SA. Results of combined therapy including HBO in salvaging diabetic limbs (abstract). Aviat Space Environ Med, 1992; May:440.

25. Wattel F, Mathieu D, Coget JM, Billard V. Hyperbaric oxygen therapy in chronic vascular wound management. Angiology, 1990; 41:59-65.

26. Oriani G, Meazza D, Favales F, et al. Hyperbaric therapy in diabetic gangrene. J Hyperbaric Medicine, 1990; 5:171-175.

27. Cianci P, Petrone G, Drager S, et al. Salvage of problem wound and potential amputation with wound care and adjunctive hyperbaric oxygen therapy: An economic analysis. J Hyperbaric Medicine, 1988, 3:127-141.

28. Britton JP, Barrie WW. Amputation in the diabetic: ten years experience in a district general hospital. Ann Royal College Surgeons, 1987; 69(3):127-129.

29. Baroni G, Porro T, Faglia E, et al. Hyperbaric oxygen in diabetic gangene treatment. Diabetes Care, 1987; 10:81-86.

30. Davis JC. The use of adjuvant hyperbaric oxygen in the treatment of the diabetic foot. Clin Podiatr Med Surg, 1987; 4:429-437.

31. Strauss MB, Villavicencio P, Hart GB, Benge C. Salvaging the difficult wound through a combined management program. In Proceedings of the Eighth International Congress on Hyperbaric Medicine. Kindwall E. ed. San Pedro, CA: Best Publishing, 1984:207-212.

32. Handbook of Emergency Cardiovascular Care for Health Care Providers, eds Hazinski ME and Cummins RD, American Heart Association, 1999, p. 3.

33. Strauss MB. Evidence review of HBO for crush injury, compartment syndrome and other traumatic ischemias. Undersea and Hyperbaric Medicine 2001; 28(Suppl):35-36.

CHAPTER 16

HYPERBARIC OXYGEN IN PLASTIC AND RECONSTRUCTIVE SURGERY

W. A. Zamboni, B.L. Persons

INTRODUCTION

HBO has become a valuable treatment modality in several areas of plastic and reconstructive surgery including problem wound management, ischemia reperfusion injury, as well as flap reconstruction and grafts. Patient selection and the timing of HBO treatment are the keys to a successful outcome.

The rationale for HBO treatment of a specific plastic surgery problem should be based on scientific research and sound physiological principles. The appropriate use of HBO for each condition will be explained based both on the authors' experience and on the latest scientific research. This chapter will focus on three plastic surgical conditions: problem wounds, flaps and grafts, and ischemia reperfusion.

HISTORY OF HBO USE IN PLASTIC SURGERY

Over the past 30 years, numerous investigators have contributed to our understanding of how HBO treatment improves wound healing and flap survival, and how it prevents ischemia reperfusion injury. Much of the original work on oxygen and wound healing was performed by Hunt who showed that elevation of oxygen tension stimulates collagen synthesis and fiberblast proliferation. [1] In 1976, studies revealed the improved ability of leukocytes to clear infected wounds of bacteria with HBO. [2,3] In 1989, we conducted a study on rats demonstrating that reduced flap necrosis afforded by HBO immediately following ischemia was a systemic phenomenon. [4] In 1993 our group showed that hyperbaric oxygen, administered immediately on reperfusion, inhibited leukocyte adherence and prevented subsequent arteolar vasoconstriction. In 1994, Hammerlund and co-workers carried out a randomized double blind study showing that the size of chronic wounds was significantly decreased over six weeks with 2.5 ATA five days a week for 30 treatments. [5] Since then, additional studies have yielded further insights into the effects and benefits of HBO therapy which are discussed in the subsequent sections.

PROBLEM WOUNDS

Problem wound management often involves prolonged hospitalizations, frequent dressing applications, and multiple surgical interventions. A thorough understanding of the basic principles of wound healing and wound pathophysiology is therefore essential in the management of problem wounds. A wound heals in three phases: inflammation (0-3 days), repair (3-21 days) and maturation (21 days to 2 years). In the inflammation phase, there are both vascular and cellular responses. Arterioles and venules dilate and then constrict. The coagulation cascade is initiated. Interleukins attract fibroblasts to the injured site and angiogenesis is initiated. Leukocytes marginate and neutrophil chemotaxis and phagocytosis take place. With resolution of the inflammation phase, the repair phase begins. Fibroblasts synthesize collagen and the wound is strengthened. During maturation, collagenase breaks down collagen and forms new stronger crosslinks.

Oxygen in Wound Healing

Wound healing can be delayed by infection, edema, anemia, poor perfusion, and improper surgical technique. These factors usually result in decreased oxygen tension. Decreased oxygen tension, in turn, affects neutrophil, macrophage, and fibroblast function. Fibroblasts and leukocytes, specifically PMNs and macrophages, require oxygen during the inflammation and repair phases of wound healing. Oxygen-dependent mechanisms are also important in the bacteriacidal functions of leukocytes. In the oxygen-dependent system known as the respiratory burst, oxygen molecules are converted to superoxide, which is an oxygen radical containing, by definition, an unpaired electron in its outermost shell. The enzyme superoxide dismutase then turns superoxide into hydrogen peroxide. Hydrogen peroxide is finally converted either into the bacteria killing molecule hydrochlorous acid (HOCl•) by myeloperoxidase or into the hydroxyl radical (OH•) extracellularly in the presence of iron. These free radicals kill bacteria by oxidizing cell membranes. The OH• radical kills bacteria effectively, but also harms surrounding cells. While hypoxia in the tissues severely inhibits or incapacitates the respiratory burst, oxygen is nonetheless also required to neutralize these free radicals.

Oxygen is also important for collagen formation by fibroblasts. Fibroblasts enter the wound environment signaled by interleukins from macrophages and begin to synthesize collagen precursors. Post-translation hydroxylation of proline and lysine forms procollagen. This process requires oxygen and vitamin C. Procollagen is then secreted from the fibroblast. Oxygen is the cofactor required for the enzyme lysyl oxydase to deaminate the lysyl or hydroxylysyl residues in procollagen so that crosslinks may form. Energy metabolism in the cell takes priority over enzyme function. In a hypoxic environment, these steps are impeded and mature collagen formation does not progress.

Hypoxia, acidosis, and elevated lactate levels in problem wounds create a gradient which is largely responsible for the influx of wound healing cells. [6] In a hypoxic wound there is a gradient of low lactate and high oxygen tension toward high lactate and low oxygen tension which stimulates angiogenesis. [7] Lactate stimulates angiogenic growth factor production *in vitro* and it up regulates vascular endothelial growth factor. The mechanisms of this effect remain uncertain. [6]

Wound Evaluation

Evaluation of a non-healing wound begins with a thorough patient history and physical exam. Important components include information about the wound duration, topical treatments, previous operative management, and co-morbid conditions such as diabetes, vascular disease, or malnutrition. Careful documentation of wound location, size, depth, and infection gives the treating physician a baseline on which to measure progress. In addition, a noninvasive vascular evaluation should be carried out to assess tissue perfusion and oxygenation (see Wound Evaluation Protocol)

The evaluation of extremity wounds should include arterial doppler studies consisting of segmental and toe pressures to evaluate perfusion and transcutaneous oxymetry ($TcPO_2$) to assess oxygenation of the wound. Normal values, greater than 50mmHg for both perfusion and oxygenation, should indicate that a wound will heal spontaneously. Toe pressures (perfusion) and $TcPO_2$ (oxygenation) values of less than 30 indicate that the wound is not likely to heal spontaneously without adjunctive treatment. After perfusion and oxygenation deficiencies are corrected, then debridement, infection control, and aggressive wound management should be carried out.

Hyperbaric Oxygen for Problem Wounds

Wound management should always include correction of perfusion and oxygenation deficiencies, debridement, infection control, aggressive wound care, and surgical closure. If a deficiency in oxygenation is found in the face of a non-healing wound, HBO may be indicated. Treatment with hyperbaric oxygen is defined breathing 100% oxygen at two to three times normal atmospheric pressure at sea level. This is designed to increase oxygen delivery and tissue partial pressure of oxygen (PO_2) by increasing arterial partial pressure of oxygen (PaO_2).

Hyperbaric oxygen therapy leads to an increase in tissue oxygen pressure which promotes wound healing in several ways. Hyperbaric oxygen therapy stimulates fibroblast proliferation and collagen synthesis, enhances leukocyte function and bacterial clearance of infected wounds, and promotes epithelialization. The increased oxygen gradient in the wound environment promotes angiogenesis. [8] In an ambient environment, oxygen delivery depends on hemoglobin's oxygen carrying capacity. In wounds, the micro-vasculature is damaged and these tissues rely largely on diffusion of oxygen. Hyperbaric oxygen at 2 ATA may raise oxygen tension from below the normal value of 30-40 mmHg to over 300 mmHg.

Supporting Data

Many clinical studies support the use of hyperbaric oxygen to treat problem wounds. In one small study, a significant number of patients with lower extremity wounds undergoing hyperbaric oxygen therapy were able to avert the need for amputations. [9] The same investigators treated 151 patients who had non-healing lower extremity wounds with HBO and 130 of the patients' wounds healed. There was, however, no control group in this study.

WOUND EVALUATION PROTOCOL
HYPERBARIC MEDICAL UNIT

Name: _____   Date: _____

MMC #: _____   Referring MD: _____

SIU #: _____   HBO MD: _____

Age: _____;   Gender: M / F ; | Labs: WBC _____; H/H _____
Ht: _____; Wt: _____; Race: C / B / O | Diff _____; TLC _____
Smoking Hx: _____; Diabetes: +   - | Pre alb _____; Alb _____
                            Insulin: +   - |
Meds: _____ | Transferrin _____; Fe ____

WOUND

Location: _____ Duration: _____
Size (cm): Length _____; Diam _____; Depth: D / SQ / Muscle / Bone
Cellulitis: +   -   ;   Tendon Exposure: +   - ;   Osteo: +   -
Arteriogram: +   -   (copy);
Quant Culture:
    Initial _____; Prev. 48h _____; Prev. 5d _____

Etiology: **Previous Tx:**
    Arterial: _____   Previous Swab: +   - (bact)
    Venous: _____   Dressings: _____
    Other: _____   Debridement: _____
                                        Vascular Reconstruction: +   -
                                        (Type, Dates)

NONINVASIVE DOPPLER STUDIES   ### WOUND DRAWING & SITES
(mm Hg)

	R	L
UE BP/MAP		
LE BP/MAP		
ABI		
Toe Pressures		

CUTANEOUS OXIMETRY (mm Hg)

Reference 2nd Interostal Space _____

	Room Air	100% O_2	HBO (2 ATA)
Site 1			
Site 2			
Other			

A closely controlled group of 18 diabetic patients with extremity gangrene showed improvement in their wounds with HBO therapy. The 10 control subjects who refused HBO wounds showed no improvement and 40% of these went on to require extremity amputation. [10] A randomized double blind study by Hammerlund and co-workers in 1994 showed that the size of chronic wounds was significantly decreased over six weeks with 2.5 ATA five days a week for 30 treatments. [5] In a later prospective randomized study, 30 patients who received hyperbaric oxygen had a significantly lower amputation rate compared with controls. [11] A prospective non-randomized study with 10 patients with diabetic lower extremity wounds showed statistically significant reduction in wound size compared with controls with seven weeks of HBO therapy. [12] Kalani et al. followed chronic diabetic foot wounds for three years in a prospective randomized study. When compared to conventionally treated wounds, HBO patients demonstrated an accelerated rate of healing, reduced rate of amputation, plus an increased rate of completely healed wounds over time. [13] Results of these relatively small studies are promising; however, in the future, additional randomized controlled studies of larger magnitude will hopefully address the remaining questions. [13]

Careful patient selection for HBO therapy is essential and should include evaluation by a vascular surgeon, and, if indicated, arteriogram. If there is no reconstructable lesion, hyperbaric oxygen therapy may be indicated. Transcutaneous oxygen tension (TcPO$_2$) values of less than 40 mmHg which increase to more than 100 mmHg while breathing 100% oxygen or to more than 200 mmHg during HBO may benefit from hyperbaric oxygen therapy. [14] Often there is no visible improvement during the early phase of HBO treatment as it usually takes 15-30 treatments to achieve healthy granulation tissue and a room air TcPO$_2$ of greater than 40 mmHg. The treatment protocol should be: 2.0-2.5 ATA for 90 minutes, five (5) days a week for thirty (30) treatments. At this point HBO may be discontinued and conventional wound care should be undertaken until the wound heals.

Problem wounds which fail to respond to traditional medical and surgical therapy can be challenging to the plastic surgeon. These wounds are often associated with exorbitant wound care costs. Indirect costs such as those related to patient productivity, disability, and premature death, can also be significant. The underlying problems in failure of a wound to heal are usually hypoxia and infecton. HBO therapy in selected patients can facilitate healing by increasing tissue oxygen tension providing the wound with a favorable environment for healing.

FLAPS AND GRAFTS

Normal skin grafts and flaps with adequate blood supply do not require HBO. Hyperbaric oxygen therapy is extremely useful where the skin grafts or flaps suffer from compromised microcirculation or hypoxia.

The benefits of HBO on flaps arise from a systemic elevation in oxygen tension rather than a local effect. [15,16,17] In addition, HBO therapy prevents neutrophil adherence and subsequent vasoconstriction following ischemia which will be discussed in the section on Ischemia Reperfusion.

Compromised Flaps

Too frequently, a compromised flap is allowed to progress over the days following surgery until visible signs of necrosis obviate the use of HBO; delayed treatment with HBO cannot revive dead tissue. The resulting disappointment, as well as the associated patient dissatisfaction, can be avoided by rapid diagnosis of the flap problem and early involvement of the hyperbaric physician.

The three keys to successful treatment of compromised flaps with HBO are:
1. Accurate diagnosis of the specific flap problem
2. Appropriate and expedient initiation of hyperbaric oxygen treatment
3. Uninhibited communication between surgeon and hyperbaric physician.

Awareness of the different etiologies of flap compromise is necessary for the treating physician to plan for effective HBO treatment. A random flap with distal necrosis is completely different from a free flap with total venous occlusion. Proper classification of flaps, different etiologies of flap compromise, and understanding which will benefit from HBO treatment is essential and will be discussed below.

Flap Types

Flap classification is based on an assessment of blood supply, tissue composition, and method of movement. Each of these elements must be evaluated, but it is blood supply that is most important. The blood supply to the flap is either axial, based on a named vessel or random, based on the subdermal plexus. Modern plastic surgery relies extensively on the availability of axial flaps and free tissue transfer utilizing named vessels for their blood supply. A random flap does not derive from a named vessel and receives its blood supply from the subdermal vascular plexus. The length to width ratio of a random flap is limited between 2 to 1 and 3 to 1. An axial flap is based on a specific arterial watershed and allows the creation of a longer flap on a narrower base or a flap isolated on the pedicle artery and vein alone. There are several causes of flap necrosis. Commonly, flap compromise occurs when the surgeon tries to mobilize tissue outside the defined arterial supply, when there is a pedicle problem, or when free flaps are exposed to prolonged ischemia.

The tissue composition of a flap may include skin, subcutaneous tissue, fascia, muscle, bone, other tissues, or a combination of these. Flap composition is very important because different tissue types have different tolerances to ischemia. For instance, a myocutaneous flap will be more susceptible to ischemia than a fasciocutaneous flap, because muscle is much more sensitive to ischemic injury than fascia and skin.

Finally, the method of movement must be considered. Local flap movement can be achieved locally by means of advancement, rotation, or transposition. Flap placement may also be distant via a pedicled, or island flap, or by means of a free tissue transfer.

Diagnosis of Flap Compromise

Compromised tissues are usually hypoxic with oxygen tensions of less than 30 mmHg. With flaps, the etiology of the flap ischemia and compromise may result from technical causes including improper flap design, closure with tension, pedicle or tissue damage, hematoma, or prolonged operative ischemia. Non-technical causes include arterial vasospasm, flap edema, postoperative infection, and patient deterioration. Specific flap problems include low arterial inflow, total arterial occlusion, partial venous congestion, and total venous occlusion.

Careful clinical evaluation of the flap is essential. An examination of color, capillary refill, temperature, and bleeding to pin prick should be performed. A flap with low arterial inflow is a pale pink color, has slow capillary refill, and is cool. With total arterial occlusion, the flap turns a pale white, capillary refill is absent, and the temperature is cold. Flaps with partial venous congestion turn dusky pink, demonstrate brisk capillary refill, and are cool. With total venous occlusion, flaps turn dark blue, capillary refill is absent, and the temperature is cold. In those circumstances where there is a prolonged primary ischemia, or any secondary ischemia resulting from vessel thrombosis and revision anastomosis, the flaps will undergo ischemia reperfusion injury. Often there is no early clinical sign of compromise. After several hours, however, dark, patchy areas develop in a random distribution. With this type of flap problem, precise knowledge of ischemia time and tissue type are very important in determining the need for adjunctive treatment.

Non-clinical means of monitoring the flap include laser doppler, transcutaneous oxymetry (TcPO$_2$) measurement, temperature and pH probes, power doppler imaging, fluorescein, and photoplethismography. Although the authors have found laser doppler monitoring of microvascular perfusion to be useful in some situations, transcutaneous oxymetry (TcPO$_2$) measurements in compromised flaps have often been unreliable and non-predictive of the response to HBO treatment. Circulation disturbances and edema within the flap may lead to an inaccurate TcPO$_2$ reading and an associated false sense of security. This experience contrasts with that of others who have found this method of monitoring useful. [18] Generally, clinical evaluation is best.

Hyperbaric Oxygen for Treatment of Compromised Flaps

When treating compromised flaps, a multimodality approach should be initiated. This approach should include the use of vasodilators if arterial vasospasm is suspected, removal of sutures if tension or compression are suspected, dextran and pentoxifylline for rheological purposes, medicinal and chemical leeching for venous congestion, and the early use of hyperbaric oxygen if blood flow can be documented.

The use of HBO therapy is appropriate only when:
1. The flap problem has been defined
2. There is documented perfusion of the flap
3. Appropriate surgical salvage measures have been considered first
4. HBO therapy can be performed in an expedient manner

The following specific flap problems and use of HBO will be discussed:

Random Flap Ischemia

Although random flaps are rarely used in plastic surgery wound closure, animal research has clearly demonstrated a modest but beneficial effect of HBO on distal random flap necrosis. [19-31] Generally the majority of these articles have shown a beneficial response of between 15-30% improvement in flap survival. This information may be useful to the plastic surgeon if the surgeon is faced with treating an axial flap that is inadvertently elevated at a length that exceeds the blood supply of a named artery. A random extension of an axial flap is produced. The treating physician can minimize loss of this distal random portion of the flap with HBO treatment. Random ischemia is usually identified within the first 24 h by a progressively dusky appearance and epidermolysis. Hyperbaric oxygen therapy should be initiated immediately if these signs are noted. The treatment regimen is 2.0-2.5 ATA, 90 min, q12 h, for 48-72 h, and then q day, 7 days a week until complete healing is noted, usually a total of 20-30 treatments.

Decreased Arterial Inflow

Intermittent vasospasms may cause low arterial inflow in pedicle and free flaps. Low inflow may result if edema in tissues around the pedicle is partially obstructing or if a hematoma is present around the pedicle. Partial obstruction appears clinically as a pale pink color with slow capillary refill. The primary treatment for this problem is surgical reexploration to ensure that a hematoma, anatomical kinking, or twisting of the pedicle is not present. If a surgical condition for the compromise is not found and the flap continues to show signs of low arterial inflow, then HBO treatment is indicated. In situations of vasospasm, the author feels that the beneficial effects of oxygenating the compromised tissue outweigh the potential for vasoconstriction within the chamber. The treatment protocol is 2.0-2.5 ATA for 90 min every q12 h, for 48-72 h, and then q day, 7 days a week until complete healing is achieved. This usually requires a total of 20-30 treatments.

Complete Arterial Occlusion

Total arterial occlusion is suspected when the flap is pale and capillary refill is absent. Etiologies include intraoperative damage to the arterial pedicle of an axial flap, mechanical compression of the artery by a hematoma, or twisting or kinking of the pedicle. Note that immediate surgical re-exploration is mandatory if there is arterial thrombosis and primary HBO treatment without surgical re-exploration is not indicated.

Once flow is surgically reestablished, HBO therapy is indicated immediately to treat ischemia reperfusion injury. If there has been a period of warm ischemia, or secondary ischemia, the treatment regimen is as follows: 2.0-2.5 ATA, 90 min, q 8 h x 24 h, then q 8-12 h x 48 h. This regimen should be initiated after a brief period of post operative recovery room observation and may be discontinued when clinical examination of the flap reveals complete viability.

Venous Congestion

Venous congestion is the most common etiology of compromise in pedicle flaps. The anatomical causes must first be ruled out including hematoma, kinking, and twisting of the pedicle vein. The venous drainage of a pedicle flap is sometimes inherently inadequate and chokes the system between capillary beds. Also, some flaps such as those having a reverse venous drainage (i.e., radial forearm flap) create a transient congestion of the flap until the venous outflow can be established through valve blowout of the venacommicantes as well as branch formation.

First line treatment should be medicinal or chemical leeching. The addition of HBO can be a useful adjunct to leeching to help oxygenate and support the flap until pedicle or peripheral venous channels can be reestablished, which usually takes 7-10 days. [32] In these instances, HBO treatment should begin within 4 hours of recognition of venous congestion at 2.0 –2.5 ATA, q 12 h until signs of venous congestion resolve.

Complete Venous Occlusion

Anatomic abnormalities can cause total venous occlusion due to compression, twisting, and kinking of the pedicle, as well as hematoma. These can lead to venous thrombosis, which is the most common cause of free flap failure. The venous anastamosis often thromboses first, causing congestion in the microcirculation and leading to arterial thrombosis and complete necrosis of the flap.

Hyperbaric oxygen therapy alone for total venous occlusion is ineffective. A study of rat axial skin flaps subjected to total venous occlusion revealed that HBO administration alone did not increase the flap survival [33]. The flaps having total venous occlusion underwent complete flap necrosis even with HBO. This result is expected since HBO therapy effects are systemic and require blood flow to the injured tissue in order to be effective. [15] However, in this same study, the combination of leeching plus HBO treatment significantly improved survival vs. leeching alone.

The primary treatment for total venous occlusion is surgical re-exploration. However, in situations where patient deterioration or refusal to reoperate are present, then leeching (to provide venous outflow) in combination with HBO therapy may result in flap salvage, provided that the artery remains patent. Treatment is at 2.0-2.5 ATA, q 8 h x 48 h, then q 12 h for approximately 7-10 days, until the flap develops adequate venous outflow.

Free Flaps

Extended primary ischemia time greater than two hours or any secondary ischemia time may result in partial or total flap necrosis. This injury is usually reversible if recognized early and treated expeditiously. Numerous research studies support the use of HBO in the salvage of compromised free tissue transfers. [15,34,35] HBO significantly improves survival when administered before and during reperfusion following 8 h of ischemia in one of our studies using an axial flap model. [15] A rat free-flap model showed similar improvement in flap survival. [34] A clinical study evaluated free flap salvage in the face of prolonged primary or any secondary ischemia. [35] Salvage was significantly better in the HBO treatment treatment group vs. controls but only if initiated within 24 hours.

Free flaps compromised by prolonged primary or secondary ischemia have responded favorably to HBO treatment with complete salvage in most cases if HBO is started early. The treatment regimen is: 2.0-2.4 ATA, 90 min q 8 h x 24 h, then q 8-12 h x 48 h. Treatment is then continued daily based on clinical evaluation.

Grafts

Skin grafts are anatomically different from flaps in that skin grafts lack an inherent blood supply. Skin grafts are composed of avascular tissue that depends entirely on the recipient bed for oxygenation. HBO is useful in preparing the recipient bed, and in promoting healthy granulation tissue to support split thickness skin grafts. One controlled study showed a significant improvement in skin graft survival from 17 to 64% with the addition of HBO treatment. The overall skin graft survival rate, however, was unusually low in this study. [36] Although there is literature to support the use of HBO for composite grafts [20], a study by our group found no significant effect of HBO on rat-ear composite grafts larger than 1 cm. [37] Further research is needed to better understand the effects of HBO on composite graft survival.

ISCHEMIA REPERFUSION INJURY

High energy trauma to the extremities can be associated with arterial injury or compartment syndrome resulting in varying degrees of tissue ischemia. Limb amputation is perhaps the most devastating form of acute traumatic ischemia. The treatment in most of these injuries is immediate restoration of blood flow. Once surgically restored, return of blood flow may actually cause accelerated tissue damage due to reperfusion injury. Ischemia times of greater than four hours will result in some degree of permanent necrosis. This section will provide a brief overview of ischemia reperfusion injury and a discussion of hyperbaric oxygen therapy, including research and clinical applications for acute traumatic ischemia.

The physiologic basis of IR injury has become better understood in recent years [38]. Most of the animal research centers around the production of oxygen free radicals. Although the endothelial xanthine oxidase pathway has received much attention in the literature [39], more recent evidence suggests that neutrophils are a more important source of oxygen free radicals via membrane NADPH oxidase and degranulation. [19] These two sources of free radicals will be discussed as well as the important role of neutrophil adhesion in IR-associated vasoconstriction.

Previous animal research centered around the intracellular xanthine oxydase free radical generating system. An oxygen radical is an unstable molecule with an unpaired electron in its outer shell. During ischemia, ATP is ultimately degraded to hypoxanthine and xanthine which are anaerobic metabolites. With reperfusion, oxygenated blood is reintroduced into the ischemic tissue, and the hypoxanthine and xanthine plus oxygen creates oxygen free radicals. Superoxide and hydroxyl radicals are formed which can cause extensive tissue damage. A rat skeletal muscle model of reperfusion after four hours of global ischemia [18] showed that neutrophil adherence to postcapillary venules is one of the earliest events associated with IR injury.

A significant increase in adherence occurs early in reperfusion, and is sustained throughout a three-hour observation period. Significant and progressive vasoconstriction occurs in arterioles adjacent to leukocyte-damaged venules. Neutrophil adherence and vasoconstriction lead to a low-flow state in the microcirculation and then vessel thrombosis, the end point in IR injury.

The leukocyte-damaged venule is thought to be responsible for the arterial vasoactive response. Because leukocyte endothelial adherence appears to be the earliest and one of the inciting events of the deleterious cascade that follows, the mechanism of this adherence function becomes important. Adhesion molecules are grouped into three families: the integrins, the selectins, and the immunoglobulin gene super family. [40] Integrins are responsible for firm neutrophil adhesion to vascular endothelium. A study [21] has provided *in vivo* quantitative proof that neutrophil adhesion function associated with IR injury is dependent on the beta-2 integrin (CD 18 chain) of the leukocyte function antigen 1 (LFA-1) on the neutrophil cell surface. This study used a transilluminated rat gracilis muscle model and administered an anti-CD 18 monoclonal antibody after 4 hours of global ischemia. The IR-induced vasoconstriction in arterioles was blocked by the monoclonal antibody. [41] The authors' group recently showed that neutrophil CD 18 expression is increased in a rat model of IR injury. CD 18 adhesion sites quantified by flow cytometry were increased in IR injury, but surprisingly, they were not reduced by HBO therapy. [42] Research currently underway suggests that the HBO effects a qualitative change in CD 18 molecule which decreases endothelial binding of neutrophils after IR injury. Neutrophil adhesion to endothelial cells has also been shown to be promoted by interleukin-1, tumor necrosis factor, endothelin, as well as by leukotriene B4, platelet activating factor, and compliment C5a.

Although neutrophil adherence has been shown to be a prerequisite to the vasoconstrictive response, the vasoactive mediators involved are still poorly understood. The authors examined the role of thromboxane A2 receptor blockade in reducing vasoconstriction. [43] TXA-2 receptor blockade does reduce but does not eliminate IR-induced vasoconstriction in this rat gracilis muscle model. There is evidence that nitric oxide may play a significant role in reperfusion injury. Thom et al. showed that HBO increased nitric oxide levels by increasing eNOS (nitric oxide synthase) in rodent cerebral cortex. [44] Jones et al. provided further evidence of HBO-induced nitric oxide-related mechanism by evaluating CD 18 polarity on neutrophils by confocal microscopy. This study showed that treatment of ischemia reperfusion plasma with HBO inhibited CD 18 polarization of neutrophils and that this effect was reversed with addition of a nitric oxide scavenger. [45] Another study by Buras et al. found that HBO decreased ICAM-1 expression which is related to a relative increase in endothelial cell nitric oxide synthase (eNOS). This could explain decreased neutrophil-endothelial adherence in IR injury with HBO. [46]

HBO Therapy for IR injury

Treatment with hyperbaric oxygen in the face of IR injury carried the concern that providing extra oxygen would increase free radical production and tissue damage. This query has been resolved by studies which have shown that HBO actually antagonizes the ill effects of IR injury in a variety of tissues. [4, 34, 47-50] One of the first studies evaluating HBO and IR injury showed that HBO immediately upon reperfusion significantly improved skin flap survival following 8 h of global ischemia in a rat axial skin flap model. [15] Laser doppler analysis of the same skin flap model showed that HBO therapy increased microvascular blood flow during reperfusion. [47] Free flaps have improved survival with HBO treatment during reperfusion even following ischemia times of up to 24 h. [34] The skin flap studies then gave rise to skeletal muscle experiments. These were germane to clinical scenarios given that traumatic ischemia usually involves skeletal muscle which is more sensitive to IR injury. Early studies demonstrated a reduction of necrosis in a rat hindlimb [51] and dog compartment syndrome [52] models.

Hyperbaric oxygen administered during and up to 1 h following 4 h global ischemia significantly reduced neutrophil endothelial adherence in venules and also blocked the progressive arteriolar vasoconstriction associated with reperfusion injury. [4] The fact that neutrophil endothelial adherence depends on CD 18 function in this model provides indirect evidence that HBO affects the neutrophil CD 18 adhesion molecule. Direct evidence of this mechanism has been demonstrated using a rat carbon monoxide model of brain IR injury by Thom and associates. [53] His experiments revealed that HBO (a) blocked *in vivo* persistent neutrophil accumulation in brain microvessels thought to be via a nitric oxide-dependent mechanism, (b) inhibited *in vitro* beta-2-integrin (CD 18)-induced neutrophil adherence function, and (c) did not alter other important neutrophil functions such as oxidative burst or stimulus-induced chemotaxis and migration. This latter finding is very important, because HBO, through its discrete action on the CD 18 adhesion molecule, blocks the neutrophil adherence associated with IR injury without interfering with other neutrophil functions which would increase the risk of infectious complications.

A rabbit hindlimb model was used to demonstrate the long term improvement in muscle function when hyperbaric oxygen is delivered during ischemia. This showed that muscle function was improved five weeks after the ischemic event. [54] This suggests that it may be useful to treat the patient with a traumatic amputation with hyperbaric oxygen while preparing to operate.

Clinical Considerations in IR Injury

Initially, the focus in acute ischemia caused by trauma should be restoration of blood supply. Replantation should be completed as soon as possible with repair of disrupted arteries and fasciotomies if necessary. Both clinical experience as well as the previously summarized research experience advocate for HBO treatment in IR injury and the results are positive and often dramatic in our experience. If muscle ischemia time is greater than four to six hours there is a significant risk of severe IR injury, muscle necrosis, and loss of the affected extremity. Skin is more resistant to IR injury but it is likely to occur after eight hours of ischemia as in the case of a digit amputation. We, therefore, recommend HBO therapy for all patients with muscle ischemia time greater than four hours and skin ischemia time greater than eight hours. Also a retrospective controlled review of compromised free flaps and replanted extremities with greater than six hours of primary ischemia and any secondary ischemia showed 100% salvage rate when HBO therapy was initiated within 24 hours of injury and 0% salvage rate when HBO therapy was initiated greater than 72 hours after the injury. [35] The major effects of IR injury are felt to occur within the first 4-7 hours of reperfusion. [52] Since some irreversible tissue damage occurs after this time it is important to take patients to receive HBO therapy immediately postoperatively, even if they are still intubated. Two ATA hyperbaric oxygen increases the tissue oxygen tension 1000 percent. Treatment protocol: 2.0-2.5 ATA for 60 min, q 8 h x 24 h, then q 8-12 h x 48 h with clinical reevaluation. If progressive signs of ischemic injury are still present, the treatment is continued at 2.0 ATA, q 12 h for 2-3 more days. Usually 72 hours of treatment is adequate as long as the first treatment is initiated within 4 hours of surgery.

SUMMARY

This chapter is designed to guide the practicing plastic surgeon and hyperbaric physician. In light of multiple studies and years of clinical experience, hyperbaric oxygen therapy should be seen as a useful adjunct to improve outcomes in a variety of problems in plastic surgery. The use of HBO must be based on specific indications formulated from a sound understanding of hyperbaric oxygen therapy. It cannot be overemphasized that patient selection and the timing of HBO treatment are the keys to a successful outcome for most conditions outlined in this chapter. Although HBO research in recent years has become more scientific and less anecdotal, there is still a need for further experimental and prospective clinical studies to more accurately define and confirm the specific role of HBO therapy for many plastic surgery conditions.

A 48-year-old male with a work related amputation of the right arm at the elbow. Successful replant of right arm, however 8 hours of primary ischemia prompted emergent HBO treatment for reperfusion injury.

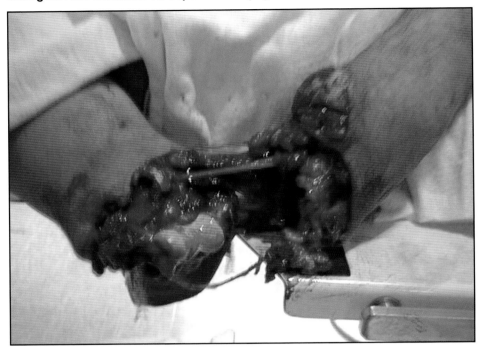

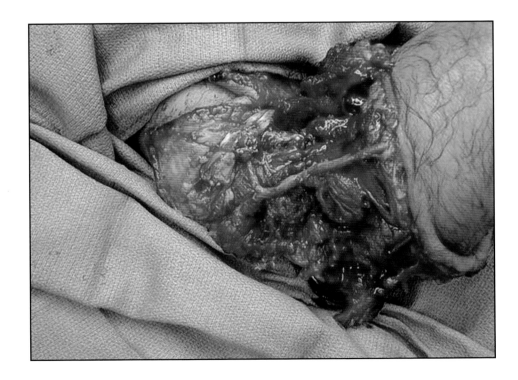

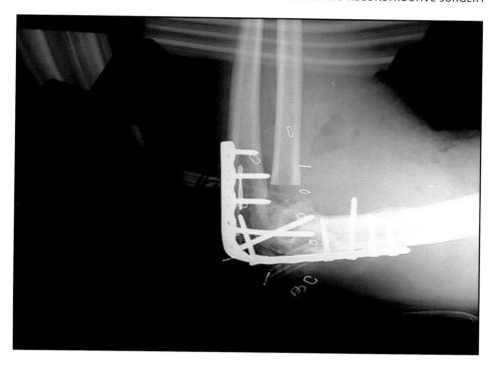

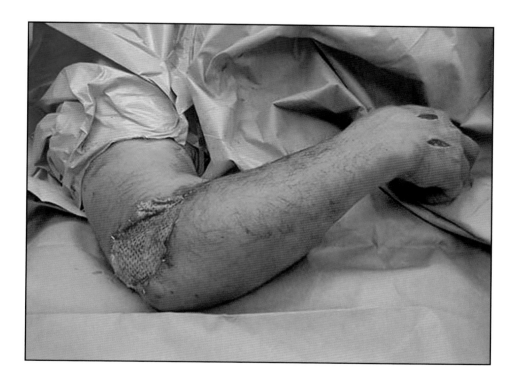

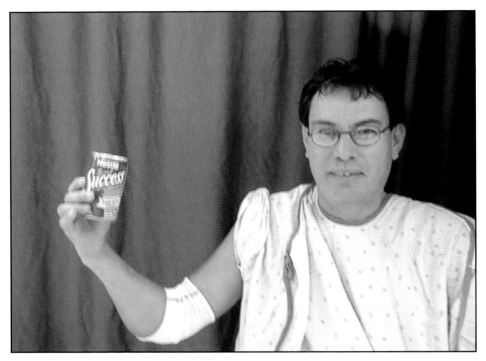

FInal results with good functional outcome.

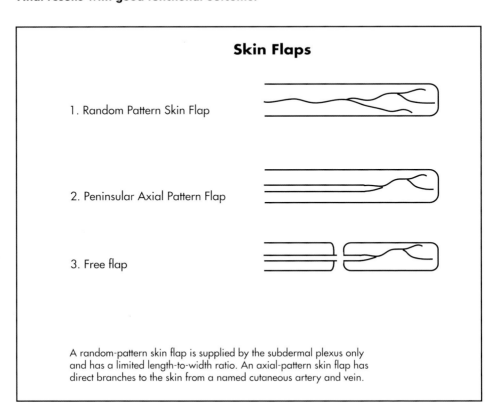

Skin Flaps

1. Random Pattern Skin Flap

2. Peninsular Axial Pattern Flap

3. Free flap

A random-pattern skin flap is supplied by the subdermal plexus only and has a limited length-to-width ratio. An axial-pattern skin flap has direct branches to the skin from a named cutaneous artery and vein.

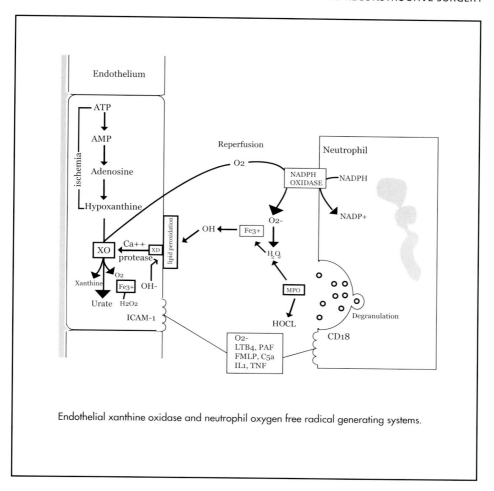

Endothelial xanthine oxidase and neutrophil oxygen free radical generating systems.

REFERENCES

1. Hunt TK, Pai MP (1972) The effect of varying ambient oxygen tensions on wound metabolism and collagen synthesis. Surg Gynecol Obstet 135:56t-567.

2. Hohn DC, Mackay RD, Halliday BJ (1976) The effect of oxygen tension on the microbial function in wounds and in vitro. Surg Forum 27:18-20.

3. Knighton DR, Halliday BJ, Hunt TK (1986) Oxygen as an antibiotic: a comparison of the effects of inspired oxygen concentration and antibiotic administration on in vivo bacterial clearance. Arch Surg 121:191-195.

4. Zamboni WA, Roth AC, Russell RC, Graham B, Suchy H, Kucan JO: Morphologic analysis of the microcirculation during reperfusion of ischemic skeletal muscle and the effect of hyperbaric oxygen. Plast Reconstr Surg 1993 May;91(6): 1110-23.

5. Hammarlund C, Sundberg T (1994) Hyperbaric oxygen reduced size of chronic leg ulcers: a randomized double-blind study. Plast Reconstr Surg 93 (4):829-833.

6. Niinikoski J, Hunt TK: Oxygen and healing wounds: Tissue Bone Repair Enhancement. In: Oriani, G, Marroni A eds. Handbook on Hyperbaric Medicine 1st ed. New York, Springer 1995.

7. Gimbel M, Hunt TK: Wound Healing and Hyperbaric Oxygen. In: Kindwall, EP, Whelan, HT, eds. Hyperbaric Medicine Practice 2nd edition. Flagstaff, Best. 1999.

8. Knighton DR, Silver IA, Hunt TK (1981) Regulation of wound healing angiogenesis – effect of oxygen gradients and inspired oxygen concentration. Surgery 90 (2):262-270.

9. Oriani G, Marroni A, eds. Handbook on Hyperbaric Medicine 1st ed. New York, Springer, 1995.

10. Baroni, G. Porro T, Faglia E, Pizzi G, Mastropasqua A, Oriani G, Pedesini G, Favales F: Hyperbaric Oxygen in Diabetes Gangrene Treatment, Diabetes Care 10:81, 1987.

11. Doctor N, Pandya S, Supe A: Hyperbaric Oxygen therapy in diabetic foot. Journal of Postgrad Med 1992; 38:112-114.

12. Zamboni WA, Wong HP, Stephenson LL, Pfeifer MA: Evaluation of hyperbaric oxygen for diabetic wounds: a prospective study. Undersea Hyperb Med 1997 Sep;24(3):175-9.

13. Kalani M, Jorneskog G, Nazanin N et al.: Hyperbaric oxygen therapy in treatment of diabetic foot ulcers: Long-term follow-up. J Diabetes Complications. 2002 Mar-Apr; 16(2):153-8.

14. Matos L, Nunez A: Enhancement of healing in selected problem wounds. In: Kindwall EP, Whelan HT eds. Hyperbaric Medicine Practice 2nd ed. Flagstaff, Best. 1999.

15. Zamboni WA, Roth AC, Russel RC, Nemiroff PM, Casas L, Smoot EC: "Hyperbaric Oxygen Improves Axial Skin Flap Survival When Administered During and After Total Ischemia." J Reconstr Micro 5:343-347, 1989.

16: Hunt TK, Pai MP: "The effect of varying ambient oxygen tensions on wound metabolism and collagen synthesis" Surg Gyn Obstet. 1972; 135:561-567.

17. Niinikoski J, Hunt TK: "Oxygen Tension in Human Wounds." J Surg Res. 1972; 12:77-82.

18. Mathieu D et al. (1993) Pedicle musculocutaneous flap transplantation: prediction of final outcome by transcutaneous oxygen measurements in hyperbaric oxygen. Plast Reconstr Surg 91:329-334.

19. Kernahan DA, Zingg W, Kay CW (1965) The effect of hyperbaric oxygen on the survival of experimental skin flaps. Plast Reconstr Surg 36:19-25.

20. McFarlane RM, Wermuth RE (1966) The use of hyperbaric oxygen to prevent necrosis in experimental pedicle flaps and composite skin grafts. Plast Reconstr Surg 37:422-430.

21. Champion WM, McSherry CK, Goulian D (1967) Effect of hyperbaric oxygen on the survival of pedicled skin flaps. J Surg Res 7:583-586.

22. Niinikoski J (1970) Viability of ischemic skin in hyperbaric oxygen. Acta Chir Scand 136: 567-568.

23. Arturson G, Khanna NN (1970) The effects of hyperbaric oxygen, dimethyl sulfoxide, and complamin on the survival of experimental skin flaps. Scand J Plast Reconstr Surg 4:8-10.

24. Jurell G, Kaijser L (1973) The influence of varying pressure and duration of treatment with hyperbaric oxygen on the survival of skin flaps. Scand J Plast Reconstr Surg 7:25-28.

25. Manson PN et al. (1980) Improved capillaries by hyperbaric oxygen in skin flaps. Surg Forum 31:564-566.

26. Tan CM et al. (1984) Effects of hyperbaric oxygen and hyperbaric air on the survival of island skin flaps. Plast Reconstr Surg 73:27-30.

27. Nemiroff PM et al. (1985) Effects of hyperbaric oxygen and irradiation on experimental skin flaps in rats. Otolaryngol Head Neck Surg 93:485-491.

28. Caffee HH, Gallagher TJ (1988) Experiments on the effects of hyperbaric oxygen on flap survival in the pig. Plast Reconstr Surg 81:751-754.

29. Nemiroff PM (1988) Synergistic effects of pentoxifylline and hyperbaric oxygen on skin flaps. Arch Otolaryngol Head Neck Surg 114:977-981.

30. Perrins DJD (1975) The effect of hyperbaric oxygen on ischemic skin flaps. In Skin flaps, W.C. Grabb and M.B. Myers, (ads). Little Brown, Boston, pp 53-63.

31. Bowersox JC, Strauss MB, Hart GB (1986) Clinical experiences with hyperbaric oxygen therapy in the salvage of ischemic skin flaps and grafts. J Hyperb Oxygen 1:141-149.

32. Lozano DD, Zamboni WA, Stephenson LL: "Effect of Hyperbaric Oxygen and Medicinal Leeching on Survival of Axial Skin Flaps Subjected to Total Venous Occlusion." Undersea and Hyperbaric Medicine suppl 24:86, 1997.

34. Kaelin CM et al. (1990) The effects of hyperbaric oxygen on free flaps in rats. Arch Surg 125:607.

35. Waterhouse MA et al. (1993) The use of HBO in compromised free tissue transfer and replantation: a clinical review. Undersea Hyperb Med 20 (Suppl):54 (Abstract).

36. Perrins DJD, Cantab MB (1967) Influence of hyperbaric oxygen on the survival of split skin grafts. Lancet 1:868-871.

37. Mazelowski MC, Zamboni WA, Haws MF, Smoot EC, Stephenson LL: "Effect of Hyperbaric Oxygen on Composite Graft Survival in a Rat Ear Model." Undersea and Hyperbaric Med Suppl 22:50 1995.

38. Kerrigan CL, Stotland MA (1993) Ischemia-reperfusion injury: a review. Microsurgery: 14:165-175.

39. Angel MF et al. (1987) Free radicals: basic concepts concerning their chemistry, patho physiology, and relevance to plastic surgery. Plast Reconstr Surg 79:990.

40. Heemann UW et al. (1994) Adhesion molecules and transplantation. Ann Surg 219 (1):4-12.

41. Zamboni WA et al. (1994) Ischemia-reperfusion injury in skeletal muscle: CD18 dependent neutrophil-endothelial adhesion. Undersea Hyperb Med 21 (Suppl): 53 (Abstract).

42. Larson JL, Stephenson LL, Zamboni WA: "Effect of hyperbaric oxygen on neutrophil CD 18 expression." Plast Reconstr Surg 2000 Apr; 105(4):1375-81.

43. Mazolewski PJ, Roth AC, Suchy H, Stephenson LL, Zamboni WA:"Role of the thromboxane A2 receptor in the vasoactive response to ischemia-reperfusion injury. Plast Reconstr Surg 1999 Oct; 104(5)1393-6.

44. Thom SR, Bhopale V, Fisher D, Manevich Y, Huang PL, Buerk DG: "Stimulation of nitric oxide synthase in cerebral cortex due to elevated partial pressures of oxygen: an oxidative stress response." J Neurobiol 2002 May;51(2):85-100.

45. Jones S, Wang WZ, Natajaraj C, Khiabani, Stephenson LL, Zamboni WA (2002) "HBO inhibits IR induced Neutrophil CD 18 Polarization by a Nitric Oxide Mechanism." Undersea Hyperb Med 35 (Suppl): 75 July 2002.

46. Buras JA, Stahl GL, Svoboda KK, Reenstra WR: "Hyperbaric oxygen downregulates ICAM-1 expression induced by hypoxia and hypoglycemia: the role of NOS." Am J Physiol Cell Physiol 2000 Feb; 278(2): C292-302.

47. Zamboni WA et al. (1992) Effect of hyperbaric oxygen on reperfusion of axial skin flaps: a laser Doppler analysis. Ann Plast Surg 28 (4):339-341.

48. Zamboni WA et al. (1989) The effect of acute hyperbaric oxygen therapy on axial pattern skin flap survival when administered during and after total ischemia. J Reconstr Microsurg 5:343-347.

42. Thom SR, Elbukin ME (1991) Oxygen dependent antagonism of lipid peroxidation. Free Radic Biol and Mail 10:413.

49. Kolski JM et al. (1994) Evaluation of HBO as treatment for testicular ischemia. Undersea Hyperb Med 21 (Suppl): 80 (Abstract).

50. Matteson K et al. (1993) The effect of hyperbaric oxygen on renal function following partial and global ischemia. Undersea Hyperb Med 20 (suppl): 61 (Abstract).

51. Nylander G et al. (1985) Reduction of post-ischemic edema with hyperbaric oxygen. Plast Reconstr Surg 76: 596.

52. Olivas, TP, Saylor, TF, Wong, HP, Stephenson, LL, "Timing of Microcirculatory Injury form Ischemia Reperfusion." Plastic Reconstructive Surgery, 107(3):785-788, 2001.

53. Thom SR (1993) Functional inhibition of leukocyte B2 integrins by hyperbaric oxygen in carbon monoxide-mediated brain injury. Toxicology and Applied Pharmacology 123:248-256.

53. Strauss MB et. al. "Reduction of skeletal muscle necrosis using intermittent hyperbaric oxygen in a model compartment syndrome." J Bone Joint Surg 65-A 656.

CHAPTER 17

HYPERBARIC OXYGEN AND RADIATION THERAPY:

TREATMENT OF LATE COMPLICATIONS
ISSUES OF CARCINOGENESIS AND RADIATION SENSITIZATION

J.J. Feldmeier

BACKGROUND AND NATURE OF RADIATION INJURY

Roentgen described his discovery of x-rays in December 1895, and within one year of his discovery radiation therapy had already been applied empirically for the treatment of cancer. In 1901, Pierre Curie applied a small amount of radium to his forearm and observed its destruction of tissue and development of a skin ulcer. This intentional application of radium followed the serendipitous development of an ulcer on the chest wall of Becquerel, who shared the Nobel Prize with the Curies for the discovery of radium. He had carried a vial of radium in a vest pocket for about two weeks and then observed skin erythema and ulceration in the tissues immediately under the radium tube on his chest wall.

In the early decades of the twentieth century, radiation therapy for cancer developed mostly empirically. The issues of total radiation dose, dose per treatment, and frequency of treatment were worked out by trial and error. Since the 1930s, based on the work of Coutard in France, the concept of daily treatment, five days per week has become the standard. Gilbert Fletcher at MD Anderson Hospital in the 1950s showed that daily doses or fractions of radiation consisting of 200 cGy (centigray or rads) per day to a total dose of 5,000 cGy were necessary to control subclinical disease for squamous cell cancer. For larger tumors or more radioresistant tumors a higher dose was required. Protracting the radiation treatment over several weeks with standard daily doses of 180 to 200 cGy spared normal tissues and reduced severe complications. Even at this slow protracted rate the tolerance of normal tissues was found to be not much more than 7,000 cGy except for very small radiation volumes. Some organs including the kidneys, spinal cord, heart, liver, and small and large bowels have much lower tolerance for serious radiation injury. Tolerance values for normal tissues to radiation are always based on volume considerations with small volumes tolerating much higher doses than if the entire organ is included within the radiation fields. With slow dose rates as in permanent seed implants for prostate cancer, the tolerance for radiation is much higher. Prostate cancers with implants receive doses in the range of 14,400 cGy, but this dose is given very slowly and continuously over about one year's time.

While clinical radiation therapy advanced empirically, great strides forward were made in the technology of radiation therapy. Low energy x-ray machines were replaced by Cobalt-60 teletherapy machines in the 1950s, and beginning in the 1960s linear accelerators became available. The high energy x-rays generated by linear accelerators have two very favorable characteristics. The first of these is "skin sparing." Low energy x-rays deposit the maximum dose along their course through tissues right at the skin surface. More energetic beams do not show the maximum accumulation of dose before several centimeters penetration below the skin surface. In this way the severe skin reactions seen with older radiation equipment can be avoided. For example, a 25mv (million-volt) beam produced by a modern linear accelerator does not deposit its maximum dose until a depth of about 4.0 cm. The second characteristic of modern high-energy radiation beams is their penetrability into tissues. For a high energy x-ray beam such as that 25 MV beam already mentioned 75% or more of the maximum dose deposited on its transit through tissues may be achieved at 15 centimeters. This depth may represent the distance of a pelvic tumor from the skin surface. By using these characteristics of modern radiation therapy beams and by designing a course of therapy consisting of multiple shaped intersecting beams, an adequate dose of radiation can be delivered to a tumor in almost any location within the body and at the same time the dose to critical nearby organs or structures can be minimized. Most recent developments in radiation therapy over the past two decades have been designed to more precisely and tightly target the tumor and its regional extensions while ensuring that the tolerance of critical normal structures is not exceeded. These efforts have moved forward hand in hand with advancements in diagnostic imaging including MRI and PET technologies.

While clinical radiation therapy advanced empirically and technical advancements progressed continuously, the understanding of the biologic mechanisms whereby radiation exerts its effects were not immediately apparent. These mechanisms have now been well studied and extensively described. Certainly, a full discussion of these mechanisms is beyond the scope of this introduction. Standard texts in radiobiology such as Hall's classic *Radiobiology for the Radiologist*[1] are available to the reader who desires a more in-depth discussion. Briefly, therapeutic radiation exerts its influence by disrupting the genetic substance of the cancer cell. If the DNA strands of the cell are adequately damaged, the cancer cells suffer a reproductive death. The cancer cells present at the time of treatment themselves will likely live out their normal life span, but they can no longer generate daughter cells. While attempting cell division in the process of mitosis, the cell's genome in its damaged state cannot reproduce successfully.

Unfortunately, both cancer cells and normal cells are impacted by the DNA damage exerted by ionizing radiation. Cells such as cancer cells that are rapidly dividing are more sensitive to radiation damage. Normal cells which are also rapidly dividing, such as skin cells and cells of the gastrointestinal mucosa, are also sensitive to acute radiation injury. This principle of radiation biology explains the acute side effects seen in the skin, oral, pharyngeal, esophageal, and enteric and colonic mucosa during radiation therapy. These and other acute radiation reactions resulting from the direct cellular impact of radiation on normal tissues are almost always self-limited and resolve within a few weeks of treatment. Their treatment consists of symptomatic support of the patient including analgesics and nutritional support. In a few tissues such as the lung and central nervous system subacute complications can be seen. These typically occur two or three months after completion of therapy. In the lung, the syndrome of radiation pneumonitis can be seen especially when high doses of radiation are delivered to large volumes of lung parenchyma. This syndrome mimics bronchitis with a dry cough and dyspnea. It generally responds to steroid therapy and is usually self-limited. In the spinal cord, a syndrome known by the eponym Lhermitte's syndrome is seen not uncommonly when a long segment of the spinal cord is treated. This syndrome is characterized by electric-like sensations shooting along the spine. It can usually be elicited when the spinal cord is stretched by forward bending of the neck. It results from a temporary demyelination of the spinal cord. It too is most frequently self-limited though some with Lhermitte's syndrome have progressed to full-blown transverse radiation myelitis. A similar syndrome due to temporary demyelination of the white matter in the brain has been described in children who receive brain irradiation. It is called the "somnolence syndrome" and as its name implies is characterized by temporary lethargy and somnolence in the children so affected. Again it is almost always self-limited.

The dreaded and dose-limiting complications or side effects of radiation are the delayed effects. These characteristically occur after a latent period of at least several months. The latent period may be many years, and late radiation complications can be triggered by other insults to tissues including surgery within the radiation field.

Within the hyperbaric community, it is widely accepted that late radiation complications including necrosis result from the vascular compromise and endarteritis, which are consistently seen in radiation-injured tissues. Although the radiation oncology community concurs that vascular changes are characteristically seen in radiation injury, one school of thought feels that the predominant cause of late injury is due to delayed cell death of parenchymal cells within the organ affected. Although this controversy continues, it does not negate the beneficial effects of hyperbaric oxygen on irradiated tissues. Probably delayed radiation injuries are the result of the combined effects of vascular damage and delayed death of parenchymal cells due to direct radiation damage. The benefits for hyperbaric oxygen may include other effects not yet identified in addition to the known beneficial effects of increasing angiogenesis and tissue oxygenation. These additional effects are likely to be moderated through certain cytokines such as TGF-ß which are active in the process of radiation damage and repair. We are just beginning to understand the impact of these cytokines in the late response of tissues to radiation.

THE EFFECTS OF HYPERBARIC OXYGEN ON RADIATED TISSUES

It is widely held that the primary beneficial effect of hyperbaric oxygen (HBO) on radiation-damaged tissues is the induction and promotion of angiogenesis. Though controversy exists within the radiation community as to the relative importance of vascular compromise failing to provide oxygen to meet the metabolic needs of irradiated tissues versus direct but delayed cellular damage to organ parenchyma, it is universally accepted that vascular damage accompanies radiation injury and contributes to its pathology. Several pieces of evidence are available to substantiate the belief that hyperbaric oxygen enhances angiogenesis in hypoxic irradiated tissues.

Marx[2] and his associates have shown in a controlled animal study the successful enhancement of angiogenesis in irradiated tissues. In this study, angiogenesis was induced in irradiated rabbits in a dose-dependent fashion. Vascular densities were assessed with angiography. These showed increasing levels of vascular density as animals were exposed to increasing levels of oxygen dose comparing 100% oxygen at ground level to hyperbaric oxygen exposure at several pressures.

Marx[3] has also demonstrated enhanced vascular density and cellularity in histologic specimens comparing post-HBO circumstances to those pre-HBO. Biopsy specimens of the same patient before and after hyperbaric oxygen demonstrate the successful induction of new vessels as well as cellularity in the same tissue bed.

Marx[4] has also published a series of serial transcutaneous measurements in patients before, during, and after hyperbaric oxygen exposures. These measurements demonstrate a continuous improvement in the measured transcutaneous levels during hyperbaric treatment with a plateau after about 20 sessions. These values approach but never achieve those of unirradiated tissues in the same patient. Follow-up in patients several years after treatment show that the improvement is maintained over time. Some have taken the occurrence of the plateau at about 20 treatments to mean that this is an adequate course of therapy and that hyperbaric oxygen can be discontinued at that time. Clinical experience has shown that for optimal outcome at least 30 treatments and more commonly 40 treatments are required in most instances for a sustained positive outcome. Occasionally more than 40 hyperbaric treatments are required. As yet the best determinant of adequate intervention is clinical judgement. No specific diagnostic tests have been developed which give specific objective guidance as to when the maximum benefit of hyperbaric oxygen therapy has been achieved. Certainly transcutaneous oxygen measurements do provide some indication.

Feldmeier[5-8] and his associates have described a series of assays done on murine tissues in a model where one half of the animals received hyperbaric oxygen seven weeks after a dose of whole abdominal irradiation. Animals were euthanized seven months after completion of radiation. A quantitative stretch assay of the small bowel was accomplished. It was designed to compare compliance in the small bowel of these animals after an identical radiation exposure. This assay showed a statistically significant increase in bowel rigidity and narrowing in those animals that received radiation alone compared to those that received hyperbaric oxygen. Quantitative morphometry using histologic staining to highlight collagenous elements was accomplished in the small bowel, rectum, and kidney of these same animals. These studies also showed a statistically significant increase in fibrosis in those organs harvested from animals that received only radiation.

HYPERBARIC OXYGEN AS TREATMENT OR PROPHYLAXIS AGAINST MANDIBULAR RADIATION NECROSIS

The best studied and most completely documented indication for hyperbaric oxygen in radiation injury is its application in the treatment and prevention of radiation necrosis of the mandible. A number of papers describing the use of hyperbaric oxygen in the treatment of mandibular necrosis have appeared in the medical literature since the 1970s.

The incidence of mandibular necrosis as a result of therapeutic radiation varies widely among several reports. Bedwinek[9] has reported a 0% incidence below doses of 6,000 cGy increasing to 1.8% at doses from 6,000 to 7,000 cGy and 9% at doses greater than 7,000 cGy. It has been reported that 85% or more of cases resulting in exposed mandibular bone will resolve spontaneously with conservative management. Unfortunately, the remaining cases generally become chronic and may become progressive, often further complicated by associated soft tissue necrosis.

Much of the early work considered radiation-induced mandibular necrosis to be a subset of mandibular osteomyelitis. Also, initially hyperbaric oxygen was delivered more or less as the sole treatment for mandibular necrosis after failure of more conservative therapy.

Robert Marx, D.D.S.[10] has provided several key principles in the understanding of the pathophysiology of mandibular necrosis and its management. He has demonstrated that infection is not the primary etiology of mandibular necrosis by obtaining deep cultures of affected bone and showing the absence of bacteria. Osteoradionecrosis is now widely accepted to be the result of avascular aseptic necrosis. Marx[11] has also shown that for hyperbaric oxygen to be consistently successful, it must be combined with surgery in the optimal fashion. Marx[11,12] has given us a staging system for mandibular necrosis. This staging system is applied to determine the severity of mandibular necrosis. It permits a plan of therapeutic intervention, which is a logical outgrowth of the stage of necrosis.

Stage I ORN (osteoradionecrosis) includes those patients with exposed bone for more than six months who have none of the serious manifestations of those in Stage III. These patients begin treatment with 30 HBO sessions with either no debridement or only minor debridement in the dental chair planned. If patients are progressing satisfactorily an additional 10 treatments are given. If patients are not progressing appropriately or if more major debridement is needed, they are advanced to Stage II and they receive the necessary surgical debridement at 30 treatments followed by 10 post-operative treatments. Surgery for Stage II patients must maintain mandibular continuity. Otherwise, they are advanced to Stage III. Patients with grave prognostic signs such as pathologic fractures, orocutaneous fistulae, or evidence of lytic involvement extending to the inferior mandibular border are treated in Stage III from the outset. Patients from Stage I or II can also be advanced to this stage if they do not make appropriate progress. In Stage III patients are entered into a reconstructive protocol where a mandibular resection is followed by a planned reconstruction. Marx has established the important surgical principle that all necrotic bone must be surgically eradicated. These patients receive the same 30 treatments prior to their resection followed by 10 post-resection treatments. Typically after a break of several weeks, the patients return to complete a reconstruction which may involve various surgical techniques including free flaps or myocutaneous flaps. In its original design, the reconstruction made use of freeze-dried cadaveric bone trays from a split rib or iliac crest combined with autologous corticocancellous bone grafting. In his original work at Wilford Hall USAF Medical Center, Marx had reconstruction patients complete a full course of an additional 30 hyperbaric treatments in support of the reconstruction. He has now shown that the vascular improvements accomplished during the initial 40 hyperbaric exposures are maintained and patients can be reconstructed without the second course of HBO.

Marx[13] has reported results in 268 patients treated according to the above protocol. In his hands applying these principles, successful resolution has been achieved in 100% of patients. Unfortunately the vast majority of patients (68%) required treatment in Stage III necessitating mandibular resection and reconstruction. Success by Marx's standards includes not only the re-establishment of mandibular continuity but also reasonable cosmetic restoration as well as success in supporting a denture. These two issues, cosmesis and re-establishment of dentition for mastication, are necessary components in improving quality of life in this group of patients.

It is widely known that extraction of teeth from heavily irradiated jaws is a common precipitating factor for mandibular necrosis. Marx[14] has published the results of a randomized prospective trial wherein patients who had received at least 6,800 cGy were randomly assigned to pre-extraction HBO versus penicillin prophylaxis. Those patients assigned to the hyperbaric group completed 20 pre-extraction HBO treatments with ten additional post-extraction hyperbaric treatments. Thirty-seven patients were treated in each group. In the penicillin group, some 29.9% of patients developed ORN while only 5.4% of patients in the hyperbaric group developed necrosis. Also the severity of ORN was more pronounced in the penicillin group with nearly three-quarters requiring treatment as Stage III patients while neither patient with ORN from the hyperbaric group required a discontinuity resection.

In summary, the principles developed by Marx in the treatment and prevention of ORN include an emphasis on pre-surgical hyperbaric oxygen to allow better tolerance to surgical wounding. The need to extirpate all necrotic bone surgically is also emphasized. In the tissue-deficient patient, myocutaneous flaps are routinely employed.

Other practitioners have applied these principles established by Marx and his colleagues and have had similar success in the prevention and treatment of mandibular necrosis. A review article now in press by Feldmeier[15] discusses the published literature related to hyperbaric oxygen for these indications. A total of 14 papers are discussed.[16-29] All but one of these shows a positive benefit for HBO. In this single negative publication, the authors fail to heed Marx's advice and do not make use of pre-operative hyperbaric oxygen.

SOFT TISSUE NECROSIS OF THE HEAD AND NECK INCLUDING LARYNGEAL NECROSIS

Fortunately laryngeal necrosis is a very rare complication of head and neck irradiation. When properly delivered, utilizing an appropriate dose-fractionation scheme, it occurs in about 1% of patients receiving radiation to the larynx. Its occurrence can be devastating and may result in laryngectomy in its most serious form. Laryngectomy necessitated by treatment complications is no less devastating for the patient than a laryngectomy done to eradicate a malignancy. It is often difficult to distinguish radiation necrosis from recurrent tumor since both often present with hoarseness, fetid breath, airway edema, and visible necrosis. Both typically occur from six months to a year after radiation is completed. Chandler[30] has established a system to grade the severity of laryngeal necrosis. Patients suffering from Grade 3 or 4 necrosis have a high likelihood of requiring laryngectomy. In fact most texts in Head and Neck Oncology recommend laryngectomy if severe symptoms of necrosis persist for more than six months. This recommendation arises from the observation that occult tumor persists in most cases and also from the belief that no effective conservative therapy is available.

Several institutions have published their experience in applying hyperbaric oxygen to the treatment of radiation laryngeal necrosis.[31-33] In these papers the outcome in a total of 35 cases is reported and only six patients were failures to treatment and required laryngectomy.

In addition to laryngeal necrosis, there are several published reports addressing the results of hyperbaric oxygen treatment in other soft tissue injuries of the head and neck. Most of these deal with soft tissue necrosis of the neck and failing flaps within irradiated fields. In the textbook *Hyperbaric Medicine*[34] edited by Dr. Kindwall, Marx has reported extensive experience in treating soft tissue radiation injuries of the head and neck. In a controlled but non-randomized report of 160 patients, he has compared wound infection, dehiscence, and delayed healing in the hyperbaric group versus a control group. He found that HBO patients experienced 6% wound infection versus 24% control; 11% dehiscence versus 48% control; and 11% delayed wound healing versus 55% control. All differences are statistically significant when the Chi square test is applied.

These results have also been duplicated by other authors. Davis[35] and his colleagues reported successful treatment in 15 of 16 patients including many with extensive necrotic wounds of the neck.

In 1997 Neovius[36] and colleagues reported a series of 15 patients treated with hyperbaric oxygen for wound complications within irradiated tissues. They compared this group to a historical control group from the same institution. Twelve of the 15 patients in the hyperbaric group healed completely with improvement in 2 and only 1 without benefit. In the control group only 7 of 15 patients healed. Two patients in the control group developed life-threatening hemorrhage and 1 of these did exsanguinate.

Any practitioner experienced in caring for head and neck cancer patients has experienced at least one patient in his or her career that exsanguinated as the result of a soft tissue necrosis of the neck which progressed to erode into the carotid artery or other major vessel.

CHEST WALL NECROSIS AND RADIATION INJURY OF THE BREAST

Radiation therapy after lumpectomy has become the preferred treatment for most early breast cancers. Radiation therapy is often used as an adjuvant treatment following mastectomy in more advanced cancers for large tumors or when axillary metastases are present. When a patient is irradiated after mastectomy, the radiation dose to the skin is high with the intent of preventing tumor in the skin or dermal lymphatics. As a result of this standard radiation technique, most women irradiated after mastectomy are subject to brisk acute radiation reactions. Hart and Mainous[17] in 1976 reported the successful application of hyperbaric oxygen as an adjunct to skin grafting in women treated for necrosis of the chest wall after mastectomy. Feldmeier and colleagues[37] in 1995 reported the outcome in applying hyperbaric oxygen as treatment of both soft tissue and bony necrosis of the chest wall. All cancer-free patients who suffered only soft tissue necrosis were treated successfully. However, only 8 of 15 patients treated for bony necrosis resolved. It appears that these patients failed at least in part because of inadequate debridement with residual necrotic bone left behind. Marx[11] had previously demonstrated the necessity of total extirpation of necrotic bone for the treatment of mandibular osteonecrosis. This general principle should apply to osteoradiaonecrosis at any site.

Carl and his colleagues[38] in Germany have reported success in applying hyperbaric oxygen to the treatment of radiation injury to the intact breast after lumpectomy in a group of 32 patients. In these patients, pain and edema were successfully treated compared to a small control group treated concurrently that refused hyperbaric treatment.

RADIATION CYSTITIS

Since 1985, a number of authors have published reports of radiation cystitis treated with hyperbaric oxygen. A recent review discovered 14 such publications.[39-52] All but one of these reported a positive outcome with resolution in the vast majority of patients. The largest series was published by Bevers and colleagues[47] and was a prospective but non-randomized trial. A total of 40 patients were treated in this report with resolution in 36. If we combine all of these reports, we find 136 patients treated with hyperbaric oxygen and resolution in 112 patients or 82.4%.

Many of the patients included in the above-cited reports had already failed conservative management including intravesical treatment with alum or formalin. Severe hemorrhagic cystitis is a life-threatening disorder. Many patients require urinary diversions or cystectomy. Cheng and Foo[53] have reported results in treating nine patients with severe radiation-induced hemorrhagic cystitis. Forty-four percent of these patients died as a result of their radiation-induced hemorrhagic cystitis in spite of aggressive surgical intervention.

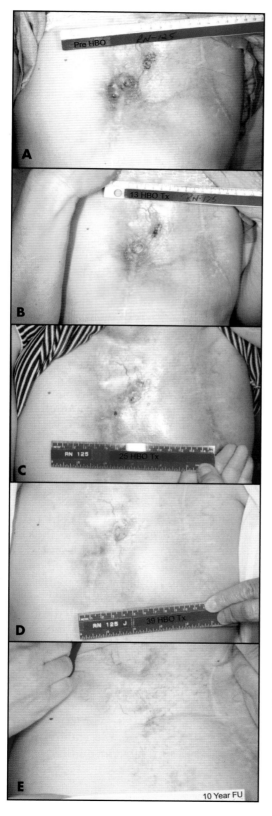

Figure 1A-1E. Chest Wall Necrosis

A-D. This patient was a 53 year old Caucasian woman who had undergone a modified radical mastectomy and adjunctive radiation therapy for breast cancer five years prior to hyperbaric oxygen. She was referred at that time for spontaneous soft tissue and bony radiation necrosis of the chest wall which had begun as small pimple like lesions over her sternum.

Prior to HBO_2, symptoms had progressed to include severe pain and open draining sinuses. Two weeks into her course of hyperbaric oxygen, she was pain free but still had small bone fragments exiting the sinus tracts.

The patient had debridement of the necrotic bone and the wound closed after 39 hyperbaric treatments without flaps or grafts.

E. A photo taken 10 years after HBO_2 shows resolution sustained over time. (Photos by David A. Davolt, C.H.T., ATMO, Inc.)

RADIATION-INDUCED PROCTITIS AND ENTERITIS

Several papers support hyperaric oxygen as treatment for radiation-induced proctitis and enteritis. Feldmeier et al[5-8] have completed several assays in an animal model of enteritis which show the benefit of hyperbaric oxygen when given prior to the expression of frank necrosis. Gross morphometry, quantitative histologic morphometry, and a study of bowel compliance show a decrease in eneropathy and a reduction of fibrosis in the bowel wall of these animals after a course of 30 hyperbaric oxygen treatments.

Nine clinical reports have been identified in a recent review by Feldmeier.[5,54-62] In these papers some 105 cases are reviewed. Thirty-four (32%) of these patients were treated with resulting complete resolution while another 67 (64%) had improved symptoms as a result of hyperbaric oxygen therapy. Only 4% of patients had no benefit from treatment.

ADDITIONAL ABDOMINAL AND PELVIC RADIATION INJURIES

In 1978 Farmer and colleagues[63] reported a case of vaginal necrosis which resolved with hyperbaric therapy. Williams et al[62] in 1992 reported their results in treating 14 patients with vaginal necrosis. Thirteen of 14 patients had complete resolution though 1 of these required a second course of HBO. In 1996 Feldmeier and his co-authors[54] published results after reviewing 44 cases with various pelvic and abdominal injury who received hyperbaric oxygen. The results in treating large and small bowel injuries were discussed in the section above. Thirty-one patients were treated for other abdominal and pelvic injuries and received at least 20 hyperbaric treatments for radiation injuries to the perineum, groin, vagina, and pelvic bone. Twenty-six of these patients had complete resolution.

If we sum those patients reported by Farmer, Williams, and Feldmeier, we find that 40 of 46 patients (87%) resolved completely with treatment. All but one patient in the three papers who suffered from soft tissue injury only had complete resolution.

NEUROLOGIC INJURIES SECONDARY TO RADIATION

In the review article previously cited, Feldmeier has identified 12 publications that report hyperbaric oxygen treatment for a variety of neurologic injuries.[15,17,64-74] These include radiation-induced transverse myelitis, brain necrosis, optic nerve injury, and brachial plexopathy.

As early as 1976, Hart and Mainous[17] reported the treatment of five cases of transverse myelitis and Glassburn and Brady[64] reported nine cases in 1977. In the report by Hart, there was no improvement in motor function while six of nine patients had improvement including motor function in Glassburn's report. In 2000 Calabro and Jinkins[72] reported a single case of transverse myelitis treated with hyperbaric oxygen who showed both clinical and MRI imaging evidence of improvement. In an animal study by Feldmeier et al[68], delay but no permanent prevention of myelitis was seen for HBO given before detectable signs of myelitis seven weeks after radiation exposure. There are no other known successful treatments for radiation-induced myelitis, and besides the obvious drastic impact on quality of life with

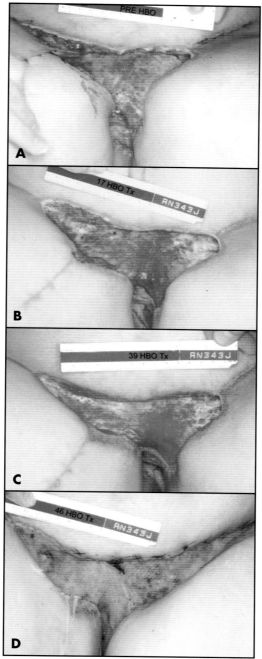

Figure 2A-2D. Soft Tissue Radiation Necrosis of the Groin

This patient was a 42-year-old Caucasian female who underwent post-operative radiation following vulvectomy and groin dissection for a recurrent anal cancer. The patient was referred for hyperbaric oxygen for non-healing necrotic wounds of the groins, reconstructed labia and skin of the suprapubic region. Her radiation had been completed about 17 months earlier. The patient had a skin graft at 40 HBO$_2$ treatments and completed another 6 post graft treatments with 100% graft take. (Photos by David A. Davolt, C.H.T, . ATMO, Inc.)

resultant paralysis, there is a high incidence of mortality as a result of this condition with two thirds of patients dying within four years of onset. Although the outcome for hyperbaric treatment has not been universally successful, given the dire consequences of fully manifest transverse myelitis, hyperbaric therapy should be considered based on humanitarian concerns.

Several publications report the use of hyperbaric oxygen for brain necrosis due to radiation. Hart and Mainous[17] in their 1976 paper report a single case of radiation-caused brain injury, which improved with HBO. Chuba and associates[70] have reported a series of ten pediatric patients with radiation-induced brain necrosis who were treated with hyperbaric oxygen. All ten improved initially. At the time of publication, four patients had died due to recurrent tumor and five of the six remaining patients had maintained their neurologic improvement after hyperbaric treatment. Leber and colleagues[71] have reported two cases of patients who experienced brain necrosis after radiosurgery procedures for arteriovenous malformations. Both of these patients had reduction in the size of necrosis after hyperbaric oxygen therapy as indicated by imaging studies and one had complete resolution. Cirafsi and Verderamae[73] have published results in a single case of brain necrosis secondary to radiation wherein the patient had no benefit with hyperbaric oxygen. The patient had also failed to respond to steroids and anticoagulants. If we combine the results from the above-cited papers, we find that eight of fourteen patients reported demonstrate improvement for brain necrosis. No other therapies short of craniotomy and resection of the necrotic focus have been successful, and intervention with hyperbaric oxygen for compassionate reasons should be considered.

Four publications discuss hyperbaric oxygen as treatment for radiation-induced optic neuritis.[65-67, 69] A total of nineteen patients are included in these publications and only four are reported to have experienced improvement. Borruat et al[69] have reported a case of a single patient with bilateral optic neuritis. After hyperbaric oxygen treatment, this patient had complete resolution of optic neuritis in the eye most recently affected and some but less than total resolution in the eye first affected. This observation reinforces the need to intervene early with HBO. The support for hyperbaric oxygen in this condition is only anecdotal at best. However, if consideration is given to the dire consequences with resulting blindness and the lack of other effective treatment, a trial of hyperbaric therapy with prompt intervention is recommended.

A randomized controlled trial by Pritchard and associates[74] has been conducted in regard to hyperbaric oxygen therapy for brachial plexopathy. Unfortunately, this trial is negative in terms of failing to show a statistically significant improvement in the hyperbaric group versus the control group. The median time of treatment after development of the neuropathy was 11 years and the injuries were certainly fixed in place over time. Though improvement was not documented, the hyperbaric group of patients had less deterioration than did the control group over time. Six patients with lymphedema in the hyperbaric group showed improvement in their arm swelling after hyperbaric oxygen with no corresponding improvement in the control group.

Taken on the whole, the supporting evidence for hyperbaric oxygen for neurologic injury is certainly only anecdotal. More study is required, but given the severe and permanent consequences of progression, especially in CNS injury, and in the complete absence of other effective treatment, serious consideration for hyperbaric treatment should be given.

RADIATION NECROSIS OF THE EXTREMITIES

This complication of radiation is really quite rare. In part, the rarity reflects the relative rarity of primary malignancies of the extremities. Radiation therapy for metastases to the extremities is not uncommon. However, in metastatic disease, radiation doses are only moderate, and patients may not survive in large numbers long enough for radiation injury to become manifest.

In the review by Feldmeier[15] only two studies were discovered which report the results of hyperbaric treatment in radiation injuries of the extremities. Farmer and associates[18] in 1978 reported a single patient treated for radiation necrosis of the foot without improvement. Feldmeier et al[75] in 2000 reported a series of 17 patients treated for extremity radiation neecrosis. Eleven of 17 patients had complete resolution. In only those patients in whom follow-up is available and who were not found to have recurrent malignancy in the wound, eleven of 13 or 85% resolved.

Certainly, the published experience in applying hyperbaric oxygen to radionecrosis of the extremities is limited. However, based on the successful treatment of radiation necrosis of both bone and soft tissues in other anatomic sites, it is reasonable to recommend hyperbaric oxygen for this indication. Oxygen in the hyperbaric setting has often been referred to as a "drug." Just as an antibiotic can be recommended for treatment of an infection of one anatomic site based on success at other sites, we can recommend hyperbaric oxygen for radiation injury of the extremities based on success in other tissues.

SPECIAL CONSIDERATIONS FOR THE SURGEON CONTEMPLATING SURGERY WITHIN AN IRRADIATED FIELD

Experienced oncologic surgeons are well aware of the difficulties in operating within an irradiated field. If pre-operative radiation is given in a planned fashion, it is common to accomplish the surgery four to six weeks after completion of the radiation. During this interval, the acute inflammatory hyperemic radiation reactions are likely to largely resolve. Radiation fibrosis and tissue hypoxia begin to become manifest after about two months and typically plateau after about one year. After endarteritis and tissue hypoxia have occurred, wound complications including delayed healing and infection increase substantially.

Marx has established the benefit for pre-extraction HBO in preventing ORN.[14] In his reported experience with soft tissue wounds of the head and neck, Marx has also emphasized the importance of delivering most of the hyperbaric treatment before the surgical intervention. The purpose of the pre-operative treatment is to enhance the quality of tissues to allow them

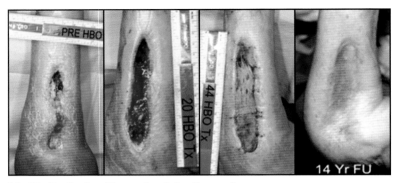

Figure 3A-3D. Radiation Necrosis of the Extremity

This patient was a 72 year old Caucasian female who had undergone radiation 5 years prior to referral for hyperbaric oxygen. She had received radiation following limb sparing surgery for a fibrosarcoma of the upper extremity. At the time of referral she had a 3X11 cm. open necrotic wound with necrotic exposed bone. After 20 hyperbaric treatments, she had debridement and bone and skin grafting. The wound closed and followup 14 years after hyperbaric oxygen shows durable resolution and a functional extremity. (Photos by David A. Davolt, C.H.T., ATMO, Inc.)

to better withstand the insult of surgical wounding. Feldmeier and his colleagues[76] have reported the successful application of a short course of hyperbaric oxygen immediately following surgery in head and neck cancer patients undergoing mostly radical resections as surgical salvage of treatment failures within the irradiated field. In this group of patients, a vast majority (87.5%) had prompt healing whereas in other reports of surgical salvage within an irradiated field, complications typically exceed 50% with fatal bleeds a not uncommon event. Both Marx and Grandstrom[77,78] have reported the benefit in supporting dental implants in radiated tissues with significant improvement in osseous integration of the dental implant in patients receiving hyperbaric oxygen. In fact, most clinicians will not attempt dental implants in heavily irradiated jaws due to the exceptionally high likelihood of failure.

In the animal model previously cited, Feldmeier and his co-investigators[5,6,8] have shown marked success in preventing reduced compliance, bowel rigidity and narrowed caliber and reduced bowel wall fibrosis when hyperbaric oxygen was given during the latent period before frank expression of bowel injury.

In a clinical series, Pomeroy[79] has delivered pre-operative hyperbaric oxygen in patients undergoing abdominal and pelvic surgery when previously irradiated. All five of the patients in this series had an uneventful postoperative course and suffered no significant complications in spite of the inherent risks of operating within the field of high dose irradiation.

Though hyperbaric oxygen is likely to be a useful adjuvant after surgery in irradiated tissues, the extensive experience by Marx and of the additional authors mentioned above as well as common sense reasoning would argue that hyperbaric oxygen should be preferentially initiated in a pre-operative mode.

HYPERBARIC OXYGEN AND CARCINOGENESIS

A frequently expressed concern by those considering hyperbaric oxygen for a patient with radiation injury is the fear that hyperbaric oxygen will somehow accelerate malignant growth or cause a dormant malignancy to be reactivated. In 1994, Feldmeier and his colleagues[80] reviewed the available literature related to this issue. An overwhelming majority of both clinical reports and animal studies reviewed in this paper showed no enhancement of cancer growth. A small number of reports actually showed a decrease in growth or rates of metastases. Feldmeier[81] updated this material for the Consensus Conference held in 2001 jointly sponsored by the European Society of Therapeutic Radiology and Oncology (ESTRO) and the European Committee for Hyperbaric Medicine (ECHM). In this update, Feldmeier emphasized the differences known in tumor and wound healing angiogenesis with similar but distinct processes operative in each case. He also showed that there are significant differences in the growth and inhibition factors, which modulate angiogenesis, in both circumstances. He summarized the literature demonstrating that tumors which are hypoxic are less responsive to treatment, less subject to death by apoptosis, and more prone to aggressive growth and lethal metastases. Most experienced practioners of hyperbaric oxygen no longer fear that hyperbaric oxygen will promote malignant growth.

HYPERBARIC OXYGEN AS A RADIOSENSITIZER

Molecular oxygen is the most potent radiosensitizer yet discovered. Well-oxygenated tumor cells are as much as three times more sensitive to radiation cell kill than are hypoxic cells. Gray[82] in 1953 described this "Oxygen Effect." In 1955 Churchill-Davidson[83] applied this principle to clinical radiation therapy by irradiating patients in hyperbaric chambers who were at 3.0 ATA breathing 100% oxygen. His positive pioneering pilot trial was followed by a series of clinical trials over the next 20 or so years. Enthusiasm for this technique was intoxicating and the early International Congress of Hyperbaric Medicine Proceedings are filled with optimistic reports of increased tumor control by hyperbaric oxygen sensitized radiation. A complete review of these works is beyond the scope of this chapter. Recently Overgaard published a very nice summary of these studies done with hyperbaric oxygen employed as a radiosensitizer for external beam radiation therapy.[84] Briefly, a review of these trials now many years after their completion continues to show enhanced local tumor control especially in Head and Neck and Cervical Cancer. This enhanced local tumor control did not consistently translate into an improved cure rate because often the advanced tumors selected for these trials had already metastasized. The metastatic disease outside the radiation field often led to the patients' demise. These trials were largely abandoned when cure rates did not live up to expectations. There were also concerns that complication rates were increased by the hyperbaric oxygen. Confounding the comparison of complications in hyperbaric oxygen radiosensitization patients to the air control patients was the tendency to use high radiation dose per treatment in the hyperbaric group. When compared to the control group the study group often experienced a higher complication rate, but as likely as not the higher complication rate was related to the radiation dose fractionation scheme with fewer radiation treatments each of a higher dose in the hyperbaric study group. The number of treatments in the radiation group was reduced because of the inconvenience and slowed through-put in busy radiation centers which resulted because patients required an additional 30 minutes or so to allow for compression, treatment, and decompression. Another difficulty was the inability to reproduce the patient's position under the treatment beam because the radiation therapists could not manually reposition a patient from outside the hyperbaric chamber.

Because of the failure in achieving the advantage expected and in spite of consistent improvements of local tumor control, hyperbaric oxygen radiosensitization was largely abandoned after the 1970s. As with many sound biologic principles, the issue of hyperbaric oxygen sensitization has now resurfaced. In 1995, a group from the Netherlands Cancer Institute reported results in treating children with intravenous infusion of MIBG (Metaiodobenzylguanidine) for neuroblastoma with hyperbaric oxygen sensitization.[85] This material is attached to radioactive Iodine131, a beta emitter. As an analogue of the neurotransmitter, norepinepherine, it has affinity for the tumor and carries the radioisotope to the malignancy. Since it is a beta source with electron only release, the patient's own body shields others from radiation exposure, and children can be taken to the hyperbaric chamber shortly after the infusion without posing a risk to any other patients or the medical staff.

Feldmeier and his colleagues[86] have demonstrated the feasability of conducting high dose rate brachytherapy treatments while a patient is in a hyperbaric chamber breathing oxygen at depth. In this treatment, a patient would have an implant device such as a catheter or needle placed prior to entering the chamber. This implant device would be accessed with catheters through an airtight port in the hyperbaric chamber wall and a computer modulated cable driven intense radioactive source would be introduced into the implant device and stepwise moved through the applicator until the desired dose was delivered.

Perhaps an even more attractive and more universally applicable technique has been pioneered by Kohshi and his collaborators.[87,88] In this approach, patients with high grade brain tumors (Grade 3 and 4 Astrocytomas) are given a hyperbaric oxygen exposure and brought from the chamber immediately to the radiation department for treatment. Kohshi has shown that high concentrations of oxygen in the brain remain for some but a finite time after exit from the chamber.[88] He has shown that improved control of these very poor prognostic tumors can be obtained if radiation occurs within 15 minutes after leaving the hyperbaric chamber. He has also shown that this advantage is lost if the delay is 30 minutes or more. Certainly this work will need to be confirmed at other centers. It is also not known whether this approach will be peculiar to brain tumors. Malignancies differentiate themselves from normal tissues by using anaerobic pathways of glycolysis for energy production even when oxygen is present. Tumor vasculature is also known to be disorganized. It may be that these factors allow oxygen tensions to be elevated in cancers for some time after hyperbaric oxygen exposure since consumption of oxygen is less than that of normal tissues and washout may be impaired by the disorganized blood supply.

Additional studies in other tumor types should be completed. If a positive and reasonable window of sensitization of at least several minutes after HBO_2 is available, such an approach would be very practical. Radiation oncology departments are accustomed to treating patients within a time window of sensitization when hyperthermia is used as a radiosensitizer or Amifostine is given as a radioprotector of normal tissues.

SUMMARY

The treatment of radiation injuries including soft tissue and bony necroses has been one of the most successful applications of hyperbaric oxygen therapy. Interventions in many tissue types and anatomic sites have been consistently positive. Prophylactic treatment prior to the manifest expression of radiation damage is very attractive outgrowth of treatment but will require the development of reliable predictive assays, which identify patients at high risk for damage. For now we can identify only certain broad groups at higher risk for injury including patients undergoing re-irradiation for recurrent tumor. An accumulating body of evidence supports pre-operative hyperbatic oxygen when surgery is contemplated within a heavily irradiated tissue bed.

The concept of hyperbaric oxygen enhanced radiation is based on sound radiobiologic principles. Innovative new approaches are developing which may permit the full clinical application of this well-established scientific observation. Oxygen is indeed the most potent radiosensitizer known and most probably the least toxic as well.

Concerns that hyperbaric oxygen somehow enhances malignant growth or awakens dormant tumor are not supported by the body of literature available on the topic. Nor does a review of the modulating growth and inhibitory factors involved in the process of tumor angiogenesis. Tumors that grow under hypoxic conditions have been shown to be resistant to death by apoptosis, to be resistant to radiation and some chemotherapy, and to have a more lethal course including more aggressive metastatic growth.

REFERENCES

1. Hall EJ. Radiology for the radiologist, Fourth edition. Philadelphia, PA, J.B. Lippincott, 1994.

2. Marx RE, Ehler WJ, Taypongsak PT, Pierce LW. Relationship of oxygen dose to angiogenesis induction in irradiated tissue. Am J Surg 1990;160:519-524.

3. Marx RE. Radiation injury to tissue. In: Kindwall EP, ed. Hyperbaric Medicine Practice, Second Edition. Flagstaff, Best Publishing, 1999, pp 669-671.

4. Marx RE. Radiation injury to tissue. In: Kindwall EP, ed. Hyperbaric Medicine Practice, Second Edition. Flagstaff, Best Publishing, 1999, pp 672-673.

5. Feldmeier JJ, Jelen I, Davolt DA, Valente PT, Meltz ML, Alecu R. Hyperbaric oxygen as a prophylaxis for radiation induced delayed enteropathy. Radiotherapy and Oncology 1995;35:138-144.

6. Feldmeier JJ, Davolt DA, Court WS, Onoda JM, Alecu R. Histologic morphometry confirms a prophylactic effect for hyperbaric oxygen in the prevention of delayed radiation enteropathy. Undersea Hyper Med 1998;25(2):93-97.

7. Feldmeier JJ, Davolt DA, Court WS, Alecu R, Onoda JM. Morphometric analysis shows decreased fibrosis in the kidneys of animals who receive hyperbaric oxygen following abdominopelvic irradiation. (Abs) Undersea and Hyperbaric Medicine, 1997;24 (supplement).

8. Feldmeier JJ, Davolt DA. Quantitative histologic morphometry confirms a prophylactic role for hyperbaric oxygen in radiation injury of the rectum. (Abs) Undersea and Hyperbaric Medicine 2000; 27 (Supplement).

9. Bedwinek JM, Shukovsky LJ, Fletcher GH, Daly TE. Osteonecrosis in patients treated with definitive radiotherapy for squamous cell cancers of the oral cavity and naso- and oropharynx. Radiology 1976;119:665-667.

10. Marx RE. Osteoradionecrosis:a new concept of its pathophsiology. J Oral Maxillofac Surg 1983;41:283-288.

11. Marx RE. A new concept in the treatment of osteoradionecrosis. J Oral Maxillofac Surg 1983;41:351-357.

12. Marx RE. Radiation injury to tissue. In: Kindwall EP, ed. Hyperbaric Medicine Practice, Second Edition. Flagstaff, Best Publishing, 1999, pp 703-715.

13. Marx RE, Johnson RP. Problem wounds in oral and maxillo-facial surgery: The role of hyperbaric oxygen. In: Davis JC, Hunt TK, eds. Problem Wounds: The Role of Oxygen. New York: Elsevier, 1988:65-123.

14. Marx RE, Johnson RP, Kline SN. Prevention of osteoradionecrosis: A randomized prospective clinical trial of hyperbaric oxygen versus penicillin. J Am Dent Assoc 1985;11:49-54.

15. Feldmeier JJ. A systematic review of the literature reporting the application of hyperbaric oxygen to the prevention and treatment of radiation injuries: an evidence based approach. Submitted to Undersea Hyper Med June 2002.

16. Mainous EG, Hart GB.Osteoradionecrosis of the mandible. Treatment with hyperbaric oxygen. Arch Otolaryngol 1975; 101(3):173-177.

17. Hart GB, Mainous EG. The treatment of radiation necrosis with hyperbaric oxygen (OHP). Cancer 1976;37:2580-5.

18. Farmer JC, Shelton DL, Bennett PD, Angelillo JD, Hudson MD. Treatment of radiation-induced injury by hyperbaric oxygen. Ann Otol 1978;87;707-15.

19. Tobey RE, Kelly JF. Osteoradionecrosis of the jaws. Otolaryngol Clin North Am 1979;12(1):183-186.

20. Davis JC, Dunn JM, Gates GA, Heimbach RD. Hyperbaric oxygen: a new adjunct in the management of radiation necrosis. Arch Otolaryngol 1979;105:58-61.

21. Marx RE. Part II: A new concept in the treatment of osteoradionecrosis. J Oral Maxillofac Surg 1983;41:351-357.

22. Marx RE. Osteoradionecrosis of the jaws: Review and update. HBO Rev 1984;5:78-126.

23. Mounsey RA, Brown DH, O'Dwyer TP, Gullane PJ, Koch GH. Role of hyperbaric oxygen therapy in the management of osteoradionecrosis. Laryngoscope 1993; 103: 605-8.

24. McKenzie MRR, Wong FLL, Epstein JBB, Lepawsky M. Hyperbaric oxygen and postradiation osteonecrosis of the mandible. European Journal of Cancer. Part B, Oral Oncology 1993; 29B: 201-7.

25. VanMerkesteyn JPP, Bakker DJJ, Borgmeijer-Hoelen AMM. Hyperbaric oxygen treatment of osteoradionecrosis of the mandible. Experience in 29 patients. Oral Surg Med Oral Pathol Oral Radiol Endod 1995;80:12-6.

26. Epstein J, van der Meij E, McKenzie M, Wong F, Lepawsky M, Stevenson-Moore P. Postradiation osteonecrosis of the mandible: a long term follow-up study. Oral Surg Med Oral Pathol Oral Radiol Endod 1997;83;657-62.

27. Maier A, Gaggl A, Klemen H, Santler G, Anegg U, Fell B, Karcher H, Smolle-Juttner FM, Friehs GB. Review of severe osteoradionecrosis treated by surgery alone or surgery with postoperative hyperbaric oxygenation. Br J Oral Maxillofac Surg 2000;38:173-6.

28. Curi MMM, Dib LLL, Kowalski LPP. Management of refractory osteonecrosis of the jaws with surgery and adjunctive hyperbaric oxygen therapy. Int J Oral Maxillofac Surg 2000;29:430-4.

29. David LA, Sandor GK, Evans AW, Brown DH. Hyperbaric oxygen therapy and mandibular osteoradionecrosis: a retrospecttive study and analysis of treatment outcomes. J Can Dent Assoc 2001;67:384.

30. Chandler JR. Radiation fibrosis and necrosis of the larynx. Ann Otol Rhinol Laryngol 1979;88:509-514.

31. Ferguson BJ, Hudson WR, Farmer JC. Hyperbaric oxygen for laryngeal radionecrosis. Ann Otol Laryngol 1987;96:1-6.

32. Feldmeier JJ, Heimbach RD, Davolt DA, Brakora MJ. Hyperbaric oxygen as an adjunctive treatment for severe laryngeal necrosis: A report of nine consecutive cases. Undersea Hyper Med 1993;20:329-335.

33. Filintisis GA, Moon RE, Kraft KL, Farmer JC, Scher RL, Piantadosi CA. Laryngeal radionecrosis and hyperbaric oxygen therapy: report of 18 cases and review of the literature. Ann Otol Rhinol Laryngol 2000;109:554-62.

34. Marx RE. Radiation injury to tissue. In: Kindwall EP, ed. Hyperbaric Medicine Practice, Second Edition. Flagstaff, Best Publishing, 1999, pp 682-689.

35. Davis JC, Dunn JM, Gates GA, Heimbach RD. Hyperbaric oxygen: a new adjunct in the management of radiation necrosis. Arch Otolaryngol 1979;105:58-61.

36. Neovius, EB, Lind MG, Lind FG. Hyperbaric oxygen for wound complications after surgery in the irradiated head and neck: a review of the literature and a report of 15 consecutive patients. Head and Neck 1997;19:315-322.

37. Feldmeier JJ, Heimbach RD, Davolt DA, Court WS, Stegmann BJ, Sheffield PJ. Hyperbaric oxygen as an adjunctive treatment for delayed radiation injury of the chest wall: a retrospective review of 23 cases. Undersea Hyperb Med 1995;22:383-393.

38. Carl UM, Feldmeier JJ, Schmitt G, Hartmann KA. Hyperbaric oxygen therapy for late sequelae in women receiving radiation after breast conserving surgery. Int J Radiat Oncol Biol Phys 2001;49:1029-31.

39. Weiss JP, Boland FP, Mori H, Gallagher M, Brereton H Preate DL. Treatment of radiation-induced cystistis with hyperbaric oxygen. J Urol 1985;134(2):352-354.

40. Schoenrock GJ, Cianci P. Treatment of radiation cystitis with hyperbaric oxygen. Urology 1986;27(3):271-272.

41. Weiss JP, Nevill EC. Hyperbaric oxygen: Primary treatment of radiation-induced hemorrhagic cystitis. J Urol 1989;142(1):43-45.

42. Rijkmans BG, Bakker DJ, Dabhoiwala NF, Kurth KH. Successful treatment of radiation cystitis with hyperbaric oxygen. European Urology 1989;16(5):354-356.

43. Norkool DM, Hampson NB, Gibbons RP, Weissman RM. Hyperbaric oxygen for radiation-induced hemorrhagic cystitis. J Urol 1993;150:332-334.

44. Lee HC, Liu CS, Chiao C, Lin SN. Hyperbaric oxygen therapy in hemorrhagic cystitis: A report of 20 cases. Undersea Hyper Med 1994;21(3):321-327.

45. Akiyama A, Ohkubo Y, Takashima R, Furugen N, Tochimoto M, Tsuchiya A. Hyperbaric oxygen in the successful treatment of two cases of radiation-induced hemorrhagic cystitis. Japanese Journal of Urology 1994;85(8):12691272.

46. Weiss JP, Mattei DM, Neville EC, Hanno PM. Primary treatment of radiation-induced hemorrhagic cystitis with hyperbaric oxygen: 10-year experience. J Urol 1994;151(6):1514-1517.

47. Bevers RF, Bakker DJ, Kurth KH. Hyperbaric oxygen treatment for haemorrhagic radiation cystitis. Lancet 1995;346:803-805.

48. Del Pizzo JJ, Chew BH, Jacobs SC, Sklar GN. Treatment of radiation induced hemorrhagic cystitis with hyperbaric oxygen: long term followup. J Urol 1998;160:731-3.

49. Miyazato T, Yusa T, Onaga T, Sugaya K, Koyama Y, Hatmabsno T, Ogawa Y. Hyperbaric oxygen for radiation-induced hemorrhagic cystitis. Japanese Journal of Urology 1998;89(5):552-556.

50. Suzuki K, Kurokawa K, Suzuki T, Okazaki H, Otake N, Imai K. Successful treatment of radiation cystitis with hyperbaric oxygen therapy: resolution of bleeding event and changes of hitopathological findings of the bladder mucosa. Int J Urol Nephrol 1998;30:267-71.

51. Mathews R, Rajan N, Josefson L, Camporesi E, Makhuli Z. Hyperbaric oxygen therapy for radiation induced hemorrhagic cystitis. J Urol 1999;161:435-437.

52. Mayer R, Klemen H, Quehenberger F, Sankin O, Mayer E, Hackl E, Smolle-Juettner FM. Hyperbaric oxygen-an effective tool to treat radiation morbidity in prostate cancer. Radiother Oncol 2001;61:151-6.

53. Cheng C, Foo KT. Management of severe chronic radiation cystitis. Ann Acad Med Singapore 1992;21:368-71.

54. Feldmeier JJ, Heimbach RD, Davolt DA, Court WS, Stegmann BJ, Sheffield PJ. Hyperbaric oxygen as an adjunctive treatment for delayed radiation injuries of the abdomen and pelvis. Undersea Hyper Med 1997;23(4):205-213.

55. Woo TCS, Joseph D, Oxer H. Hyperbaric oxygen treatment for radiation proctitis. Int J Radiat Oncol Biol Phys 1997;38(3):619-622.

56. Warren DC, Feehan P, Slade JB, Cianci PE. Chronic radiation proctitis treated with hyperbaric oxygen. Undersea Hyper Med 1997;24(3):181-184.

57. Bredfeldt JE, Hampson NB. Hyperbaric oxygen (HBO) therapy for chronic radiation enteritis. Am J Gastroenterol 1998;93(9):1665.

58. Feldmeier JJ and Davolt DA, Court WS, Onoda JM, Alecu R. Histologic morphometry confirms a prophylactic effect for hyperbaric oxygen in the prevention of delayed radiation enteropathy. Undersea and Hyperbaric Medicine 1998;25;93-7.

59. Carl UM, Peusch-Dreyer D, Frieling T, Schmitt G, Hartmann KA. Treatment of radiation proctitis with hyperbaric oxygen: what is the optimal number of HBO treatments? Strahlenther Onkol 1998;174:482-3.

60. Gouello JP et al. Interet de l'oxygenotherapie hyperbare dans la pathologie digestive post-radique. 36 observations. Presse Med 1999;28:1053-7.

61. Bem J, Bem S, Singh A. Use of hyperbaric oxygen chamber in the management of radiation-related complications of the anorectal region: report of two cases and review of the literature. Dis Colon Rectum 2000;43:1435-8.

62. Williams JAA, Clarke D, Dennis WAA, Dennis EJJ, Smith STT. Treatment of pelvic soft tissue tadiation necrosis with hyperbaric oxygen. Am J Obstet Gynecol 1992;167:415-6.

63. Farmer JC, Shelton DL, Bennett PD, Angelillo JD, Hudson MD. Treatment of radiation-induced injury by hyperbaric oxygen. Ann Otol 1978;87;707-15.

64. Glassburn JR, Brady LW. Treatment with hyperbaric oxygen for radiation myelitis. Proc. 6th Int Cong on Hyperbaric Medicine 1977:266-77.

65. Guy J, Schatz NJJ. Hyperbaric oxygen in the treatment of radiation-induced optic neuropathy. Ophthalmology 1986;93:1083-8.

66. Roden D, Bosley TM, FowbleB, Clark J, Savino PJ, Sergott RC, Schatz NJ. Delayed radiation injury to the retrobulbar optic nerves and chiasm. Clinical syndrome and treatment with hyperbaric oxygen and corticosteroids. Ophthalmolgy 1990;97:346-51.

67. Fontanesi J, Golden EB, Cianci PC, Heideman RL. Treatment of radiation-induced optic neuropathy in the pediatric population. Journal of Hyperbaric Medicine 1991;6(4): 245-248.

68. Feldmeier JJ, Lange JD, Cox SD, Chou L, Ciaravino V. Hyperbaric oxygen as a prophylaxis or treatment for radiation myelitis. Undersea Hyper Med 1993;20(3) :249-255.

69. Borruat FXX, Schatz NJJ, Glaser JSS, Feun LGG, Matos L. Visual recovery from radiation-induced optic neuropathy. The role of hyperbaric oxygen therapy. J Clin Neuroophthalmol 1993;13:98-101.

70. Chuba PJ, Aronin P, Bhambhani K, Eichenhorn M, Zamarano L, Cianci P, Muhlbauer M, Porter AT, Fontanesi J. Hyperbaric oxygen therapy for radiation-induced brain injury in children. Cancer 1997;80:2005-2012.

71. Leber KA, Eder HG, Kovac H, Anegg U, Pendl G. Treatment of cerebral radionecrosis by hyperbaric oxygen therapy. Sterotact Funct Neurosurg 1998;70(Suppl 1):229-36.

72. Calabro F, Jinkins JR. MRI of radiation myelitis: a report of a case treated with hyperbaric oxygen. Eur Radiol 2000;10:1079-84.

73. Cirafisi C, Verderame F. Radiation-induced rhomboencephalopathy. Ital J Neurol Sci 1999;20:55-8.

74. Pritchard J, Anand P, Broome J, Davis C, Gothard L, Hall E, Maher J, McKinna F, Millington J, Misra VPP, Pitkin A, Yarnold JRR. Double-blind randomized phase II study of hyperbaric oxygen in patients with radiation-induced brachial plexopathy. Radiother Oncol 2001;58:279-86.

75. Feldmeier JJ, Heimbach RD, Davolt DA, McDonough MJ, Stegmann BJ, Sheffield PJ. Hyperbaric oxygen in the treatment of delayed radiation injuries of the extremities Undersea Hyper Med 2000;27(1):15-19.

76. Feldmeier JJ, Newman R, Davolt DA, Heimbach RD, Newman NK, Hernandez LC. Prophylactic hyperbaric oxygen for patients undergoing salvage for recurrent head and neck cancers following full course irradiation (abstract). Undersea Hyper Med 1998;25(Suppl):10.

77. Granstrom G, Jacobsson M, Tjellstrom A. Titanium implants in irradiated patients: benefits from hyperbaric oxygen. Int J Oral maxillofac Implants 1992;7:15-25.

78. Marx RE. Radiation injury to tissue. In: Kindwall EP, ed. Hyperbaric Medicine Practice, Second Edition. Flagstaff, Best Publishing, 1999, pp 693-693.

79. Pomeroy, BD, Keim LW, taylor RJ. Preoperative hyperbaric oxygen therapy for radiation induced injuries. J Urol 1998;159:1630-1632.

80. Feldmeier JJ, Heimbach RD, Davolt DA, Brakora MJ, Sheffield PJ, Porter AT. Does hyperbaric oxygen have a cancer causing or promoting effect? A review of the pertinent literature. Undersea Hyper Med 1994;21:467-475.

81. Feldmeier JJ. Hyperbaric oxygen: does it have a cancer causing or growth enhancing effect. In: Proceedings of the Consensus Conference sponsored by the European Society for Therapeutic Radiology and Oncology and the European Committee for Hyperbaric Medicine. Portugal 2001:129-146.

82. Gray KH, Conger AD, Ebert M, Hornsey S and Scott OCA: The concentration of oxygen dissolved in tissues at the time of irradiation as a factor in radiotherapy. Br J Radiol 26:638-648, 1953.

83. Churchill-Davidson I, Sanger C and Thomlinson RH: High-pressure oxygen and radio therapy. Lancet 1:1091-1096, 1955.

84. Overgaard J and Horsman MR: Modification of hypoxia-induced radioresistance in tumors by the use of oxygen and sensitizers. Seminars in Radiation Oncology. 6;1:10-21, 1996.

85. Voute PA, van der Kliej AJ, De Kraker J, Hoefnagel CA et al: Clinical experience with radiation enhancement by hyperbaric oxygen in children with recurrent neuroblastoma stage IV: Eur J Cancer 31A;4:596-600, 1995.

86. Feldmeier JJ, Court WS, Alecu R, Davolt DA and Porter AT: High dose rate brachytherapy with hyperbaric oxygen sensitization: a feasibility study (abs). Undersea and Hyperbaric Medicine 23:80, 1996.

87. Kohshi K, Kinoshita Y, Terashima H et al: Radiotherapy after hyperbaric oxygenation for malignant gliomas: a pilot study. J Cancer Res Clin Oncol 122:676-678, 1996.

88. Kohshi K, Kinoshita Y, Imada H et al:Effects of radiotherapy after hyperbaric oxygenation on malignant gliomas. Br J Ca 80:236-241, 1999.

CHAPTER **18**

HYPERBARIC OXYGEN AND WOUND HEALING

T.K. Hunt, M.L. Gimbel

INTRODUCTION AND HISTORY

Oxygen plays a unique and central role in the mechanisms of wound healing no less than in life itself. Inadequate oxygen is perhaps the most common cause of complicated healing. Simple therapies based on new knowledge of oxygen supply and delivery can restore healing that has failed, can accelerate healing that is slow, and can prevent wound complications. Unfortunately, obtaining widespread recognition of this fact has been a slow and painful process.

Surgeons have noted for centuries that wounds in poorly perfused tissues heal poorly or not at all and, furthermore, are excessively prone to infection. In Andean lore, descending to the lower winter habitats is the appropriate therapy for wounds that fail to heal in the high summer pastures. A Russian experimentalist measured inadequate epithelization at high altitude six decades ago. My grandmother told me many years ago to use warmth for wounds and infection because warmth improves the circulation. These ideas have taken a long time in coming to the medical profession.

Medical interest in oxygen in wound healing began the 1960s when practitioners noted that hyperbaric oxygen therapy given for other reasons stimulated growth of granulation tissue in ischemic and irradiated wounds. Even more important, judging from the rapid spread, Jacques Cousteau's divers noted that their work-wounds healed most rapidly when they lived in their undersea habitat at thirty feet under water. When the senior author of this chapter began his work on measuring oxygen in tissues in 1964, however, tissue oxygen was thought to be unchangeable. His senior medical colleagues felt that he was wasting his time, that the only way to increase oxygen delivery was to increase hemoglobin. That is, they thought that dissolved oxygen was insignificant in oxygen transport.

A small group of physiologists and physicians thought differently. Their observations stimulated three questions concerning wounds: 1) What is the concentration of oxygen in injured and healing tissue? 2) If it is low, as they expected, might it be raised? 3) If it can be raised, will the increase be beneficial to healing?

Technology to measure oxygen concentration, PO_2, in tissue, newly refined at that time, soon proved that wound PO_2 (1) is low, (2) can be raised by oxygen supplementation, and 3) significantly benefits healing when elevated.

In the process of answering these questions, a large amount of conflicting data accumulated, and from this confusion, a number of obstacles to maintaining and elevating PO_2 in tissue were found. We had to learn how oxygen travels from the vessels to its point of use and how vulnerable PO_2 in tissue is to vasoconstriction. Little of this was actually new. It simply had not been adopted into clinical usage.

OXYGEN IN TISSUE

To understand the behavior of oxygen in tissue, one needs first to understand some terminology and how tissue PO_2 is regulated.

The usual clinical use of the term "*oxygen delivery*," the cardiac output multiplied by the oxygen carrying capacity of a liter of blood, has little reference to wounded tissue. For reference to healing, we need to know the oxygen delivery to the wound, the wound perfusion rate times the carrying capacity plus an added factor, arterial PO_2. Cardiac output has some relationship to wound perfusion only in that high is usually better. Unfortunately, wound "*perfusion*," the blood flow in a wound per unit time, is not usually quantifiable. Indirect approaches must be used.

Wound "*tissue PO_2*" is a measure of oxygen concentration in a given tissue, in other words, an expression of oxygen "availability." It is not equivalent to "oxygen delivery." For present purposes, it is expressed as millimeters of mercury. It can also be expressed as moles or millimoles per unit volume. The "concentration" in tissue is important because substrate concentrations control the rate of enzymatic reactions. PO_2 is specifically important because the relative lack of oxygen often controls the rate of important enzymes that use it as a substrate, and several such enzymes are critical to healing.

How much oxygen a given enzyme can use at a given substrate concentration depends upon the avidity, the "*passion*," with which the enzyme and the substrate combine. The avidity is expressed as the Km for that enzyme, that is, the concentration of the substrate (oxygen in this case) that allows the enzyme to produce its end product at half the maximal rate. Cytochrome oxidase, one of the most avid for oxygen, produces its product at half-maximal rate even when PO_2 is less than 1 mm Hg. That is, it is so avid for oxygen that PO_2 must fall to lethal levels before its rate is affected. On the other hand, collagen prolyl hydroxylase, which is vital in healing, has a Km of about 25 mm Hg. Its product, extracellular collagen, depends on PO_2 throughout the entire physiologic range. Wound cells survive well at low PO_2 by glycolysis alone, but function poorly.

Oxygen concentration in tissue represents the oxygen reserve, what is left over after consumption has been subtracted from delivery, and often most importantly is the driving force to diffusion of oxygen into poorly vascularized tissues.

Oxygen movement into tissue is limited by diffusion pressure, capillary PO_2. Tissue PO_2 can never be higher than the arterial PO_2. Arterial blood at low PO_2 can deliver considerable oxygen if there is enough hemoglobin, but lacking concentration, it can penetrate only short distances.

How much oxygen is used depends on the PO_2 at the point of use. High local tissue concentrations can be reached even in anemic subjects if arterial PO_2 and blood flow are high and oxygen consumption is relatively low, as it is in most wounds. Though PO_2 is vital in wounds, wounds use relatively little oxygen.

Tissue oxygen consumption is highly variable according to local PO_2 and the cell or organ in question. Cardiac myocytes, for example, are generously equipped with enzymes (cytochrome oxidase, for instance) that have a high affinity for oxygen; i.e., they consume oxygen and function well at low PO_2. Working muscle, with its high oxygen consumption, relies upon a high hemoglobin content and high flow as well as a relatively high PO_2. On the other hand, reparative cells, i.e., fibroblasts, endothelial cells, and inflammatory cells, have relatively few mitochondria. Their enzymes have a lower affinity for oxygen, and they function poorly at low PO_2. For this reason, as PO_2 falls, wound healing fails well before tissue viability is in danger.

Perfusion, the rate at which blood perfuses a <u>tissue</u>, can be critical to its functions. Medicine has long been interested in cardiac output and the state of the arteries, but commonly, the perfusion of wounded and healing tissue is reduced (often unnecessarily) by the vasoconstriction that occurs as a result of low blood volume, cold, pain, and vasoconstrictive drugs. Wounds on the surface of the body and in those tissues whose vessels contract under "stress" are particularly vulnerable. In practical terms, for wound healing, this is an enormously important item! As perfusion falls, the fraction of delivered oxygen that is consumed increases, and PO_2 in capillary blood and tissue fall, and wounds fail.

OXYGEN IN INJURED TISSUE

Injury diminishes perfusion and oxygen delivery by damaging the microvasculature. Subsequent coagulation deepens the injury and further reduces perfusion. Inflammatory cells, primed and activated on entering the wound, begin to consume large amounts of oxygen by converting it to superoxide and thence to other oxidants. This sequence dominates healing if there is any space to heal (Figure 1). The energy for the conversion comes from aerobic glycolysis (i.e., does not require oxygen). Lactate is produced as a by-product. The result is hypoxia in a highly oxidative, highly lactated environment. This condition serves well as a metabolic definition of a "*healing wound*."

The extent of vascular injury and inflammation are highly variable. However, even "insignificant" wounds contain areas of ischemia where the healing cells exist in microscopic units, such as a few macrophages, a few fibroblasts, and perhaps no vessels. (For instance, patients have developed tetanus without displaying any sign of a wound.)

Collagen must be deposited in this ischemic, relatively hypoxic environment. One of the challenges to healing, then, is to develop new vessels to support the added new tissues, i.e., angiogenesis. New vessels need collagenous support. Indeed, they supply their own, but collagen can be deposited only in the presence of a considerable concentration of oxygen. Until these new vessels acquire blood flow, the necessary oxygen for collagen deposition must diffuse toward the wound, a considerable distance from the last free-flowing vessel. This requires a high arterial PO_2 so that diffusion can overcome the distance.

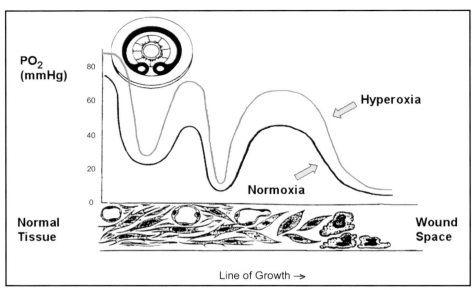

Figure 1. PO$_2$ in Wounds

A hole has been made in a rabbit's ear and filled with an "ear chamber" that traps the growing wound between two membranes. The cells within always progress in the same order, from left to right. Polymorphonuclear cells are omitted for clarity. At the growing edge are macrophages followed by replicating and young fibroblasts. New blood vessels follow. Using an oxygen microprobe, the PO$_2$ has been measured with the animal breathing normal air (heavy line) and normobaric oxygen (lighter line). Note the long gradient to low levels in wound space. At this point, macrophages convert molecular oxygen to oxidants. This causes the central hypoxia.

The relationship between the wound and the arterial PO$_2$ has been measured and is predictable in uncomplicated wounds provided that circulatory conditions are normal and there are no sources of vasoconstriction. In turn, wound PO$_2$ has been measured and correlated to collagen deposition, infectability, and angiogenesis in human, animal, and cellular experiments. The PO$_2$ in the center of a dead space wound can be quite low; 10 to 15 mm Hg has been measured in normal wounds with dead spaces in them. As the space gets smaller, the PO$_2$ rises. Clearly, oxygen is being used in the space. As the space approaches zero, the PO$_2$ rises to about 40 or 50 (if the arterial PO$_2$ is normal), a figure one can accept as an estimate of normal at the wound edge. One hundred percent oxygen at 1 ATA raises it to the region of 150 to 200. Hyperbaric oxygen at 2 ATA raises it to about 400 or above with a wide variation. The PO$_2$ of the dead space itself may rise only to 90 or so during HBO depending on the size of the space.

Large variability in PO$_2$ and collagen deposition has been found seven to ten days postoperatively in human surgical patients. Statistically most of the variability is due to vasoactivity and arterial PO$_2$. Most of the differences in collagen production are due to the variation in local PO$_2$. The simple fact is that when more oxygen is made available to healing tissue, more is used, and some of the added consumption contributes to accelerated healing. However, the amount of benefit one can get depends on the difference between baseline and elevated oxygen levels according to the following graph (Figure 2) which was constructed on the basis of arterial PO_2 levels.

While it is relatively easy to enhance normal healing with continuous, long-term oxygen therapy, periodic hyperbaric exposure is not as effective. Hyperbaric is used mainly for severely hypoxic wounds and complicated wounds in which its effect on oxidant signaling and infection become important features. In those circumstances,periodic hyperoxia is more effective.

The findings in Figure 2 predict that increased local PO_2 must also accelerate angiogenesis, i.e., the ingress of new vasculature. Increased angiogenesis in ischemic tissue due to hyperbaric oxygen and flow has more recently been confirmed by sophisticated methods in several laboratories. Sheffield probably was the first to note increasing PO_2 in human wounds after hyperbaric treatment. This confirms clinical observations made during treatment of wounded patients with hyperbaric oxygen.

It is intuitive that ischemia and hypoxia should be the stimulus to angiogenesis and collateral blood flow. To some extent it is true, but other studies have confirmed that hypoxia is detrimental to angiogenesis. This may seem counter-intuitive and will be discussed in more detail later.

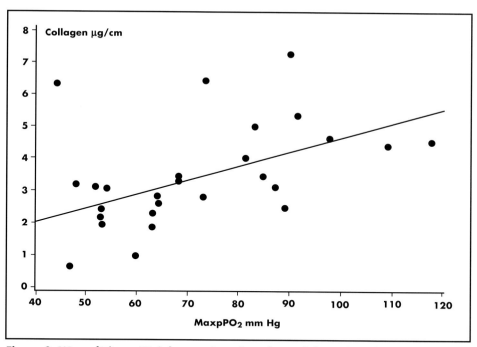

Figure 2. Wound Tissue Weight as a Function of Arterial PO_2 in Rabbit Wire Mesh Cylinders

Collagen deposition in implanted Gortex tubes that were implanted in the subcutaneous tissue of the upper arm in patients at the time of surgery. MaxPO$_2$ refers to the maximum wound PO$_2$ reached with the patient breathing 50% oxygen. The slope is highly significant (p<0,01). More extensive experiments in rabbits show a curve rather than a straight line, and the curve is asymptotic to about 250 mm Hg, agreeing with the Km for prolyl hydroxylase.

A <u>major</u> portion of the infectability noted in ischemic wounds is also related to wound/tissue PO_2! Studies in animals show that bacteria placed in wounds are cleared at an order of magnitude faster when the subjects breathe oxygen and the added oxygen is transmitted to tissue. Human studies confirm this in terms of the incidence of postoperative wound infections. One must realize, however, that some ischemic tissue, including tissue that has healed (scarred) repeatedly cannot be oxygenated by any means and must be debrided surgically and radically, that is, back to bleeding tissue, before healing can be expected. This is particularly true of osteomyelitis in which oxygen therapy must be considered only part of a combined therapy with <u>surgical</u> debridement.

In summary, decreased perfusion, increased diffusion distances, and a rising demand for oxygen in wounds due to inflammation all lead to local hypoxia, an oxidative environment, and local lactacidosis. Provision of oxygen to wounded tissue, where circulation is sufficient, raises tissue concentration (PO_2) in wounds and profoundly influences healing. The mechanisms, as far as they are known, are strikingly similar.

MECHANISMS

Immunity to Infection

The mechanism by which wounds resist bacterial infection is the most direct entry to the explanation of how oxygen works in wounds. Ischemic wounds are notoriously vulnerable to infection. This undoubtedly involves many mechanisms, but impaired bactericidal oxidant production by leukocytes appears to be the major one, at least to surgeons.

Leukocytes are "activated" by phagocytosis and/or by entry into wounds. They adopt many functions when they are "activated." For one, they consume oxygen in large quantities by converting it to oxidants that are inserted into the phagosomes where they kill engulfed bacteria by oxidizing their membranes. The equation is:

$$O_2 + glucose \longrightarrow O_2^- + lactate + H^+$$

The Km is about 75 mm Hg.

The oxygenase converts oxygen first to superoxide, in what is called the "*oxidative burst*" (Figure 3). The term oxidative "burst" comes from the fact that oxygen consumption rises as much as 50-fold upon activation. About 98% of the oxygen consumed is converted to superoxide. The superoxide is then converted to hydrogen peroxide and other oxidants, including peroxynitrite.

The enzyme that adds the electron to oxygen is the NADPH-linked oxygenase, often called PHOX. Its Km, that is, the oxygen concentration necessary to support superoxide formation at half the maximum rate, is about 75 mm Hg. The PO_2 at the wound edge is rarely above 50 mm Hg if the subject is breathing air at one atmosphere. In surgical patients breathing air, therefore, this system operates at significantly less than half its potential. Reduced PO_2 markedly reduces bacterial killing. Raising PO_2 from a reduced value restores the loss and is capable of adding an increment, which may

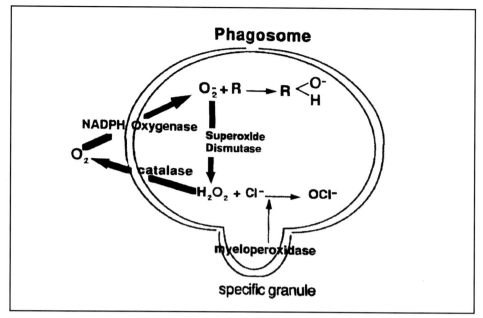

Figure 3. The Pathway for Oxygen in Wound Immunity

When bacteria a phagocytosed, the NADPH oxygenase is assembled in the phagosome membrane. Oxygen is converted to superoxide which is injected into the phagosome. Various enzymes convert the superoxide to other bactericidal oxidants. Antioxidants in the granular membrane protect the cell.

increase the killing rate to well above normal. Many studies show that bacteria are cleared more rapidly from hyperoxic as opposed to hypoxic wounds, and it is clear that assurance of adequate oxygen tension in wounds is an excellent means of preventing wound infections and is approximately as powerful as specific antibiotics.

The absence of any of the PHOX genes can produce a profound, often fatal susceptibility to the same organisms that infect wounds. As oxygen tensions fall into the 20 mm Hg range, wounds approach this degree of vulnerability. It is now generally accepted that hypoxia of the magnitude seen clinically in human wounds is a major source of vulnerability to infection. For example, ensuring an adequate PO_2 in wounds simply by warmth, oxygen breathing, and blood volume support lowers wound infections in surgical patients by more than half! The effect is proved to be specific to elevated PO_2 (which, on occasion, may require hyperbaric oxygen to achieve).

Nitric oxide, NO, is also bactericidal. It is formed from arginine and molecular oxygen by nitric oxide synthetase:

$$O_2 + arginine ----> NO + citrulline$$

As noted above, the rate of NO production is proportional to local oxygen concentration. The Km is uncertain and may be tissue specific, but for most purposes it appears to be about 15 mm Hg.

Collagen Synthesis

Oxygen concentration influences collagen synthesis, deposition, and cross-linking in at least three places in the synthetic pathway—gene transcription, post-translational modification, and extracellular cross-linking.

In a mechanism that is still not fully understood, the combination of oxygen and lactate and transition metals leads to oxidant production, and this in turn stimulates collagen gene transcription.

Although hypoxia is said to induce collagen gene transcription, the experimental conditions that were used in the experiments were actually hypoxia-followed-by-reoxygenation, a sequence that is now known as hypoxia/reoxygenation that is well known to cause release of oxidants. The process is known as "oxidant stress" when excessive, or as "oxidant signaling" when in the physiologic range. The emerging view is that among many other ways (TGFbeta etc.), oxidant signaling enhances collagen transcription (Figure 4).

Oxidant signaling, which occurs intermittently or at very low concentrations, is an established concept, but so is oxidant damage that occurs after very high or constant exposures. There is a balance, and wounds are well able to defend themselves against excess being well protected by protein carboxylation and nitration, thiols, superoxide dismutase, catalase, and others.

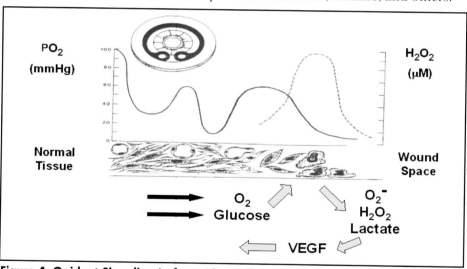

Figure 4. Oxidant Signaling (refer to Figure 4)

Oxygen is consumed in the signaling zone, next to the wound space, by conversion to oxidants. Oxidants (dashed and dotted lines) are rather quickly used. Note: Lack of quantification. Hydrogen peroxide level in the wound space is 2 to 6 micro moles. Molecular oxygen and glucose, neither angiogenic, are converted to oxidants, lactate and hypoxia, all angiogenic. Molecular oxygen, however, supports vessel growth at the response zone where the new vessels grow. Other growth factors emanating from the macrophages also converge on the response zone, the sum total increasing cell replication, collagen production, etc.

Contrary to conventional concepts, many biologic processes other than energy metabolism depend upon PO_2. Three oxygenases (enzymes that consume oxygen as a substrate) are critically important in collagen deposition. They are prolyl-hydroxylase, lysyl-hydroxylase and lysyl-oxidase.

The reason for the oxygen dependence of collagen secretion from the fibroblast is well understood. (Figure 5) Proline, not hydroxyproline, is incorporated into the procollagen peptides before they leave the cell. Later, in a post-translational step that occurs in the endoplasmic reticulum, prolyl hydroxylase inserts an oxygen atom into selected prolines converting some of them to hydroxyprolines. The oxygen atom can be obtained only from molecular oxygen. At this point, collagen peptides can assume their normal triple helical structure within the cell and can be exported into the extracellular space. Regardless of the rate of peptide synthesis, collagen is not released from cells, i.e., deposited, until prolyl hydroxylase and molecular oxygen hydroxylate it. There is no dispute about this. Since enzymatic reaction rates are hyperbolic with respect to the concentrations of their substrates, collagen deposition is 0 at $PO_2=0$, half-maximal at $PO_2=25$ (the Km) and maximal only at above 200 mm Hg. This is the entire physiologic range of PO_2 and beyond! These numbers may be tissue specific for some organs and/or cells. The Km for endothelial cells may be as low as 5 mm Hg.

Similarly, hydroxylated lysines, by the same type of mechanism (lysyl-hydroxylase), assist extracellular cross-linking of collagen monomers into collagen fibrils. This step also requires oxygen and is analogous to proline hydroxylation. Its half-maximal rate also occurs at a PO_2 of approximately 25 mm Hg. If this step is incomplete, collagen fibers are weak.

Lastly, lysines in the collagen molecule are condensed by lysyl oxidase, yet another oxygen-requiring enzyme, in the extracellular polymerization of collagen. The Km of enzyme is not well defined but appears to be

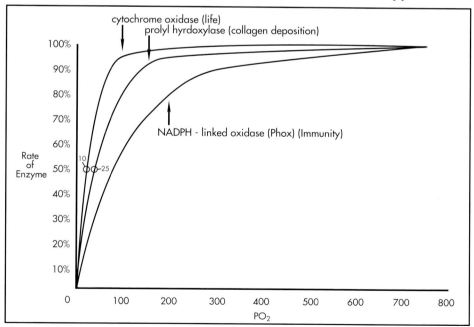

Figure 5.

Kinetics curves for prolyl hydroxylase and cytochrome oxidase showing that as oxygen concentration falls (right to left), collagen deposition due to prolyl hydroxylation and bactericidal oxidant production will fall long before cell viability is threatened.

higher than 25 mm Hg and thus collagen cross-linking is probably even more susceptible to hypoxia than its deposition. If these steps are incomplete, collagen fibers are sparse and weak.

"Hypoxia" stimulates the release of several growth factors and cytokines that induce collagen synthesis, particularly hypoxia inducible factor (hif-1alpha), tumor necrosis factor, transforming growth factor beta, interleukin-1, and vascular endothelial growth factor. However, these functions appear to be duplicated, at least to some extent, by lactate and oxidant signaling. On the other hand, hypoxia suppresses IGF-1 synthesis between $PO_2=0$ and $PO_2=35$. IGF-1 deficiency is one of the few growth factors whose absence has been demonstrated to suppress collagen deposition in actual wounds. The mechanism is unknown, but lack of IGF-1 probably contributes to the problems of hypoxia.

In summary, collagen deposition and both intra- and extra-cellular cross-linking are oxygen dependent. They are decelerated when perfusion and/or arterial PO_2 are below normal and accelerated when they are higher. As noted in Figure 5, this difference can be several fold. The clinically important lesson is that collagen synthesis, cell replication, and oxidant production can be easily optimized by simple clinical means such as warming to increase perfusion and breathing oxygen to increase arterial PO_2.

Collagen deposition is also powerfully controlled by lactate. Adding lactate to animal wounds to raise lactate concentration by only about 20% increases collagen deposition by 50%. As noted above, lactate is generated by leukocytes. They are also <u>aerobically</u> glycolytic and contribute to the accumulation of lactate. This comes about also in two other ways. Smooth muscle cells and most cancer cells also generate lactate aerobically (that is, in the presence of oxygen). Lastly, lactate is the by-product of anaerobic metabolism.

Lactate accumulation in wounds is also important because the <u>lactate stimulates collagen gene transcription by stimulating its promoter and by activating prolyl hydroxylase, i.e., collagen deposition</u>. These appear to occur through a mechanism involving the pool of reduced NAD^+. The mechanism is complex. High lactate concentrations shift the equilibration ratio of $NAD^+/NADH$ in favor of NADH through the familiar action of lactate dehydrogenase that transfers hydrogens from accumulated lactates to NAD^+ with the production of NADH.

The diminished NAD^+, in turn, has a vital consequence, namely that its metabolites, particularly adenosine diphosphoribose (ADPR) production are diminished. This term describes the molecule that results when the "N" is removed from NAD^+.

ADPR has an important <u>normal</u> role. It suppresses both collagen gene transcription in the nucleus and prolyl hydroxylase activity in the cytoplasm thus (in the absence of lactate) inhibiting collagen synthesis and deposition when they are not "needed." Injury, with its consequent accumulated lactate and lowered NAD^+, therefore overcomes a repressive mechanism. Exposing fibroblasts to lactate, in the presence of oxygen, reduces NAD^+ in favor of NADH. The net result is increased collagen deposition, which we know to be further accelerated by increased PO_2. Thus, simultaneous elevation of lactate and PO_2 leads to increased collagen synthesis. (See **Angiogenesis**)

All this runs contrary to classic thought. The standard questions which arise are 1) Shouldn't hyperoxia decrease lactate? and 2) Isn't hypoxia necessary for lactate production? The demonstrated fact is that hyperoxygenation of wounded animals does not lower wound lactate levels. Furthermore, addition of lactate, in the presence of oxygen to fibroblasts in culture and/or wounds in animals, enhances collagen production significantly. Adding NAD^+ increases ADPR production and suppresses collagen production even in lactated fibroblast cultures.

Angiogenesis

The logic of parsimony suggests that since macrophages, new blood vessels, and fibroblasts exist close together in wounds and act cooperatively (Figures 1, 4, 6), the mechanisms of angiogenesis should be similar to those of collagen synthesis and deposition and should involve oxidants. Angiogenesis is dependent upon collagen deposition (by endothelial cells) to give physical support to growing vessels. In fact, the mechanisms of angiogenesis and collagen synthesis and deposition are strikingly similar.

It is well accepted that hypoxia leads to release of vascular endothelial growth factor (VEGF) from many cell types. It is not well known, but is nevertheless also true, that lactate stimulates VEGF release from macrophages even in the presence of oxygen (Figure 6). The mechanism currently appears to involve oxidant formation from oxygen, iron, and lactate.

This fact is particularly useful because the assumption that hypoxia is the single cause of VEGF release in wounds is incompatible with the fact that angiogenesis occurs best in well- or even hyper-oxygenated wounds and is accelerated during hyperbaric oxygen therapy. Hyperbaric oxygen exposure enhances angiogenesis in matrigel in implants in animal wounds. Furthermore, hypoxia truncates angiogenesis both clinically and experimentally. There are several putative mechanisms for this. Hyperoxia enhances endothelial response through oxidants. Small increases of peroxide, consistent with hyperoxia, also increase release of VEGF. Oxygen is required for vessel formation. Therefore hyperoxia secures both a release of VEGF and a response from the endothelial cells. This argues for the central importance of lactate in healing and fits the clinical facts. Both hypoxia and hyperoxia enhance VEGF release, and VEGF release is lowest at normal tissue oxygen concentrations. Although a number of angiogenic substances are found in wound fluid, VEGF seems to be the major player.

Of all the wound mechanisms, angiogenesis is by far the most important for take of skin grafts. Elevating oxygen tension, whether to normal or above normal, is the only known angiogenic strategy that is effective in ischemic tissue.

Epithelization

Though several animal studies have shown that epithelization is accelerated in the presence of oxygen, the mechanism is unknown. Epithelial cells synthesize collagen just as endothelial cells do. By analogy with the above, it should be expected that oxygen and oxidants should be involved.

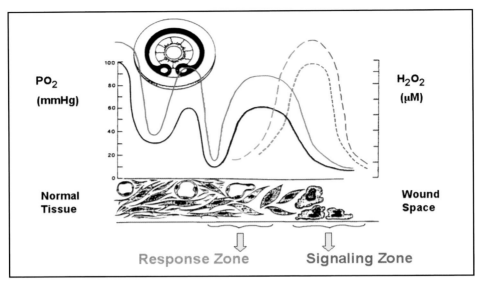

Figure 6. Arterial Hyperoxia (refer to Figures 1 and 2)

In hyperoxia, oxidants are increased while the PO$_2$ in the macrophage layer (signaling zone) remains quite low. Increased hypoxia signals coexist with unchanged hypoxia signal.

Epithelial cells can extract oxygen directly from the ambient air and/or other gases as well as from blood. No quantification is available. However, major differences in epithelization are observed in some patients during oxygen breathing. Epithelization has also been enhanced dramatically in some patients by <u>topical</u> application of oxygen!

CHRONIC WOUNDS

There are a number of sources of chronic (impeded) wounds: trauma, arteriosclerosis, venous, diabetes, hypertension, arteritis, osteomyelitis, pressure necrosis, etc.

With some exceptions, chronic wounds are less well oxygenated than acute wounds. Most are on the lower extremity and are associated with arterial or venous insufficiency and/or excessive inflammation, all of which produce local hypoxia.

The healing potential of a lower extremity wound is directly related to its circulation. The circulation is currently best assessed by the transcutaneous PO$_2$ (TcPO$_2$) in its vicinity. This measurement, however, must be carefully done in order to isolate the physiologic and vasoactive variables. It must be done with the leg warmed under a cover of water vapor-impermeable substance and a blanket. The skin temperature must be recorded. The ideal method is to start with a well-hydrated, pain-free patient and then to obtain stability with the patient supine. One hundred percent oxygen is then added by mask. Once stability is again reached, the leg is raised 30 degrees. Stability is reached again, and the patient is measured sitting or standing. In this manner, artifact due to dehydration, pain, and cold are avoided and the effects of arterial and venous disease are isolated. A slight fall on elevation is normal; a large one is due to obstructive arterial disease. A rise above the supine value with standing is normal, but a large rise followed by a fall is indicative of venous disease.

If the baseline $TcPO_2$ is over 30 mm Hg, especially if a plentiful response to oxygen occurs, the ulceration is not due to hypoxia. If it is less, hypoxia is a likely contributor. Fifteen mm Hg or less (remember that cold alone even with normal arteries can cause this level) without a rise due to oxygen spells a grave prognosis unless vascular surgery can be done. A low PO_2 that responds to oxygen breathing suggests that hyperbaric oxygen will be helpful. Preferably, these values should be obtained after infection is controlled. The capacity of oxygen to heal an ischemic wound is not estimated until the patient and wound are uninfected and warm, and the patient is hydrated and without pain.

The degree of hypoxia in venous wounds has been debated, but the majority of evidence now supports the theory that chronic, intermittent ischemia and hypoxia followed by reperfusion causes tissue death. The ischemia is caused by poor flow during prolonged standing. The reoxygenation occurs when bringing the leg up toward heart level restores the A/V pressure gradient. Prevention of stasis by pressure wrappings, the first treatment of choice, prevents the rise of venous pressure and accomplishes that same objective. Surgical interruption of venous perforators in or near the ulcer, thus preventing local ischemia/reperfusion, can be very helpful, but the healing time is still prolonged. Hyperbaric oxygen therapy is not usually a choice for venous ulcers unless they are hypoxic for other reasons as well.

By far the most effective therapy for hypoxic wounds is revascularization, reduction of oxygen consuming inflammation and infection, warmth, and stopping use of (vasoconstricting) tobacco. All of these have the potential to raise the tissue oxygen concentration. If they are corrected, breathing oxygen can often be expected to raise wound PO_2 to recovery levels. Few hyperbaric units observe all these conditions.

We are also persuaded that medical therapy is effective. Use of warmth in patients with active sympathetic nervous systems is usually helpful. Vasodilation with Clonidine and/or calcium channel blockers, or possibly by ACE inhibitors is also helpful in some cases. One of the best uses of transcutaneous oximetry is in proving (or disproving) the efficacy of such therapies, since it is a system in which failure can be detected in hours or days rather than waiting weeks in vain for a result.

CLINICAL STRATEGIES

Correcting tissue hypoxia is more complex than simply breathing oxygen. Using wound oximeters, we have seen many surgical patients whose wound PO_2 is low and totally unaffected by breathing oxygen. Even their vascular anatomy is normal and arterial PO_2 is significantly raised. Yet when given adequate fluid and warmed, their oximetry profile becomes normal. This emphasizes the importance of local perfusion. The most important causes of vasoconstriction are dehydration, blood volume loss, cold, pain, smoking, and fear. Expansion of blood volume is more important than increasing red cell mass. The essential observation, however, is that for optimal results, all of these elements must be corrected all at the same time because any one is sufficient to cause maximal vasoconstriction. Think of what happens to your peripheral perfusion when you are relaxed, not smoking, not in pain, but cold! You have white fingers and toes.

Warmth has been regarded as potentially harmful to chronic wounds for many years. Sympathetic innervation is supposed to be inoperative in diabetic legs. Nevertheless, warming often aids perfusion as measured by transcutaneous PO_2. Furthermore, external warmth penetrates to the subcutaneous tissue, and usually vasodilates and increases tissue PO_2. We have not seen warmth lowering it. A response to warmth predicts a therapeutic potential. Sympathetic overactivity is a frequent property of chronic wounds, and preventing cold-mediated vasoconstriction is almost always beneficial.

Similarly, pain activates vasoconstriction. It is necessary to avoid the vicious cycle of pain/vasoconstriction/more pain, etc. Beta adrenergic blockade, diuretics, and smoking compound hypoxic problems and should be regulated. As nearly as anyone can tell, their harmful effects are due to limitation of oxygen supply. Many postoperative patients are blood volume depleted, in pain, and cold, and beta blocked (as they probably should be). Correcting these vasoconstrictive stimuli, particularly cold and smoking, has led to significant decrements in postoperative wound infections—60% in the case of warming during surgery and oxygen in the immediate postoperative period. Wound PO_2 can also be elevated through the use of the alpha antagonist clonidine in the patch dosage form because blood volume changes and vasoconstriction occur very rapidly and the need for protection is constant. Many anesthesiologists like to use this strategy, and the drug is excellent medication for hypertension.

These strategies can be put into place arbitrarily in most cases. Some, particularly those involving chronic wounds, are best planned on the basis of transcutaneous oximetry which should be available in all non-invasive vascular laboratories.

HYPERBARIC OXYGEN

The most precise indication for hyperbaric therapy is a chronic wound in which peri-wound transcutaneous PO_2 is low and responds to oxygen breathing in a hyperbaric chamber with the ulcerated part warm and at heart level.

Hyperbaric oxygen has remained a controversial issue for many years mainly because of our inability to effectively stratify chronic wounds and, therefore, predict responders. Transcutaneous oxygen measurement, while not perfect, has largely changed that. The authors have not had hyperbaric capability, but our experience, also not blinded, has been almost uniformly favorable when the above conditions are met. From all existing data, the beneficial effect on angiogenesis appears to be the most important of the several components that are affected inasmuch as prevention of major amputations in human ischemic diseases has now been documented.

As experience with oximetry has expanded, the success rate of hyperbaric therapy has risen, and indications have been clarified. Several prospective and blinded studies have recently been completed, and despite their size, the data seems quite clear that if the problem is ischemia (periwound hypoxia), and oxygen breathing raises periwound PO_2, hyperbaric oxygen can save limbs. On the basis of the enzyme kinetics noted above, hyperbaric oxygen would bring little benefit to normoxic wounds, and it doesn't.

One might also predict that hyperbaric oxygen would be of little benefit for venous ulcers, which have not healed before, since it adds little to the oxygen tension that can be obtained by rest, elevation, and compression. This has been the general experience. The major exception would be in venous ulcers that have healed many times and are chronically scarred thus setting up an oxygen diffusion block. (It is well known that capillary density decreases with each subsequent healing.) In this case, a judgement would have to be made as to whether hyperbaric oxygen or radical debridement is the best choice.

One of its most fruitful applications has been in osteoradionecrosis. The data is convincing. (Marx et al.) Several authors, including Marx, have noted a favorable influence on angiogenesis.

The usual daily therapy is short. How can such a short exposure have a significant effect? Though the current explanations may not be all-inclusive, they are helpful. First, tissue hyperoxia of a 90-minute exposure actually lasts about two hours longer than that. Second, during the exposure, bacterial killing is increased. The effect of eliminating large numbers of bacteria probably has "down stream" significance just as one would expect from a bolus of antibiotic. Third, as angiogenesis, collagen synthesis, and epithelization are enhanced for three to four hours, the degree of infection becomes correspondingly less as treatment cycles add up. In fact, the very periodicity of hyperbaric administration may be responsible for its success. If oxygen at that tension were continued for long, wound oxidants become lethal.

It is fascinating that hyperbaric and growth factor therapy for problem wounds have suffered from the same obstacles to clinical verification. In contrast, hyperbaric oxygen has been regarded with far more skepticism despite the fact that its rationale is more complete and its capacities include problems that are not helped by growth factors!

CONCLUSIONS

Hypoxia is the most common deficiency found in failed wounds, and restoration of oxygen concentration in tissue allows wound cells to deposit collagen, to resist infection, to epithelize, and to develop new vasculature.

Although tissue hypoxia can stimulate the assembly of many mechanisms of healing, it frustrates each of them in the end. Lactate accumulation mimics hypoxia in most if not all wounds, and leaves the clinician in a position to increase oxygen concentration (PO_2) in both acute and chronic ischemic wounds with benefits to almost all aspects of healing as well as resistance to infection.

The following are important, practical rules for mitigating the hypoxia:

- PO_2 in wounds is profoundly influenced by the rate at which blood perfuses them. Perfusion is reduced by vasoconstriction. Vasoconstriction is a response to low blood volume, pain, fear, smoking, cold, etc.
- Vasoconstriction can almost always be overcome using warmth, fluids, or medications even in the hyperbaric chamber.

- Wound PO_2 also varies with arterial PO_2 and falls as the distance that oxygen has to diffuse to get to the healing wound cells increases.
- Surgical debridement, infection control, and hyperbaric oxygen are useful to overcome diffusion obstacles and excessive demand for oxygen due to inflammation.

Oxygen has a surprising diversity of effects in wounds. The rates of angiogenesis, collagen deposition, epithelization, and the ability of wounds to resist infection are all dependent on oxygen concentration.

REFERENCES

Overview

1. Ahn ST, Mustoe TA. Effects of ischemia on ulcer wound healing: a new model in the rabbit ear. Ann Plast Surg. 24 (1): 17-23, 1990.

2. Aro H, Eerola E, Aho AJ, Niinikoski. Tissue oxygen tension in externally stabilized tibial fractures in rabbits during normal healing and infection. J Surg Res. 37 (3): 202-7, 1984.

3. Davis JC, Hunt TK. Problem Wounds: The Role of Oxygen. Elsevier Science Publishing Co., Inc., New York, 1988.

4. Zhao LL DJ, Wee SC, Roth SI, Mustoe TA. Effect of Hyperbaric Oxygen and Growth Factors on Rabbit Ear Ischemic Ulcers. Arch Surg. 129 1043-1049, 1994.

5. Sheffield, Mitra A, Stueber K, Smith YR. The effects of nicotinamide and hyperbaric oxygen on skin flap survival. Scand J Plast Reconstr Surg Hand Surg. 25 (1): 5-7, 1991.

6. Hammarlund C, Svedman C, Svedman P. Hyperbaric oxygen treatment of healthy volunteers with ultraviolet-irradiated blister wounds. Burns. 17 (4): 296-301, 1991.

7. Heppenstall RB, Goodwin CW, Brighton CT. Fracture healing in the presence of chronic hypoxia. J Bone Joint Surg [Am]. 58 (8): 1153-6, 1976.

8. Kase F, D'Amico JC. A literature search for the methods and materials used to stimulate osteogenesis. J Am Podiatry Assoc. 66 (8): 604-17, 1976.

9. Kivisaari J, Vihersaari T, Renvall S, Niinikoski J. Energy metabolism of experimental wounds at various oxygen environments. Ann Surg. 181 (6): 823-8, 1975.

10. Moelleken B, Mathes S, Amerhauser A et al. An adverse wound environment activates leukocytes prematurely. Arch Surg 1991; 126:225.

11. Meltzer T, Myers B. The effect of hyperbaric oxygen on the bursting strength and rate of vascularization of skin wounds in the rat. Am Surg. 52 (12): 659-62, 1986.

12. Niinikoski J, Rajamaki A, Kulonen E. Healing of open wounds: effects of oxygen, disturbed blood supply and hyperemia by infrared irradiation. Acta Chir Scand. 137 (5): 399-401, 1971.

13. Niinikoski J. Oxygen and wound healing. Clin Plast Surg. 4 (3): 361-74, 1977.

14. Stillman RM. Effects of hypoxia and hyperoxia on progression of intimal healing. Arch Surg. 118 (6): 732-7, 1983.

Infection

15. Babior BM. Oxygen-dependent microbial killing by phagocytes. N Engl J Med. 198 659, 1978.

16. Hohn DC. Oxygen and leukocyte microbial killing in Hyperbaric Oxygen Therapy. Davis JC, Hunt TH. Undersea Medical Society, Bethesda, 1977. p. 101-110.

17. Hopf HW, Hunt TK, West JM, Blomquist P, Goodson III WH, Jensen JA et al. Wound tissue oxygen tension predicts the risk of wound infection in surgical patients. Arch Surg 1997; 132:997-1004.

18. Hunt TK, Hopf HW. Wound healing and wound infection. What the surgeon and anesthesiologist can do. Surg Clin N Amer 1997; 77:587.

19. Hunt TK, Linsey M, Grislis H, Sonne M, Jawetz E. The effect of differing ambient oxygen tensions on wound infection. Ann Surg. 181 (1): 35-9, 1975.

20. Allen DB, Maguire JJ, Mani M, Wicke C, Marcocci L et al. Wound hypoxia and acidosis limit neutrophil bacterial killing mechanisms. Arch Surg 1997; 132:991-6.

21. Jonsson K, Hunt T, Mathes S. Oxygen as an isolated variable influences resistance to infection. Ann Surg. 208 (6): 783-7, 1988.

22. Benhaim P, Hunt TK. Natural resistance to infection: leukocyte functions. J Burn Care Rehabil. 13 (2 Pt 2): 287-92, 1992.

23. Knighton DR, Halliday BJ, Hunt TK. Oxygen as an antibiotic: a comparison of the effects of inspired oxygen concentration and antibiotic administration on in vivo bacterial clearance. Arch Surg 1986; 121(2):191.

24. Kurtz A, Sessler D, Lenhardt R et al. Perioperative normothermia to reduce the incidence of surgical-wound infection and shorten hospitalization. N Engl J Med. 1996; 334:1209-1215.

Tissue Oxygen Concentration and Perfusion

25. Piasecki C. First experimental results with oxygen electrode as a local blood flow sensor in canine colon. Br J Surg. Vol 72 (no. 6): 452-3, 1985.

26. Rabkin JM, Hunt TK. Local heat increases blood flow and oxygen tension in wounds. Arch Surg. 122 (2): 221-5, 1987.

27. Sheffield, Hopf H, Sessler D, Schroeder M, Hunt T, West J. Local heat reverses the decrease in subcutaneous oxygen tension produced by thermoregulatory vasoconstriction. Anesth Analg. 76 S389, 1993.

28. Remensnyder JP, Majno G. Oxygen gradients in healing wounds. Am J Pathol. 52 (2): 301-23, 1968.

29. Sheffield PJ. Tissue oxygenation measurements, in Davis JC, Hunt TK, editors: Problem wounds: the role of oxygen, Elsevier, New York, 1988.

30. Ameli FM, Byrne P, Provan JL. Selection of amputation level and prediction of healing using transcutaneous tissue oxygen tension (PtcO2). J Cardiovasc Surg (Torino). 30 (2): 220-4, 1989. 2 (1): 72, 1994.

31. Ballard JL, Eke CC, Bunt TJ, Killeen JD. A prospective evaluation of transcutaneous oxygen measurements in the management of diabetic foot problems. J Vasc Surg. 22 (4): 485-90; discussion 490-2, 1995.

32. Brighton CT, Krebs AG. Oxygen tension of nonunion of fractured femurs in the rabbit. Surg Gynecol Obstet. 135 (3): 379-85, 1972.

33. Silver IA. The measurement of oxygen tension in healing tissue. Prog Resp Res. 3 124-135, 1969.

34. Sheffield CW, Hopf HW, Sessler DI, Hunt TK, West JM. Thermoregulatory vasoconstriction decreases subcutaneous oxygen tension in anesthetized volunteers. Anesthesiology. 77 A96, 1992.

35. Chang N, Goodson WH, Gottrup F, Hunt TK. Direct measurement of wound and tissue oxygen tension in postoperative patients. Ann Surg. 197 (4): 470-8, 1983.

36. Conlon KC, Sclafani L, DiResta GR, Brennan MF. Comparison of transcutaneous oximetry and laser Doppler flowmetry as noninvasive predictors of wound healing after excision of extremity soft-tissue sarcomas. Surgery. 115 (3): 335-40, 1994.

37. Gottrup F, Firmin R, Rabkin J, Halliday BJ, Hunt TK. Directly measured tissue oxygen tension and arterial oxygen tension assess tissue perfusion. Crit Care Med. 15 (11): 1030-6, 1987.

38. West J, Hopf H, Sessler D, Hunt T. The effect of rapid postoperative rewarming on tissue oxygen. Wound Repair and Regeneration. 1 (2): 93, 1993.

39. Hopf H, Hunt T, Jensen J. Calculation of Subcutaneous Tissue Blood Flow. Surgical Forum. 39 33-36, 1988.

40. Hartmann M, Jonsson K, Zederfeldt B. Effects of dextran and crystalloids on subcutaneous oxygen tension and collagen accumulation. A randomized study in surgical patients. Eur Surg Res. 25 (5): 270-7, 1993.

41. Heughan C, Niinikoski J, Hunt TK. Effect of excessive infusion of saline solution on tissue oxygen transport. Surg Gynecol Obstet. 135 (2): 257-60, 1972.

42. Hopf HW, Glass-Heidenreich L, Silva J, Pearce F, Ochsner MG, Rozycki G, Frankel H, Upton R, Champion H, Drucker W, Hunt TK. Subcutaneous tissue oxygen tension in "well-resuscitated" trauma patients. Crit Care Med. 22 (1): A59, 1994.

43. Jonsson K, Jensen JA, Goodson W Hd, Scheuenstuhl H, West J, Hopf HW, Hunt TK. Tissue oxygenation, anemia, and perfusion in relation to wound healing in surgical patients. Ann Surg. 214 (5): 605-13, 1991.

44. Kamler M, Lehr HA, Barker JH, Saetzler RK, Galla TJ, Messmer K. Impact of ischemia on tissue oxygenation and wound healing: intravital microscopic studies on the hairless mouse ear model. Eur Surg Res. 25 (1): 30-7, 1993.

45. Heughan C, Zederfeldt B, Grislis G, Hunt TK. Effect of dextran solutions on oxygen transport in wound tissue. An experimental study in rabbits. Acta Chir Scand. 138 (7): 639-43.

46. Jensen JA, Goodson WHd, Omachi RS, Lindenfeld SM, Hunt TK. Subcutaneous tissue oxygen tension falls during hemodialysis. Surgery. 101 (4): 416-21, 1987.

47. Hartmann M, Jonsson K, Zederfeldt B. Effects of dextran. Jonsson K, Jensen JA, Goodson WHd, West JM, and Hunt TK. Assessment of perfusion in postoperative patients using tissue oxygen measurements. Br J Surg. 74 (4): 263-7, 1987.

48. Hartmann M, Jonsson K, Zederfeldt B. Perfusion and oxygenation on accumulation of collagen in healing wounds. Randomized study in patients after major abdominal operations. Eur J Surg. 158 (10): 521-6, 1992.

49. Jonsson K, Jensen SA, Goodson WHd et al. Tissue oxygenation, anemia and perfusion in relation to wound healing in surgical patients. Ann Surg 1991; 214:605.

50. Jensen JA, Goodson WH, Hopf HW, Hunt TK. Cigarette smoking decreases tissue oxygen. Arch Surg. 126 (9): 1131-4, 1991.

51. Komoto Y, Nakao T, Sunakawa M, Yorozu H. Elevation of tissue PO2 with improvement of tissue perfusion by topically applied CO2. Adv Exp Med Biol. 222 637-45, 1988.

MECHANISMS

Collagen

52. Skover GR. Cellular and biochemical dynamics of wound repair. Wound environment in collagen regeneration. Clin Podiatr Med Surg. 8 (4): 723-56, 1991.

53. Myalla R, Ruderman LL, Kiviriko KI. Kinetic analysis of the reaction sequences. Mechanism of prolyl hydroxylase. Eur J Biochem 1977; 80:349-57.

54. Hussain MZ, Ghani QP, Hunt TK. Inhibition of prolyl hydroxylase by poly(ADP-ribose) and phosphoribosyl AMP. Possible role of ADP-ribosylation in intracellular prolyl hydroxylase regulation. J Biol Chem 264:7850-7855, 1989.

55. Ghani QP, Hussain MZ, Zhang J, Hunt TK. Control of procollagen gene transcription and prolyl hydroxylase activity by poly(ADP-ribose). In: Poirier and Moreaer, (eds). ADP-Ribosylation. Springer-verlag, New York, 1991.

56. Dinkins GA, Scheuenstuhl H, Hussain MZ, Spencer EM, Hunt TK. The effect of oxygen tension on insulin-like growth factor production by fibroblasts. Surg Forum. 47:676-678, 1995.

57. Zabel DD, Feng JJ, Scheuenstuhl H, Hunt TK, Hussain MZ. Lactate stimulation of macrophage-derived angiogenic activity is associated with inhibition of poly(ADP-ribose) synthesis. Lab Invest. 74:644-649, 1996.

58. Hunt TK, Dunphy JE. Effects of increasing oxygen supply to healing wounds. Br J Surg. 56 (9): 1969.

59. Helfman T, Falanga V. Gene expression in low oxygen tension. Am J Med Sci. 306 (1): 37-41, 1993.

60. Kirkeby L, Hussain Z, Hunt TK. Stimulation of collagen synthesis in fibroblasts by hydrogen peroxide. Mol Biol Cell. 1991 6(44).

Angiogenesis

61. Knighton DR, Hunt TK, Scheuenstuhl H, Halliday BJ, Werb Z, Banda MJ. Oxygen tension regulates the expression of angiogenesis factor by macrophages. Science. 221:1283-1285, 1983.

62. Knighton DR, Silver IA, Hunt TK. Regulation of wound-healing angiogenesis-effect of oxygen gradients and inspired oxygen concentration. Surgery. 90 (2): 262-70, 1981.

63. Knighton DR, Hunt TK, Scheuenstuhl H, Halliday BJ, Werb Z, Banda MJ. Oxygen tension regulates the expression of angiogenesis factor by macrophages. Science. 221 (4617): 1283-5, 1983.

64. Knighton DR, Fiegel VD. Macrophage-derived growth factors in wound healing: regulation of growth factor production by the oxygen microenvironment. Am Rev Respir Dis. 140 (4): 1108-11, 1989.

65. Marx et al. Relationship of oxygen dose to angiogenesis induction in irradiated tissue. Am J Surg 1990; 160:519.

66. Zabel DD, Feng JJ, Scheuenstuhl H et al. Lactate stimulation of macrophage-derived angiogenic activity is associated with inhibition of poly(ADP-ribose) synthesis. Lab Invest. 1996; 74:644-9.

67. Ketchum SAd, Thomas AN, Hall AD. Effect of hyperbaric oxygen on small first, second, and third degree burns. Surg Forum. 18 65-7, 1967.

68. Hunt TK, Knighton DR, Thakral KK et al. Studies on inflammation and wound healing: Angiogenesis and collagen synthesis stimulated in vivo by resident and activated wound macrophages. Surg. 96 48-54, 1984.

69. Feng JJ, Hussain MZ, Constant J, Hunt TK. Angiogenesis in wound healing. J Surg Pathol. 1998; 3:1-8.

70. Gibson JJ, Angeles A, Hunt TK. Increased oxygen tension potentiates angiogenesis. Surg Forum. 1997; 48:696.

71. Sheikh AY, Hussain Z, Hunt TK. Effect of hyperoxia on vascular endothelial growth factor levels in a wound model Arch Surg. 2000. 135(11) 1293-7.

72. Cho M, Hunt TK, Hussain MZ. Hydrogen Peroxide Stimulates Macrophage Vascular Endothelial Growth Factor Release. Cho M, Hunt TK, Hussain MZ. Am J Physiol Heart Circ Physiol. 2001 May;280(5):H2357-63.

73. Constant JS, Feng JJ, Zabel DD, Yuan H, Suh DY, Scheuenstuhl H, Hunt TK, Hussain Z. Lactate Elicits vascular endothelial growth factor from macrophages: a possible alternative to hypoxia. Wd. Rep and Regen. 8:353-360; 2000.

Epithelization

74. Winter GD. Oxygen and epidermal wound healing. Adv Exp Med Biol. 94 673-8, 1977.

75. Kaufman T, Alexander JW, Nathan P, Brackett KA, MacMillan BG. The microclimate chamber: the effect of continuous topical administration of 96% oxygen and 75% relative humidity on the healing rate of experimental deep burns. J Trauma. 23 (9): 806-15, 1983.

76. Pentland AP, Marcelo CL. Modulation of proliferation in epidermal keratinocyte cultures by lowered oxygen tension. Exp Cell Res. 145 (1): 31-43, 1983.

ERICSSON

Contraction

77. Kivisaari J, Niinikoski J. Effects of hyperbaric oxygenation and prolonged hypoxia on the healing of open wounds. Acta Chir Scand. 141 (1): 14-9, 1975.

Oxidants

78. Kaufman T, Neuman RA, Weinberg A. Is postburn dermal ischaemia enhanced by oxygen free radicals? Burns. 15 (5): 291-4, 1989. Note, This reports the dark side of oxidants, too much for too long.

79. Sen CK, Khanna S, Venojarvi M, Trikha P, Ellison EC, Hunt TK, Roy S. Copper-induced vascular endothelial growth factor expression and wound healing. Am J Physiol Heart Circ Physiol 282:H000-H000,2002.

80. Sen CK, Khanna S, Babior BM, Hunt TK, Ellison EC, Roy S. Oxidant induced vascular endothelial growth factor expression in human keratinocytes and cutaneous wound healing. J Biol Chem. 2002 Jun 14 [epub ahead of print] PMID: 12068011 3.

81. Sen CK, et al. Oxygen, oxidants, and antioxidants in wound healing: an emerging paradigm. Ann NY Acad Sci, 2002. 957: p 239-49.

82. Sen CK, et al. Oxidant induced vascular endothelial growth factor experssion in human keratinocytes and cutaneous wound healing J Biol Chem, 2002. 14: p 14.

83. Lelkes PI, Hahn KL, Sukovich DA, Karmiol S, Schmidt DH. On the possible role of reactive oxygen species in angiogenesis. Adv Exp Med Biol 1998; 454:295-310.

Miscellaneous

84. 1972 Heughan C, Grislis G, Hunt TK. The effect of anemia on wound healing. Ann Surg. 179 (2): 163-7, 1974.

85. Hopf H, Swanson D, Hunt T. Moderate anemia does not decrease tissue oxygen in rabbits. Wound Repair and Regen. 1 (2): 107, 1993.

NOTES

APPENDIX

BIO MEDICAL SYSTEMS GROUP
Environmental Tectonics

GULF COAST HYPERBARICS
Medical Systems

REIMERS SYSTEMS

AMRON INTERNATIONAL

PROTEUS HYPERBARIC SYSTEMS

HAUX-LIFE-SUPPORT

OXYHEAL HEALTH GROUP

SECHRIST INDUSTRIES

VMW INDUSTRIES

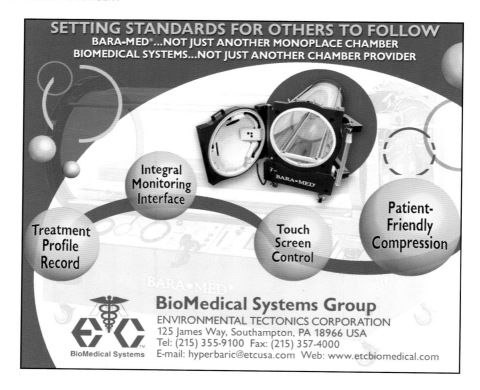

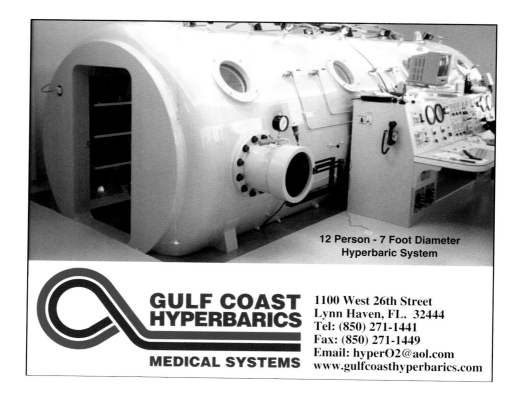

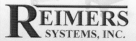
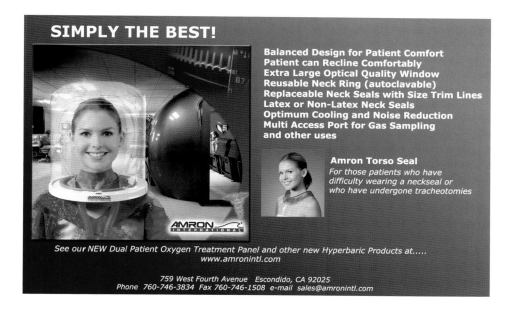

PROTEUS

For the first time **PROTEUS** combines all of the "hands-on" patient management and inherent safety advantages of a multiple chamber with the simplicity, mobility, and economy of a monoplace system:

- Ready access to the patient whenever desired without patient depressurization.
- Monitoring, recording, and patient support functions can be performed simultaneously from outside and inside the chamber regardless of pressure level.
- High degree of patient comfort—an internal space more than twice (2X) that of a monoplace design.
- Large full-size view port in the access doors and ample view ports on both sides.
- Instant Oxygen / Air delivery unique system assures patient is breathing 100% Oxygen, yet can be instantly changed to air breathing for patient safety.
- Oxygen can be utilized only for patient breathing reducing Oxygen consumption and considerable cost.
- Stainless steel pressure vessel alone assures unlimited life and durability, 6 ATA (Atmosphere Absolute) treatment capability, fulfilling all Navy table requirements. This structuring lends to impact, heat and corrosion resistance.
- Triple Lock Feature

Proteus Hyperbaric Systems, Inc.
223 East Thousand Oaks Blvd - Suite 407
Thousand Oaks, CA 91360

Tele: (800) 808-4276
Fax: (805) 446-4278
Website: www.hyperbaric.com

An access compartment allows for an additional patient treatment or care-givers rapid access to patients without interrupting therapy.

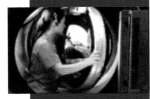

Attendant enters forward Cabin via Center Locking Door.

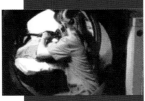

She attends patient

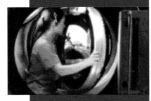

and then locks out.

This same attendant lock is utilized as a patient lock when attendant is not required.

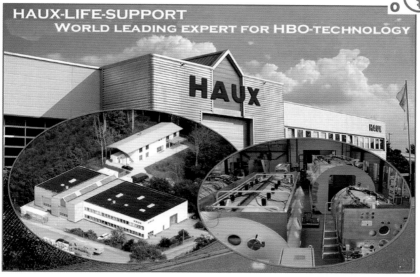
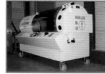
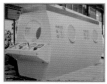
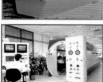
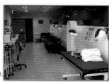
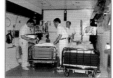
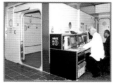

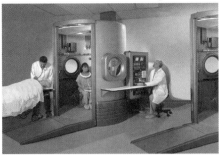
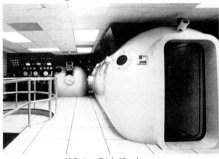
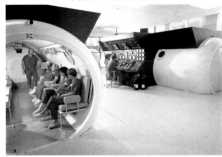
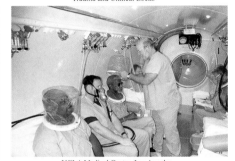

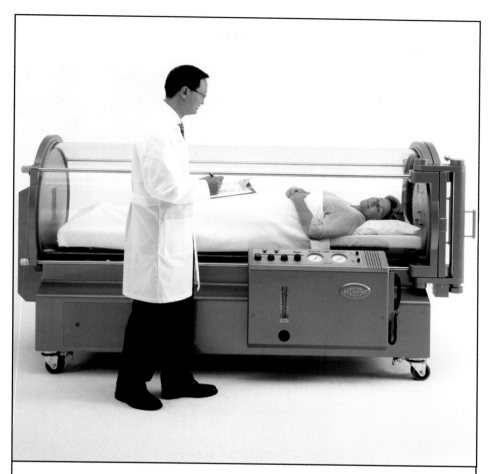

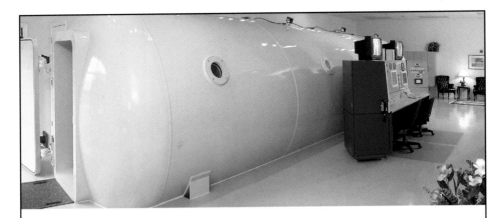
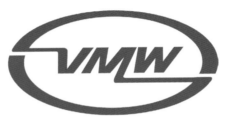
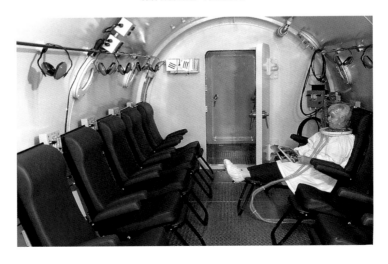

NOTES

NOTES